Neuroglia

Neuroglia

Selected Articles Published by MDPI

MDPI • Basel • Beijing • Wuhan • Barcelona • Belgrade

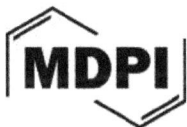

MDPI

This is a reprint of articles published online by the open access publisher MDPI in 2018 (available at: www.mdpi.com/journal/brainsciences). The responsibility for the book's title and preface lies with MDPI, who compiled this selection.

For citation purposes, cite each article independently as indicated on the article page online and as indicated below:

LastName, A.A.; LastName, B.B.; LastName, C.C. Article Title. *Journal Name* **Year**, *Article Number*, Page Range.

ISBN 978-3-03897-990-6 (Pbk)
ISBN 978-3-03897-991-3 (PDF)

Contents

neuroglia

MDPI

Perspective

Interlaminar Glia and Other Glial Themes Revisited: Pending Answers Following Three Decades of Glial Research

Jorge A. Colombo

Unit of Applied Neurobiology (UNA, CEMIC-CONICET), Buenos Aires 1053, Argentina;
drjacolombo@yahoo.com

Received: 23 January 2018; Accepted: 22 February 2018; Published: 1 March 2018

Abstract: This review aims to highlight the various significant matters in glial research stemming from personal work by the author and associates at the Unit of Applied Neurobiology (UNA, CEMIC-CONICET), and some of the pending questions. A reassessment and further comments on interlaminar astrocytes—an astroglial cell type that is specific to humans and other non-human primates, and is not found in rodents, is presented. Tentative hypothesis regarding their function and future possible research lines that could contribute to further the analysis of their development and possible role(s), are suggested. The possibility that they function as a separate entity from the "territorial" astrocytes, is also considered. In addition, the potential significance of our observations on interspecies differences in in vitro glial cell dye coupling, on glial diffusible factors affecting the induction of this glial phenotype, and on their interference with the cellular toxic effects of cerebrospinal fluid obtained from L-DOPA treated patients with Parkinson´s disease, is also considered. The major differences oberved in the cerebral cortex glial layout between human and rodents—the main model for studying glial function and pathology—calls for a careful assessment of known and potential species differences in all aspects of glial cell biology. This is essential to provide a better understanding of the organization and function of human and non-human primate brain, and of the neurobiological basis of their behavior.

Keywords: interlaminar astrocytes; role(s) of interlaminar astrocytes; control of interlaminar glia development; thalamic regulation of interlaminar glia; comparative dye coupling; glial diffusible factors

---

1. Introduction

Following retirement from active laboratory work, a change in the experimental line of research at the Unit of Applied Neurobiology (UNA, CEMIC-CONICET) laboratories—at present aimed at studying more decisively neurocognitive issues—has provided the opportunity to propose this sort of brief account and reassessment of unresolved and pending questions on "glial issues" that were dealt with in our neurobiological laboratory in recent decades. This personal viewpoint is intended to stress and revisit several aspects of our own observations on glial physiology and comparative studies, which are aimed at encouraging further research in the field.

Thorough updates, comprehensive reviews, and inspirational thoughts on other related aspects of glial physiology can be found in Kettenmann and Ransom (2005), Verkhratsky and Butt (2013), and Verkhratsky and Nedergaard (2018) [1–3], as well as in numerous individual articles, for it, seems evident that experimental research on neuroglia has entered an era of further fertile analysis. Yet, as it will be considered later, caution and weighed decisions should be exerted in attempting interspecies extrapolations—in the present context referred to brain glia—and building our understanding of human and non-human primate brain organization and phyisology based on what can be considered "general mammalian" characteristics, stemming from non-comparative Rodentia approaches. This may limit our views on the neurobiological basis of primate brain evolution and behavior.

2. Interlaminar Astrocytes and Primate Brain Evolution

Interlaminar glia or interlaminar astrocytes (Figure 1) essentially represent a primate evolutionary development [4–8] linked to the split between prosimians and Anthropoidea. They are characterized by a cell soma placed in lamina I—in general next to the glia limitans—of the cerebral cortex, and long, descending, cell processes that could extend for about 1 mm, thus traversing more than one cortical laminae. Remaining characteristics are mentioned below.

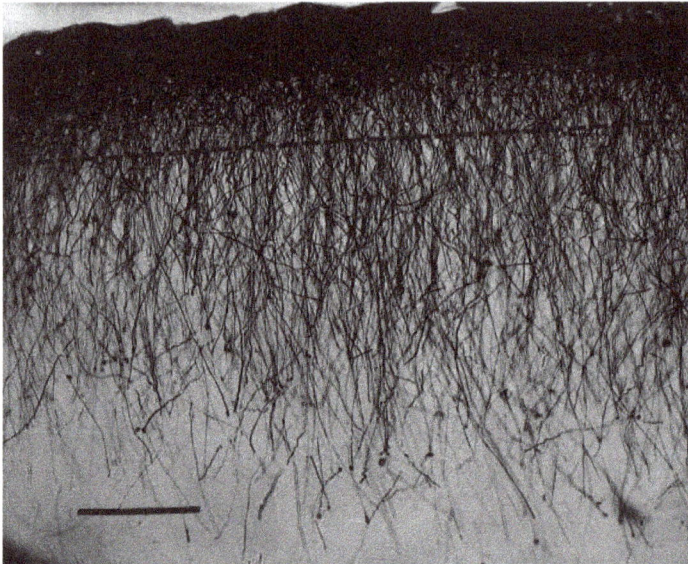

Figure 1. Coronal section from the striate cerebral cortex obtained from an adult *Saimiri boliviensis*. Note dense packing of glial fibrillary acidic protein-immunoreactivity (GFAP-IR) astroglial processes, the relative height of the band of processes and the frequent appearance of slender bulbous endings. Broken line indicates the limit of lamina I. Scale bar: 100 μm. Adapted from Figure 1 in [9].

The expression of interlaminar glia among orders and species, according to our screening of available samples and histological identification procedures, is incipient—they take form of isolated events—in the prosimian lemur (no brain samples were available at that time from galago and tarsier), it is absent in Callithricidae (marmosets and the tamarins), constant and yet variable in its palisade expression in Ceboidea (New World monkeys), and fully expressed in Cercopithecidae (Old World monkeys) and Hominoidea (great apes and humans) [4–8]. Their original development in primates possibly relates to point mutation or epigenesis—predating some of the factors that are hypothetically linked to the later increase in brain size (e.g., expensive tissue hypothesis of Aiello and Wheeler [10]; socio-ecological hypothesis of Dunbar [11] and other convergent hypotheses on brain size evolution in humans). The author considers that its emergence is probably associated with the less promoted—in terms of evolutionary impact on brain function—development of columnar organization of the cerebral cortex, which remains to be further comparatively explored in terms of distributed neural circuits (or modules) and of its impact on cerebral cortex information efficiency (response speed, unit assembly synchrony, cognitive fluidity). In this respect, the possibility that they contribute to a "non-territorial" management of the cerebral cortex intercellular space and intercellular interactions should be analyzed. Consequently, whether they are coupled or not to "local–territorial–astrocytes" could add to the characterization of their physiological role(s) and integration into the cerebral cortex processing.

It seems apparent that brain evolution among anthropoid primates has proceeded in a series of continuous structural and functional—neurotransmitter and receptor dynamics for once—deletions and aggregates, which were not exclusively confined to neurons (see e.g., [12]). Among them, appearance of interlaminar astrocytes would represent an evolutionary—"primate-specific"—brain cell trait added to the "general mammalian" brain glial cell family, as suggested by Colombo and colleagues [4,7,8]. Although functional insertion of interlaminar astrocytes into cerebral cortex organization remains highly speculative (see below), their ontogenetic development and some interactions and responses following experimental procedures and pathologies, provide grounds for further research inquiries and analysis.

One important obstacle to experiments aimed at advancing into the general understanding of human brain evolution and organization, resides in the limited access to extant anthropoid species for comparative research purposes—for interlaminar astrocytes are not a "general mammalian" event. In order to minimize the need for more general invasive protocols, perhaps the use of biopsic material would help to bypass such limitation, besides the possibility of novel methodological imaging approaches. Overcoming these problems is imperative, because the positive selection of interlaminar glia in the primate order calls for a full characterization and understanding of its role in cerebral cortex function.

It may be opportune to state upfront that although other laboratory species provide valuable insights into "general mammalian" brain organization and evolution, the above-mentioned limitation generates an unavoidable and objective conceptual "gap" when extrapolating results from non-primate mammals to primates. Such consideration arises since the subtle, bioelectric, ionic/molecular dynamic interactions with cellular receptors operating in a particular brain organization is what provides the finely tuned scaffolding—besides structural or hardware connectivity—for the generation and expression of the characteristic complex and fluid human cognitive and emotional (manifest or introspective) behaviors. In this regard, further advances in the comparative—neuronal and glial—analysis within the primate order—specifically with genetically close extant species—seems critically needed. Perhaps, following the historically theoretical preeminence of the "neuronal doctrine", most studies have been performed on these cells in anthropoid species, generating a clear gap with respect to advances made on glial cells.

In such respect, although not intended to be reviewed here, numerous studies regarding associated neuronal and behavioral issues have been performed in primates by several authors. In particular, for example, some recent studies on the comparative distribution of neurotransmitter receptors in the brains of humans and extant primate species were reported by Zilles and colleagues [13,14], as well as comparative genetic studies by Pu et al. [15], Muntané et al. [16] and Mitchell and Silver [17]. Yet, the ethical limitations on the experimental use of primate species, and the needed minimization of invasive actions to be taken on them, as well as added limitations imposed on the inclusion in experimental protocols of extant species of great apes—mostly those genetically closer as *Pan troglodytes* and *Pan paniscus* (chimpanzee and bonobo, respectively)—calls for developing imaginative and minimally invasive research tools and procedures. The "handicap" of glial cells in terms of lacking readily in situ detectable bioelectric signals adds to the limitations on this field of the neurosciences.

At any rate, as pointed out by several authors (e.g., [4,12,18]), it has become unavoidable to include the spectrum of glial cells into theoretical constructions of brain evolution and organization. Certainly, this stage has been built following studies based on the access to laboratory rodent species. But time has come to work on new approaches and theoretical models to avoid known limitations to expand glial research into primates.

Developmental studies tracing the ontogenetic cellular origin of interlaminar glia remain missing. In the human brain, the developmental expression of interlaminar glia takes place during early postnatal life, following a period of "physiological astrogliosis" by 20–40 days of postnatal life, and attaining the adult-like configuration of interlaminar astrocytes by the second month of life [19]. Genetic analysis following the isolation of these cells could instigate detailed studies of their evolutionary origin and cell lineage.

The soma of interlaminar glial cells is closely apposed to the glia limitans and its short superficial processes are probably functionally associated with the subarachnoid space [9]. This layout suggests that their most superficial aspect could be linked to exchange with the pial vasculature/subarachnoid space, while their distal ending—usually a slender bulbous formation—has been shown [20] to be connected to a blood vessel (Figure 2) or "floating" in the intercellular space. Hence, a role in "fast sink" operations appears as a possibility, besides ion exchange through the membrane of its long interlaminar processes. This glial morphotype rather than engulfing synaptic terminals and intimately interacting with them as the type of layout reported by Grosche et al. [21] for parenchymal astroglia, interlaminar processes would appear to "navigate" in the extracellular space, perhaps monitoring and regulating ionic/molecular imbalances. In this regard, their membrane dynamic characteristics remain to be determined. It would be of significant interest to establish whether this type of glia is independent from the astroglial syncytia, and whether they form a parallel network that is perhaps interconnected at the subpial level. However, our attempts to analyze possible dye coupling of interlaminar glia—in samples from a non-human primate—failed due to technical reasons (previous exposure to an antifreeze medium for transport of fresh sections affected membrane permeable characteristics), and the limited number of sections to work with.

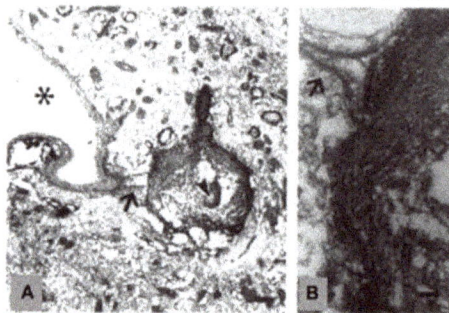

Figure 2. Interlaminar bulbous ending in an aged human cerebral cortex sample. Note in (**A**) a mitochondrion, and bridge (arrow) connecting with blood vessel (asterisk) (also in (**B**)). In (**B**), note the multilamellar structure. Scale bar: 50 μm in (**A**) and 200 nm in (**B**). Adapted from Figure 4 in Colombo et al. [20].

The possibility of vesicular transport as reported by Potokar et al. [22] for rodent glia should also be considered.

Attainment of final length, density and palisade display of interlaminar processes (Figure 1) depends on species and subspecies characteristics: for example, some New World monkeys could present a non-systematic, patchy and more scattered or unpredictable palisade, such as is the case of *Cebus paella* (tufted capuchin), while a more typical palisade occurs in *Saimiri boliviensis* (black-capped squirrel monkey). According to experimental data, the presence and length of interlaminar processes are significantly affected by interaction with thalamic cortical afferents, at least in areas that are related to the visual system [23] and spinal cord somatosensory input [24].

What are the signals involved in determining the characteristics of the palisade? Physiological signals driving morphological changes of interlaminar processes under the reported conditions remain undetermined. Whether effects on interlaminar glia (Figures 3 and 4) represent a trophic or regulatory role of thalamic afferents, or an indirect one through their cerebral cortex projections on neuronal activity [25,26], remains an open question. The disruption of the interlaminar cortical palisade after 11–13 months following spinal cord transection—with a lack of evidence of additional astrogliosis—and a somewhat "wavy" individual process display [24], suggests a rather long-term impact on the rearrangement of the local neuropil, or that it acquired a new steady state condition following lesioning, with loss or perturbation of the original columnar arrangement, and perhaps sharing an expanded spatial monitoring due to local disruption of the columnar modules.

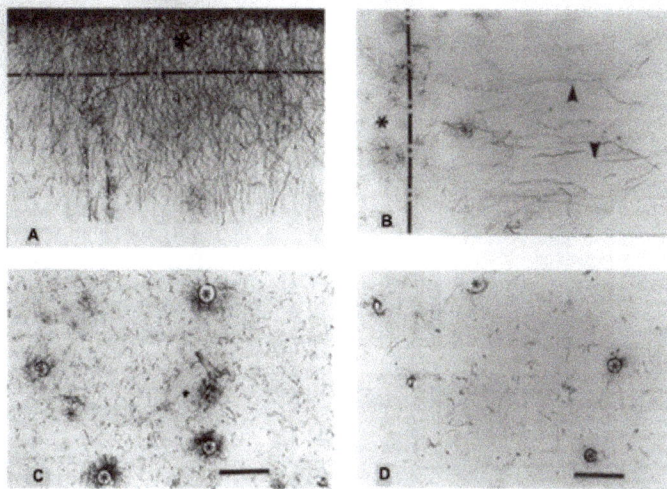

Figure 3. Interlaminar GFAP-IR events observed in coronal (**A,B**) and tangential (flattened) (**C,D**) sections of the striate cortex from control, intact (**C**) and three months visually deprived (**D**) adult *Cebus apella* monkey. Asterisk and broken line in (**A**) indicate the limit of lamina I. Vascular elements in (**C,D**) are marked by an asterisk. Note paucity of events in sections on the right side. Scale bar: 100 µm. Adapted from Colombo et al. [23].

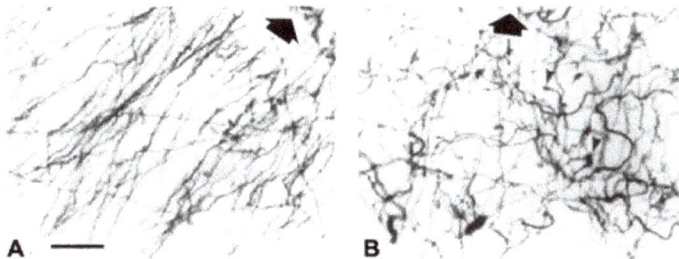

Figure 4. Morphology and spatial arrangement of GFAP-IR interlaminar processes in the somatosensory cortex of control and long-term spinal cord-transected *Macaca* individuals. (**A**) Control; (**B**) Operated. Note extreme departure from the rectilinear trajectory and several "terminal masses" (arrowheads). Large arrow indicates direction of the cortical surface. Scale bar: 40 µm. Adapted from Reisin and Colombo [24].

Quite interestingly, following cortical lesioning or, most clearly, under cerebral cortex pathological conditions (such as Alzheimer's disease or advanced Down's syndrome), or aging, interlaminar glia do not show reactive forms (in contrast to parenchymal astrocytes), but rather disappear [19,27], tending to lose their characteristic, ordered, lay out of long interlaminar processes, or to acquire increased bulbous endings (Figures 3 and 4, and [28]).

The description of the "wavy" terminal (15–30 μm in length) segment [5,19] in interlaminar glia (Figures 5–7) usually shows a tortuous "corkscrew" shape that was tentatively interpreted as a local increase in membrane surface, as it also was considered to be its normally slender bulbous ending (10–15 μm in diameter), in some cases being associated to blood vessels [20]. The presence of a mitochondrion embedded in its terminal implies a specific local energy requirement associated with ionic/molecular exchange mechanisms or possibly general terminal structural maintenance. These bulbous terminals acquire larger and sometimes even "massive" proportions (30 μm in diameter) with ageing and in Alzheimer´s disease, thus possibly representing a maladaption to such conditions, also observed, for example, in Albert Einstein´s brain samples [6,29].

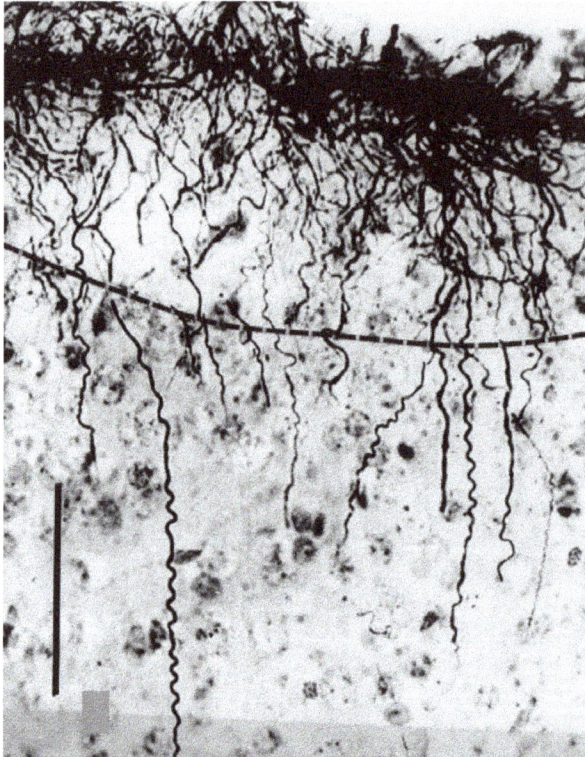

Figure 5. Striate cerebral cortex sample from 2.5-months-old *Saimiri boliviensis*. Glial fibrillary acidic protein immunostaining with Nissl stain. Scale bar: 100 μm. Adapted from Figure 2 in [9]. Note marked wavy configuration of the long (interlaminar) cellular processes.

Attempts to immunohistochemically label interlaminar processes with other cytoskeletal or neurotrasmitter markers, besides glial fibrillary acidic protein (GFAP), failed systematically in our hands, except at early postnatal ages, as illustrated (Figure 6), in which they could be labelled with a-vimentin.

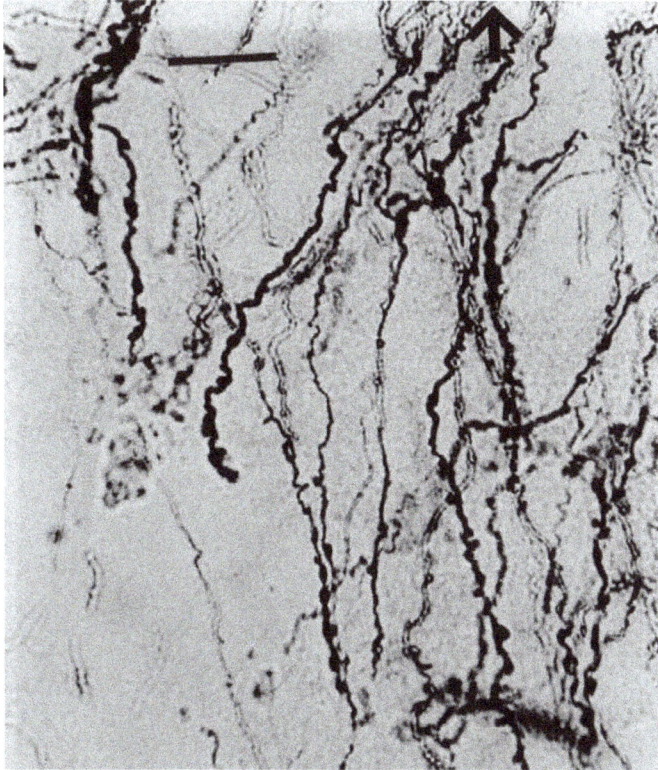

Figure 6. Intrasurgical sample. Human frontal cerebral cortex from a seven-year-old. Vimentin immunohistochemistry. Long processes with "corkscrew" appearance. Pia mater is towards the top of the figure asterisk indicates cortical surface. Scale bar: 20 μm. Adapted from Figure 5 in [9].

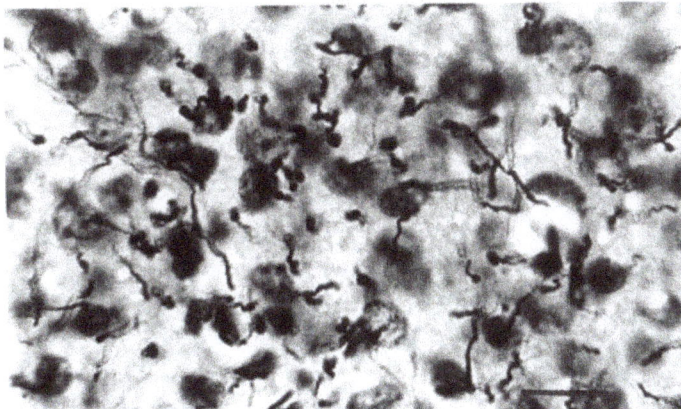

Figure 7. Tangential section of striate cortex from an adult *Saimiri boliviensis* monkey, reacted for GFAP with Nissl counterstain, note wavy terminal segments and slender bulbous terminals decorating them. Scale bar: 20 μm. Adapted from Figure 5 in [5].

The role of interlaminar glia in the regulation of the extracellular space and intercellular interactions is also unknown, although some speculative hypotheses were proposed by Reisin and Colombo [30], which were linked to the columnar organization of the neocortex "as proposed by Jakob and Onelli (1913), and later formalized by Lorente de No (1938) and electrophysiologically characterized by Powell and Mountcastle (1959) and Hubel and Wiesel (1965)" cf. [30]. To take this work forward requires studies on fresh tissue sections and/or using procedures, such as "tissue printing". We have successfully applied tissue printing procedures aimed at developing a new approach to analyze the ionic/molecular dynamics of single interlaminar processes [31], based on previous procedures developed in rats [32]. Unfortunately, these studies could not be continued, but this less invasive procedure—if based on surgical biopsies—could partially overcome the limited access to human and non-human primate brain samples.

3. Analysis of Astroglia in the In Vitro Conditions

Applying lucifer yellow dye coupling procedures comparative studies were performed in human, non-human primate, and rat cerebral cortex astroglial cell cultures. Their hypothetical role in cerebral cortex modularity was analyzed following initial observations on cell coupling in the cerebral cortical and striatal cells from *Cebus apella* (tufted capuchin) monkeys, demonstrating its functional preservation following freezing and thawing procedures [33]. Later, a comparison between rat, monkey, and human cell cultures from regional brain samples that were obtained at early ages and stored deep frozen, was undertaken by Lanosa et al. [34]. Rat striatum and cerebral cortex showed different coupling characteristics. Significant differences were observed in dye coupling between rodent and human brain cortical cells in in vitro conditions (Figure 8), which were suggestive of a comparatively reduced diffusion of dye coupling in human samples. It remains to be proven that these observations hold true in situ using brain slices. Should it be confirmed, it could be speculated that in *Homo* there is less tendency to spread cell coupling, which would aid in limiting spatial compromise of ionic/molecular perturbations and hence contribute more precise spatial (modular) characteristics, through reduction of glial territories.

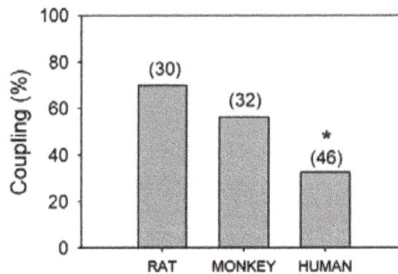

Figure 8. Interspecies analysis of astroglial coupling levels following lucifer yellow pressure injections in astroglia-enriched cultures from rat, monkey and human cerebral cortex, expressed as the percentage of cells coupled out of the total cells essayed (percentage of cell coupling). Numbers in parentheses indicate sample size. Significant differences were detected using Pearson's chi-square test (* $p = 0.006$). Adapted from Figure 3 in [34].

For the aforementioned experiments, the ages that were examined were developmentally early, as determined by the availability of samples from human and non-human primates, using cerebral cortex astroglial culture stocks of rat (five-day-old male), monkey (three-month-old male) and human (six-month-old female; intrasurgical sample) from postnatal origin, kept frozen under N_2-atmosphere until they were used [34]. Hence, an effect of age cannot be overlooked. Yet, the results open up an intriguing additional potential difference in glial functional (coupling) characteristics among mammalian species.

4. Glial Cells in Subcortical White Matter: Elements of a Subcortical, Distributed Information Neural Control Circuit?

An additional issue regarding the roles of glial cells in the regulation of information transfer is whether the so called subcortical "interstitial" (neuronal and glial) cells are solely residual (neurons) and maintenance (glia) of projection and association fibers, or they are part of regionally distributed, subcortical, neuron–glial networks, with a role in the control of information transfer probability through such axonal fibers. This matter has been further discussed in [35,36], and the regulation of timing and signal transfer probability in the subcortical white matter alternatively considered. This possibility calls for adequate experimental testing.

5. Diffusible Factors Released by Astroglia

According to observations by Colombo and Napp [37,38], and Hunter and Hatten [39], conditioned medium by confluent embryonic cell cultures of astroglia showed evidence of releasing diffusible inducers of radial glia and neuritogenesis in the in vitro settings. Our contribution further stressed the compatibility and potential usefulness of this in vitro model for the ex vivo analysis of factors affecting the molecular dynamics that are involved in neuronal migration. Figure 9 illustrates characteristic neuronal adhesion to radial glia and their leading and trailing processes. These radial glial cells expressed laminin and 401-R antigens.

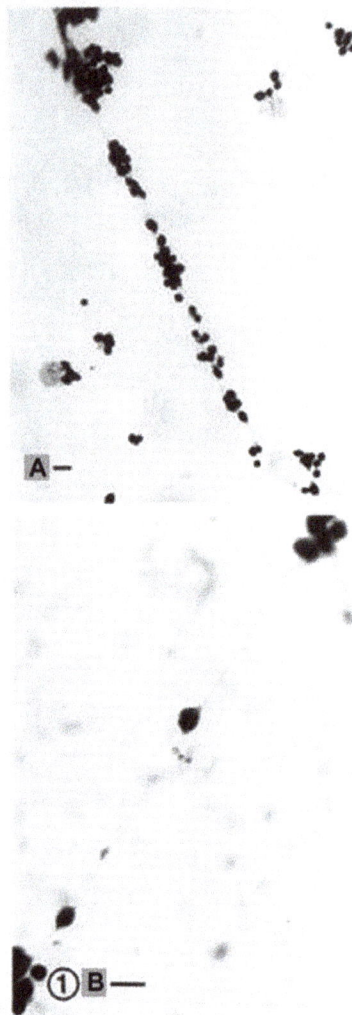

Figure 9. (**A**) Adhesion of cerebral cortex primary fetal (embryonic day 17 (E17)) cells onto elongated ("radial-like") processes of subcultured cerebral cortex glia exposed to cerebral cortex astroglial conditioned medium during 24 h, 3 h after seeding primary cells. Note in (**B**) evidence of leading and trailing processes of primary cells, adherent to a cell process. Induced processes were laminin-positive and Rat-401 antisera-positive. Adapted from Figure 1 in [37]. Scale bar: 10 µm (**A,B**).

In pathological conditions, such as Parkinson's disease, when considering that cerebrospinal fluid (CSF) from L-DOPA treated Parkinson's disease patients is dystrophic to neuronal cultures, possible diffusible messengers released into the CSF affecting astroglial cells [40] may intervene in the progression of associated brain pathology. Figure 10 illustrates the effect of CSF preincubation with cultured control glia on the otherwise deleterious effects of cerebrospinal fluid from patients with Parkinson's disease treated with L-DOPA.

The reported trophic influences of glia [37–41] prompted its implementation in a cell transplantation chymera in a non-human primate in the in vivo system, based on the intracarotid administration of the neurotoxin1-methyl-1-4-phenyl-1,2,3,6-tetrahydropyridine (MPTP)-induced parkinsonism in *Cebus apella* monkeys [42]. Following bilateral astroglial transplantation, significant performance improvement in a spatial delayed response task was observed, although it failed to modify perseveration in an object retrieval detour task, or to improve motor clinical rating. These observations suggest the possibility of dissociating brain circuits that are subserving various motor and cognitive performances. It should be added that the experimental design should take into consideration cognitive premorbid training effects, to avoid any interference with the interpretation of changes due to transplantation proper [43].

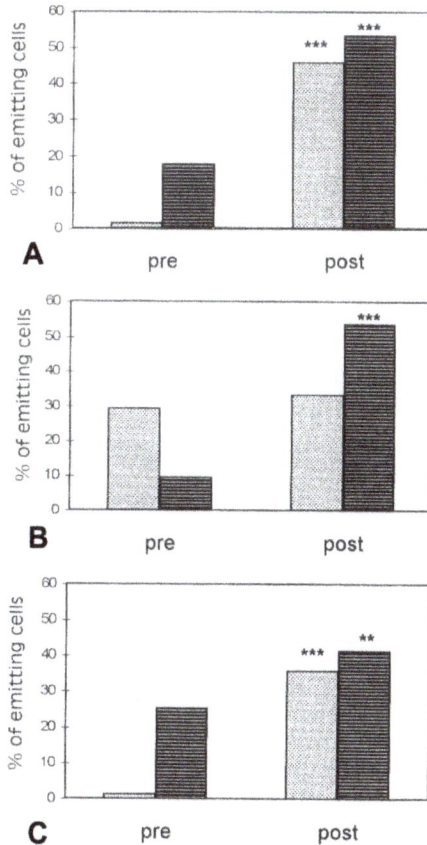

Figure 10. (A–C) Effect of astroglial conditioning of three different sources of cerebrospinal fluid (CSF) from Parkinson's disease patients on neuronal processes. Percentage of emitting cells in rat primary cultures of striatum (dotted bars) or ventral mesencephalon (horizontally dashed bars) after 24 h in culture with CSF before (pre) glial conditioning or after (post) 24 h conditioning with fetal mesencephalic astroglia. Pearson's chi-square test; ** $p < 0.01$; *** $p < 0.001$. Adapted from Figure 6 in [40].

6. Environmental Effects on Glial Response to Injury and Dye Coupling

The reported effects of environmental enrichment (EE) on neuronal events [44–46] suggested the need to analyze glial cell responses to such contingencies. We have studied this in two different protocols. One, in terms of recovery after cortical mechanical lesioning [47], with results suggesting that the exposure to EE conditions prior to injury attenuates the post-lesional astroglial GFAP-response in the perilesional cortex of rats, and, hence, could modulate post-lesional reactive components. This requires further studies to characterize the mechanisms that are involved.

In the second protocol, we analyzed glial dye coupling in fresh tissue sections from rat motor cortex, after varying periods of EE. These studies reported several observations, but in terms of EE on cell coupling in cortical laminae II–III, 30 days of EE resulted in a significant increase in the area of cell coupling, but not in the number of coupled cells, with a concomitant decrease in cell density, suggesting a volume increase in intercellular—gliopil—space [48]. These results can be interpreted as a spatial expansion of the glial net, perhaps involving an increase in glial connectivity. Further studies should clarify the mechanisms underlying such gliopil expansion (e.g., astrocyte hypertrophy), and whether changes in neuronal and vascular elements also take part in the process following EE.

7. Summary and Conclusions

Significant recent advances have been made in our understanding of general mammalian characteristics of glial cells and their roles in brain functional organization. However, care must be taken when extrapolating data to primate species. The absence of interlaminar glia in rodent species is an excellent case in point of such limitations. Critical functional knowledge must be based on primate species if we are to understand the role of glia in the complex organization of human and primate brains. In particular, "general mammalian" glial functional characteristics need to be critically assessed in light of interspecies differences in order to appreciate their significance in the cognitive and emotional processes that underlie primate and human behavior. For this purpose, continuously improved experimental procedures in primate species, such as in vitro cell culture, ex vivo organotypic brain slice preparations, and in vivo functional brain imaging and limited brain sampling procedures, would provide efficient means to accomplish such critical aims in highly protected species.

Acknowledgments: Contribution by Fundación Conectar to the development of the present review is gratefully acknowledged. Dedicated research involvement of colleagues and technical support personnel at the Unit of Applied Neurobiology (UNA, CEMIC-CONICET) during several demanding years, and sustained financial suport to the UNA research projects by various local and foreign granting agencies, is also gratefully acknowledged.

Conflicts of Interest: The author declares no conflict of interest.

References

1. Kettenmann, H.; Ransom, B.R. *Neuroglia*; Oxford University Press: New York, NY, USA, 2005; ISBN 0-19-515222-0.
2. Verkhratsky, A.; Butt, A. *Glial Physiology and Pathophysiology*; Wiley-Blackwell: Oxford, UK, 2013; ISBN 978-0-470-97852-8.
3. Verkhratsky, A.; Nedergaard, M. Physiology of Astroglia. *Physiol. Rev.* **2018**, *98*, 239–389. [CrossRef] [PubMed]
4. Colombo, J.A. Interlaminar astroglial processes in the cerebral cortex of adult monkeys but not of adult rats. *Acta Anat.* **1996**, *155*, 57–62. [CrossRef] [PubMed]
5. Colombo, J.A. A columnar-supporting mode of astroglial architecture in the cerebral cortex of adult primates? *Neurobiology* **2001**, *9*, 1–16. [CrossRef] [PubMed]
6. Colombo, J.A. The interlaminar glia: From serendipity to hypothesis. *Brain Struct. Funct.* **2017**, *222*, 1109–1129. [CrossRef] [PubMed]
7. Colombo, J.A.; Fuchs, E.; Härtig, W.; Marotte, L.R.; Puissant, V. "Rodent-like" and "primate-like" types of astroglial architecture in the adult cerebral cortex of mammals: A comparative study. *Anat. Embryol.* **2000**, *201*, 111–120. [CrossRef] [PubMed]
8. Colombo, J.A.; Sherwood, C.; Hof, P. Interlaminar astroglial processes in the cerebral cortex of great apes. *Anat. Embryol.* **2004**, *429*, 391–394. [CrossRef] [PubMed]
9. Colombo, J.A.; Lipina, S.; Yáñez, A.; Puissant, V. Postnatal development of interlaminar astroglial processes in the cerebral cortex of primates. *Int. J. Dev. Neurosci.* **1997**, *15*, 823–833. [CrossRef]
10. Aiello, L.C.; Wheeler, P.T. The Expensive-Tissue Hypotesis: The brain and the digestive system in human and primate evolutiom. *Curr. Anthropol.* **1995**, *36*, 199–221. [CrossRef]

11. Dunbar, R.I.M. The social brain hypothesis and its implications for social evolution. *Ann. Hum. Biol.* **2009**, *36*, 562–572. [CrossRef] [PubMed]

12. Robertson, J.M. Astrocytes and the evolution of the human brain. *Med. Hypotheses* **2014**, *82*, 236–239. [CrossRef] [PubMed]

13. Zilles, K.; Schlaug, G.; Matelli, M.; Luppino, G.; Schleicher, A.; Qü, M.; Dabringhaus, A.; Seitz, R.; Roland, P.E. Mapping of human and macaque sensorimotor areas by integrating architectonic, transmitter receptor, MRI and PET data. *J. Anat.* **1995**, *187*, 515–537. [PubMed]

14. Zilles, K.; Palomero-Gallagher, N. Multiple transmitter receptors in regions and layers of the human cerebral cortex. *Front. Neuroanat.* **2017**, *11*, 1–26. [CrossRef] [PubMed]

15. Pu, M.M.; Yao, J.; Cao, X. Genomics: Disclose the influence of human specific genetic variation on the evolution and development of cerebral cortex. *Hereditas* **2016**, *38*, 957–970. [PubMed]

16. Muntané, G.; Santpere, G.; Verendeev, A.; Sherwood, C. Interhemispheric gene expression differences in the cerebral cortex of humans and macaque monkeys. *Brain Struct. Funct.* **2017**, *222*, 3241–3254. [CrossRef] [PubMed]

17. Mitchell, C.; Silver, D.L. Enhancing our brains: Genomic mechanisms underlying cortical evolution. *Semin. Cell Dev. Biol.* **2017**. [CrossRef] [PubMed]

18. Oberheim, N.A.; Takano, T.; Han, X.; He, W.; Lin, J.H.; Wang, F.; Xu, Q.; Wyatt, J.D.; Pilcher, W.; Ojemann, J.G.; et al. Uniquely hominid features of adult human astrocytes. *J. Neurosci.* **2009**, *29*, 3276–3287. [CrossRef] [PubMed]

19. Colombo, J.A.; Reisin, H.D.; Jones, M.; Bentham, C. Development of interlaminar astroglial processes in the cerebral cortex of control and Down's syndrome human cases. *Exp. Neurol.* **2005**, *193*, 207–217. [CrossRef] [PubMed]

20. Colombo, J.A.; Gayol, S.; Yáñez, A.; Marco, P. Immunocytochemical and electron microscope observations on astroglial interlaminar processes in the primate neocortex. *J. Neurosci. Res.* **1997**, *48*, 352–357. [CrossRef]

21. Grosche, J.; Matyash, V.; Moller, T.; Verkhratsky, A.; Reichenbach, A.; Kettenmann, H. Microdomains for neuron–glia interaction: Parallel fiber signaling to Bergmann glial cells. *Nat. Neurosci.* **1999**, *2*, 139–143. [CrossRef] [PubMed]

22. Potokar, M.; Kreft, M.; Andersson, J.D.; Pangrsic, T.; Chowdhury, H.H.; Pekny, M.; Zorec, R. Cytoskeleton and vesicle mobility in astrocytes. *Traffic* **2007**, *8*, 12–20. [CrossRef] [PubMed]

23. Colombo, J.A.; Yáñez, A.; Lipina, S. Disruption of immunoreactive glial fibrillary acidic protein patterns in the *Cebus apella* striate cortex following loss of visual input. *J. Brain Res.* **1999**, *39*, 447–451.

24. Reisin, H.; Colombo, J.A. Glial changes in primate cerebral cortex following long-term sensory deprivation. *Brain Res.* **2004**, *1000*, 179–182. [CrossRef] [PubMed]

25. Peters, A.; Feldman, M.L. The projection of the lateral geniculate nucleus to area 17 of the rat cerebral cortex. IV Terminations upon spiny dendrites. *J. Neurocytol.* **1977**, *6*, 669–689. [CrossRef] [PubMed]

26. Biane, J.S.; Takashima, Y.; Scanziani, M.; Conner, J.M.; Tuszynski, M.H. Thalamocortical projections onto behaviorally relevant neurons exhibit plasticity during adult motor learning. *Neuron* **2016**, *89*, 1173–1179. [CrossRef] [PubMed]

27. Colombo, J.A.; Quinn, B.; Puissant, V. Disruption of astroglial interlaminar processes in Alzheimer's disease. *Brain Res. Bull.* **2002**, *58*, 235–242. [CrossRef]

28. Colombo, J.A.; Yañez, A.; Lipina, S. Interlaminar astroglial processes in the cerebral cortex of non-human primates: Response to injury. *J. Brain Res.* **1997**, *38*, 503–512.

29. Colombo, J.A.; Reisin, H.D.; Miguel-Hidalgo, J.J.; Rajkowska, G. Cerebral cortex astroglia and the brain of a genius: A propos of A. Einstein's. *Brain Res. Rev.* **2006**, *52*, 257–263. [CrossRef] [PubMed]

30. Reisin, H.D.; Colombo, J.A. Considerations on the astroglial architecture and the columnar organization of the cerebral cortex. *Cell. Mol. Neurobiol.* **2002**, *22*, 633–644. [CrossRef] [PubMed]

31. Colombo, J.A.; Napp, M.I.; Yañez, A.; Reisin, H. Tissue printing of astroglial interlaminar processes from human and non-human primate cerebral cortex. *Brain Res. Rev.* **2001**, *55*, 561–565. [CrossRef]

32. Barres, B.A.; Koroshetz, W.J.; Chun, L.L.Y.; Corey, D.P. Ion channel expression by white matter glia: The type 1 astrocyte. *Neuron* **1990**, *5*, 527–544. [CrossRef]

33. Gayol, S.; Pannicke, T.; Reichenbach, E.; Colombo, J.A. Cell–cell coupling in cultures of striatal and cortical astrocytes of the monkey *Cebus apella*. *J. Brain Res.* **1999**, *4*, 473–478.

34. Lanosa, X.A.; Reisin, H.D.; Santacroce, I.; Colombo, J.A. Astroglial dye-coupling: An in vitro analysis of regional and interspecies differences in rodents and primates. *Brain Res.* **2008**, *1240*, 82–86. [CrossRef] [PubMed]
35. Colombo, J.A.; Bentham, C. Immunohistochemical analysis of subcortical white matter astroglia of infant and adult primates, with a note on resident neurons. *Brain Res.* **2006**, *1100*, 93–103. [CrossRef] [PubMed]
36. Colombo, J.A. Cellular complexity in subcortical white matter: A distributed control circuit? *Brain Struct. Funct.* **2018**, *223*, 981–985. [CrossRef] [PubMed]
37. Colombo, J.A.; Napp, M.I. Ex vivo astroglial-induced radial glia express in vivo markers. *J. Neurosci. Res.* **1996**, *46*, 674–677. [CrossRef]
38. Colombo, J.A.; Napp, M.I. Forebrain and midbrain astrocytes promotes neuritogenesis in cultured chromaffin cells. *Restor. Neurol. Neurosci.* **1994**, *7*, 111–117. [PubMed]
39. Hunter, K.E.; Hatten, M.E. Radial glial cell transformation to astrocytes in bidirectional regulation by a diffusible factor in embryonic forebrain. *Proc. Natl. Acad. Sci. USA* **1995**, *92*, 2061–2065. [CrossRef] [PubMed]
40. Colombo, J.A.; Napp, M.I. Cerebrospinal fluid from L-dopa-treated Parkinson's disease patients is dystrophic for various neural cell types ex vivo: Effects of astroglia. *Exp. Neurol.* **1998**, *154*, 452–463. [CrossRef] [PubMed]
41. Uceda, G.; Colombo, J.A.; Michelena, P.; López, M.G.; García, A.G. Rat striatal astroglia induce morphological and neurochemical changes in adult bovine, adrenergic-enriched adrenal chromaffin cells in vitro. *Restor. Neurol. Neurosci.* **1995**, *8*, 129–136. [PubMed]
42. Lipina, S.J.; Colombo, J.A. Dissociated functional recovery in parkinsonian monkeys following transplantation of astroglial cells. *Brain Res.* **2001**, *911*, 176–180. [CrossRef]
43. Lipina, S.J.; Colombo, J.A. Premorbid exercising in specific cognitive tasks prevents impairment of performance in parkinsonian monkeys. *Brain Res.* **2007**, *1134*, 180–186. [CrossRef] [PubMed]
44. Diamond, M.C.; Krech, D.; Rosenzweig, M.R. The effects of an enriched environment on the histology of the rat cerebral cortex. *J. Comp. Neurol.* **1964**, *123*, 111–120. [CrossRef] [PubMed]
45. Globus, A.; Rosenzweig, M.R.; Bennett, E.L.; Diamond, M.C. Effects of differential experience on dendritic spine counts in rat cerebral cortex. *J. Comp. Physiol. Psychol.* **1973**, *82*, 175–181. [CrossRef] [PubMed]
46. Sirevaag, A.M.; Greenough, W.T. Differential rearing effects on rat visual cortex synapses. III. Neuronal and glial nuclei, boutons, dendrites, and capillaries. *Brain Res.* **1987**, *424*, 320–332. [CrossRef]
47. Lanosa, X.A.; Santacroce, I.; Colombo, J.A. Exposure to environmental enrichment prior to a cerebral cortex stab wound attenuates the postlesional astroglia response in rats. *Neuron Glia Biol.* **2011**, *7*, 1–13. [CrossRef] [PubMed]
48. Santacroce, I. Plasticity of Astroglial Networks in the Cerebral Cortex of the Rat: Response to Environmental Enrichment and Physicochemical Variables. Ph.D. Thesis, University of Buenos Aires, Buenos Aires, Argentina, 2017.

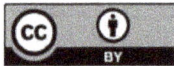

neuroglia

MDPI

Commentary

The Special Case of Human Astrocytes

Alexei Verkhratsky [1,2,3,*] [ID], Nancy Ann Oberheim Bush [4], Maiken Nedergaard [3,5]
and Arthur Butt [6,*] [ID]

1   Faculty of Biology, Medicine and Health, University of Manchester, Manchester, M13 9PT, UK
2   Center for Basic and Translational Neuroscience, Faculty of Health and Medical Sciences, University of
     Copenhagen, 2200 Copenhagen, Denmark
3   Achúcarro Basque Center for Neuroscience, 48940 Leioa, Spain; Maiken_Nedergaard@URMC.Rochester.edu
4   Division of Neuro-Oncology, Department of Neurological Surgery, University of California,
     San Francisco, CA 92093, USA; NancyAnn.OberheimBush@ucsf.edu
5   Center for Translational Neuromedicine, University of Rochester Medical Center, Rochester, NY 14642, USA
6   Institute of Biomedical and Biomolecular Sciences, School of Pharmacy and Biomedical Science, University
     of Portsmouth, Portsmouth PO1 2UP, UK
*   Correspondence: Alexej.Verkhratsky@manchester.ac.uk (A.V.); Arthur.butt@port.ac.uk (A.B.)

Received: 19 February 2018; Accepted: 19 February 2018; Published: 1 March 2018

✓ check for updates

Abstract: In this first issue of *Neuroglia*, it is highly appropriate that Professor Jorge A. Colombo at the Unit of Applied Neurobiology (UNA, CEMIC-CONICET) in Buenos Aires, Argentina, writes a perspective of idiosyncrasies of astrocytes in the human brain. Much of his work has been focused on the special case of *interlaminar astrocytes*, so-named because of their long straight processes that traverse the layers of the human cerebral cortex. Notably, interlaminar astrocytes are primate-specific and their evolutionary development is directly related to that of the columnar organization of the cerebral cortex in higher primates. The human brain also contains *varicose projection astrocytes* or *polarized astrocytes* which are absent in lower animals. In addition, classical protoplasmic astrocytes dwelling in the brains of humans are ≈15-times larger and immensely more complex than their rodent counterparts. Human astrocytes retain their peculiar morphology even after grafting into rodent brains; that is, they replace the host astrocytes and confer certain cognitive advantages into so-called 'humanised' chimeric mice. Recently, a number of innovative studies have highlighted the major differences between human and rodent astrocytes. Nonetheless, these differences are not widely recognized, and we hope that Jorge Colombo's *Perspective* and our associated *Commentary* will help stimulate appreciation of human astrocytes by neuroscientists and glial cell biologists alike.

Keywords: astroglia; protoplasmic astrocytes; interlaminar astrocytes; varicose projection astrocytes; human brain; astroglial domains

---

The widespread notion of neuroglia as the "neglected cells of neuroscience" is far from reality. The introduction of the concept of neuroglia as the connective tissue of the brain by Virchow [1] was followed by a steady flow of discoveries on glial cells and their roles in health and disease. All of the prominent neuroanatomists and neuropathologists of the second half of the 19th and early 20th century studied neuroglia (see for example [2–14]). These great minds laid the foundation of our knowledge of glial cells, mainly based on observation of human tissue.

It was the invention of "*La reazione nera*" by Golgi [15,16] and the many other staining techniques that it instigated which widened the visualisation and characterisation of diverse types of glia in the human brain. Prior to this, several types of glial cells had been described, most notably specialised types of radial astrocytes called the retinal Müller cells [17,18] and the cerebellar Bergmann glia [19]. In the following 50 years, the profuse use of Golgi staining resulted in the description of multiple morphological phenotypes of parenchymal glia (Figures 1 and 2), which were named "astroglia" in 1895 [20] (for further details on glial history, see [21–23]). The absolute majority of the original histological characterisation of glial cells was performed on human tissue, and there was little attempt to compare with smaller mammals, which were of little interest to classical neuroanatomists. This is diametrically opposed to the heavy reliance of modern neuroscience on rodent models.

A   B

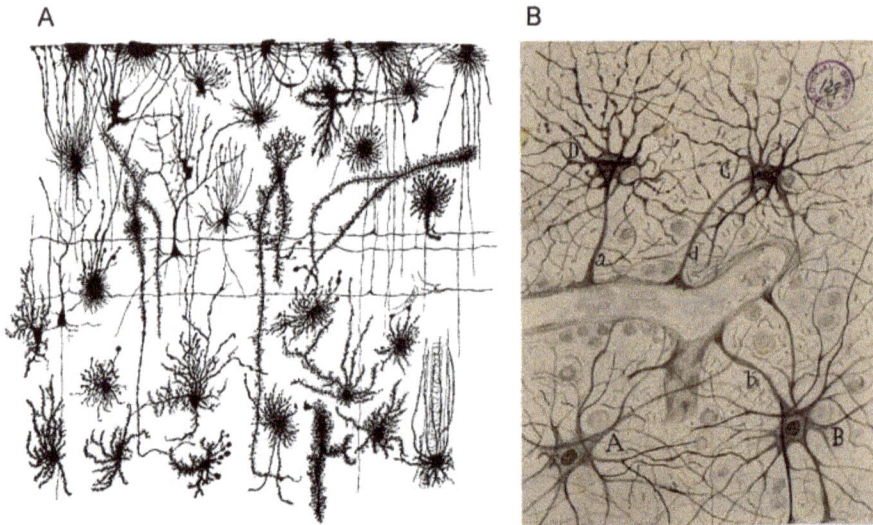

Figure 1. Early images of human astroglia. (**A**) Glial polymorphism in human foetal cortex as seen by Gustav Retsius [24]. (**B**) Perivascular astrocytes drawn by Santiago Ramón y Cajal; the image is from the collection of the Cajal Legacy at the Cajal Institute of the Spanish Research Council (CSIC). "®CAJAL INSTITUTE, CSIC", Madrid, Spain.

The early advances in glial morphology inspired abundant speculation on glial function. Some argued that glia existed merely to fill the otherwise empty spaces and provide a structural matrix, within which neurones are embedded [9], whereas some, however, went much further and assigned glia fundamental homeostatic functions [25] , whilst still others, most notably Carl Ludwig Schleich and Santiago Ramón y Cajal, suggested that glial cells control local blood flow, initiate sleep, and regulate information transfer in neuronal networks [8,14,26]. It is now apparent that astrocytes fulfil all of these operations and more, including the most fundamental neuronal attribute of synaptogenesis [27–30]. Similarly, the fundamental role of neuroglia in neurological diseases was highlighted by the most prominent neuropathologists, such as Franz Nissl, Carl Frommann, Ludwig Merzbacher, Alois Alzheimer, and Nicolas Achucarro [13,31–34]. At the turn of the 20th century, William Ford Robertson identified what he called "mesoglia" and proposed that they underwent pathological transformation in the diseased brain [35,36]. These mesoglia were Cajal's "third element", and they were characterised in detail by Pio del Rio Hortega, who identified them as oligodendrocytes and microglia. Del Rio Hortega clearly perceived microglia as having a defensive function [37–39] and that of oligodendrocytes in axonal myelination [40], which are indispensable in moulding the human brain connectome. Robertson's mesoglia almost certainly also incorporated the last addition to the glial family, namely NG2-glia, which were clearly identified by William Stallcup and his colleagues [41] and are also known as polydendrocytes or synantocytes [42].

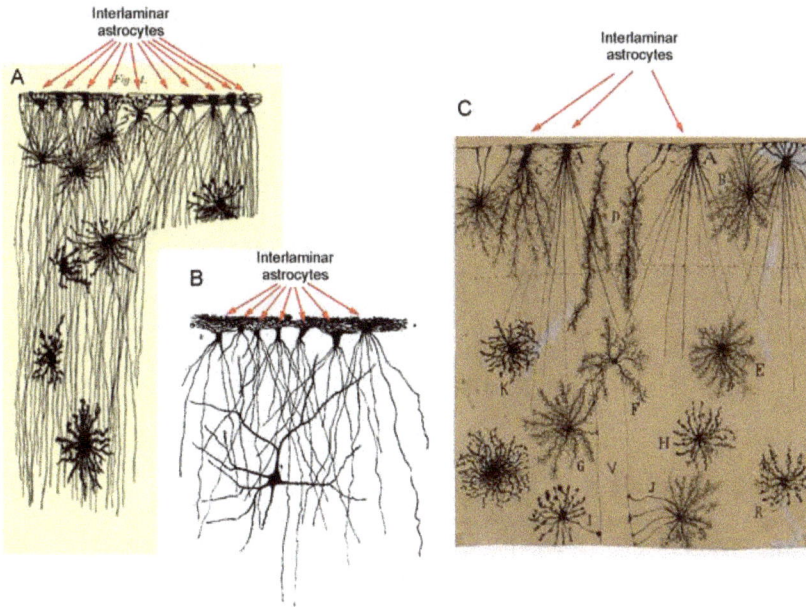

Figure 2. Early images of interlaminar astrocytes. (**A**) Glial cells from cerebral cortex of a one-year-old child drawn by Gustav Retzius [24]; numerous interlaminar astrocytes are clearly seen. (**B**) Interlaminar astrocytes as observed by William Lloyd Andriezen in 1893 [43]. (**C**) Golgi impregnated glia from human cortex (two-month-old child) in the plexiform layer (A–D), second and third layers (E–H and K, R, respectively) and perivascular glia (I, J). V, blood vessel. Cells labelled with A are interlaminar astrocytes. The image is from the collection of the Cajal Legacy at the Cajal Institute of the Spanish Research Council (CSIC). "®CAJAL INSTITUTE, CSIC", Madrid, Spain.

The golden age of neuroglial research resulted in the detailed characterisation of human glial types. Much less was known about glial cell physiology until the 1950s, when the first microelectrode studies were performed on the brains of cats, dogs, and subsequently amphibians and rodents [44–48]. The latter soon became the experimental paradigm of choice, and human neuroglia were largely neglected for a long time. However, the comprehensive analyses performed during the last decade have revealed extraordinary differences between human and rodent glia, in particular, differences in their astrocytes [49–53].

First and foremost, astrocytes are many times larger and much more complex in the human brain than their rodent counterparts. Human protoplasmic astrocytes have about 10 times more primary processes and a more complex secondary process arborisation, with an average volume that is about 16.5 times larger than the corresponding domain in a rat brain (Figure 3) [50]. The larger human protoplasmic astrocytes have also extended outreach onto neuronal structures, on average contacting and encompassing up to two million synapses residing in their territorial domains. This is significantly more than the integrating capacity of rodent protoplasmic astrocytes, which cover ≈20,000–120,000 synaptic contacts [50,54]. Similarly, human fibrous astrocytes have a domain 2.14-fold larger than that in rodents [50].

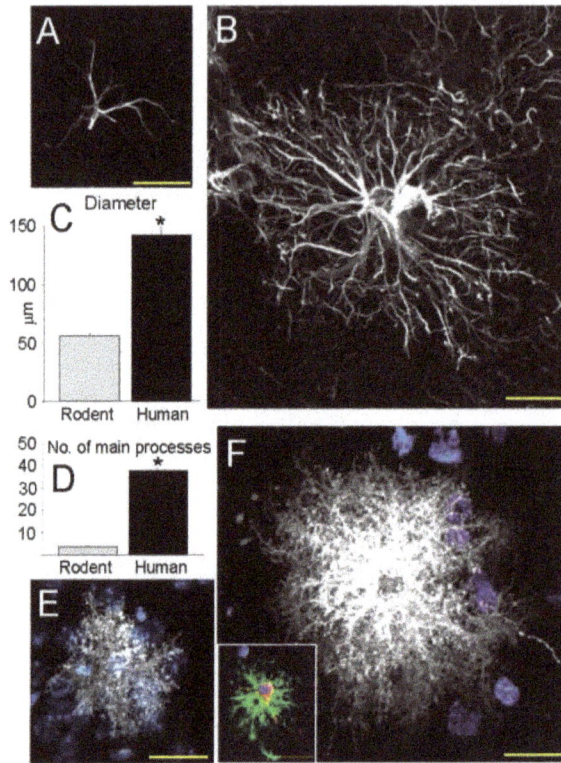

Figure 3. Comparison of rodent and human protoplasmic astrocytes. (**A**) Typical mouse protoplasmic astrocyte. Glial fibrillary acidic protein (GFAP) staining is shown in white. Scale bar: 20 μm. (**B**) Typical human protoplasmic astrocyte in the same scale. Scale bar: 20 μm. (**C,D**) Human protoplasmic astrocytes are 2.55-fold larger and have 10-fold more main GFAP processes than mouse astrocytes (human, n = 50 cells from seven patients; mouse, n = 65 cells from six mice; mean ± standard error mean (SEM); *$p < 0.005$, t-test). (**E**) Mouse protoplasmic astrocyte diolistically labelled with lypophilic dye DiI (white staining) and sytox (blue staining) revealing the full structure of the astrocyte, including its numerous fine processes. Scale bar: 20 μm. (**F**) Diolistically-labelled human astrocyte demonstrates the highly complicated network of fine process that defines the human protoplasmic astrocyte. Scale bar: 20 μm. Inset: Diolistically-labelled human protoplasmic astrocyte, also immunolabelled for GFAP (green staining), demonstrating colocalization. Scale bar: 20 μm. Reproduced with permission from [50].

In addition to the principal types of astroglia being particularly large and complex, the brains of higher primates and humans also contain several types of glia that do not exist in lower animals. The first type of uniquely human astrocyte that came under scrutiny was the class of *interlaminar astrocytes*, so-named by Jorge Colombo [55], whose historic and personal perspective is published in *Neuroglia* [56]. Notably, these cells were also seen by early neuroanatomists (Figure 2). Interlaminar astrocytes account for a rather substantial population of all astrocytes in the human cortex, while their functional role still remains enigmatic. The small (≈10 μm in diameter) spheroid cell bodies of interlaminar astrocytes dwell in cortical layer I (supragranular), and several short and one or two very long (up to 1 mm) processes emanate from these somata (Figure 4A,B). The processes of interlaminar astrocytes penetrate through the cortex, ending in deeper layers, from layer II to IV. These processes sometimes contact with blood vessels, while their terminal portions end with peculiar bouton-like structures, generally known as *terminal masses* or *end bulbs*. The processes of interlaminar astrocytes run parallel to each other, giving an appearance of a palisade.

The second type of astrocyte peculiar to the human brain are the *varicose projection astrocytes* or *polarized astrocytes*, which send several very long (up to 1 mm) unbranched processes with varicosities that extend in all directions through the deep cortical layers (Figure 4C–H) [51]. Apart from their long varicose processes, these cells otherwise look similar to classical protoplasmic astrocytes, but can be distinguished by their immunopositivity to CD44, also known as the homing cell adhesion molecule [52]. The density of these cells demonstrate remarkable individual variation, and their appearance is somehow related to age; that is, they have never been detected in the neonatal human brain, and it has been speculated that the appearance of these cells may reflect age-dependent adaptive changes and reflect individual life experiences [52].

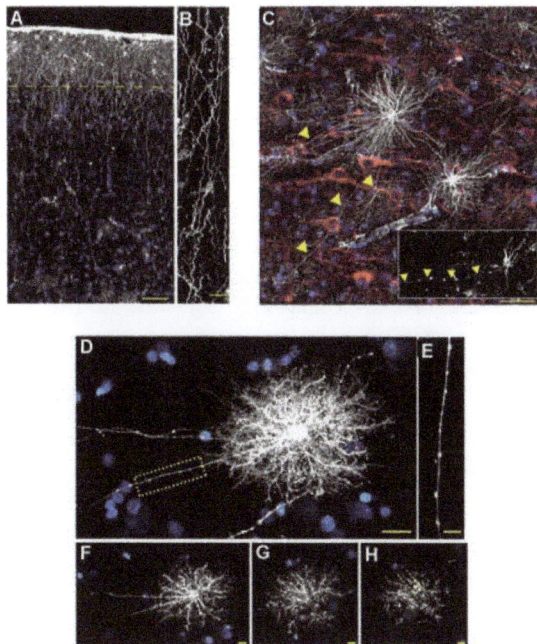

Figure 4. Interlaminar and varicose projection astrocytes in human cortex. (**A**) Pial surface and layers I–II of human cortex. GFAP staining is in white; 4′,6-diamidino-2-phenylindole (DAPI) staining is in blue. Scale bar: 100 μm. Yellow line indicates border between layer I and II. (**B**) Interlaminar astrocyte processes. Scale bar: 10 μm. (**C**) Varicose projection astrocytes reside in layers V–VI6 and extend long processes characterised by evenly-spaced varicosities. Inset: Varicose projection astrocyte from chimpanzee cortex. GFAP staining is in white, microtubule-associated protein 2 (MAP2) staining is in red and DAPI staining is in blue. Yellow arrowheads indicate varicose projections. Scale bar: 50 μm. (**D**) Diolistic labelling (in white) of a varicose projection astrocyte whose long process terminates in the neuropil, sytox staining is in blue. Scale bar: 20 μm. (**E**) High-power image of the yellow box in (**B**) highlighting the varicosities seen along the processes. Scale bar: 10 μm. (**F–H**) Individual z-sections of the astrocyte in (E) demonstrating long processes, straighter fine processes, and association with the vasculature. Reproduced with permission from [49,50].

The evolutionary development of human astrocytes, with processes that span multiple cortical layers, is directly related to the evolution of a highly complex columnar cortical organisation in higher primates. Moreover, developmental studies indicate that ontogeny recapitulates phylogeny;

for example, interlaminar astrocytes are first apparent at the end of the first month postnatal, and they reach their adult-like configuration by the second month of life [57]. It is tempting to speculate that the remarkably idiosyncratic morphology of human astrocytes translates into specific higher primate functions associated with information processing and intelligence. The theme of 'intelligent astrocytes' resurfaces sporadically; already in the 1960s, Robert Galambos proclaimed that "Glia is . . . conceived as genetically charged to organize and program neuron activity so that the best interests of the organism will be served; the essential product of glia action is visualized to be what we call innate and acquired behavioural responses. In this scheme, neurons in large part merely execute the instructions glia give them" [58]. This heretic and yet inspiring idea, which defines glia as a central element for information processing in the brain, has galvanized many followers [59–63], although it is still in need of credible experimental corroboration.

To attempt this corroboration, the chimeric model of 'humanised' mice was developed, in which the brains of neonatal animals were injected with human foetal glial cell progenitors. These human cells survived implantation and expanded to populate large areas of brain tissue and replace native rodent astrocytes. Moreover, mice bearing human astrocytes outperformed their wild type relatives in learning and memory tasks, while the threshold for long-term potentiation was reduced in these chimeras. Does this experiment indeed point out the intelligence potential of human astroglia? Or does the better performance of humanised mouse nervous tissue reflect a much higher capacity of human astrocytes to provide homeostatic and metabolic support? These points are not mutually exclusive, and the question remains open.

We hope that our *Commentary* has highlighted some key differences between astrocytes in the human brain and their simpler brethren in rodents. Currently, mice are the main animal model for studying brain function and pathology. Going forward, it is important to recognise the singularity of human astrocytes and interpret data from mice and other species appropriately. Jorge Colombo's perspective of his career studying interlaminar astrocytes helps bring these cells to the attention of neurobiologists who might otherwise be unfamiliar with them, and it will hopefully help stimulate future studies on these remarkable cells.

Acknowledgments: We are grateful to Ricardo Martínez Murillo (Instituto Cajal, Spain) for providing images of Cajal's drawings.

Author Contributions: All authors participated equally in writing this commentary.

Conflicts of Interest: The authors declare no conflict of interest.

References

1. Virchow, R. *Die Cellularpathologie in ihrer Begründung auf Physiologische and Pathologische Gewebelehre. Zwanzig Vorlesungen Gehalten Während der Monate Februar, März und April 1858 im Pathologischen Institut zu Berlin*, First ed.; August Hirschwald: Berlin, Germany, 1858; 440p.

2. Deiters, O. *Untersuchungen über Gehirn und Rückenmark des Menschen und der Säugethiere*; Vieweg: Braunschweig, Germany, 1865.

3. Besser, L. Zur histiogenese der nervösen elementarteile in den centralorganen der neugeborenen menschen. *Arch. Pathol. Anat. Physiol. Klin. Med.* **1866**, *36*, 305–333. [CrossRef]

4. Jastrowitz, M. Encephalitis und myelitis des ersten kindersalters. *Arch. Psychiatr.* **1870**, *2*, 389–414. [CrossRef]

5. Butzke, V. Studien über den feineren bau der grosshirnrinde. *Arch. Psych. Nervenkr.* **1871**, *3*, 575–601. [CrossRef]

6. Rindfleisch, E. *Handbuch der Pathologischen Gewebelehre. 3 aufl*; Engelmann: Leipzig, Germany, 1873.

7. Nansen, F. *The Structure and Combination of the Histological Elements of the Central Nervous System*; Bergens Museum Aarbs: Bergen, Norway, 1886.

8. Ramón y Cajal, S. Algunas Conjeturas sobre el Mecanismo Anatómico de la Ideación, Asociación y Atención. Imprenta y Libreria de Nicolas Moya: Madrid, Spain, 1895.

9. Weigert, C. *Kenntnis der Normalen Menschlichen Neuroglia*; Moritz Diesterweg: Frankfurt am Main, Germany, 1895; 213p.

10. Kölliker, A.v. *Handbuch der gewebelehre des menschen. 6 aufl*; Engelmann: Leipzig, Germany, 1896.
11. Held, H. Über die neuroglia marginalis der menschlichen grosshirnrinde. *Monatschr. Psychol. Neurol* **1909**, *26*, 360–416. [CrossRef]
12. Ramón y Cajal, S. Histologie du Système Nerveux de l'Homme et des Vertébrés. Maloine: Paris, France, 1909.
13. Achucarro, N. De l'évulotion de la névroglie, et spécialement de ses relations avec l'appareil vasculaire. *Trab. Lab. Invest. Biol. (Madrid)* **1915**, *13*, 169–212.
14. Ramón y Cajal, S. Contribution a la connaissance de la nevroglia cerebrale et cerebeleuse dans la paralyse generale progressive. *Trab. Lab. Invest. Biol. Univ. Madrid* **1925**, *23*, 157–216.
15. Golgi, C. *Opera omnia*; Hoepli: Milan, Italy, 1903.
16. Golgi, C. Suella struttura della sostanza grigia del cervello (comunicazione preventiva). *Gazzetta Medica Italiana Lombardia* **1873**, *33*, 244–246.
17. Müller, H. Zur histologie der netzhaut. *Z. Wissenschaft. Zool* **1851**, *3*, 234–237.
18. Schulze, M. *Observationes de retinae structura penitiori*; Published lecture; University of Bonn: Bonn, Germany, 1859.
19. Bergmann, K. Notiz über einige strukturverhältnisse des cerebellums und rükenmarks. *Z. Med.* **1857**, *8*, 360–363.
20. Lenhossék, M.v. *Der Feinere Bau des Nervensystems im Lichte Neuester Forschung*, 2nd ed.; Fischer's Medicinische Buchhandlung H. Kornfield: Berlin, Germany, 1895.
21. Verkhratsky, A.; Nedergaard, M. Physiology of astroglia. *Physiol. Rev.* **2018**, *98*, 239–389. [PubMed]
22. Kettenmann, H.; Verkhratsky, A. Neuroglia: The 150 years after. *Trends Neurosci.* **2008**, *31*, 653–659. [CrossRef] [PubMed]
23. Verkhratsky, A.; Butt, A.M. *Glial Physiology and Pathophysiology*; Wiley-Blackwell: Chichester, UK, 2013; 560p, ISBN 978-0-470-97852-8.
24. Retzius, G. *Biologische Untersuchungen. Neue Folge*; Volume vi. Mit 32 tafeln; Von Gustav Fischer: Stockholm, Sweden, 1894; 87p.
25. Lugaro, E. Sulle funzioni della nevroglia. *Riv. Patol. Nerv. Ment.* **1907**, *12*, 225–233.
26. Schleich, C.L. *Schmerzlose Operationen: Örtliche Betäubung mit Indiffrenten Flüssigkeiten. Psychophysik des Natürlichen und Künstlichen Schlafes*; Julius Springer: Berlin, Germany, 1894; 256p.
27. Butt, A.M.; Nedergaard, M.; Verkhratsky, A. Remembering Ben Barres. *Neuroglia* **2018**, *1*, 2. [CrossRef]
28. Verkhratsky, A.; Nedergaard, M. Astroglial cradle in the life of the synapse. *Philos. Trans. R Soc. Lond. B Biol. Sci.* **2014**, *369*, 20130595. [CrossRef] [PubMed]
29. Pfrieger, F.W.; Barres, B.A. Synaptic efficacy enhanced by glial cells in vitro. *Science* **1997**, *277*, 1684–1687. [CrossRef] [PubMed]
30. Eroglu, C.; Barres, B.A. Regulation of synaptic connectivity by glia. *Nature* **2010**, *468*, 223–231. [CrossRef] [PubMed]
31. Frommann, C. *Untersuchungen über die Gewebsveränderungen bei der Multiplen Sklerose des Gehirns und Rückenmarks*; Verlag von Gustav Fischer: Jena, Germany, 1878.
32. Nissl, F. Ueber einige beziehungen zwischen nervenzellerkrankungen und gliissen erscheinungen bei verschiedenen psychosen. *Arch. Psychiat.* **1899**, *32*, 1–21.
33. Merzbacher, L. *Untersuchungen über die Morphologie und Biologie der Abräumzellen im Zentralnervensystem*; Fischer-Verlag: Stuttgart, Germany, 1909.
34. Alzheimer, A. Beiträge zur kenntnis der pathologischen neuroglia und ihrer beziehungen zu den abbauvorgängen im nervengewebe. In *Histologische und Histopathologische Arbeiten über die Grosshirnrinde mit Besonderer Berücksichtigung der Pathologischen Anatomie der Geisteskrankheiten*; Verlag von Gustav Fischer: Jena, Germany, 1910; Volume 3, Band 3.
35. Robertson, W. A microscopic demonstration of the normal and pathological histology of mesoglia cells. *J. Mental Sci.* **1900**, *46*, 724. [CrossRef]
36. Robertson, W.F. *A Textbook of Pathology in Relation to Mental Disease*; William F. Clay: Edinburgh, UK, 1900.
37. Del Rio-Hortega, P. Poder fagocitario y movilidad de la microglia. *Bol. de la Soc. Esp. de Biol.* **1919**, *9*, 154.
38. Metz, A.u.S.H. Die hortegaschen zellen, das sogenannte "dritte element" und uber ihre funktionelle bedeutung. *Z. Neur.* **1924**, *100*, 428–449.

39. Del Rio-Hortega, P. Microglia. In *Cytology and Cellular Pathology of the Nervous System*; Penfield, W., Ed.; Hoeber: New York, NY, USA, 1932; Volume 2, pp. 482–534.

40. Del Río-Hortega, P. Estudios sobre la neuroglia. La glia de escasas radiaciones oligodendroglia. *Biol. Soc. Esp. Biol.* **1921**, *21*, 64–92.

41. Stallcup, W.B. The NG2 antigen, a putative lineage marker: Immunofluorescent localization in primary cultures of rat brain. *Dev. Biol.* **1981**, *83*, 154–165. [CrossRef]

42. Butt, A.M.; Hamilton, N.; Hubbard, P.; Pugh, M.; Ibrahim, M. Synantocytes: The fifth element. *J. Anat.* **2005**, *207*, 695–706. [CrossRef] [PubMed]

43. Andriezen, W.L. The neuroglia elements of the brain. *Br. Med. J* **1893**, *2*, 227–230. [CrossRef] [PubMed]

44. Wardell, W.M. Electrical and pharmacological properties of mammalian neuroglial cells in tissue-culture. *Proc. R. Soc. Lond. B Biol. Sci.* **1966**, *165*, 326–361. [CrossRef] [PubMed]

45. Hild, W.; Chang, J.J.; Tasaki, I. Electrical responses of astrocytic glia from the mammalian central nervous system cultivated in vitro. *Experientia* **1958**, *14*, 220–221. [CrossRef] [PubMed]

46. Tasaki, I.; Chang, J.J. Electric response of glia cells in cat brain. *Science* **1958**, *128*, 1209–1210. [CrossRef] [PubMed]

47. Kuffler, S.W.; Nicholls, J.G. The physiology of neuroglial cells. *Ergeb. Physiol.* **1966**, *57*, 1–90. [CrossRef] [PubMed]

48. Orkand, R.K.; Nicholls, J.G.; Kuffler, S.W. Effect of nerve impulses on the membrane potential of glial cells in the central nervous system of amphibia. *J. Neurophysiol.* **1966**, *29*, 788–806. [CrossRef] [PubMed]

49. Oberheim, N.A.; Goldman, S.A.; Nedergaard, M. Heterogeneity of astrocytic form and function. *Methods Mol. Biol.* **2012**, *814*, 23–45. [PubMed]

50. Oberheim, N.A.; Takano, T.; Han, X.; He, W.; Lin, J.H.; Wang, F.; Xu, Q.; Wyatt, J.D.; Pilcher, W.; Ojemann, J.G.; et al. Uniquely hominid features of adult human astrocytes. *J. Neurosci.* **2009**, *29*, 3276–3287. [PubMed]

51. Oberheim, N.A.; Wang, X.; Goldman, S.; Nedergaard, M. Astrocytic complexity distinguishes the human brain. *Trends Neurosci.* **2006**, *29*, 547–553. [CrossRef] [PubMed]

52. Sosunov, A.A.; Wu, X.; Tsankova, N.M.; Guilfoyle, E.; McKhann, G.M.; Goldman, J.E. Phenotypic heterogeneity and plasticity of isocortical and hippocampal astrocytes in the human brain. *J. Neurosci.* **2014**, *34*, 2285–2298.

53. Zhang, Y.; Sloan, S.A.; Clarke, L.E.; Caneda, C.; Plaza, C.A.; Blumenthal, P.D.; Vogel, H.; Steinberg, G.K.; Edwards, M.S.; Li, G.; et al. Purification and characterization of progenitor and mature human astrocytes reveals transcriptional and functional differences with mouse. *Neuron* **2016**, *89*, 37–53. [PubMed]

54. Bushong, E.A.; Martone, M.E.; Jones, Y.Z.; Ellisman, M.H. Protoplasmic astrocytes in ca1 stratum radiatum occupy separate anatomical domains. *J. Neurosci.* **2002**, *22*, 183–192. [PubMed]

55. Colombo, J.A. Interlaminar astroglial processes in the cerebral cortex of adult primates: Further characterization. In Proceedings of the 1st Int Conference on Glial Contributions to Behaviour, Belfast, Ireland, 28 August–1 September 1995; pp. 117–118.

56. Colombo, J.A. Interlaminar glia and other glial themes revisited: Pending answers following three decades of glial research. *Neuroglia* **2018**, *1*, 3.

57. Colombo, J.A.; Reisin, H.D.; Jones, M.; Bentham, C. Development of interlaminar astroglial processes in the cerebral cortex of control and Down's syndrome human cases. *Exp. Neurol.* **2005**, *193*, 207–217.

58. Galambos, R. A glia-neural theory of brain function. *Proc. Natl. Acad. Sci. USA* **1961**, *47*, 129–136. [CrossRef] [PubMed]

59. Bellini-Leite, S.; Pereira, A.J. Is global workspace a cartesian theater? How the neuro-astroglial interaction model solves conceptual issues. *J. Cogn. Sci.* **2013**, *14*, 335–360.

60. Caudle, R.M. Memory in astrocytes: A hypothesis. *Theor. Biol. Med. Model* **2006**, *3*, 2. [CrossRef] [PubMed]

61. Pereira, A., Jr.; Dos Santos, R.P.; Barros, R.F. The calcium wave model of the perception-action cycle: Evidence from semantic relevance in memory experiments. *Front. Psychol.* **2013**, *4*, 252. [CrossRef] [PubMed]

62. Pereira, A., Jr.; Furlan, F.A. Astrocytes and human cognition: Modeling information integration and modulation of neuronal activity. *Prog. Neurobiol.* **2010**, *92*, 405–420. [CrossRef] [PubMed]
63. Robertson, J.M. Astrocyte domains and the three-dimensional and seamless expression of consciousness and explicit memories. *Med. Hypotheses* **2013**, *81*, 1017–1024. [CrossRef] [PubMed]

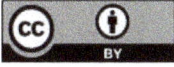

neuroglia

MDPI

Article

Cooperation between NMDA-Type Glutamate and P2 Receptors for Neuroprotection during Stroke: Combining Astrocyte and Neuronal Protection

Philipp Vermehren [1,†], Melissa Trotman-Lucas [2,†] (ID), Beatrice Hechler [3,4], Christian Gachet [3,4], Richard J. Evans [5], Claire L. Gibson [2] and Robert Fern [6,*] (ID)

[1] Department of Cell Physiology and Pharmacology, University of Leicester, Leicester LE1 9BH, UK; pvermehren@hotmail.co.uk

[2] Department of Neuroscience, Psychology & Behaviour, University of Leicester, Leicester LE1 9BH, UK; mt307@leicester.ac.uk (M.T.-L.); cg95@leicester.ac.uk (C.L.G.)

[3] UMR_S949, Institut National de la Santé et de la Recherche Médicale (INSERM), F-67065 Strasbourg, France; Beatrice.Hechler@efs-alsace.fr, (B.H.); christian.gachet@efs-alsace.fr (C.G.).

[4] Établissement Français du Sang-Alsace (EFS-Alsace), F-67065 Strasbourg, France

[5] Department of Molecular and Cell Biology, University of Leicester, Leicester LE1 9BH, UK; rje6@le.ac.uk

[6] Peninsula School of Medicine and Dentistry, University of Plymouth, John Bull Building, Research Way, Plymouth PL6 8BU, UK

* Correspondence: Robert.fern@plymouth.ac.uk; Tel.: +44-1572-383-202

† These authors contributed equally to this work.

Received: 13 February 2018; Accepted: 8 March 2018; Published: 14 March 2018

Abstract: Excitotoxicity is the principle mechanism of acute injury during stroke. It is defined as the unregulated accumulation of excitatory neurotransmitters such as glutamate within the extracellular space, leading to over-activation of receptors, ionic disruption, cell swelling, cytotoxic Ca^{2+} elevation and a feed-forward loop where membrane depolarisation evokes further neurotransmitter release. Glutamate-mediated excitotoxicity is well documented in neurons and oligodendrocytes but drugs targeting glutamate excitotoxicity have failed clinically which may be due to their inability to protect astrocytes. Astrocytes make up ~50% of the brain volume and express high levels of P2 adenosine triphosphate (ATP)-receptors which have excitotoxic potential, suggesting that glutamate and ATP may mediate parallel excitotoxic cascades in neurons and astrocytes, respectively. Mono-cultures of astrocytes expressed an array of P2X and P2Y receptors can produce large rises in $[Ca^{2+}]i$; mono-cultured neurons showed lower levels of functional P2 receptors. Using high-density 1:1 neuron:astrocyte co-cultures, ischemia (modelled as oxygen-glucose deprivation: OGD) evoked a rise in extracellular ATP, while P2 blockers were highly protective of both cell types. GluR blockers were only protective of neurons. Neither astrocyte nor neuronal mono-cultures showed significant ATP release during OGD, showing that cell type interactions are required for ischemic release. P2 blockers were also protective in normal-density co-cultures, while low doses of combined P2/GluR blockers where highly protective. These results highlight the potential of combined P2/GluR block for protection of neurons and glia.

Keywords: astrocyte; ATP; excitotoxicity; glutamate; NMDA; neuron; P-2 receptor; stroke

1. Introduction

Stroke involves the sudden onset of cerebral ischemia, producing cellular injury and loss of function, leading to permanent disability [1,2]. The principle mechanism underlying acute cell injury is excitotoxicity, involving the toxic build of extracellular neurotransmitters. Work towards an effective prophylactic intervention for patients at stroke risk has focused on ionotropic glutamate receptors (GluRs) and the neuro-protective promise of blocking excitotoxic over-activation of N-methyl-D-aspartate (NMDA)-type GluRs (see [3]). We have recently demonstrated, for example, that many of the contraindications of this approach can be resolved by using a low-dose prophylactic strategy employing the clinically approved drug memantine hydrochloride [4], and that selective targeting of Nr2C/D NMDA subunits is highly protective of both grey and white matter. However, ~50% of the brain parenchymal volume is made of astrocytes, essential neural partner cells that are required for neuronal survival and function. Astrocytes generally express low levels of GluRs (e.g., [5]) but robustly express P2 nucleotide adenosine triphosphate (ATP) receptors (see [6]). ATP can also act as an excitotoxin via activation of P2 receptors [7,8] and extracellular ATP is significantly elevated both in vitro and in vivo under hypoxic and ischemic conditions [9–16]. Prolonged application of ATP or ATP analogues produces necrotic and delayed cell damage in both neurons and astrocytes in vitro and in vivo [17–21]. The harmful effects of ATP may be enhanced during ischemia by a reduced efficiency of ATP-degrading ecto-nucleotidases, which will reduce the capacity of the brain to clear extracellular ATP [22,23].

Astrocytes play important roles in the acute injury and survival of neurons affected by ischemia, including the release/uptake of neurotransmitters, regulation/dysregulation of extracellular ionic homeostasis and the production/buffering of reactive species. In addition to their essential support role in neural function, astrocyte cell death is a prerequisite for the evolution of necrotic stroke infarction [24]. Astrocyte protection may also be directly beneficial to neighbouring neuronal elements; for example, astrocyte glycogen storage can have a powerful influence upon the survival chances of neighbouring axons [25]. In the present study, we use neuron-enriched, astrocyte-enriched and 50/50 co-cultures where the two cell types can be distinguished to probe the effects of P2 receptor block on oxygen-glucose deprivation (OGD)-induced neurotransmitter release and associated cell death. We report that, even at very low concentrations, P2 receptor block is a highly effective pathway to astrocyte protection from acute ischemia which, unlike GluR block, reduces both neuron and glia injury. Combined block of P2 and GluRs effectively prevented cell death, the first time a combined pharmacological strategy has been identified to block acute ischemic cell death in both neurons and glia.

2. Materials and Methods

2.1. Cell Culture

Normal-density primary cortical neuron and astrocyte co-cultures were prepared from the cerebral cortices of C57BL/6 mouse gestation day 15–17 embryos (Charles river, Margate, UK), following humane cervical dislocation under UK Home Office Schedule 1 regulations. Cortices were removed and placed into Hank's balanced salt solution (HBSS), trypsinised (1% trypsin/DNAse) at 37 °C for 10 min, triturated and then centrifuged (1500 rpm/5 min). Cells were subsequently re-suspended in growth media (Dulbeco's minimum essential medium (DMEM), containing 4500 mg/L glucose, Glutamax-I, 110 mg/L pyruvate, penicillin/streptomycin and 10% foetal bovine serum (FBS)), and plated onto 175 cm^2 flasks. At two days in vitro (DIV), excess microglia were removed by gentle tapping and swirling of the flask prior to 100% DMEM media change. At six DIV, unwanted oligodendrocytes and microglia were removed by multiple agitations and washing steps until the lower-most astrocyte layer remained. Astrocytes were removed from the flask by trypsin action (0.5% Trypsin/5.3 mM EDTA), centrifuged and re-suspended in DMEM. Astrocytes were counted and plated at 0.15×10^6 cells/mL onto previously poly-L-lysine (100 µg/mL) coated coverslips. At eight DIV cortical neurons were prepared from E16 embryos in the same fashion as astrocytes up to the initial re-suspension where the media used was Neurobasal (Neurobasal medium, penicillin/streptomycin, B27 supplement, Glutamax-I). Cells were passed through a 100 µm cell strainer prior to counting. Neurons were plated at 0.15×10^6 cells/mL directly on top of previously plated astrocytes and the media was changed to Neurobasal. Cultures were used from 12 DIV. High-density neuronal-enriched, astrocyte-enriched and 1:1 co-cultures were prepared from BALBc mice in a similar fashion to the above but using higher plating densities (see [4] for details). These high-density cultures were useful for characterising receptor responses and measuring neurotransmitter release.

2.2. Distinguishing Neurons and Astrocytes in Co-Culture

Co-cultured astrocytes and neurons are morphologically distinct under phase contrast. To distinguish between the co-cultured cells, pseudo-fluorescent images were overlaid on the corresponding phase-contrast images for identification. Astrocytes form a continuous layer of flat low phase-contrast cells, whereas neuronal cells are high contrast showing pyramidal, fusiform or multipolar characteristics; these identifying characteristics have recently been confirmed in sister cultures [4]. Unidentifiable cells were excluded from subsequent analysis.

2.3. Cell Imaging (Viability and $[Ca^{2+}]_i$)

For imaging of cell viability, cell death was assessed using an intracellular green CellTracker^{TM} probe, 5-chloromethylfluorescein diacetate (CMFDA) (Fisher, Loughborough, UK), AM loaded at 2.5 µM. CMFDA-loaded cultures were mounted into an atmosphere perfusion chamber (Warner Instruments, Hamden, CT, USA), perfused at 2 mL/min (artificial cerebro-spinal fluid (aCSF) mM: 153 Na$^+$, 3 K$^+$, 2 Mg^{2+}, 2 Ca^{2+}, 131 Cl$^-$, 26 HCO$_3^-$, 2 H$_2$PO$_4^{4-}$ and 10 dextrose (bubbled with O$_2$ 95%/CO$_2$ 5%), 317–319 milliosmoles) and maintained at 37 °C. Temperature was monitored and regulated via flow-through, objective and room heaters (see [26]). Once mounted onto the stage of an epi-fluorescence microscope (Nikon, Tokyo, Japan), oil immersion ×20 images were collected at 508 nm via appropriate filter sets (Chroma Technology Corporation, Bellows Falls, VT, USA) following excitation at 489 nm (optoscan, Cairn Research, Faversham, UK). Images were captured by a coolSNAP HQ camera (Roper Scientific, Vianen, The Netherlands) controlled via MetaFluor (Molecular Devices, San Jose, CA, USA) with background signal subtracted. OGD conditions were induced by switching from aCSF to aCSF-zero glucose (OGD mM: 153 Na$^+$, 3 K$^+$, 2 Mg^{2+}, 2 Ca^{2+}, 131 Cl$^-$, 26 HCO$_3^-$, 2 H$_2$PO$_4^{4-}$ (bubbled with N$_2$ 95%/CO$_2$ 5%) and switching the chamber atmosphere from 95% O$_2$/5%CO$_2$ to 95%N$_2$/5%CO$_2$. Cultures were perfused with aCSF for 10 min before switching to OGD. Two sets of image data were collected from each CMFDA experiment. Quadrant images were taken at 0 and 100 min of perfusion where initial cell and surviving cell counts were taken in the four complete adjacent fields of view contiguous with the imaged field in the centre. These quadrant images were used to determine total cell death over the whole time-course of the experiment, and also acted as a control to ensure that fluorescent excitation illumination was not affecting cell viability (these cells were not exposed to illumination during the course of the experiment). Fluorescent images were taken every 30 s from the central field of view where cell death was characterised by a sudden collapse of the fluorescent signal as previously described (see [4]). These data were used to calculate cell death rates with time within the field of view. Cell death data are plotted as a time course represent the real time recordings from the central field of view, while total cell death data include the cells from the surrounding quadrants.

For $[Ca^{2+}]_i$ imaging during OGD, cultures were loaded with FURA-2FF (Invitrogen, Carlsbad, CA, USA), a low affinity dye that does not affect cell viability during ischemia [27]. The more sensitive FURA-2 was used for agonist responses. In both cases, cells were AM-loaded (see [26] for more details of imaging methods). A rapid exchange perfusion system was used for short application agonist experiments (ValveBank8.2, AutoMate Scientific, Berkeley, CA, USA). Oil immersion ×20 images were collected at 520 nm using appropriate filter sets (Chroma Technology Corporation, Bellows Falls, VT, USA). Cells were illuminated at 340, 360, and 380 nm (Optoscan, Cairn Research, Faversham, UK). For FURA-2 imaging, 340:380 was converted to $[Ca^{2+}]_i$ using a calcium calibration kit (Invitrogen). Cell death was characterized by sudden collapse of the fluorescent signal to the background level and this phenomenon was used to calculate cell death rates and precise time points of cell death for all cells within the field of view.

2.4. Biosensors

ATP and glutamate microelectrode biosensors (Sarissa Biomedical, Coventry, UK) [28], amplified via a Duo-Stat ME-200$^+$ potentiostat (Sycopel International Ltd., Tyne & Wear, UK), were used to record real time glutamate or ATP concentration changes in vitro from the unstirred fluid layer surrounding cells in high-density cultures. Signals were recorded differential to a null electrode and both active and null electrodes were carefully inserted into a modified atmosphere chamber until the sensor tips rested directly on the cell layer (see [4]). An Ag/AgCl reference electrode was introduced at a distal site. OGD and control experiments were performed as described above for cell imaging. Sensors were recalibrated in the chamber at the end of the OGD period after retraction from the cell layer. Values from the null, sensor, and sensor-minus-null outputs were recorded at 0.5 Hz and subsequently converted into Δ ATP or Δ glutamate, rather than absolute concentrations. Experiments were repeated a minimum of three times, all values collected for a time point during a specific condition/experiment were averaged using Prism software (GraphPad, Prism Software, Droitwich, UK).

2.5. Statistics

Experiments were repeated a minimum of three times on three separate culture preparations. Results are presented as mean ± standard error of the mean (SEM). Statistical analysis for comparison of experimental groups was undertaken using one-way analysis of variance (ANOVA) with Tukey's post-hoc test for multiple comparisons. For all data, differences of $p < 0.05$ were deemed significant.

3. Results

3.1. Functional P2 Receptors and GluR in Astrocyte-Enriched and Neuron-Enriched Cultures

Functional GluR and P2 ATP receptor expression was examined in neuron- and astrocyte-enriched cultures, using Ca^{2+} micro-fluorimetry. Resting $[Ca^{2+}]_i$ was significantly higher in astrocyte cultures compared to neurons (98.0 nM ± 3.0 n = 554 vs. 65.0 nM ± 1.5, n = 739, respectively; $p < 0.001$), and in both cases was affected by tonic application of various receptor antagonists used in this study. For this reason, $[Ca^{2+}]_i$ changes have been used for the statistical comparison of drug effects, rather than absolute $[Ca^{2+}]_i$ levels. To confirm the presence of functional P2 receptors on astrocytes, cells were exposed to a series of P2 receptor agonists. One hundred percent of astrocytes responded to 100 µM ATP, with a mean $[Ca^{2+}]_i$ increase of 722.9 ± 29.2 nM (n = 341; Figure 1A–C). All receptor sub-type selective agonists tested (100 µM adenosine diphosphate (ADP), 100 µM ATPγS, 10 nM MRS-2365, 100 µM BzATP) had response rates approaching 100% and produced smaller $[Ca^{2+}]_i$ responses than those produced by ATP, in the 328–539 nM range (Figure 1A–C). A second application of 100 µM ATP at the end of the experiment produced a $[Ca^{2+}]_i$ rise of a similar amplitude to the initial response, but a degree of response run-down was found during multiple sequential applications of ATP (falling to 84.9% of the first response after six repeats, 5 min apart, n = 62). Small amplitude glutamate responses were observed in a sub-set of cultured astrocytes (e.g., Figure 1A), as reported in a companion study [4].

The presence of ionotropic glutamate receptors is well documented in cultured neurons (see [4] for studies on sister cultures), P2 receptor responses less so. The proportion of cells in neuronal cultures responding to sequential exposure to a series of P2 agonists ranged from 58.0 ± 4.2% for ATP down to 26.4 ± 7.1% for BzATP (Figure 1D,E), in all cases significantly lower than the corresponding response rate in astrocyte cultures. The maximal $[Ca^{2+}]_i$ rises evoked by P2 agonists were also smaller than in astrocytes, between 110.0 ± 4.6 nM for ATP and 56.9 ± 4.3 nM for BzATP (Figure 1F). In general, neurons responded to either the majority of P2 agonists or none at all, although the amplitude of responses varied within cells. As with astrocytes, a degree of hysteresis in the ATP response was observed in cultured neurons with a second application evoking a significantly smaller response (Figure 1F).

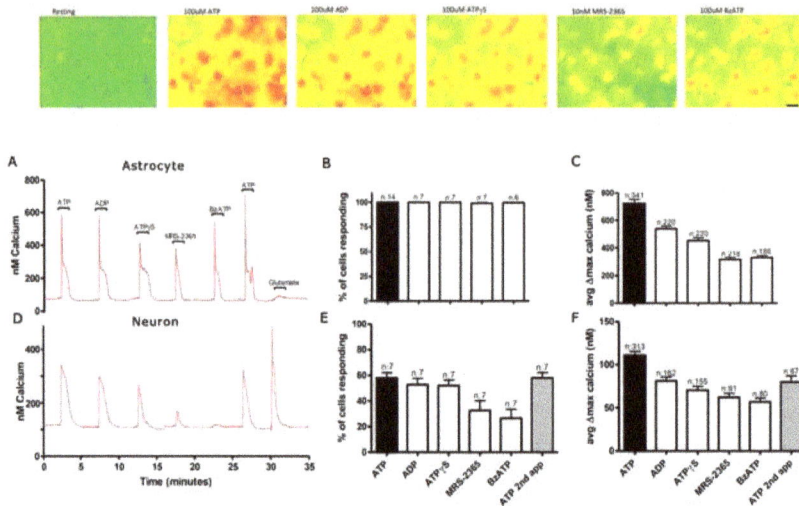

Figure 1. P2 receptor-mediated responses in astrocyte and neuronal cultures. (**A**) [Ca^{2+}]$_i$ recorded from a typical individual astrocyte showing baseline and agonist-evoked responses. Raw pseudo-colour images from this experiment are shown at the top, demonstrating cell responses to each of the agonists (each colder spot in the resting image is a single cell). Scale = 10 μm. (**B**) Mean number of astrocytes which respond to individual agonists (*n* = number of individual cultures). (**C**) Mean change in [Ca^{2+}]$_i$ evoked by agonists (*n* = individual astrocytes). (**D–F**) Similar series to (**A–C**), in this case for cultured neurons. ATP: adenosine triphosphate, ADP: adenosine diphosphate.

Since neurons express both functional GluR and P2 receptors, the effects of combined P2 + GluR block were examined on agonist-induced responses in neuronal cultures. Combined block of GluR and P2 receptors (60 min pre-treatment with 30 μM NBQX + 10 μM MK-801 + 100 μM PPADS) reduced the proportion of neurons responding to glutamate (under zero-Mg^{2+} conditions) from 100% to 72.0 ± 3.2%, with response amplitude falling by 73.1% (*p* < 0.001; *n* = 107; Figure 2A–D). Responses to specific NMDA- and non-NMDA-type ionotropic glutamate receptor agonists were suppressed to a greater extent than those to glutamate, indicating a significant metabotropic component to the glutamate response in cultured neurons. The cellular ATP response rate fell to 13.7 ± 6.6% (*p* < 0.001; *n* = 231) in the presence of the antagonist cocktail, but the amplitude of [Ca^{2+}]$_i$ rises in the remaining responding cells was not significantly affected (Figure 2C,D).

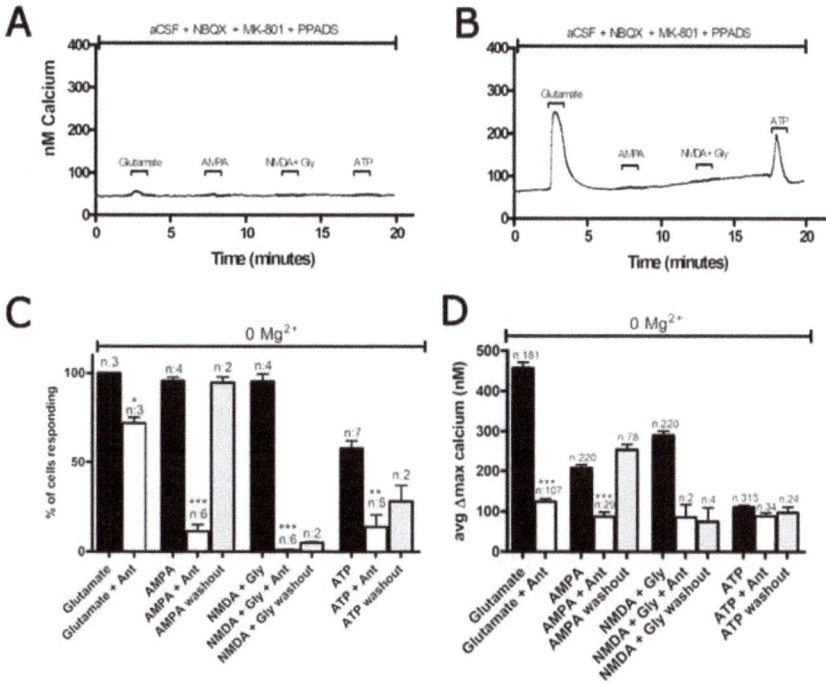

Figure 2. Combined P2 and ionotropic glutamate receptor block of neuronal responses. (**A,B**) $[Ca^{2+}]_i$ changes evoked by serial application of the receptor agonists glutamate (100 µM), AMPA (100 µM), NMDA (100 µM) + glycine (10 µM) and ATP (100 µM) in two cultured neurons from the same culture in the combined presence of 30 µM NBQX + 10 µM MK-801 + 100 µM PPADS (pre-applied for 60 min, all in zero-Mg^{2+}). These two cells show the range of responses observed. Note that, while all responses are small or blocked in the cell shown in (**A**), robust glutamate and ATP responses are retained in (**B**). (**C,D**) Mean number of responding cells (**C**) and mean $[Ca^{2+}]_i$ changes (**D**).

Astrocytes express a wide range of P2 receptors and to differentiate P2X- and P2Y-mediated responses the Ca^{2+}-dependence of P2 responses in these cells was investigated [29]. Astrocyte cultures were pre-treated with 1 µM thapsigargin for 60 min to block sarcoplasmic/endoplasmic reticulum Ca^{2+}-ATPase (SERCA) and deplete Ca^{2+} stores prior to sequential exposure to ATP and ADP in the presence and then the absence of extracellular Ca^{2+} (Figure 3). In normal aCSF, thapsigargin treatment reduced the proportion of ATP-responding cells from 100% to 60.1 ± 13.0% and response amplitude to 7.3% of control (both $p < 0.001$). All responses were eliminated by the removal of extracellular Ca^{2+} (Figure 3B,C). The data suggest that ~60% of astrocytes express functional P2X receptors but that these contribute less than 10% to the Ca^{2+} rises evoked by ATP. ADP, which is a selective agonist for a sub-set of P2Y receptors, produced only limited responses following thapsigargin treatment, consistent with this hypothesis. The P2Y receptor compliment on astrocytes included a significant $P2Y_1$ component since ~30% of the $[Ca^{2+}]_i$ response to ATP was lost when experiments were conducted on astrocyte cultures prepared from $P2Y_1$ −/− mice (Figure 4). The $[Ca^{2+}]_i$ responses to ADP were also reduced in these cells (by over 80%), and all effects of the selective $P2Y_1$ agonist MRS-2365 were abolished (Figure 4). As a corollary, this experiment demonstrates the purity of the ATP used since some cells responded to ATP but not ADP; ADP impurity has been a major concern in commercially available ATP [30].

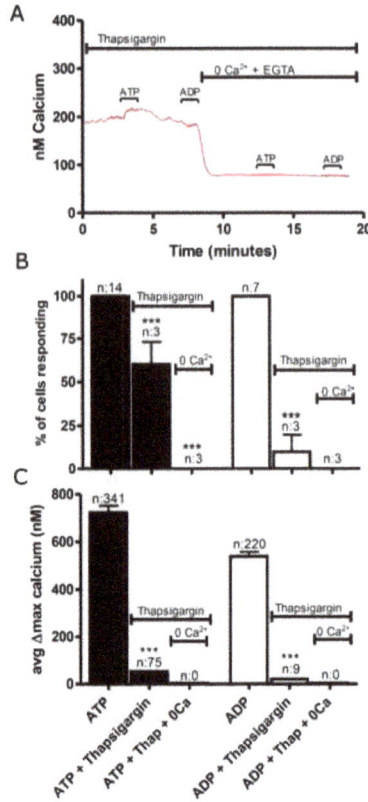

Figure 3. P2X and P2Y receptors are expressed in cultured astrocytes. (**A**) Representative data showing the effects of 100 μM ATP and 100 μM ADP perfusion following depletion of Ca^{2+}_i stores by treatment with 1 μM thapsigargin in the presence and then the absence of extracellular Ca^{2+}. (**B,C**) Mean number of responding cells (n = cover slips) (**B**) and mean $[Ca^{2+}]_i$ changes (n = cells responding) (**C**) showing the major contribution to ATP responses by P2Y receptors in these cells.

In astrocyte cultures, pre-incubation for 60 min with the broad-spectrum P2 antagonists suramin (100 μM, Figure 5A,B) or PPADS (100 μM, Figure 5C,D) reduced the mean $[Ca^{2+}]_i$ response to ATP by 43.9 ± 1.4% and 55.9 ± 1.8% of control, respectively. ADP responses, which should be largely P2Y-mediated, were reduced by 59.5 ± 1.9% and 39.5 ± 1.9%, respectively. Drug washout was incomplete over the time-course of the experiment. Neither drug significantly reduced the 100% response rate of the cells to either agonist. The concentration-dependence of PPADS was investigated during shorter exposure periods (Figure 5E,F). Sixty-minute pre-incubation with combined application of the selective P2Y$_1$ antagonist MRS-2179 and the P2X$_7$ antagonist KN-62 was also tested (Figure 5G,H). This protocol significantly reduced the amplitude of the $[Ca^{2+}]_i$ responses to ATP to 69.4 ± 2.2% of control ($p < 0.001$, $n = 119$), with limited reversibility after 5 min wash-out. Somewhat larger effects of this antagonist combination was found upon the responses evoked by the selective P2Y$_1$ and P2X$_7$ agonists MRS-2365 and BzATP (Figure 5G,H).

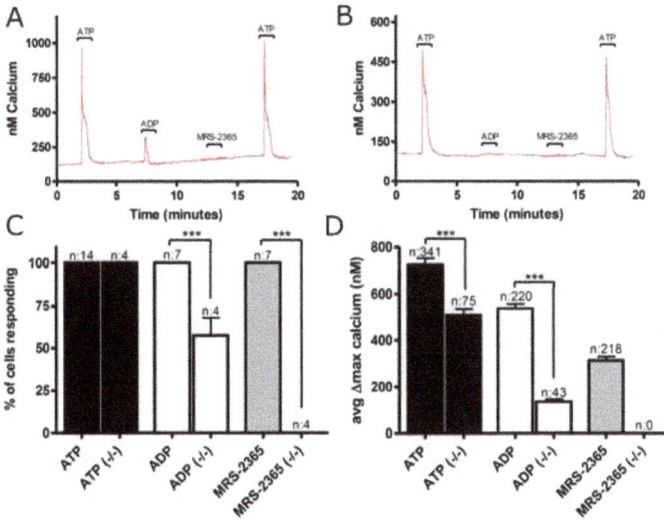

Figure 4. $P2Y_1$ receptors in astrocytes. (**A,B**) Representative responses in two astrocytes in cultures prepared from $P2Y_1$ $-/-$ mice. (**C,D**) Mean number of responding cells (n = cover slips) (**C**) and mean $[Ca^{2+}]_i$ changes (n = cells responding) (**D**) showing lower amplitude $[Ca^{2+}]_i$ rises in response to ATP and ADP in the knock-out cells, and no response to the selective agonist MRS-2365.

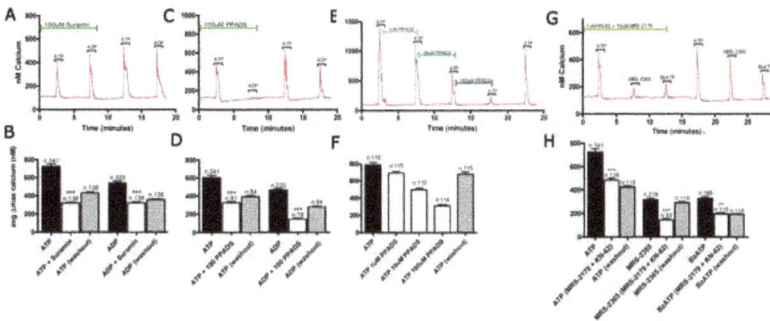

Figure 5. P2 receptor block in cultured astrocytes. (**A–D**) The effect of pre-perfusion for 60 min with 100 µM suramin or 100 µM PPADS upon ATP and ADP evoked $[Ca^{2+}]_i$ changes. (**E,F**) Concentration-dependence of the effect of PPADS during shorter antagonist exposures. (**G,H**) The effect of combined exposure to the selective $P2Y_1$ antagonist 10 µM MRS-2179 and the $P2X_7$ antagonist 1 µM KN-62 upon ATP-evoked $[Ca^{2+}]_i$ changes.

3.2. Oxygen-Glucose Deprivation in High-Density Neuron/Astrocyte Co-Cultures

Ischemic conditions in the brain were modelled by exposing high-density co-cultures to OGD with a similar neuron:astrocyte ratio to that found in the CNS (1:1). OGD evoked a gradual rise in extracellular ATP measured in the unstirred media layer surrounding cells [4] (Figure 6A,B). The mean extracellular ATP increase reached 8.9 ± 3.1 µM during the 80–90 min period of OGD ($p < 0.01$ relative to control perfused cultures). A significant elevation in ATP concentration was apparent in the 60–70 min epoch ($p < 0.05$), but the data trend suggests that ATP release started soon after the initiation of OGD (Figure 6A). Activation of P2 receptors during OGD was subsequently found to contribute to acute cell death in this preparation (See below). To test the hypothesis that P2 receptor antagonists act independently of glutamate release, glutamate was measured in the mixed high density cultures during OGD in the presence and absence of 10 μM PPADS (Figure 6C,D). OGD evoked an early increase in extracellular glutamate in this preparation, and this was not significantly affected by block of P2 receptors.

The effect of a range of ionotropic glutamate and P2 receptor blockers in isolation and in combination (see Tables 1 and 2 for selectivity of P2 antagonists) were tested upon the degree of cell death produced by 90 min of OGD in high-density co-cultures, assessed via CFMDA cell-tracker imaging (Figure 7). This approach allowed neurons and astrocytes to be differentiated using unambiguous morphological criteria [4]. The non-selective P2 antagonist PPADS (10 μM) was highly protective of both neurons and astrocytes, with neuronal death reduced to $2.8 \pm 1.7\%$ and astrocyte death to $9.4 \pm 4.5\%$ ($n = 10$; $p < 0.001$); PPADS (100 μM) (sufficient to block all P2 receptor types) reduced total cell death to a level below that found in control perfused cultures ($0.9 \pm 0.5\%$; $p < 0.001$). Suramin (100 μM) has been reported to block P2X 2, 3, 5, 6 and 7 in addition to P2Y 1, 2, 6, 12 and 13 types, produced significant protection of neurons but not astrocytes, reducing over-all cell death as a result. In contrast, reactive blue-2, which at the concentration used (100 μM) has been reported to block P2X 1–3 and 5 and P2Y 1, 4, 6 and 11–12, was without effect. The P2X$_7$ selective antagonist KN-62 (1 μM) did not have a significant effect upon either cell type, while the P2Y$_1$ antagonist MRS-2179 (10 μM) significantly protected both astrocytes and neurons from cell death, and reduced total cell death to $15.5 \pm 6.3\%$. Consistent with prior reports, block of non-NMDA or NMDA GluRs (NBQX 30 μM or MK-801 10 μM, respectively), was protective of neurons. The most significant protection was found during combined application of both antagonists; no glutamate receptor blocking protocol had any significant effect upon astrocyte survival. Combined block of P2 and glutamate receptors with 100 μM suramin + 10 μM MK-801 + 30 μM NBQX (100S10M30N) completely abolished all cell death in both astrocytes and neurons. Combined perfusion with low agonist concentrations was also tested. PPADS (1 μM) + mk-801 (1 μM) + NBQX (1P1M3N) (3 μM) was highly protective of both neurons ($1.1 \pm 0.9\%$ cell death) and astrocytes ($8.5 \pm 3.9\%$ cell death), with total cell death reduced from $13.2 \pm 1.6\%$ to $5.0 \pm 2.9\%$ ($p < 0.001$).

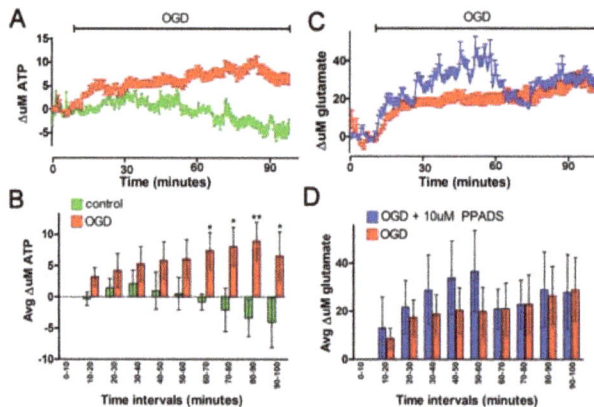

Figure 6. Neurotransmitter release from mixed cultures. (**A**) ATP concentration in the media surrounding cultured neurons and astrocytes rises gradually during a 90 min period of OGD (red data) compared to control recordings (green). Means +/− standard error mean are shown. (**B**) Mean data for each 10 min interval showing statistical significant between control and OGD at later time points. (**C**) Glutamate in the extracellular media is elevated during OGD, an effect that is not affected by co-perfusion with 10 μM PPADS to block P2 receptors. (**D**) Mean data for 10 min intervals, showing no statistical significant effect of PPADS.

Table 1. Antagonists at P2X receptors.

	Suramin	PPADS	KN-62	Highly Selective Antagonists [a,h,p,s]
P2X$_1$	No, >1 mM [g] (mouse) 0.01–0.3, 0.851 [e,t] (human)	0.4 [g] (mouse) 0.01–0.3, 1.29 [a,t] (human)	No	NF449, NF864, RO-1
P2X$_2$	33.1 [e] (rat) 1-32 [m,p,t] (human)	3.8 [e] (rat) 0.4–20.4 [a,m,p,t] (human)	No	-
P2X$_3$	0.776 [e] (rat) 14.9, 15.8, >100 [e,n,p,t] (human)	3.63 [e] (rat) 1.7–5.13 [e,n,t] (human)	No	-
P2X$_4$	>100 [q] (mouse) 178.1–200 [e,o,p] (human)	10.5 [q] (mouse) 10–25,27.5, >100 [a,o,p] (human)	No, >3 [q] (mouse)	Benzofuro-1,4-diazepin-2-ones
P2X$_5$	4.5 [r] (rat) 0.199 [p,t] (human)	2 [r] (rat) 0.01-0.3, 3.16 [p,t] (human)	No	-
P2X$_6$	No, >30 [r] (rat)	No, >30 [r] (rat) >0.3 [t] (human)	No	-
P2X$_7$	40 [f] (mouse)No, >100 [e,t] (human)	*Cation pore opening* 14.79 [a] (mouse) 3.24 [a] (human) *Large pore formation* 7, 9, >100 [a,b] (mouse) 0.015 [b] (human)	*Cation pore opening* 0.389 [a] (mouse) 0.38 [a] (human) *Large pore formation* 0.18, 1.17 [a,b] (mouse) 0.011 [b] (human)	1A-438079 ** 1A-740003 ** A-804590 GSK314181A AZ11645373 1AZ10606120
P2X$_{2/3}$	33.1 [e] (rat)	1.26 [e] (rat) 16.6 [a] (human)	No	A-317491 RO-3
P2X$_{1/5}$	1.58 [p] (rat)	0.5–8.6 [h] (mouse)	No	-
P2X$_{4/6}$	Some activity [u] (rat)	Some activity [u] (rat)	No	-

Numbers represent IC$_{50}$ values, in μM. Murine data are presented where available. **: antagonists with good oral bioavailability. References: [a] (Donnelly-Roberts et al., 2009), [b] (Chessell et al., 1998), [e] (Bianchi et al., 1999), [f] (Watano et al., 2002), [g] (Ikeda, 2007), [h] (Lalo et al., 2008), [m] (Lynch et al., 1999), [n] (Garcia-Guzman et al., 1997a), [o] (Garcia-Guzman et al., 1997b), [p] (Gever et al., 2006), [q] (Jones et al., 2000), [r] (Collo et al., 1996), [s] (Jarvis and Khakh, 2009), [t] (Burnstock and Knight, 2004), [u] (Le et al., 1998a).

Table 2. Antagonists at P2Y receptors.

	Suramin	PPADS	MRS-2179	Highly Selective Antagonists [h]
P2Y$_1$	Effective at 100uM [d] (mouse) 1.67 [t] (turkey) 3.16 [a] (human)	Effective at 30 uM [d] (mouse) 1.05 [t] (turkey) 2 [b] (human)	Effective at 10 uM [f,g] (mouse) 0.015–0.331 [f,h,p,q] (human)	MRS-2279 MRS-2179 MRS-2500 A3P5P
P2Y$_2$	47.86 [t] (human)	No [b,t] (human)	No [a,s,u]	AR-C126313 MRS-2576
P2Y$_4$	No [n,o] (mouse/human)	45 [n] (mouse) 15 [o] (human)	No [a,s,u]	MRS-2577
P2Y$_6$	Effective at 100uM [d] (mouse)	Effective at 30uM [d] (mouse)	No [a,s,u]	MRS-2578 MRS-2575
P2Y$_{12}$	3.6 [r] (human)	No [r] (human)	No [a,s]	MeSAMP AZD6140 INS50589 Clopidogrel
P2Y$_{13}$	2.3 [e] (human)	11.7 [e] (human)	>100 [e] (human)	MRS-2211

Numbers represent IC$_{50}$ values, in μM; Murine data are presented where available. References: [a] (Fischer and Krugel, 2007), [b] (Donnelly-Roberts et al., 2009), [d] (Calvert et al., 2004), [e] (Marteau et al., 2003), [f] (Baurand et al., 2001), [g] (Atterbury-Thomas et al., 2008), [h] (Jacobson et al., 2009), [n] (Suarez-Huerta et al., 2001), [o] (Communi et al., 1996b), [p] (Waldo and Harden, 2004), [q] (Moro et al., 1998), [r] (Abbracchio et al., 2006), [t] (Charlton et al., 1996b), [u] (Boyer et al., 1998).

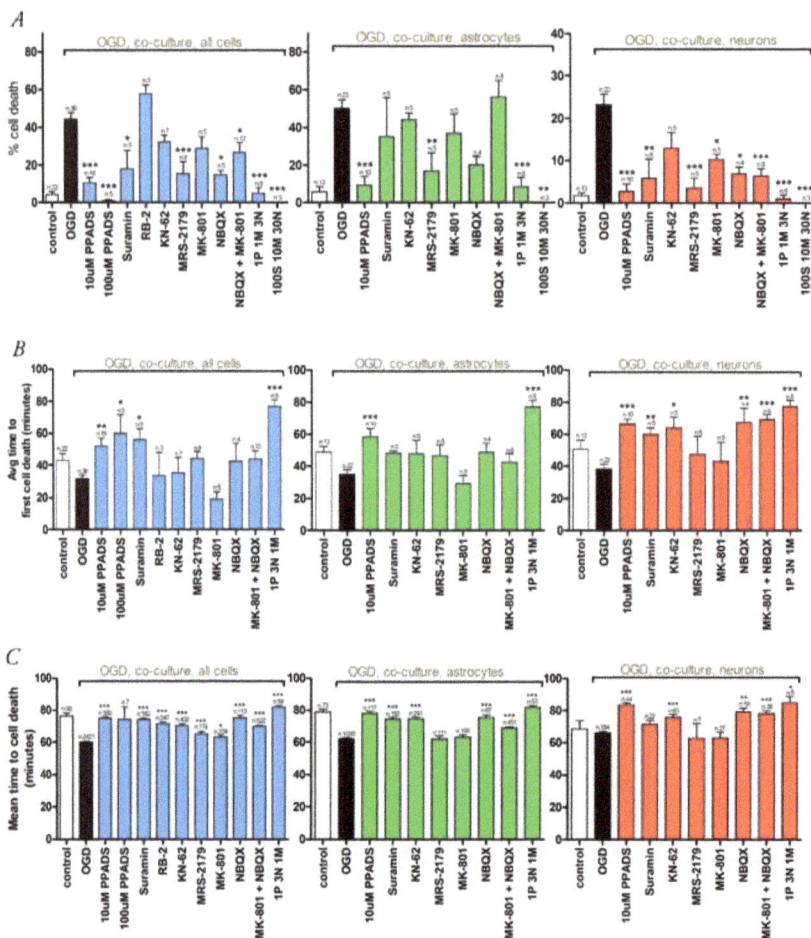

Figure 7. The effects of various receptor agonists on OGD-induced cell death in mixed cultures. (**A**) The per cent cell death of all cells (blue), astrocytes (green) and neurons (red) under control perfused (white), control OGD (black) and OGD in the presence of single or combined receptor antagonist (coloured). (**B**) Analysis showing the mean time to the first cell death event in each culture. (**C**) Mean time to cell death. * $p < 0.05$, ** $p < 0.005$, *** $p < 0.001$ vs. cell death under control OGD conditions. "1P" = 1 μM PPADS; "1M" = 1 μM MK-801; "3N" = 3 μM NBQX; "100S" = 100 μM suramin; "n" = number of cultures.

3.3. Oxygen-Glucose Deprivation in Normal-Density Neuron/Astrocyte Co-Cultures

To test whether the highly protective nature of combined P2 and GluR block was limited to the high-density cultures required for biosensor recording of neurotransmitter release, we examined the effect of combined blockade in normal density 50:50 neuron:astrocyte cultures using low doses of clinically applicable drugs. Control levels of total cell death was higher in these normal-density cultures, an effect that was countered by low concentrations of PPADS which acted by reducing astrocyte death (Figure 8A). PPADS at 0.5 μM reduced total cell death under control normoxic conditions from 13.2 ± 1.6% to 3.1 ± 0.5% over the 100 min recording protocol ($p < 0.001$), suggesting tonic ATP release and low levels of on-going P2 receptor-mediated excitotoxicity in these cultures. Ninety-minute OGD evoked a significantly lower level of overall cell death (22.0 ± 1.6%; Figure 8B) than it did in the high density cultures (see Figure 7), the difference accounted for by a reduced level of astrocyte death. This phenomenon is potentially related to lower levels of ischemic neurotransmitter release associated with lower cell density. Very low levels of PPADS significantly reduced OGD-induced astrocyte and total cell death, with 0.5 μM reducing overall cell death during OGD to $16.7 \pm 5.8\%$ ($p < 0.02$ vs. OGD alone). PPADS (1 μM) reduced total cell death to $11.2 \pm 1.6\%$ ($p = 0.01$), with only the highest concentration tested (10 μM) having any protective effect upon neurons ($8.4 \pm 2.2\%$, $p = 0.002$). The time-course of cell death under control perfused and during OGD are shown in Figure 8C,D.

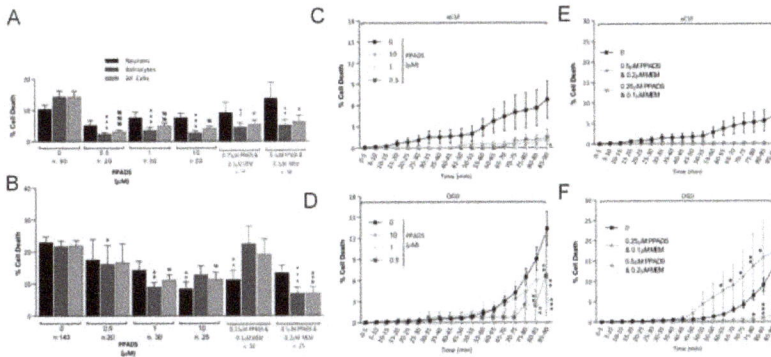

Figure 8. The effects of P2 and GluR antagonists on OGD-induced cell death in normal-density co-cultures. (**A**) The extent of cell death during a 100 min period of control imaging, showing neuron, astrocyte and neuron death. Note the relatively high level of baseline cell death in the absence of antagonists and the protective effect of even low concentrations of PPADS or combined low dose PPADS + memantine. (**B**) Cell death during 90 min of OGD and the protective effects of low concentrations of PPADS or low dose PPADS + memantine. (**C–F**) The time-course of total cell death for the two sets of conditions shown in "A" and "B". * $p < 0.05$, ** $p < 0.005$, *** $p < 0.001$ vs. no drugs present.

To test combined block of NMDA-type GluR and P2 receptors in this preparation, cultures were exposed to 0.2 μM memantine + 0.5 μM PPADS. Current and established data show that these concentrations given individually are not protective of total cell death in this preparation [4]. Following application of this combination a significant protective effect against astrocyte ($7.0 \pm 2.0\%$, $p < 0.0001$) and total cell death ($7.0 \pm 2.0\%$, $p < 0.0001$; Figure 8B) was found. However, no significant effect was seen upon neuronal death ($13.3 \pm 2.4\%$, $p = 0.0772$). Memantine (0.2 μM) + PPADS (0.5 μM) significantly decreased cumulative cell death at 75 min onwards compared to OGD-only conditions (Figure 8F; $p < 0.001$). A further low concentration combination was investigated. PPADS (0.25 μM) and MEM (0.1 μM) significantly reduced neuronal death ($11.3 \pm 3.0\%$; $p < 0.01$), with no effect on astrocyte or all cell death (Figure 8D). This combination showed an increased cumulative level of cell death in continually-imaged cells compared to OGD-only conditions (Figure 8F).

4. Discussion

The focus for acute stroke intervention research has been on re-vascularization therapies, reactive species buffering or excitotoxicity interruption via NMDA-type GluR blockers [31]. Drugs directed toward glutamate-mediated excitotoxicity have shown particular promise in animals, but have not translated into clinical practice. Neural function is dependent upon the homeostatic relationship between neurons and astrocytes, and any successful stroke intervention must protect both cell types if functional improvement is to be achieved. Since the NMDA-type GluRs which largely mediate glutamate excitotoxicity are either absent or expressed at low levels in astrocytes (e.g., [5]), one shortfall of targeting glutamate excitotoxicity may be a lack of astrocyte protection. Astrocytes express a high density of P2 ATP receptors [6], and brain ischemia produces significant rises in extracellular ATP concentration [16]; targeting ATP-mediated excitotoxicity may therefore be necessary for stroke neuroprotection.

For ATP and glutamate mediated excitotoxic cascades to co-exist, cells must release excessive ATP and glutamate during ischaemic conditions, events which we have confirmed in high-density cultures using biosensor microelectrodes. Neurotransmitter release was apparent soon after the onset of OGD, although ATP levels were lower and reached statistical significance later than glutamate. In this preparation, astrocytes rather than neurons contributed the majority of glutamate release during OGD, since significant glutamate release only occurred from astrocyte cultures and co-cultures. Glutamate release from co-cultures was not attenuated by the non-selective P2 blocker PPADS, suggesting that P2 receptor activation does not contribute to ischaemic glutamate release. Excessive ischemic ATP release was only consistently detected in co-cultures, indicating that astrocytes and neurons interact/co-operate by an unknown mechanism to release ATP or enhance extracellular ATP accumulation during ischaemia.

A second pre-requisite for ATP and glutamate mediated excitotoxicity is the functional expression of P2 and GluRs on neural cells. Functional receptor responses were examined via Ca^{2+} imaging, revealing widespread ionotropic and metabotropic GluR responses in neuronal cultures, while only a small percentage of cultured astrocytes expressed functional (mostly metabotropic) GluRs. Cultured neurons and astrocytes expressed a variety of functional P2 receptors, with 100% of astrocytes and approximately 60% of neurons responding to ATP. In both cell types, there was a dominant contribution of metabotropic P2Y over ionotropic P2X receptors. A P2 receptor subtype expression profile obtained using multiple P2 agonists/antagonists and $P2Y_1 -/-$ astrocytes found expression on neurons and astrocytes of $P2Y_1$ and $P2Y_6$, with a possibility of $P2Y_2$ and/or $P2Y_4$, while astrocytes in particular also expressed functional $P2X_7$ receptors.

4.1. GluR Antagonists Protect Neurons but Not Astrocytes

Blocking NMDA and/or AMPA/kainate GluRs reduced OGD-induced cell death in neurons but not astrocytes. A similar differential effect has been previously documented in cell cultures, and correlates with the largely neuronal pattern of GluR expression [4,32–35]. Analysis of the time course of cell lysis revealed that the reduction in neuronal death produced by the NMDA blocker MK-801 reached statistical significance after 90 min of OGD, and did not reduce the mean time to cell death. NBQX (alone or in combination with MK-801) significantly reduced cell death after 60–65 min of OGD, and significantly delayed the mean time to cell death. Consistent with this, NMDA GluR antagonists are less effective than AMPA/kainate receptor antagonists during prolonged and/or more severe ischaemia.

4.2. Broad-Spectrum P2 Antagonists Protect Neurons and Astrocytes

Of the broad-spectrum P2 antagonists tested, PPADS is selective for P2 receptors while suramin and RB-2 have non-specific effects including activity at GluRs [36–43] (see Tables 1 and 2). RB-2 did not significantly affect cell death, although it did delay the mean time to cell death of all cells combined. Suramin significantly reduced neuronal but not astrocyte death, and also increased the average time to first death of neurons. PPADS was the most protective of the antagonists tested, significantly reducing death of both neurons and astrocytes. PPADS (100 µM) almost eliminated cell death during the 90 min OGD period, while 10 µM reduced astrocyte and neuron death by ~80% and significantly delaying the average time to first death and mean time to cell death for both cell types.

Suramin or PPADS reduce neuronal death in primary neuron and brain slice cultures exposed to glucose deprivation or OGD (injury assessed ≥ 20 h) [44–46]; protection with low (PPADS, 5 µM) concentrations of has been reported in hippocampal slice cultures [47]. The current findings are the first to demonstrate that P2 antagonists can protect neurons during acute ischaemia, and that PPADS protects both neurons and astrocytes. The absence of protection afforded by RB-2 in the current results contradicts reports that have measured injury at delayed time-points [45,48,49], and may indicate an effect of this blocker only on delayed injury. The selective P2X$_7$ antagonist KN-62 also produced no significant protection in high-density cultures, consistent with results with other P2X$_7$ antagonist and receptor knock-out animals where infarct volume following middle cerebral artery occlusion is not significantly affected [50,51]. The size of excitotoxic lesions induced by the NMDA receptor agonist methano-glutamate in vivo are not reduced in P2X$_7$ −/− animals or by three different selective P2X$_7$ antagonists, suggesting that these receptors are not involved in glutamate neurotoxicity [50,51].

P2Y$_1$ receptor block was highly protective in high-density cultures. P2Y$_1$ receptor block delays anoxic depolarization in hippocampal slices [52], but the current data are consistent with reports that P2Y$_1$ block is effective against ischemic injury in vivo [53–55]. P2Y$_1$ receptor activation stimulates glutamate release from cultured hippocampal and spinal cord astrocytes but not neurons, while P2Y$_1$ receptor antagonists reduce ATP induced glutamate release from astrocytes [56–58]. P2Y$_1$ antagonists may therefore act to mitigate glutamate excitotoxicity via reduced glutamate release, although the current finding that PPADS did not reduce ischaemic glutamate efflux from the co-culture argues against this. Furthermore, glutamate receptor antagonists only significantly reduced neuronal ischaemic death without protecting astrocytes. Heteromeric functional coupling of P2Y$_1$ and A$_1$ receptors has been demonstrated in neurons and astrocytes [59,60], resulting in A$_1$ receptor desensitization following P2Y$_1$ activation. Since A$_1$ receptor activation is protective, P2Y$_1$ blockers may afford neural protection via this alternative mechanism. However, the most likely mechanisms is reduced Ca^{2+} over-loading during OGD following receptor block; P2Y$_1$ receptors are shown to mediate a significant component of the Ca^{2+}-rise evoked by ATP and since elevated [Ca^{2+}]$_i$ is central to acute ischemic cell injury, block of any receptor mediating [Ca^{2+}]$_i$ elevation is predicted to be protective. The data relating to receptor-mediated excitotoxic injury during acute ischemic conditions in mixed neuron-astrocyte environments are summarized in Figure 9.

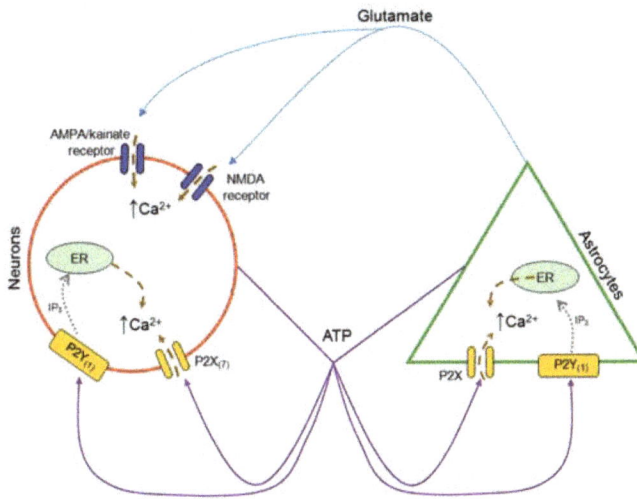

Figure 9. A model of purinergic and glutamatergic events involved in astrocyte and neuronal death during OGD. Glutamate and ATP accumulate in the extracellular space following the onset of OGD: glutamate is released by astrocytes, while the source of ATP is not clear. Glutamate evokes neuronal death by gating AMPA/kainate and NMDA receptors, leading to cytotoxic Ca^{2+} influx. ATP activates P2 receptors on both astrocytes and neurons, leading to Ca^{2+} release from intracellular stores (P2Y receptors) and/or Ca^{2+} influx through P2X ion channels. P2Y$_1$ receptors in particular are present on both cell types and contribute to cell death. P2X$_7$ receptors may be involved in early neuronal but not astrocyte death.

4.3. Synergistic Effect of P2 and Glutamate Receptor Antagonists

Initially, suramin (100 μM) + NBQX (30 μM) + MK-801 (10 μM) were added to high-density cultures: this combination completely prevented cell death during 90 min of OGD and was significantly more protective than either suramin or NBQX + MK-801 paradigms. To further probe this synergism, PPADS (1 μM) + NBQX (3 μM) + MK-801 (1 μM) was tested. This combination, less likely to produce non-selective effects, reduced acute astrocyte and neuron lysis by 83% and 95%, respectively, and significantly delaying the onset and mean time to cell death more than any other antagonist combination. The synergistic effect was significantly greater than that produced by either class of antagonist alone, even when applied at high concentrations. A similar combined protective effect was suggested in a study by Runden-Pran and colleagues [47], where the combination of suramin (200 μM) + MK-801 (100 μM) significantly attenuated cell death in hippocampal slice cultures exposed to 32 min OGD followed by up to 48 h of re-oxygenation [47]. However, this was not significantly more protection than either antagonist on its own, and this suramin concentration is poorly specificity. Low concentrations of PPADS or PPADS + the clinically approved NMDA GluR blocker memantine were tested in normal density co-cultures. PPADS at 1 μM and combined 0.5 μM PPADS + 0.2 μM memantine were protective against acute OGD-induced lysis in neurons and astrocytes, and also reduced background levels of cell death in these cultures. The current data are the first to confirm that a combinatorial approach blocking P2 and ionotropic glutamate receptors provides synergistic protection against ischaemic death of astrocytes and neurons in vitro. Thus, a combinatorial approach may be relevant to test in vivo but this will require the development of selective PPADS antagonists which are able to cross the blood brain barrier.

Acknowledgments: This work was supported by the BBSRC (RF: BB/J016969/1) and by MediSearch (Leicester: RF).

Author Contributions: R.F. conceived and designed the experiments; P.V. and M.T.-L. performed the experiments and analyzed the data; B.H., C.G. and R.J.E. contributed the P2Y$_1$−/− mouse; C.L.G. and R.F. supervised the project; and R.F. wrote the paper.

Conflicts of Interest: The authors declare no conflict of interest.

References

1. Ginsberg, M.D. Current status of neuroprotection for cerebral ischemia: Synoptic overview. *Stroke* **2009**, *40*, S111–S114. [CrossRef] [PubMed]
2. Dirnagl, U.; Iadecola, C.; Moskowitz, M.A. Pathobiology of ischaemic stroke: An integrated view. *Trends Neurosci.* **1999**, *22*, 391–397. [CrossRef]
3. Pringle, A.K. In, out, shake it all about: Elevation of [Ca^{2+}]i during acute cerebral ischaemia. *Cell Calcium* **2004**, *36*, 235–245. [CrossRef] [PubMed]
4. Trotman, M.; Vermehren, P.; Gibson, C.L.; Fern, R. The dichotomy of memantine treatment for ischemic stroke: Dose-dependent protective and detrimental effects. *J. Cereb. Blood Flow Metab.* **2015**, *35*, 230–239. [CrossRef] [PubMed]
5. Lalo, U.; Pankratov, Y.; Kirchhoff, F.; North, R.A.; Verkhratsky, A. NMDA receptors mediate neuron-to-glia signaling in mouse cortical astrocytes. *J. Neurosci.* **2006**, *26*, 2673–2683. [CrossRef] [PubMed]
6. Butt, A.M. Atp: A ubiquitous gliotransmitter integrating neuron-glial networks. *Semin. Cell Dev. Biol.* **2011**, *22*, 205–213. [CrossRef] [PubMed]
7. Franke, H.; Illes, P. Involvement of P2 receptors in the growth and survival of neurons in the CNS. *Pharmacol. Ther.* **2006**, *109*, 297–324. [CrossRef] [PubMed]
8. Sperlagh, B.; Zsilla, G.; Baranyi, M.; Illes, P.; Vizi, E.S. Purinergic modulation of glutamate release under ischemic-like conditions in the hippocampus. *Neuroscience* **2007**, *149*, 99–111. [CrossRef] [PubMed]
9. Hisanaga, K.; Onodera, H.; Kogure, K. Changes in levels of purine and pyrimidine nucleotides during acute hypoxia and recovery in neonatal rat brain. *J. Neurochem.* **1986**, *47*, 1344–1350. [CrossRef] [PubMed]
10. Phillis, J.W.; O'Regan, M.H.; Perkins, L.M. Adenosine 5′-triphosphate release from the normoxic and hypoxic in vivo rat cerebral cortex. *Neurosci. Lett.* **1993**, *151*, 94–96. [CrossRef]

11. Phillis, J.W.; Smith-Barbour, M.; O'Regan, M.H. Changes in extracellular amino acid neurotransmitters and purines during and following ischemias of different durations in the rat cerebral cortex. *Neurochem. Int.* **1996**, *29*, 115–120. [CrossRef]

12. Lutz, P.L.; Kabler, S. Release of adenosine and ATP in the brain of the freshwater turtle (*Trachemys scripta*) during long-term anoxia. *Brain Res.* **1997**, *769*, 281–286. [CrossRef]

13. Juranyi, Z.; Sperlagh, B.; Vizi, E.S. Involvement of P_2 purinoceptors and the nitric oxide pathway in [3H]purine outflow evoked by short-term hypoxia and hypoglycemia in rat hippocampal slices. *Brain Res.* **1999**, *823*, 183–190. [CrossRef]

14. Parkinson, F.E.; Sinclair, C.J.; Othman, T.; Haughey, N.J.; Geiger, J.D. Differences between rat primary cortical neurons and astrocytes in purine release evoked by ischemic conditions. *Neuropharmacology* **2002**, *43*, 836–846. [CrossRef]

15. Melani, A.; Turchi, D.; Vannucchi, M.G.; Cipriani, S.; Gianfriddo, M.; Pedata, F. ATP extracellular concentrations are increased in the rat striatum during in vivo ischemia. *Neurochem. Int.* **2005**, *47*, 442–448. [CrossRef] [PubMed]

16. Dale, N.; Frenguelli, B.G. Release of adenosine and ATP during ischemia and epilepsy. *Curr. Neuropharmacol.* **2009**, *7*, 160–179. [CrossRef] [PubMed]

17. Ferrari, D.; Chiozzi, P.; Falzoni, S.; Dal Susino, M.; Collo, G.; Buell, G.; Di Virgilio, F. ATP-mediated cytotoxicity in microglial cells. *Neuropharmacology* **1997**, *36*, 1295–1301. [CrossRef]

18. Amadio, S.; D'Ambrosi, N.; Cavaliere, F.; Murra, B.; Sancesario, G.; Bernardi, G.; Burnstock, G.; Volonte, C. P2 receptor modulation and cytotoxic function in cultured CNSs neurons. *Neuropharmacology* **2002**, *42*, 489–501. [CrossRef]

19. Ryu, J.K.; Kim, J.; Choi, S.H.; Oh, Y.J.; Lee, Y.B.; Kim, S.U.; Jin, B.K. ATP-induced in vivo neurotoxicity in the rat striatum via P2 receptors. *Neuroreport* **2002**, *13*, 1611–1615. [CrossRef] [PubMed]

20. Volonte, C.; Amadio, S.; Cavaliere, F.; D'Ambrosi, N.; Vacca, F.; Bernardi, G. Extracellular ATP and neurodegeneration. *Curr. Drug Targets CNS Neurol. Disord.* **2003**, *2*, 403–412. [CrossRef] [PubMed]

21. Matute, C.; Torre, I.; Perez-Cerda, F.; Perez-Samartin, A.; Alberdi, E.; Etxebarria, E.; Arranz, A.M.; Ravid, R.; Rodriguez-Antiguedad, A.; Sanchez-Gomez, M.; et al. P2x7 receptor blockade prevents ATP excitotoxicity in oligodendrocytes and ameliorates experimental autoimmune encephalomyelitis. *J. Neurosci.* **2007**, *27*, 9525–9533. [CrossRef] [PubMed]

22. Zimmermann, H. Biochemistry, localization and functional roles of ecto-nucleotidases in the nervous system. *Prog. Neurobiol.* **1996**, *49*, 589–618. [CrossRef]

23. Robson, S.C.; Kaczmarek, E.; Siegel, J.B.; Candinas, D.; Koziak, K.; Millan, M.; Hancock, W.W.; Bach, F.H. Loss of ATP diphosphohydrolase activity with endothelial cell activation. *J. Exp. Med.* **1997**, *185*, 153–163. [CrossRef] [PubMed]

24. Swanson, R.A.; Farrell, K.; Stein, B.A. Astrocyte energetics, function, and death under conditions of incomplete ischemia: A mechanism of glial death in the penumbra. *Glia* **1997**, *21*, 142–153. [CrossRef]

25. Fern, R. Ischemic tolerance in pre-myelinated white matter: The role of astrocyte glycogen in brain pathology. *J. Cereb. Blood Flow Metab.* **2015**, *35*, 951–958. [CrossRef] [PubMed]

26. Fern, R. Intracellular calcium and cell death during ischemia in neonatal rat white matter astrocytes in situ. *J. Neurosci.* **1998**, *18*, 7232–7243. [PubMed]

27. Bondarenko, A.; Chesler, M. Rapid astrocyte death induced by transient hypoxia, acidosis, and extracellular ion shifts. *Glia* **2001**, *34*, 134–142. [CrossRef] [PubMed]

28. Dale, N.; Hatz, S.; Tian, F.; Llaudet, E. Listening to the brain: Microelectrode biosensors for neurochemicals. *Trends Biotechnol.* **2005**, *23*, 420–428. [CrossRef] [PubMed]

29. Centemeri, C.; Bolego, C.; Abbracchio, M.P.; Cattabeni, F.; Puglisi, L.; Burnstock, G.; Nicosia, S. Characterization of the Ca^{2+} responses evoked by ATP and other nucleotides in mammalian brain astrocytes. *Br. J. Pharmacol.* **1997**, *121*, 1700–1706. [CrossRef] [PubMed]

30. Reifel Saltzberg, J.M.; Garvey, K.A.; Keirstead, S.A. Pharmacological characterization of P2Y receptor subtypes on isolated tiger salamander muller cells. *Glia* **2003**, *42*, 149–159. [CrossRef] [PubMed]

31. Hoyte, L.; Barber, P.A.; Buchan, A.M.; Hill, M.D. The rise and fall of NMDA antagonists for ischemic stroke. *Curr. Mol. Med.* **2004**, *4*, 131–136. [CrossRef] [PubMed]

32. Goldberg, M.P.; Weiss, J.H.; Pham, P.C.; Choi, D.W. N-methyl-D-aspartate receptors mediate hypoxic neuronal injury in cortical culture. *J. Pharmacol. Exp. Ther.* **1987**, *243*, 784–791. [PubMed]

33. Choi, D.W.; Rothman, S.M. The role of glutamate neurotoxicity in hypoxic-ischemic neuronal death. *Annu. Rev. Neurosci.* **1990**, *13*, 171–182. [CrossRef] [PubMed]
34. Goldberg, M.P.; Choi, D.W. Combined oxygen and glucose deprivation in cortical cell culture: Calcium-dependent and calcium-independent mechanisms of neuronal injury. *J. Neurosci.* **1993**, *13*, 3510–3524. [PubMed]
35. Newell, D.W.; Barth, A.; Papermaster, V.; Malouf, A.T. Glutamate and non-glutamate receptor mediated toxicity caused by oxygen and glucose deprivation in organotypic hippocampal cultures. *J. Neurosci.* **1995**, *15*, 7702–7711. [PubMed]
36. Balcar, V.J.; Dias, L.S.; Li, Y.; Bennett, M.R. Inhibition of [3H]CGP 39653 binding to NMDA receptors by a P2 antagonist, suramin. *Neuroreport* **1995**, *7*, 69–72. [CrossRef] [PubMed]
37. Nakazawa, K.; Inoue, K.; Ito, K.; Koizumi, S.; Inoue, K. Inhibition by suramin and reactive blue 2 of GABA and glutamate receptor channels in rat hippocampal neurons. *Naunyn-Schmiedeberg's Arch. Pharmacol.* **1995**, *351*, 202–208. [CrossRef]
38. Price, C.J.; Raymond, L.A. Evans blue antagonizes both alpha-amino-3-hydroxy-5-methyl-4-isoxazolepropionate and kainate receptors and modulates receptor desensitization. *Mol. Pharmacol.* **1996**, *50*, 1665–1671. [PubMed]
39. Peoples, R.W.; Li, C. Inhibition of NMDA-gated ion channels by the P2 purinoceptor antagonists suramin and reactive blue 2 in mouse hippocampal neurones. *Br. J. Pharmacol.* **1998**, *124*, 400–408. [CrossRef] [PubMed]
40. Lambrecht, G. Agonists and antagonists acting at P2X receptors: Selectivity profiles and functional implications. *Naunyn-Schmiedeberg's Arch. Pharmacol.* **2000**, *362*, 340–350. [CrossRef]
41. Zona, C.; Marchetti, C.; Volonte, C.; Mercuri, N.B.; Bernardi, G. Effect of P2 purinoceptor antagonists on kainate-induced currents in rat cultured neurons. *Brain Res.* **2000**, *882*, 26–35. [CrossRef]
42. Suzuki, E.; Kessler, M.; Montgomery, K.; Arai, A.C. Divergent effects of the purinoceptor antagonists suramin and pyridoxal-5'-phosphate-6-(2'-naphthylazo-6'-nitro-4',8'-disulfonate) (PPNDS) on α-amino-3-hydroxy-5-methyl-4-isoxazolepropionic acid (AMPA) receptors. *Mol. Pharmacol.* **2004**, *66*, 1738–1747. [CrossRef] [PubMed]
43. Lammer, A.; Gunther, A.; Beck, A.; Krugel, U.; Kittner, H.; Schneider, D.; Illes, P.; Franke, H. Neuroprotective effects of the P2 receptor antagonist PPADS on focal cerebral ischaemia-induced injury in rats. *Eur. J. Neurosci.* **2006**, *23*, 2824–2828. [CrossRef] [PubMed]
44. Cavaliere, F.; D'Ambrosi, N.; Ciotti, M.T.; Mancino, G.; Sancesario, G.; Bernardi, G.; Volonte, C. Glucose deprivation and chemical hypoxia: Neuroprotection by P2 receptor antagonists. *Neurochem. Int.* **2001**, *38*, 189–197. [CrossRef]
45. Cavaliere, F.; Florenzano, F.; Amadio, S.; Fusco, F.R.; Viscomi, M.T.; D'Ambrosi, N.; Vacca, F.; Sancesario, G.; Bernardi, G.; Molinari, M.; et al. Up-regulation of p2x₂, p2x₄ receptor and ischemic cell death: Prevention by p2 antagonists. *Neuroscience* **2003**, *120*, 85–98. [CrossRef]
46. Cavaliere, F.; Dinkel, K.; Reymann, K. Microglia response and P2 receptor participation in oxygen/glucose deprivation-induced cortical damage. *Neuroscience* **2005**, *136*, 615–623. [CrossRef] [PubMed]
47. Runden-Pran, E.; Tanso, R.; Haug, F.M.; Ottersen, O.P.; Ring, A. Neuroprotective effects of inhibiting N-methyl-D-aspartate receptors, P2X receptors and the mitogen-activated protein kinase cascade: A quantitative analysis in organotypical hippocampal slice cultures subjected to oxygen and glucose deprivation. *Neuroscience* **2005**, *136*, 795–810. [CrossRef] [PubMed]
48. Cavaliere, F.; D'Ambrosi, N.; Sancesario, G.; Bernardi, G.; Volonte, C. Hypoglycaemia-induced cell death: Features of neuroprotection by the P2 receptor antagonist basilen blue. *Neurochem. Int.* **2001**, *38*, 199–207. [CrossRef]
49. Melani, A.; Amadio, S.; Gianfriddo, M.; Vannucchi, M.G.; Volonte, C.; Bernardi, G.; Pedata, F.; Sancesario, G. P2X₇ receptor modulation on microglial cells and reduction of brain infarct caused by middle cerebral artery occlusion in rat. *J. Cereb. Blood Flow Metab.* **2006**, *26*, 974–982. [CrossRef] [PubMed]
50. Le Feuvre, R.; Brough, D.; Rothwell, N. Extracellular ATP and P2X₇ receptors in neurodegeneration. *Eur. J. Pharmacol.* **2002**, *447*, 261–269. [CrossRef]
51. Le Feuvre, R.A.; Brough, D.; Touzani, O.; Rothwell, N.J. Role of P2X₇ receptors in ischemic and excitotoxic brain injury in vivo. *J. Cereb. Blood Flow Metab.* **2003**, *23*, 381–384. [CrossRef] [PubMed]
52. Coppi, E.; Pedata, F.; Gibb, A.J. P2Y₁ receptor modulation of Ca²⁺-activated K⁺ currents in medium-sized neurons from neonatal rat striatal slices. *J. Neurophysiol.* **2012**, *107*, 1009–1021. [CrossRef] [PubMed]

53. Kuboyama, K.; Harada, H.; Tozaki-Saitoh, H.; Tsuda, M.; Ushijima, K.; Inoue, K. Astrocytic P2Y$_1$ receptor is involved in the regulation of cytokine/chemokine transcription and cerebral damage in a rat model of cerebral ischemia. *J. Cereb. Blood Flow Metab.* **2011**, *31*, 1930–1941. [CrossRef] [PubMed]

54. Chin, Y.; Kishi, M.; Sekino, M.; Nakajo, F.; Abe, Y.; Terazono, Y.; Hiroyuki, O.; Kato, F.; Koizumi, S.; Gachet, C.; et al. Involvement of glial P2Y$_1$ receptors in cognitive deficit after focal cerebral stroke in a rodent model. *J. Neuroinflamm.* **2013**, *10*, 95. [CrossRef] [PubMed]

55. Carmo, M.R.; Simoes, A.P.; Fonteles, A.A.; Souza, C.M.; Cunha, R.A.; Andrade, G.M. ATP P2Y$_1$ receptors control cognitive deficits and neurotoxicity but not glial modifications induced by brain ischemia in mice. *Eur. J. Neurosci.* **2014**, *39*, 614–622. [CrossRef] [PubMed]

56. Domercq, M.; Brambilla, L.; Pilati, E.; Marchaland, J.; Volterra, A.; Bezzi, P. P2Y$_1$ receptor-evoked glutamate exocytosis from astrocytes: Control by tumor necrosis factor-α and prostaglandins. *J. Biol. Chem.* **2006**, *281*, 30684–30696. [CrossRef] [PubMed]

57. Zeng, J.W.; Liu, X.H.; He, W.J.; Du, L.; Zhang, J.H.; Wu, X.G.; Ruan, H.Z. Inhibition of ATP-induced glutamate release by MRS2179 in cultured dorsal spinal cord astrocytes. *Pharmacology* **2008**, *82*, 257–263. [CrossRef] [PubMed]

58. Zeng, J.W.; Liu, X.H.; Zhang, J.H.; Wu, X.G.; Ruan, H.Z. P2Y$_1$ receptor-mediated glutamate release from cultured dorsal spinal cord astrocytes. *J. Neurochem.* **2008**, *106*, 2106–2118. [CrossRef] [PubMed]

59. Tonazzini, I.; Trincavelli, M.L.; Storm-Mathisen, J.; Martini, C.; Bergersen, L.H. Co-localization and functional cross-talk between A1 and P2Y$_1$ purine receptors in rat hippocampus. *Eur. J. Neurosci.* **2007**, *26*, 890–902. [CrossRef] [PubMed]

60. Tonazzini, I.; Trincavelli, M.L.; Montali, M.; Martini, C. Regulation of A1 adenosine receptor functioning induced by P2Y$_1$ purinergic receptor activation in human astroglial cells. *J. Neurosci. Res.* **2008**, *86*, 2857–2866. [CrossRef] [PubMed]

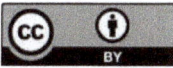

neuroglia

MDPI

Article

L-Dopa and Fluoxetine Upregulate Astroglial 5-HT$_{2B}$ Receptors and Ameliorate Depression in Parkinson's Disease Mice

Dan Song [1,†], Kangli Ma [1,†], Alexei Verkhratsky [2,3] and Liang Peng [1,*]

1   Laboratory of Metabolic Brain Diseases, Institute of Metabolic Disease Research and Drug Development,
    China Medical University, 110122 Shenyang, China; sd_nature@hotmail.com (D.S.);
    springlili233@163.com (K.M.)
2   Faculty of Biology, Medicine and Health, The University of Manchester, Manchester, M13 9PT, UK;
    Alexej.Verkhratsky@manchester.ac.uk
3   Achucarro Center for Neuroscience, IKERBASQUE, Basque Foundation for Science, 48011 Bilbao, Spain
*   Correspondence: sharkfin039@163.com
†   These authors contributed equally to this work.

Received: 19 March 2018; Accepted: 13 April 2018; Published: 23 April 2018

Abstract: Here, we report the association between depressive behavior (anhedonia) and astroglial expression of 5-hydroxytryptamine receptor 2B (5-HT$_{2B}$) in an animal model of Parkinson's disease, induced by bilateral injection of 6-hydroxydopamine (6-OHDA) into the striatum. Expression of the 5-HT$_{2B}$ receptor at the mRNA and protein level was decreased in the brain tissue of 6-OHDA-treated animals with anhedonia. Expression of the 5-HT$_{2B}$ receptor was corrected by four weeks treatment with either L-3,4-dihydroxyphenylalanine (L-dopa) or fluoxetine. Simultaneously, treatment with L-dopa abolished 6-OHDA effects on both depressive behavior and motor activity. In contrast, fluoxetine corrected 6-OHDA-induced depression but did not affect 6-OHDA-induced motor deficiency. In addition, 6-OHDA downregulated gene expression of the 5-HT$_{2B}$ receptor in astrocytes in purified cell culture and this downregulation was corrected by both L-dopa and fluoxetine. Our findings suggest that 6-OHDA-induced depressive behavior may be related to the downregulation of gene expression of the 5-HT$_{2B}$ receptor but 6-OHDA-induced motor deficiency reflects, arguably, dopamine depletion. Previously, we demonstrated that fluoxetine regulates gene expression in astrocytes by 5-HT$_{2B}$ receptor-mediated transactivation of epidermal growth factor receptor (EGFR). However, the underlying mechanism of L-dopa action remains unclear. The present work indicates that the decrease of gene expression of the astroglial 5-HT$_{2B}$ receptor may contribute to development of depressive behavior in Parkinson's disease.

Keywords: 5-HT$_{2B}$ receptor; astrocytes; depressive behavior; Parkinson's disease; fluoxetine

1. Introduction

Parkinson's disease (PD) is characterized by a progressive degeneration of dopaminergic midbrain neurons in the substantia nigra pars compacta (SNpc) [1] and becomes clinically manifest when more than 50% of SNpc neurons are lost. In addition to motor symptoms, which include resting tremor, slowness of movement, rigidity, and postural instability, the non-motor symptoms, such as cognitive deficits and behavioral abnormalities, have been recognized as integral part of the clinical presentation of PD [2]. Depression is the frequent psychiatric signature of the PD and it is one of the most significant factors affecting the quality of life of patients [3]. Whether L-3,4-dihydroxyphenylalanine (L-dopa) treatment improves depression in PD is controversial (see [4] for review). Nevertheless, the serotonergic system is affected in PD patients and in some animal models [4], while 5-hydroxytryptamine (5-HT) depletion may contribute to motor and non-motor symptoms of PD [5].

The role of astroglia in pathological evolution of PD remains to be revealed in detail, although both astroglial reactivity and astrodegeneration with loss of function and compromised neuroprotective capacity are documented [6,7]. It is generally acknowledged that the morbid changes associated with depression include profound remodeling of neuroglia, and furthermore, the contribution of astrocytes to the pathogenesis of various neuropsychiatric disorders is well appreciated [8,9]. Previously, we reported that fluoxetine, a selective serotonin reuptake inhibitor (SSRI) activates astroglial 5-hydroxytryptamine receptor 2B (5-HT$_{2B}$) receptors which results in transactivation of epidermal growth factor receptor (EGFR) [10]. We also found that expression of 5-HT$_{2B}$ receptors as well as other signaling molecules is suppressed in astrocytes but not in neurons in the cerebral cortex of anhedonic animals, which experienced chronic mild stress (CMS) [11,12]. Chronic treatment with fluoxetine eliminated both decrease in expression of astroglial 5-HT$_{2B}$ receptors and anhedonia [11]. These findings corroborate the role for astrocytic 5-HT$_{2B}$ receptor in depressive behavior. Recently, we also found a decrease in gene expression of astrocytic but not neuronal 5-HT$_{2B}$ receptor in animals that received 1-methyl-4-phenyl-1,2,3,6-tetrahydropyridine (MPTP) and became anhedonic. Fluoxetine corrected MPTP-induced decrease of 5-HT$_{2B}$ receptor expression and depressive behavior [13]. These findings indicate that changes in gene expression of 5-HT$_{2B}$ receptors in astroglia may be associated with pathophysiological evolution of depression in PD.

Another animal model of PD is induced by a bilateral injection of 6-hydroxydopamine (6-OHDA) into the striatum. 6-Hydroxydopamine has high affinity to dopamine transporter and the structure of 6-OHDA is similar to that of dopamine, but the presence of an additional hydroxyl group makes it toxic to dopaminergic neurons [14]. Injection of 6-OHDA into the striatum induces retrograde degeneration of tyrosine hydroxylase (TH)-positive terminals in the striatum which instigated death of TH positive neurons in the SNpc, similarly to PD in humans [14]. Using the 6-hydroxydopamine animal model of PD, this study aimed to examine effects of L-dopa and fluoxetine on the gene expression of the 5-HT$_{2B}$ receptor in primary cultures of astrocytes and in the brain of animals treated with 6-OHDA and correlates these changes with the depressive behavior and motor deficits.

2. Materials and Methods

All experimental techniques were essentially similar to those employed in our previous studies of astroglial 5-HT$_{2B}$ receptors [11–13]. All experiments were carried out in accordance with the USA National Institutes of Health Guide for the Care and Use of Laboratory Animals (NIH Publication No. 8023) and its 1978 revision, and all experimental protocols were preregistered and approved by the Institutional Animal Care and Use Committee of China Medical University.

2.1. Animals

CD-1 mice (Charles River, Beijing, China), weighing 30–40 g, male C57BL/6 mice (Chang Sheng Biotechnology, Benxi, China), weighing 22–26 g and mice with fluorescently tagged astrocytes and neurons (males FVB/NT-g(GFAP-GFP)14Mes/J or B6.Cg-Tg(Thy1-YFPH)2 Jrs/J, respectively; the Jackson Laboratory, Bar Harbor, ME, USA), weighing 20–25 g were kept at standard housing conditions with light/dark cycle of 12 h. Water and food were provided at libitum.

2.2. 6-OHDA Treatment

C57BL/6 mice were anesthetized with pentobarbital and mounted in a stereotaxic frame. Each mouse received a bilateral injection of 1 µL 6-OHDA (5 µg/µL in saline containing 0.02% ascorbic acid) into the dorsal-lateral striatum, according to the following coordinates (mm): antero-posterior + 0.5, medio-lateral ± 2, and dorso-ventral −3. Control sham-lesioned mice were injected with the same volume of vehicle (saline). After surgery, the animals were allowed to recover for three weeks.

2.3. Drug Treatment

After three-week recovery from the 6-OHDA lesions, anhedonic mice were daily injected intraperitoneally with fluoxetine (10 mg/kg/d dissolved in saline) or L-dopa (20 mg/kg/d in saline and combined with 12 mg/kg/d of benserazide) for four weeks. In the present study, mice were separated into six groups: (1) sham-lesioned animals treated with saline (Control); (2) sham-lesioned animals treated with fluoxetine (Flu); (3) sham-lesioned animals treated with L-dopa (L-dopa); (4) 6-OHDA-lesioned animals treated with saline (6-OHDA); (5) 6-OHDA-lesioned animals treated with fluoxetine (6-OHDA + Flu); (6) 6-OHDA-lesioned animals treated with L-dopa (6-OHDA + L-dopa).

Prior to surgery, three and seven weeks thereafter, mice underwent behaviour tests for motor function and mood. After three weeks of 6-OHDA treatment, only mice with depressive behavior (around 60%) were selected for L-dopa or fluoxetine treatment for another four weeks. At the end of the experiments (seven weeks), mice were sacrificed and cerebral cortex was dissected out for gene expression analysis of 5-HT$_{2B}$ receptor. FVB/NT-g(GFAP-GFP)14Mes/J or B6.Cg-Tg(Thy1-YFPH)2 Jrs/J mice were sacrificed after three-week recovery from the 6-OHDA lesions.

2.4. Behavioral Tests

Several behavioral tests were applied to 6-OHDA-treated mice to assess motor activity (pole test and rotarod test) and depression behavior (sucrose preference test, forced swim, tail suspension and open field tasks).

The pole test was performed as previously described [15] with minor modifications. The mouse was placed head-upward on the top of a vertical rough-surfaced pole (diameter 1 cm; height 55 cm). The time to turn downward from the top (T-turn time) and to descend to the floor (locomotor activity time, T-LA time) were measured. The total time was recorded with a maximum duration of 30 s.

Motor coordination was assessed with rotarod test. Mice were positioned on a rotating bar set to a rotation speed of up to 18 rpm during the test. The time spent on the rotating bar, known as the latent period, was recorded. Latency to fall was recorded with a stopwatch, with a maximum of 90 s. The test was repeated twice and mean latencies were analyzed.

The depressive behavior was assessed with despair-based tests represented by the tail suspension test and forced swimming test, as well as with anxiety-based open field test. In tail suspension test mice were individually suspended from their tails at the height of 20 cm using a piece of adhesive tape wrapped around the tail 2 cm from the tip. Behavior was videotaped for 6 min. The duration of immobility was measured by an observer blinded to the treatment groups. Mice were considered immobile only when completely motionless and mice that climbed their tails were excluded from the data.

In the forced-swimming test, animals were dropped into glass cylinders (20 × 20 cm) containing 20 cm deep water maintained at 25 ± 1 °C and kept in water for 6 min. The time of immobility was recorded during the last 4 min of the 6 min testing period, followed by 2 min of habituation.

In the open field test, mice were placed in the central square of the open field box (60 × 60 × 40 cm) divided in to nine squares. Behavior was videotaped for 5 min. The parameters used for analysis included number of squares crossed, frequency of rearing, and time spent in the central area.

The sucrose preference test is a reward-based test and provides a measure of anhedonia, the lack of interest in pleasant activities. Anhedonia is a characteristic symptom of major depression [11]. Baseline sucrose preference was measured before lesion. After 20 h of food and water deprivation, mice were placed in individual cages and presented with two pre-weighted bottles, one containing 2.5% sucrose solution and another filled with water for 2 h. Percent preference was calculated according to the following equation: % preference = (sucrose intake/(sucrose + water intake)) × 100. A decrease of sucrose preference below 65% was taken as the criterion for anhedonia. This criterion was based on the fact that none of the control mice exhibited less than or equal to 65% preference for sucrose at that time point of the experiment.

2.5. Acute Isolation of Cells

For identification of acutely isolated cells, we used transgenic mice expressing a fluorescent marker under control of a cell-specific promoter (glial fibrillary acidic protein (GFAP) for astrocytes or cell surface glycoprotein Thy1 for neurons) thus allowing fluorescence-activated sorting of specified cell fractions; for detailed description of the technique see [12,16,17]. After isolation, cells were sorted by fluorescence-activated cell sorting (FACS) using the BD FACSAria Cell Sorting System (35 psi sheath pressure, FACSDiva software S/W 2.2.1; BD Biosciences, San José, CA, USA). Cell identity and purity were verified by mRNA expression of cell markers of astrocytes, neurons, and oligodendrocytes, analyzed by reverse-transcription polymerase chain reaction (RT-PCR), in astrocytic and neuronal cell preparations. As shown previously [17], there is no contamination with neuronal or oligodendrocytic genes in the samples of astrocytes or of astrocytic or oligodendrocytic genes in the neuronal samples.

2.6. Primary Cultures of Astrocytes

Primary cultures of mouse astrocytes were prepared from the neopallia of the cerebral hemispheres of newborn CD-1 mice as previously described [18,19], sparsely seeded and grown in Dulbecco's minimum essential medium (DMEM) with 7.5 mM glucose. After two weeks in vitro, 0.25 mM dibutyryl cyclic adenosine monophosphate (dBcAMP) was included in the medium. These cultures are highly enriched in astrocytes as assessed by GFAP and glutamine synthetase expression [20]. Incubation with dBcAMP promotes morphological and functional differentiation as evidenced by the extension of cell processes and increases in several metabolic and functional activities characteristic of astrocytes in situ [21]. 6-Hydroxydopamine at 20 μM was added to the culture after three weeks of culturing and continued for 6, 12, 24, and 48 h.

2.7. Reverse Transcription-Polymerase Chain Reaction

For determination of the mRNA expression of the 5-HT$_{2B}$ receptor by RT-PCR, all samples from the cerebral cortex or astrocyte cultures were homogenized in Trizol (Invitrogen, Carlsbad, CA, USA). The RNA pellet was precipitated with isopropanol, washed with 75% ethanol, and dissolved in 10 μL sterile, distilled water and an aliquot was used for determination of the amount of RNA [22].

Reverse transcription was initiated by a 5 min incubation at 65 °C of 1 μg RNA extract with Random Hexamer (TaKaRa, Daliang, China) at a final concentration of 12.5 ng/L and deoxy-ribonucleoside triphosphates (dNTPs) at a final concentration of 0.5 mM. The mixture was rapidly chilled on ice and briefly spun and 4 μL 5 × First-Strand Buffer, 2 μL 0.1 M dithiotreitol and 1 μL RNaseOUT Recombinant RNase Inhibitor (40 U/μL) (TaKaRa) were added. After the mixture had been incubated at 42 °C for 2 min, 1 μL (200 U) of Superscript II was added and the incubation at 42 °C continued for another 50 min. Subsequently the reaction was inactivated by heating to 70 °C for 15 min and the mixture was chilled and briefly centrifuged.

Polymerase chain reaction amplification was performed in a Robocycler thermocycler (Biometra, Westburg, The Netherlands) with 0.2 μM of sense or antisense and 0.375 U of Taq polymerase for 5-HT$_{2B}$ receptor (forward, 5′-CTCGGGGGTGAATCCTCTGA-3′; reverse, 5′-CCTGCTCATCACCCTCTCTCA-3′) [22], for TATA box-binding protein (TBP), used as a housekeeping gene (forward, 5′-CCACGGACAACTGCGTTGAT-3′; reverse, 5′-GGCTCATAGCTACTGAACTG-3′) [23]. Initially, the template was denatured by heating to 94 °C for 2 min, followed by 2.5 min amplification cycles, each consisting of two 45 s periods and one 60 s period, the first at 94 °C, the second at 61 °C for 5-HT$_{2B}$ receptor and at 55 °C for TBP and the third at 72 °C. The final step was extension at 72 °C for 10 min. The PCR products were separated by 1% agarose gel electrophoresis, stained with 0.5 μg/mL ethidium bromide, and captured by Fluorchem 5500 (Alpha Innotech Corporation, San Leandro, CA, USA). The sizes of the PCR product of 5-HT$_{2B}$ receptor was 370 bp and that of TBP 236 bp.

2.8. Western Blotting

Protein content was determined by the Lowry method [24], using bovine serum albumin as the standard. Samples containing 50 μg protein were applied on slab gels of 10% polyacrylamide and electrophoresed. After transfer to polyvinylidene fluoride (PVDF) membranes, the samples were blocked by 5% skim milk powder in TBS-T (30 mM Tris-HCl, 125 mM NaCl, 0.1% Tween 20) for 1 h. The PVDF membranes were incubated with the primary antibody, specific to 5-HT$_{2B}$ receptor overnight at 4 °C or β-actin for 2 h at room temperature. After washing, the blots were incubated with peroxidase-conjugated affinity-purified goat anti-rabbit or goat anti-mouse horseradish peroxidase (HRP) antibody for 2 h. Staining was visualized by enhanced chemiluminescence (ECL) detection reagents. Digital images were obtained using Gel-Imaging System (Tanon 4200, Shanghai, China). Optical density for each band was assessed using the Window AlphaEase TM FC 32-bit software (Genetic Technologies, Miami, FL, USA). Ratios were determined between scanned 5-HT$_{2B}$ receptor and β-actin, the latter used as housekeeping protein.

2.9. Statistics

Differences between multiple groups were evaluated by two-way analysis of variance (ANOVA) followed by Fisher's least significant difference (LSD) multiple comparison test for unequal replications. The level of significance was set at $p < 0.05$.

2.10. Materials

Most chemicals, including 6-OHDA, fluoxetine, L-dopa, benserazide, DNase I, propidium iodide, 6,7-dinitroquinoxaline-2,3-dione (DNQX), 2-amino-5-phosphonovalerate (APV), and first antibodies and the first β-actin antibody were purchased from Sigma (St. Louis, MO, USA). BD Biosciences (Franklin Lakes, NJ, USA) supplied the first antibody, raised against 5-HT$_{2B}$ receptor. The second antibody goat anti-mouse IgG HRP conjugate was from Promega (Madison, WI, USA) and goat anti-rabbit IgG HRP conjugate from Santa Cruz Biotechnology (Santa Cruz, CA, USA). Enhanced chemiluminescence detection reagents were from Amersham Biosciences (Buckinghamshire, UK). Random Hexamer, deoxyribonucleotide triphosphates (dNTPs) and Taq-polymerase for RT-PCR were purchased from TaKaRa Biotechnology Co., Ltd. and Superscript II from Gibco Life Technology Invitrogen (Grand Island, NY, USA). Chemicals for preparation of culturing medium were purchased from Sigma and horse serum from Invitrogen.

3. Results

3.1. Depressive Behavior

Intrastriatal injection of 6-OHDA resulted in development of depressive behavior in mice. The consumption of sucrose, indicative of 6-OHDA-induced anhedonia, is presented in Figure 1A. In the three weeks after 6-OHDA treatment, sucrose consumption decreased significantly, reflecting progressive anhedonia. (Figure 1A; Control: $72.14 \pm 2.23\%$, $n = 18$; 6-OHDA: $55.05 \pm 3.43\%$, $n = 18$; $p < 0.05$). Glucose consumption was further decreased after seven weeks (Figure 1A; Control $72.79 \pm 1.33\%$, $n = 6$; 6-OHDA: $51.68 \pm 3.37\%$, $n = 6$; $p < 0.05$). Administration of fluoxetine and L-dopa for four weeks ameliorated 6-OHDA-induced decrease of sucrose consumption, albeit only partially (Flu: $76.05 \pm 4.55\%$, $n = 6$; 6-OHDA + Flu: $65.18 \pm 3.17\%$, $n = 6$; L-dopa: $75.43 \pm 2.74\%$, $n = 6$; 6-OHDA + L-dopa: $63.03 \pm 3.95\%$, $n = 6$; $p < 0.05$).

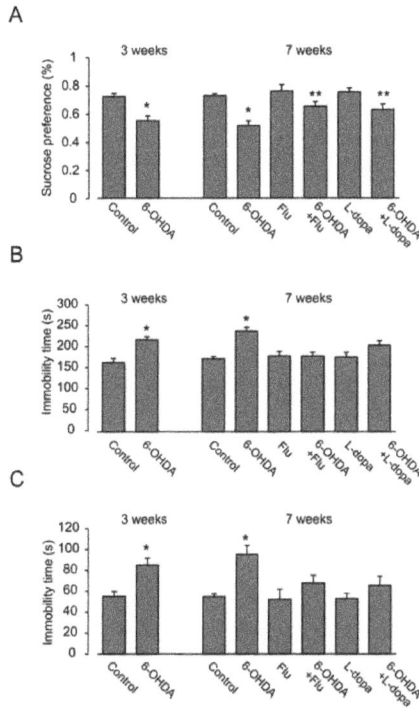

Figure 1. Effects of L-dopa and fluoxetine on depressive behavior (sucrose preference test, tail suspension test, and forced swimming test) induced by 6-Hydroxydopamine (6-OHDA). After three weeks recovery from the 6-OHDA lesions, mice with anhedonia were daily injected intraperitoneally with fluoxetine (10 mg/kg/d) or L-dopa (20 mg/kg/d in saline and combined with 12 mg/kg of benserazide) for four weeks. Behavior tests were performed just before or after L-dopa or fluoxetine treatment. (**A**) Percentage of sucrose preference in sucrose preference test. Values were expressed as the mean ± standard error of the mean (SEM). * Indicates statistically significant ($p < 0.05$) difference from other groups at the same treatment period. ** Indicates statistically significant ($p < 0.05$) difference from control, 6-OHDA, fluoxetine (Flu) and L-dopa group after four-weeks treatment of fluoxetine or L-dopa. (**B**) The duration of immobility in tail suspension test. Values are expressed as the mean ± SEM. * Indicates statistically significant ($p < 0.05$) difference from other groups at the same treatment period. (**C**) The duration of immobility in forced swimming test. Values are expressed as the mean ± SEM. * Indicates statistically significant ($p < 0.05$) difference from other groups at the same treatment period.

The duration of immobility of tail suspension test is presented in Figure 1B. Three weeks after 6-OHDA treatment, the duration of immobility increased significantly (Control: 165.14 ± 10.01 s, $n = 18$; 6-OHDA: 219.29 ± 7.70 s, $n = 18$; $p < 0.05$) and it was further increased after seven weeks (Control: 173.75 ± 5.45%, $n = 6$; 6-OHDA: 240.00 ± 8.80%, $n = 6$; $p < 0.05$). Administration of fluoxetine and L-dopa for four weeks removed 6-OHDA-induced increase of duration of immobility (Flu: 180.40 ± 10.87 s, $n = 6$; 6-OHDA + Flu: 180.20 ± 9.30 s, $n = 6$; L-dopa: 177.60 ± 11.76 s, $n = 6$; 6-OHDA + L-dopa: 206.33 ± 10.59 s, $n = 6$; $p < 0.05$).

In the forced-swimming test (Figure 1C), injection of 6-OHDA significantly increased the time of immobility at three weeks after surgery (Control: 55.08 ± 4.55 s, $n = 18$; 6-OHDA: 85.16 ± 6.85 s, $n = 18$; $p < 0.05$). Immobility time was further increased after seven weeks (Control: 54.75 ± 2.84 s, $n = 6$; 6-OHDA: 95.40 ± 8.41 s, $n = 6$; $p < 0.05$). Administration of fluoxetine and L-dopa for four weeks corrected 6-OHDA-induced increase of time of immobility (Flu: 52.00 ± 9.99 s, $n = 6$; 6-OHDA + Flu: 67.80 ± 7.59 s, $n = 6$; L-dopa: 52.80 ± 5.23 s, $n = 6$; 6-OHDA + L-dopa: 65.67 ± 8.71 s, $n = 6$; $p < 0.05$).

The results of time spent in the central area in the open field test are presented in Figure 2A. Three and seven weeks after exposure to 6-OHDA, there was no change in time spend in the central in open field. However, the drug decreased the number of squares crossed (three weeks: Control: 85.12 ± 15.27, $n = 18$; 6-OHDA: 51.53 ± 5.44, $n = 18$; $p < 0.05$; seven weeks: Control: 46.60 ± 5.96, $n = 6$; 6-OHDA: 27.00 ± 3.69, $n = 6$; $p < 0.05$) and frequency of rearing (three weeks: Control: 15.11 ± 2.24, $n = 185$; 6-OHDA: 10.79 ± 1.44, $n = 18$; $p < 0.05$; seven weeks: Control: 14.40 ± 1.86, $n = 6$; 6-OHDA: 8.20 ± 0.97, $n = 6$; $p < 0.05$) after three and seven weeks of treatment (Figure 2B,C). Administration of fluoxetine and L-dopa for four weeks corrected 6-OHDA-induced decrease of square crossed (Flu: 46.00 ± 4.46, $n = 6$; 6-OHDA + Flu: 45.00 ± 6.27, $n = 6$; L-dopa: 44.00 ± 3.22, $n = 6$; 6-OHDA + L-dopa: 44.80 ± 8.41, $n = 6$; $p < 0.05$) and frequency of rearing (Flu: 14.40 ± 1.17, $n = 6$; 6-OHDA + Flu: 15.00 ± 2.24, $n = 6$; L-dopa: 13.80 ± 1.85, $n = 6$; 6-OHDA + L-dopa: 15.80 ± 2.71, $n = 6$; $p < 0.05$).

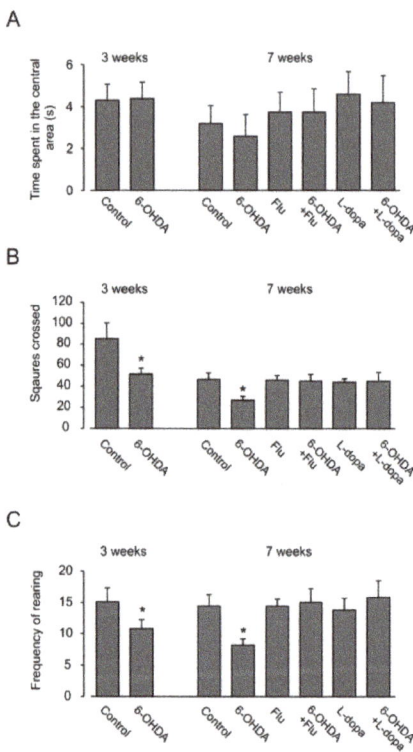

Figure 2. Effects of L-dopa and fluoxetine on open field test in mice treated with 6-OHDA. After three-weeks recovery from the 6-OHDA lesions, mice with anhedonia were daily injected intraperitoneally with fluoxetine (10 mg/kg/d) or L-dopa (20 mg/kg/d in saline and combined with 12 mg/kg of benserazide) for four weeks. Behavior tests were performed just before or after L-dopa or fluoxetine treatment. (**A**) The time spent in the central square in the open field test. The values are expressed as the mean $\pm$ SEM. (**B**) The number of squares crossed in open field test. The values are expressed as the mean $\pm$ SEM. * Indicates statistically significant ($p < 0.05$) difference from other groups at the same treatment period. (**C**) Frequency of rearing in open field test. The values are expressed as the mean $\pm$ SEM. * Indicates statistically significant ($p < 0.05$) difference from other groups at the same treatment period.

3.2. Motor Activity

In the rotarod performance test, the latency of fall (Figure 3A) in mice treated with 6-OHDA was significantly shorter than in control groups after three weeks (Control: 69.30 ± 4.27 s, n = 18; 6-OHDA: 57.13 ± 4.58 s, n = 18; p < 0.05) and after seven weeks (Control: 53.10 ± 6.26 s, n = 6; 6-OHDA: 31.90 ± 2.04 s, n = 6; p < 0.05) of 6-OHDA treatment. Although L-dopa corrected 6-OHDA-induced decrease of latency of fall after seven weeks, fluoxetine had no effect (Flu: 49.10 ± 6.19 s, n = 6; 6-OHDA + Flu: 29.20 ± 5.84 s, n = 6; L-dopa: 50.70 ± 8.74 s, n = 6; 6-OHDA + L-dopa: 49.90 ± 9.43 s, n = 6; p < 0.05).

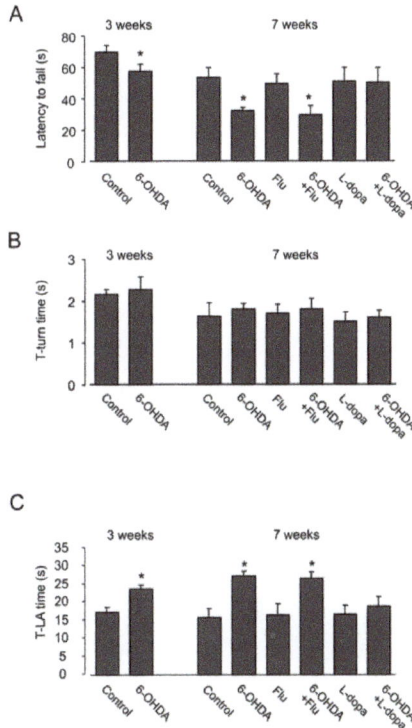

Figure 3. Effects of L-dopa and fluoxetine on motor activity (the rotarod test and the pole test) in mice treated with 6-OHDA. After three-weeks recovery from the 6-OHDA lesions, mice with anhedonia were daily injected intraperitoneally with fluoxetine (10 mg/kg/d) or L-dopa (20 mg/kg/d in saline and combined with 12 mg/kg/d of benserazide) for four weeks. Behavior tests were performed just before or after L-dopa or fluoxetine treatment. (**A**) The latency to fall off the rotarod in the rotarod test. The values are expressed as the mean ± SEM. * Indicates statistically significant (p < 0.05) difference from other groups at the same treatment period. (**B**) T-turn time in the pole test. The values are expressed as the mean ± SEM. (**C**) Time to descend to the floor T-LA time in the pole test. The values are expressed as the mean ± SEM. * Indicates statistically significant (p < 0.05) difference from other groups at the same treatment period.

The time taken by the mice to turn completely downward (Figure 3B; T-turn time) was not significantly affected by 6-OHDA after three weeks (Control: 2.15 ± 0.12 s, n = 18; 6-OHDA: 2.27 ± 0.30 s, n = 18; p > 0.05) and seven weeks (Control: 1.62 ± 0.32 s, n = 6; 6-OHDA: 1.80 ± 0.13 s, n = 6; p > 0.05). However, the time taken by the mice to reach the floor (Figure 3C; T-LA time) was significantly increased after three (Control: 17.36 ± 1.32 s, n =18; 6-OHDA: 23.92 ± 0.99 s, n = 18; $p < 0.05$) and seven weeks (Control: 15.75 ± 2.56 s, n = 6; 6-OHDA: 27.33 ± 1.36 s, n = 6; $p < 0.05$). Again, L-dopa corrected 6-OHDA-induced increase of T-turn time after seven weeks, but fluoxetine had no effect (Flu: 16.50 ± 3.13 s, n = 6; 6-OHDA + Flu: 26.70 ± 1.76 s, n = 6; L-dopa: 16.80 ± 2.44 s, n = 6; 6-OHDA + L-dopa: 18.90 ± 2.83 s, n = 6; $p < 0.05$).

3.3. Expression of mRNA and Protein of 5-HT$_{2B}$ Receptor

In cerebral tissue of mice treated with 6-OHDA, the mRNA level of 5-HT$_{2B}$ receptor decreased to 43.8 ± 4.7% of control groups (n = 3, $p < 0.05$) and protein expression to 67.3 ± 4.3% (n = 3, $p < 0.05$) seven weeks after lesion (Figure 4A,B). Experiments with freshly isolated astrocytes and neurons from transgenic mice demonstrated that the decrease of 5-HT$_{2B}$ receptor mRNA expression in the in vivo brain was confined to astrocytes and was not detected in neurons (Figure 4C). However, this downregulation was corrected by L-dopa (Figure 4A,B) or fluoxetine (Figure 4D,E) that was injected three weeks after 6-OHDA treatment and continued for four weeks.

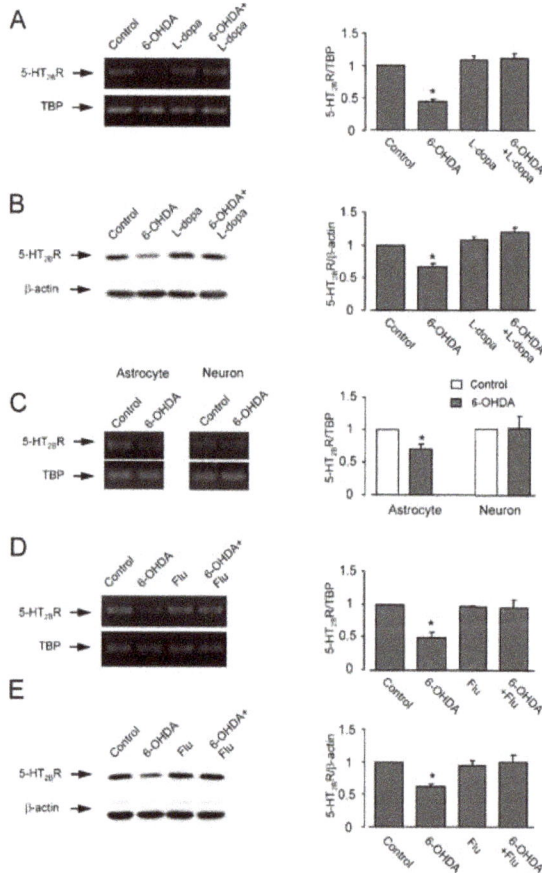

Figure 4. Effects of L-dopa and fluoxetine on expression of mRNA and protein of 5-HT$_{2B}$ receptor in brains of anhedonia mice induced by 6-OHDA. After three-weeks recovery from the 6-OHDA lesions, mice with anhedonia were daily injected intraperitoneally with fluoxetine (10 mg/kg/d) or L-dopa (20 mg/kg/d in saline and combined with 12 mg/kg/d of benserazide) for four weeks.

In some experiments, (**C**) freshly isolated astrocytes and neurons from transgenic mice were used for determination of 5-HT$_{2B}$ receptor mRNA expression. (**A,C,D**) mRNA expression measured by reverse transcription-polymerase chain reaction (RT-PCR) of (**A**) 5-HT$_{2B}$ receptor in cerebral cortex in vivo from anhedonia mice treated with L-dopa for four weeks, (**C**) in freshly isolated astrocytes and neurons from transgenic mice, or (**D**) in cerebral cortex in vivo from anhedonia mice treated with fluoxetine for four weeks. A representative experiment showing mRNA for 5-HT$_{2B}$ receptor and for TATA box-binding protein (TBP), as a housekeeping gene. The size of PCR product of 5-HT$_{2B}$ receptor is 370 bp and that of TBP 236 bp. Similar results were obtained in three independent experiments. Average mRNA expression was quantified as the ratio between 5-HT$_{2B}$ receptor and the housekeeping TBP gene. Ratios between 5-HT$_{2B}$ receptor and TBP in control group were designated a value of one. Standard error of the mean (SEM) values are indicated by vertical bars. * Indicates statistically significant ($p < 0.05$) difference from all other groups. (**B,E**) Protein expression measured by immunoblotting of 5-HT$_{2B}$ receptor in cerebral cortex in vivo from anhedonia mice treated with (**B**) L-dopa or fluoxetine (**E**) for four weeks. Immunoblots from representative experiments. Bands of 55 kDa and 42 kDa represent 5-HT$_{2B}$ receptor (5-HT$_{2B}$R) and β-actin, respectively. Similar results were obtained in three independent experiments. Average protein level was quantified as ratios between 5-HT$_{2B}$R and β-actin. Ratios between 5-HT$_{2B}$ receptor and β-actin in control group were designated a value of one. Standard error of the mean values are indicated by vertical bars. * Indicates statistically significant ($p < 0.05$) difference from all other groups.

The time course of expression of 5-HT$_{2B}$ receptor mRNA during 6-OHDA treatment in cultured astrocytes is shown on Figure 5A. At 6 h and 12 h, there was no difference in 5-HT$_{2B}$ receptor expression in control and 6-OHDA groups. However, after 24 h treatment, mRNA of 5-HT$_{2B}$ receptor decreased to $64.7 \pm 6.2\%$ of control groups ($n = 3$, $p < 0.05$). It was further decreased to $57.1 \pm 9.6\%$ after 48 h of treatment ($n = 3$, $p < 0.05$). Expression of 5-HT$_{2B}$ receptor protein showed similar pattern as mRNA (Figure 5B). After 24 h-exposure to 6-OHDA, cultures were treated with L-dopa or fluoxetine for another two weeks. Both L-dopa at 10 μM and fluoxetine at 1 μM abolished effect of 6-OHDA (Figure 5C–F).

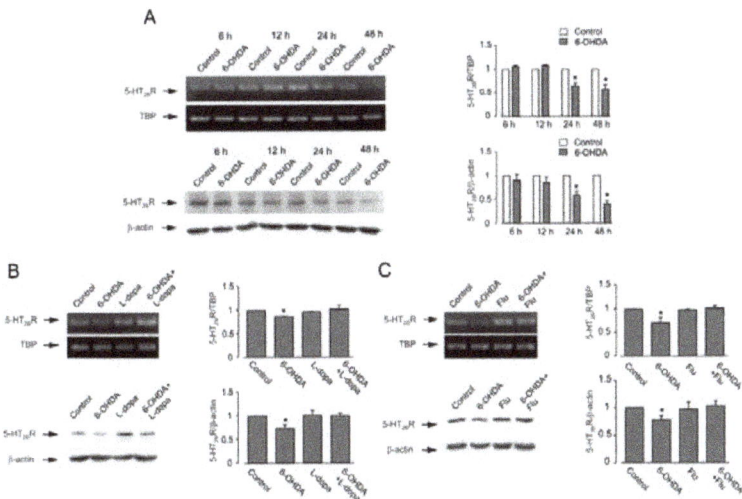

Figure 5. Effects of L-dopa and fluoxetine on 6-OHDA induced downregulation of expression of mRNA and protein of 5-HT$_{2B}$ receptor in primary cultures of astrocytes. (**A**) Effects of 6-OHDA on mRNA and protein expression of 5-HT$_{2B}$ receptor in primary cultures of astrocytes. Cells were treated with saline (Control) or 6-OHDA (50 μM) for 6 h, 12 h, 24 h and 48 h. (**B**) Effects of L-dopa on 6-OHDA induced downregulation of expression of mRNA and protein of 5-HT$_{2B}$ receptor in primary cultures of astrocytes.

Cells were treated with L-dopa (10 µM) for two weeks after 24 h 6-OHDA exposure. (C) Effects of fluoxetine on 6-OHDA induced downregulation of expression of mRNA and protein of 5-HT$_{2B}$ receptor in primary cultures of astrocytes. Cells were treated with fluoxetine (1 µM) for two weeks after 24 h 6-OHDA exposure. Representative experiments show mRNA expression for 5-HT$_{2B}$ receptor and for TBP, as a housekeeping gene (top panels). The size of PCR product of 5-HT$_{2B}$ receptor is 370 bp and that of TBP 236 bp. Similar results were obtained in three independent experiments. Average mRNA expression was quantified as ratio between 5-HT$_{2B}$ receptor and the housekeeping TBP gene. Ratios between 5-HT$_{2B}$ receptor and TBP in control group were designated a value of one. Immunoblots show bands of 55 kDa and 42 kDa representing 5-HT$_{2B}$ receptor and β-actin, respectively. Similar results were obtained in three independent experiments. Average protein level was quantified as ratios between 5-HT$_{2B}$R and β-actin. Ratios between 5-HT$_{2B}$ receptor and β-actin in the control group were designated a value of one. Standard error of the mean values are indicated by vertical bars. * Indicates statistically significant ($p < 0.05$) difference from other groups at the same treatment period.

4. Discussion

Astrocytes, being intimately associated with synaptic structures, regulate neurotransmission, synaptic plasticity, and integration in neuronal networks through multiple mechanisms that control synaptogenesis, maintain ion and neurotransmitter homeostasis in the synaptic cleft, provide neuronal terminals with neurotransmitter precursors, and contribute to synaptic extinction [25–29]. Pathological changes to astroglia, therefore, may significantly affect brain function and lead to neurological disorders [30]. In particular, astrocytopathies, mainly in the form of atrophy, decrease in astroglial densities, and possibly loss in astroglia homeostatic function, contribute to major neuropsychiatric diseases such as major depression and schizophrenia [8,9,31,32]. Expression of astroglial serotonin receptors, which mediate neuronal–glial interactions, are modified in major depression and bipolar disorders; and antidepressants correct these pathological changes [33,34].

Previously, we reported that the decrease of gene expression of astrocytic 5-HT$_{2B}$ receptor parallels the development of depressive behavior in the MPTP mouse model of PD, while fluoxetine ameliorates both the decrease in 5-HT$_{2B}$ receptor expression and anhedonia [13]. In this study, we describe similar results obtained in 6-OHDA mouse model of PD. These new findings further corroborate the notion that the decrease in gene expression of astroglial 5-HT$_{2B}$ receptors may be associated with pathophysiological evolution of PD-associated depression.

The MPTP is a lipidophilic compound able to penetrate the blood–brain barrier (BBB). Consequently, MPTP can be injected systemically to induce a bilateral parkinsonism, or, when infused through the carotid artery, to induce hemiparkinsonism [35]. In the latter settings, contralateral hemisphere can be used as control [36]. After crossing the BBB, MPTP (which by itself is non-toxic) is accumulated in astrocytes, where monoaminoxidase-B converts it to the toxic metabolite, MPP+. The latter is released from astrocytes and is accumulated by dopaminergic neurons through the dopamine transporter. In neurons, the MPP+ inhibits mitochondrial complex I, thus affecting adenosine triphosphate (ATP) synthesis, boosting production of reactive oxygen species (ROS), and leading to cell death [37]. After intraperitoneal injection (which we used in a previous study), MPTP spreads throughout the brain. Astrocytes thus may be affected directly by the drug as we have seen in cultured astrocytes [13], irrespective to the deficiency of dopaminergic system. In this study, we used 6-OHDA, a compound that cannot cross the BBB. 6-Hydroxydopamine enters dopaminergic neurons by dopamine transporter and thereafter triggers the production of neurotoxic ROS [36]. In contrast to MPTP, which is converted in neurotoxic agent by astrocytes, 6-OHDA enters neurons causing their demise. The usage of the 6-OHDA model therefore excludes possible direct damage to astrocytes which might be present in MPTP-treated animals. 6-Hydroxydopamine induces nigral dopamine cell loss and dopamine depletion. However, it does not seem to affect other brain regions, such as olfactory structures, lower brain stem areas, or locus coeruleus [14]. Therefore, the decrease of 5-HT$_{2B}$ receptor in the brain in vivo may be related to the aberrations in serotonergic, adrenergic, or dopaminergic neurotransmission [38], although we cannot exclude the possibility of direct drug effect on astrocytes in cerebral hemispheres since 6-OHDA also decreases gene expression of 5-HT$_{2B}$ receptor in cultured astrocytes.

L-Dopa is a precursor of dopamine; L-dopa crosses the BBB and is converted to dopamine by aromatic amino acid decarboxylase [39]. In the clinical treatment of PD, L-dopa is used to replenish dopamine pool and is therapeutically effective in both PD patients and animal models of the disease [40]. However, it is controversial whether L-dopa has effect on PD depression. The clinical data show that L-dopa has no effect or accelerates depression or anxiety (see [4] and references therein). Similar results were obtained from animal models of PD [4]. Our data show that treatment with L-dopa for four weeks ameliorates both 6-OHDA-induced decrease of 5-HT$_{2B}$ receptor expression in the brain in vivo and 6-OHDA-induced depressive behavior, suggesting the link between 5-HT$_{2B}$ receptors and 6-OHDA-induced depression. Astrocytes express neutral amino acid transporter (LAT/SLC7A5) and dopamine transporter (DAT/SLC6A3) [41–45]; astroglia mainly function as a reservoir of L-dopa that regulates the uptake or release of L-dopa depending on extracellular L-dopa concentration, but are less capable of converting L-dopa to dopamine [46]. The effect L-dopa on ROS production is debatable. When L-dopa is decarboxylated to dopamine (DA) by aromatic L-amino acid decarboxylase (AADC), ROS are generated that could ultimately lead to cell death [47]. Nevertheless, L-dopa in some in vivo and in vitro experiments had no toxic effects, or even showed antioxidant capabilities [48–51]. Oxidative stress in peripheral blood mononuclear cells from patients with PD is negatively correlated with L-dopa dosage [48]. Experiments with catecholaminergic human neuroblastoma cells showed that L-dopa may have a protective effect on dopaminergic cells [49]. Similar results were also obtained in PC12 cells [52]. In the perinatal 6-OHDA lifelong model of PD, elevated basal levels of ROS occurring in denervated dopaminergic striatum are suppressed by L-dopa treatment [50]. L-Dopa in follicular fluid is an antioxidant factor and exerts positive influences on cultured human granulosa cells, whereas DA derived from L-dopa has opposite actions [51]. In the present work, we have found that L-dopa corrects 6-OHDA-induced decrease of 5-HT$_{2B}$ receptor in astrocytes in primary cultures, suggesting L-dopa that may protect cells by its antioxidant effects.

In contrast to L-dopa, fluoxetine has no effect on 6-OHDA-induced motor deficiency, suggesting the effect of L-dopa on motor activity is dependent on DA replenishment. However, the effect of fluoxetine on depressive behavior develops in parallel with its effect on the gene expression of the 5-HT$_{2B}$ receptor [10]. The effects of fluoxetine on astrocytes are mediated by the 5-HT$_{2B}$ receptor. The affinity 5-HT to the astroglial 5-HT$_{2B}$ receptor is substantially higher than to 5-HT$_{2C}$ receptor [53]. Different SSRIs bind to and activate astroglial 5-HT$_{2B}$ receptors, which induce EGFR transactivation [54]. Stimulation of EGFR-dependent signaling cascades regulates expression of multiple genes (for a review, see [55,56]). In mice that develop anhedonia following chronic stress, expression of astroglial 5-HT$_{2B}$ receptor is significantly suppressed; at the same time, expression of 5-HT$_{2B}$ receptor does not change in mice which do not develop anhedonia [11]. Chronic treatment with fluoxetine rescues this deficit and increases expression of 5-HT$_{2B}$ receptors in astrocytes in the brains of anhedonic animals [12]. Similarly, astrocytic 5-HT$_{2B}$ receptor is downregulated only in anhedonic mice, but not in those that do not develop anhedonia in MPTP-induced PD model animals. This is in agreement with our present findings that astrocytic 5-HT$_{2B}$ receptor is decreased in depressed animals in 6-OHDA PD model.

Pathophysiology of depression associated with PD is not clear. We have shown that downregulation of the gene expression of 5-HT$_{2B}$ receptors occurs specifically in astrocytes in parallel with the development of depressive behavior in both 6-OHDA and MPTP animal models of PD. The relevance of 5-HT$_{2B}$ receptors to depression is corroborated by (1) the decrease of its gene expression in the nervous tissue of animals developing depressive behavior under the CMS [11,57], in the MPTP PD animal model [13], and in the 6-OHDA PD animal model; (2) the upregulation of 5-HT$_{2B}$ receptor gene expression by chronic treatment with fluoxetine in astrocytes in cultures and freshly isolated from the in vivo brains [11,57]; and (3) the dependence of antidepressant effect of fluoxetine on 5-HT$_{2B}$ receptors in vivo [58]. Since both drugs directly decrease expression of 5-HT$_{2B}$

receptors in cultured astrocytes, there is still a possibility that this phenomenon may only occur in PD animal models. To make a conclusion, postmortem examination of 5-HT$_{2B}$ receptors in PD patients' brains is needed.

Acknowledgments: This study was supported by Grant No. 31400925 to D.S. from the National Natural Science Foundation of China.

Author Contributions: L.P. conceptualized the study and supervised experimental work; D.S. and K.M. performed the experiments and analyzed the data; A.V. and L.P. wrote the paper.

Conflicts of Interest: The authors declare no conflict of interest.

References

1. Hornykiewicz, O.; Kish, S.J. Biochemical pathophysiology of Parkinson's disease. *Adv. Neurol.* **1987**, *45*, 19–34. [PubMed]
2. Chiu, W.H.; Depboylu, C.; Hermanns, G.; Maurer, L.; Windolph, A.; Oertel, W.H.; Ries, V.; Höglinger, G.U. Long-term treatment with L-DOPA or pramipexole affects adult neurogenesis and corresponding non-motor behavior in a mouse model of Parkinson's disease. *Neuropharmacology* **2015**, *95*, 367–376. [CrossRef] [PubMed]
3. Costa, F.H.; Rosso, A.L.; Maultasch, H.; Nicaretta, D.H.; Vincent, M.B. Depression in Parkinson's disease: Diagnosis and treatment. *Arq. Neuropsiquiatr.* **2012**, *70*, 617–620. [CrossRef] [PubMed]
4. Eskow Jaunarajs, K.L.; Angoa-Perez, M.; Kuhn, D.M.; Bishop, C. Potential mechanisms underlying anxiety and depression in Parkinson's disease: Consequences of L-DOPA treatment. *Neurosci. Biobehav. Rev.* **2011**, *35*, 556–564. [CrossRef] [PubMed]
5. Fox, S.H.; Chuang, R.; Brotchie, J.M. Serotonin and Parkinson's disease: On movement, mood and madness. *Mov. Disord.* **2009**, *24*, 1255–1266. [CrossRef] [PubMed]
6. Booth, H.D.E.; Hirst, W.D.; Wade-Martins, R. The role of astrocyte dysfunction in Parkinson's disease pathogenesis. *Trends Neurosci.* **2017**, *40*, 358–370. [CrossRef] [PubMed]
7. Verkhratsky, A.; Steardo, L.; Parpura, V.; Montana, V. Translational potential of astrocytes in brain disorders. *Prog. Neurobiol.* **2016**, *144*, 188–205. [CrossRef] [PubMed]
8. Verkhratsky, A.; Rodríguez, J.J.; Steardo, L. Astrogliopathology: A central element of neuropsychiatric diseases? *Neuroscientist* **2014**, *20*, 576–588. [CrossRef] [PubMed]
9. Verkhratsky, A.; Parpura, V. Astrogliopathology in neurological, neurodevelopmental and psychiatric disorders. *Neurobiol. Dis.* **2016**, *85*, 254–561. [CrossRef] [PubMed]
10. Li, B.; Zhang, S.; Zhang, H.; Nu, W.; Cai, L.; Hertz, L.; Peng, L. Fluoxetine-mediated 5-HT$_{2B}$ receptor stimulation in astrocytes causes EGF receptor transactivation and ERK phosphorylation. *Psychopharmacology* **2008**, *201*, 443–458. [CrossRef] [PubMed]
11. Li, B.; Dong, L.; Wang, B.; Cai, L.; Jiang, N.; Peng, L. Cell type-specific gene expression and editing responses to chronic fluoxetine treatment in the in vivo mouse brain and their relevance for stress-induced anhedonia. *Neurochem. Res.* **2012**, *37*, 2480–2495. [CrossRef] [PubMed]
12. Dong, L.; Li, B.; Verkhratsky, A.; Peng, L. Cell type-specific in vivo expression of genes encoding signalling molecules in the brain in response to chronic mild stress and chronic treatment with fluoxetine. *Psychopharmacology* **2015**, *232*, 2827–2835. [CrossRef] [PubMed]
13. Zhang, X.; Song, D.; Gu, L.; Ren, Y.; Verkhratsky, A.; Peng, L. Decrease of gene expression of astrocytic 5-HT$_{2B}$ receptors parallels development of depressive phenotype in a mouse model of Parkinson's disease. *Front. Cell. Neurosci.* **2015**, *9*, 388. [CrossRef] [PubMed]
14. Blesa, J.; Phani, S.; Jackson-Lewis, V.; Przedborski, S. Classic and new animal models of Parkinson's disease. *J. Biomed. Biotechnol.* **2012**, *2012*, 845618. [CrossRef] [PubMed]
15. Matsuura, K.; Kabuto, H.; Makino, H.; Ogawa, N. Pole test is a useful method for evaluating the mouse movement disorder caused by striatal dopamine depletion. *J. Neurosci. Methods* **1997**, *73*, 45–48. [CrossRef]
16. Lovatt, D.; Sonnewald, U.; Waagepetersen, H.S.; Schousboe, A.; He, W.; Lin, J.H.; Han, X.; Takano, T.; Wang, S.; Sim, F.J.; et al. The transcriptome and metabolic gene signature of protoplasmic astrocytes in the adult murine cortex. *J. Neurosci.* **2007**, *27*, 12255–12266. [CrossRef] [PubMed]
17. Fu, H.; Li, B.; Hertz, L.; Peng, L. Contributions in astrocytes of SMIT1/2 and HMIT to myo-inositol uptake at different concentrations and pH. *Neurochem. Int.* **2012**, *61*, 187–194. [CrossRef] [PubMed]

18. Hertz, L.; Peng, L.; Lai, J.C. Functional studies in cultured astrocytes. *Methods* **1998**, *16*, 293–310. [CrossRef] [PubMed]

19. Hertz, L.; Bock, E.; Schousboe, A. GFA content, glutamate uptake and activity of glutamate metabolizing enzymes in differentiating mouse astrocytes in primary cultures. *Dev. Neurosci.* **1978**, *1*, 226–238. [CrossRef]

20. Hertz, L.; Juurlink, B.H.J.; Szuchet, S. Cell cultures. In *Handbook of Neurochemistry*; Lajtha, A., Ed.; Plenum Press: New York, NY, USA, 1985.

21. Meier, E.; Hertz, L.; Schousboe, A. Neurotransmitters as developmental signals. *Neurochem. Int.* **1991**, *19*, 1–15. [CrossRef]

22. Kong, E.K.; Peng, L.; Chen, Y.; Yu, A.C.; Hertz, L. Up-regulation of 5-HT2B receptor density and receptor-mediated glycogenolysis in mouse astrocytes by long-term fluoxetine administration. *Neurochem. Res.* **2002**, *27*, 113–120. [CrossRef] [PubMed]

23. El-Marjou, A.; Delouvée, A.; Thiery, J.P.; Radvanyi, F. Involvement of epidermal growth factor receptor in chemically induced mouse bladder tumour progression. *Carcinogenesis* **2000**, *21*, 2211–2218. [CrossRef] [PubMed]

24. Lowry, O.H.; Rosebrough, N.J.; Farr, A.L.; Randall, R.J. Protein measurement with the Folin phenol reagent. *J. Biol. Chem.* **1951**, *193*, 265–275. [PubMed]

25. Verkhratsky, A.; Nedergaard, M. Astroglial cradle in the life of the synapse. *Philos. Trans. R. Soc. Lond. B Biol. Sci.* **2014**, *369*, 20130595. [CrossRef] [PubMed]

26. Verkhratsky, A.; Nedergaard, M. Physiology of astroglia. *Physiol. Rev.* **2018**, *98*, 239–389. [CrossRef] [PubMed]

27. De Pitta, M.; Brunel, N.; Volterra, A. Astrocytes: Orchestrating synaptic plasticity? *Neuroscience* **2016**, *323*, 43–61. [CrossRef] [PubMed]

28. Dallerac, G.; Rouach, N. Astrocytes as new targets to improve cognitive functions. *Prog. Neurobiol.* **2016**, *144*, 48–67. [CrossRef] [PubMed]

29. Zorec, R.; Horvat, A.; Vardjan, N.; Verkhratsky, A. Memory formation shaped by astroglia. *Front. Integr. Neurosci.* **2015**, *9*, 56. [CrossRef] [PubMed]

30. Pekny, M.; Pekna, M.; Messing, A.; Steinhäuser, C.; Lee, J.M.; Parpura, V.; Hol, E.M.; Sofroniew, M.V.; Verkhratsky, A. Astrocytes: A central element in neurological diseases. *Acta Neuropathol.* **2016**, *131*, 323–345. [CrossRef] [PubMed]

31. Rajkowska, G.; Stockmeier, C.A. Astrocyte pathology in major depressive disorder: Insights from human postmortem brain tissue. *Curr. Drug Targets* **2013**, *14*, 1225–1236. [CrossRef] [PubMed]

32. Niciu, M.J.; Henter, I.D.; Sanacora, G.; Zarate, C.A., Jr. Glial abnormalities in substance use disorders and depression: Does shared glutamatergic dysfunction contribute to comorbidity? *World J. Biol. Psychiatry* **2014**, *15*, 2–16. [CrossRef] [PubMed]

33. Peng, L.; Verkhratsky, A.; Gu, L.; Li, B. Targeting astrocytes in major depression. *Expert Rev. Neurother.* **2015**, *15*, 1299–1306. [CrossRef] [PubMed]

34. Peng, L.; Li, B.; Verkhratsky, A. Targeting astrocytes in bipolar disorder. *Expert Rev. Neurother.* **2016**, *16*, 649–657. [CrossRef] [PubMed]

35. Bankiewicz, K.S.; Oldfield, E.H.; Chiueh, C.C.; Doppman, J.L.; Jacobowitz, D.M.; Kopin, I.J. Hemiparkinsonism in monkeys after unilateral internal carotid artery infusion of 1-methyl-4-phenyl-1,2,3,6-tetrahydropyridine (MPTP). *Life Sci.* **1986**, *39*, 7–16. [CrossRef]

36. Bové, J.; Perier, C. Neurotoxin-based models of Parkinson's disease. *Neuroscience* **2012**, *211*, 51–76. [CrossRef] [PubMed]

37. Meredith, G.E.; Totterdell, S.; Potashkin, J.A.; Surmeier, D.J. Modeling PD pathogenesis in mice: Advantages of a chronic MPTP protocol. *Parkinsonism Relat. Disord.* **2008**, *14* (Suppl. S2), S112–S115. [CrossRef] [PubMed]

38. Ossowska, K.; Lorenc-Koci, E. Depression in Parkinson's disease. *Pharmacol. Rep.* **2013**, *65*, 1545–1557. [CrossRef]

39. Mura, A.; Jackson, D.; Manley, M.S.; Young, S.J.; Groves, P.M. Aromatic L-amino acid decarboxylase immunoreactive cells in the rat striatum: A possible site for the conversion of exogenous L-DOPA to dopamine. *Brain Res.* **1995**, *704*, 51–60. [CrossRef]

40. Nagatsua, T.; Sawadab, M. L-Dopa therapy for Parkinson's disease: Past, present and future. *Parkinsonism Relat. Disord.* **2009**, *15* (Suppl. 1), S3–S8. [CrossRef]

41. Inyushin, M.Y.; Huertas, A.; Kucheryavykh, Y.V.; Kucheryavykh, L.Y.; Tsydzik, V.; Sanabria, P.; Eaton, M.J.; Skatchkov, S.N.; Rojas, L.V.; Wessinger, W.D. L-DOPA uptake in astrocytic endfeet enwrapping blood vessels in rat brain. *Parkinson's Dis.* **2012**, 321406. [CrossRef] [PubMed]

42. Kim, D.K.; Kim, I.J.; Hwang, S.; Kook, J.H.; Lee, M.C.; Shin, B.A.; Bae, C.S.; Yoon, J.H.; Ahn, S.G.; Kim, S.A. System L-amino acid transporters are differently expressed in rat astrocyte and C6 glioma cells. *Neurosci. Res.* **2004**, *50*, 437–446. [CrossRef] [PubMed]

43. Tsai, M.J.; Lee, E.H. Characterization of L-DOPA transport in cultured rat and mouse astrocytes. *J. Neurosci. Res.* **1996**, *43*, 490–495. [CrossRef]

44. Inazu, M.; Kubota, N.; Takeda, H.; Zhang, J.; Kiuchi, Y.; Oguchi, K.; Matsumiya, T. Pharmacological characterization of dopamine transport in cultured rat astrocytes. *Life Sci.* **1999**, *64*, 2239–2245. [CrossRef]

45. Inazu, M.; Takeda, H.; Ikoshi, H.; Uchida, Y.; Kubota, N.; Kiuchi, Y.; Oguchi, K.; Matsumiya, T. Regulation of dopamine uptake by basic fibroblast growth factor and epidermal growth factor in cultured rat astrocytes. *Neurosci. Res.* **1999**, *34*, 235–244. [CrossRef]

46. Asanuma, M.; Miyazaki, I.; Murakami, S.; Diaz-Corrales, F.J.; Ogawa, N. Striatal astrocytes act as a reservoir for L-DOPA. *PLoS ONE* **2014**, *9*, e106362. [CrossRef] [PubMed]

47. Stansley, B.J.; Yamamoto, B.K. L-Dopa-induced dopamine synthesis and oxidative stress in serotonergic cells. *Neuropharmacology* **2013**, *67*, 243–251. [CrossRef] [PubMed]

48. Prigione, A.; Begni, B.; Galbussera, A.; Beretta, S.; Brighina, L.; Garofalo, R.; Andreoni, S.; Piolti, R.; Ferrarese, C. Oxidative stress in peripheral blood mononuclear cells from patients with Parkinson's disease: Negative correlation with levodopa dosage. *Neurobiol. Dis.* **2006**, *23*, 36–43. [CrossRef] [PubMed]

49. Colamartino, M.; Padua, L.; Meneghini, C.; Leone, S.; Cornetta, T.; Testa, A.; Cozzi, R. Protective effects of L-dopa and carbidopa combined treatments on human catecholaminergic cells. *DNA Cell Biol.* **2012**, *31*, 1572–1579. [CrossRef] [PubMed]

50. Kostrzewa, J.P.; Kostrzewa, R.A.; Kostrzewa, R.M.; Brus, R.; Nowak, P. Perinatal 6-hydroxydopamine to produce a lifelong model of severe Parkinson's disease. *Curr. Top. Behav. Neurosci.* **2015**. [CrossRef]

51. Blohberger, J.; Buck, T.; Berg, D.; Berg, U.; Kunz, L.; Mayerhofer, A. L-DOPA in the human ovarian follicular fluid acts as an antioxidant factor on granulosa cells. *J. Ovarian Res.* **2016**, *9*, 62. [CrossRef] [PubMed]

52. Zhong, S.Y.; Chen, Y.X.; Fang, M.; Zhu, X.L.; Zhao, Y.X.; Liu, X.Y. Low-dose levodopa protects nerve cells from oxidative stress and up-regulates expression of pCREB and CD39. *PLoS ONE* **2014**, *9*, e95387. [CrossRef] [PubMed]

53. Li, B.; Zhang, S.; Li, M.; Hertz, L.; Peng, L. Serotonin increases $ERK_{1/2}$ phosphorylation in astrocytes by stimulation of $5\text{-}HT_{2B}$ and $5\text{-}HT_{2C}$ receptors. *Neurochem. Int.* **2010**, *57*, 432–439. [CrossRef] [PubMed]

54. Zhang, S.; Li, B.; Lovatt, D.; Xu, J.; Song, D.; Goldman, S.A.; Nedergaard, M.; Hertz, L.; Peng, L. $5\text{-}HT_{2B}$ receptors are expressed on astrocytes from brain and in culture and are a chronic target for all five conventional 'serotonin-specific reuptake inhibitors'. *Neuron Glia Biol.* **2010**, *6*, 113–125. [CrossRef] [PubMed]

55. Peng, L.; Huang, J. Astrocytic $5\text{-}HT_{2B}$ receptor as in vitro and in vivo target of SSRIs. *Recent Pat. CNS Drug Discov.* **2012**, *7*, 243–253. [CrossRef] [PubMed]

56. Hertz, L.; Rothman, D.L.; Li, B.; Peng, L. Chronic SSRI stimulation of astrocytic $5\text{-}HT_{2B}$ receptors change multiple gene expressions/editings and metabolism of glutamate, glucose and glycogen: A potential paradigm shift. *Front. Behav. Neurosci.* **2015**, *9*, 25. [PubMed]

57. Li, B.; Zhang, S.; Li, M.; Hertz, L.; Peng, L. Chronic treatment of astrocytes with therapeutically relevant fluoxetine concentrations enhances cPLA2 expression secondary to $5\text{-}HT_{2B}$-induced, transactivation-mediated $ERK_{1/2}$ phosphorylation. *Psychopharmacology* **2009**, *207*, 1–12. [CrossRef] [PubMed]

58. Diaz, S.L.; Doly, S.; Narboux-Nême, N.; Fernández, S.; Mazot, P.; Banas, S.M.; Boutourlinsky, K.; Moutkine, I.; Belmer, A.; Roumier, A.; et al. $5\text{-}HT_{2B}$ receptors are required for serotonin-selective antidepressant actions. *Mol. Psychiatry* **2012**, *17*, 154–163. [CrossRef] [PubMed]

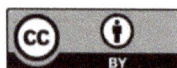

neuroglia

MDPI

Review

To Be or Not to Be: Environmental Factors that Drive Myelin Formation during Development and after CNS Trauma

Nicole Pukos [1,2,†], Rim Yoseph [1,2,†] and Dana M. McTigue [2,3,*]

[1]   Neuroscience Graduate Program, Ohio State University, Columbus, OH 43210, USA;
      pukos.1@buckeyemail.osu.edu (N.P.); yoseph.5@buckeyemail.osu.edu (R.Y.)
[2]   Center for Brain and Spinal Cord Repair, Ohio State University, Columbus, OH 43210, USA
[3]   Department of Neuroscience, Ohio State University, Columbus, OH 43210, USA
*   Correspondence: mctigue.2@osu.edu; Tel.: +1-614-292-5523
†   These authors contributed equally to this manuscript.

Received: 7 May 2018; Accepted: 4 June 2018; Published: 11 June 2018

Abstract: Oligodendrocytes are specialized glial cells that myelinate central nervous system (CNS) axons. Historically, it was believed that the primary role of myelin was to compactly ensheath axons, providing the insulation necessary for rapid signal conduction. However, mounting evidence demonstrates the dynamic importance of myelin and oligodendrocytes, including providing metabolic support to neurons and regulating axon protein distribution. As such, the development and maintenance of oligodendrocytes and myelin are integral to preserving CNS homeostasis and supporting proper functioning of widespread neural networks. Environmental signals are critical for proper oligodendrocyte lineage cell progression and their capacity to form functional compact myelin; these signals are markedly disturbed by injury to the CNS, which may compromise endogenous myelin repair capabilities. This review outlines some key environmental factors that drive myelin formation during development and compares that to the primary factors that define a CNS injury milieu. We aim to identify developmental factors disrupted after CNS trauma as well as pathogenic factors that negatively impact oligodendrocyte lineage cells, as these are potential therapeutic targets to promote myelin repair after injury or disease.

Keywords: development; spinal cord injury; myelination; growth factor; cytokine; oligodendrocyte progenitor cells

1. Introduction

The central nervous system (CNS) provides an excellent model to study cellular interactions because of the intimate association of its main parenchyma—neurons and glia. Neurons conduct action potentials and communicate to other neurons and cells throughout the body. Glia, representing the majority of the cells in the CNS, were originally referred to as helper cells, but studies have verified their importance in proper CNS functions, including communication between neurons. An essential component for rapid neuron signaling, especially for larger axons, is axon ensheathment by myelin. Oligodendrocytes (OLs) produce CNS myelin, which was first described by van Leeuwenhoek in 1717 [1]. Myelin does not just passively wrap axons, however. Extensive molecular interactions between OLs and axons regulate axon structure, including cytoskeletal maturation and restricting ion channels to nodal regions [2,3]. Evolutionarily, myelin first appeared when animals formed jaws and increased in physical size; myelin allowed increased axon conduction speed, which in turn allowed for faster escape from predators [4]. This huge evolutionary advantage separates vertebrates from invertebrates, who have supporting cells around axons rather than compact myelin [4].

Oligodendrocytes terminally differentiate from distinct cellular domains within the developing neural tube. As cells transition from an embryonic stem cell to oligodendrocyte progenitor cells (OPCs), OL lineage specific markers are upregulated; as cells continue to mature, they differentiate into OLs that engage axons and form compact myelin [5]. Interestingly, the adult CNS maintains a large population of OPCs throughout the white and gray matter whose OL progenitor role is retained (for recent review, see [6]). Indeed, the response of adult OPCs after experimental demyelination is well-documented and includes proliferation, migration into the demyelinated lesions and differentiation into remyelinating OLs [7,8]. However, their role in endogenous myelin repair after other types of CNS damage such as trauma is not fully understood. This is, in part, due to the complex biochemical cascades that are unique to the trauma milieu, which are initiated immediately after injury but then fluctuate over time. This review will begin by outlining some key factors in normal myelin development and then discuss how these and other factors affect the response of OPCs to CNS trauma.

2. Development: OPC Migration, Proliferation, and Differentiation

Gans and Northcutt theorized that vertebrates exist because of the neural crest, a source of diverse cell lineages derived from the embryonic ectoderm [9]. These multipotent neural stem cells give rise to OPCs, the majority of which arise from the motor neural progenitor (pMN) domain of ventral ventricular zone in the spinal cord, although ≈20% originate in the dorsal ventricular zone [10–13]. Both intraspinal progenitor populations have the same electrophysiological properties, but dorsal progenitors arise later and myelinate dorsal spinal tracts whereas ventral progenitors migrate dorsally and laterally to populate the entire white matter of the spinal cord; a similar wave of ventral to dorsal OPCs populate the brain developmentally [13–16]. During the first few postnatal weeks, a subset of OPCs extends branches to contact surrounding axons and terminally differentiate into mature OLs. Each developmental step is strictly regulated by a multitude of extracellular and intracellular signaling molecules that cooperate and coordinate to ensure proper CNS assembly (for recent review, see [5]).

2.1. Migration

Successful myelination of the CNS is contingent upon proper OPC migration. In the spinal cord, migration is strongly regulated by sonic hedgehog (Shh) and bone morphogenic protein (BMP). Sonic hedgehog is a ventral inductive signal secreted by the notochord that induces OPC specification in the ventral neural tube, whereas dorsal progenitors are Shh-independent and rely on local stimuli like BMP for induction [12,17–19]. Once formed, OPCs migrate in waves from the ventricular zone to distribute equally throughout the grey and white matter, with each cell occupying its own non-overlapping domain with neighboring OPCs [12,20,21]. For this to occur, OPCs need a mechanism to spatially locate neighboring OPCs. Indeed, dynamic filopodia from OPCS continuously surveil their environment to locate adjacent OPCs and guide cell trajectory [21]. In vivo imagining of OPCs in zebrafish shows OPCs exhibit contact-mediated inhibition in which they retract and change direction upon contacting filopodia from neighboring cells [21,22]. While all cellular signals causing retraction are not entirely known, Nogo-A is one factor thought to be involved in OPC spacing [23].

2.1.1. Growth Factors

Platelet-derived growth factor (PDGF) is secreted by astrocytes [24], which first form at embryonic day 16 in mice [25]. Similar to Shh, PDGF is secreted early during OPC migration and functions as a chemoattractant through activating the extracellular-regulated-kinase (ERK) signaling pathway [26]. Initially, PDGF acts a mobilizer to enhance cell mobility, and competes with Netrin-1, a laminin-like guidance molecule expressed in the floor plate [27]. Oligodendrocyte progenitor cells express Platelet-derived growth factor receptor alpha (PDGFRα) and netrin receptors, allowing both ligands to act as migratory cues in which netrin opposes PDGF-induced migration [25,28–31]. As OPCs migrate to their final target, they encounter various extracellular matrix ligands to which they are responsive [32]. Of particular importance are integrins, cell surface receptors that facilitate bidirectional signaling between the intracellular and extracellular environment. PDGF binds to integrin $\alpha_v\beta_3$, which stimulates OPC migration and proliferation [33]. Despite its crucial role, however, PDGF does not act as solitary migratory factor but instead cooperates with other environmental cues for proper signaling.

Fibroblast growth factor 2 (FGF-2) is also produced by astrocytes [34] and stimulates OPC migration, although not as strongly as PDGF. For instance, transient exposure to FGF-2 has no effect on OPC migration, whereas OPCs show long-term migration when exposed to PDGF-A under the same conditions [26]. Treating cells with both growth factors leads to faster migration compared to either alone, and also converts progenitors from slowly to rapidly dividing cells [26,35–38]. Similar to PDGF-A, FGF-2 promotes OPC migration via the ERK1/2 signaling pathway after binding to its receptors FGFR1, which is necessary for FGF-2-induced migration [27,37,39,40]. Overall, FGF-2 is crucial for OPC migration, but the combinatory effects of PDGF and FGF-2 far surpass that of either factor alone, indicating proper OL development is contingent upon signaling from multiple factors.

2.1.2. Chemokines

Chemokines are secreted "chemotactic cytokines" best known for their role in regulating immune cell migration. Interestingly, chemokines in the C–X–C family also promote OPC proliferation and migration.

CXCL1 (also known as Gro-α) is expressed by astrocytes and binds to CXCR2 on OPCs to inhibit PDGF-stimulated migration [41–44]. CXCL1 signals through CXCR2 and serves as a stop signal for developmental OPC migration [43,45]. The importance of CXCL1 for proper OPC distribution is seen when it is absent, which results in continued OPC migration to the pial surface with extensive OPC migration into the periphery [46]. Most OPC proliferation occurs in the white matter as PDGF and CXCL1 work synergistically to inhibit migration while simultaneously promoting proliferation [41]. Eliminating CXCR2 expression diminishes OPC proliferation and reduces OL numbers, thereby reducing myelination and overall white matter area [43,45]. These studies highlight the importance of CXCL1 in localizing cells to allow for proper patterning of the white matter and efficient myelination.

CXCL12, also known as stromal cell-derived factor 1, binds to its receptor CXCR4, a G-protein coupled receptor highly conserved in evolution. Detection of CXCL12 and its receptor expression begins around E7.5 in the ventral neural tube, and expands to various cell types including OLs and neurons as the CNS matures [46–48]. The diverse expression of CXCL12 is crucial for proper CNS development, as the knockout of its receptor is embryonic lethal due to complications in the immune and central nervous systems [49]. For OPCs, CXCL12 acts a chemoattractant that promotes migration, proliferation, and survival in the brain and spinal cord [50,51]. Oligodendrocyte progenitor cells in CXCR4-deficient mice fail to migrate dorsally from the ventral neural tube since they are unresponsive to CXCL12. CXCR4 expression peaks during OPC migration, then decreases as OPCs differentiate in OLs, indicating CXCL12 and its receptor are important during early CNS development [50]. Overall, chemokines regulate the outward migration of OPCs from the neural tube to allow for proper CNS patterning.

2.2. Proliferation

2.2.1. Three Major Mitogens

In addition to promoting OPC migration, PDGF also acts a mitogen and is crucial for glial progenitor cell survival [24,29,52]. However, unlike migration, PDGF proliferation is mediated by the phosphatidylinositol-3-kinase (PI3K)-Akt and Wnt-β-catenin signaling pathways instead of the ERK pathway [53]. Interestingly, a population of proliferating OPCs is maintained into adulthood in the CNS [54,55]. Since OPCs in culture do not mimic this proliferative response, it suggests the balance between OPC self-renewal and differentiation is regulated by intrinsic and extrinsic signaling molecules [56–58]. Indeed, OPCs supplemented with astrocytes or PDGF, in traditional and new culture assays, proliferate steadily for weeks [38,59–62]. Blocking PDGF in the developing optic nerve reduces proliferation by 70% and progenitors immediately differentiate into OLs [60], findings that were later confirmed in vivo [25,29,63,64]. Complete PDGFRα knockout mice die in utero due to complications in patterning and cell survival throughout the body [65]. However, PDGF-deficient mice survive into adulthood but present with fewer OPCs and OLs, with the largest loss in the spinal cord and cerebellum; as would be expected, PDGF over-expression results in hyper-proliferation of OPCs [66–68]. Together, these experiments illustrate that PDGF and its receptor are important for controlling the timing and rate of proliferation. However, since inhibiting PDGF in the optic nerve eliminates only 70% of mitogenic activity, other signaling molecules must also play a role.

PDGFRα expression peaks on OPCs, then decreases as cells differentiate. However, adding FGF-2 reverses this effect by increasing PDGFRα expression, amplifying its response and stimulating long-term proliferation [63,69,70]. OPCs exposed to combined PDGF and FGF-2 continuously proliferate and self-renew, whereas if exposed to either PDGF or FGF-2 individually, progenitors exit the cell cycle [35], revealing these factors work synergistically to induce division and inhibit differentiation in a timely manner [71].

When acting alone, FGF-2 is a less potent mitogen than PDGF but still blocks OPC differentiation [38,72,73]. Developmentally, FGF-2 expression increases during proliferation and peaks during OL formation when it functions to regulate the number of mature OLs [74,75]. FGF-2 binds with high affinity to all four FGF receptors, but only fibroblast growth factors receptors 1–3 (FGFR1-3) affect OPC proliferation. In OPCs, FGFR-1 levels continually rise, therefore exposure to FGF-2 increases OPC migration and proliferation [75,76]. As early OPCs transition to late stage OPCs and FGRF-1 levels continue to rise, FGF-2 switches to inhibiting differentiation. Fibroblast growth factor receptor 1 small interfering RNA (siRNA) blocks this inhibition leading to a higher number of differentiated OLs, revealing that FGFR-1 halts OL differentiation [77]. Similar to FGFR-1, FGFR-3 expression also peaks in the late OL progenitor stage to further block OL differentiation. Later in development, FGF-2 severely disrupts myelin production by dysregulating myelin gene expression [78–80]. Overall, FGF-2 promotes the proliferation of OPCs by stimulating DNA synthesis and inhibiting OL lineage progression during all stages of development.

Insulin-like growth factor-1 (IGF-1) works in concert with PDGF and FGF-2 to promote OPC proliferation through binding the type 1 IGF receptor (IGFR1) [81,82]. PDGF increases IGFR1 expression, thereby potentiating IGF-1 effects and maximizing OPC proliferation [83]. Adding IGF-1 to OPCs isolated from perinatal rat cerebrum increases OPC proliferation six-fold [84,85]. Moreover, developmental IGF-1 overexpression accelerates the cell cycle and increases neuronal and OPC proliferation, leading to larger brain size and weight [86,87].

The effects of IGF-1 depend on PI3K-Akt signaling, which promotes OPC survival and proliferation by inhibiting apoptosis and preventing the degradation of cyclin-D1 [88]. In addition, IGF-1 works synergistically with FGF-2 to activate the ERK1/2 pathway to stimulate cell growth and proliferation by upregulating nuclear cyclin-D expression [88–91]. Together, the PI3K/Akt and ERK1/2 pathways enhance G1/S progression, therefore IGF-1 shortens the cell cycle to allow increased cell proliferation [92]. In normal conditions, PDGF and FGF-2 trigger cells to enter G1 from the G0 phase. However, in conjunction with IGF-1, cells rapidly progress through G1 to the S phase due to upregulation of G1 cyclins, positive regulators of the cell cycle [83,87,88,91,92]. IGF-1-regulated PI3K-Akt signaling also functions as a survival signal by both protecting OPCs from tumor necrosis factor (TNF)α-induced cell death and preventing apoptosis [86,93–95]. Thus, overall, IGF-1 acts as a progression factor that accelerates the cell cycle, and a survival factor that maintains OPC levels.

2.2.2. Neurotrophic Factors

Neurotrophins are soluble growth factors crucial for nervous system development. These factors, consisting of nerve growth factor (NGF), brain-derived neurotrophic factor (BDNF), neurotrophin-3

(NT-3), and neurotrophin-4/5 (NT-4/5), are synthesized as precursor proteins, then cleaved into mature molecules. Mature neurotrophins signal through two distinct classes of receptors: the high-affinity receptor tyrosine kinase tropomyosin-related kinase (Trk), and the pan-neurotrophin receptor (p75NTR), a member of the TNFα receptor subfamily [96–98]. All neurotrophins bind with similar low affinity to p75NTR, but are selective in activating Trk receptors. Specifically, NGF binds TrkA, BDNF and NT-4/5 binds TrkB, and NT-3 binds TrkC [99,100].

Neurotrophins exhibit mitogenic effects on OPCs, although BDNF effects appear to be region-dependent. For instance, BDNF is a potent mitogen for OPCs in the basal forebrain while having no effect on optic nerve OPCs [94,101]. Once TrkB is bound by BDNF, its cytoplasmic domain becomes phosphorylated, leading to mitogen-activated protein kinase (MAPK) activation and increased DNA synthesis [97,101,102].

Like BDNF, the proliferative effects of NT-3 are mediated through MAPK signaling, after binding to TrkC receptors [33,103]. In the optic nerve, NT-3 is a stronger mitogen than PDGF, although NT-3 requires IGF-1 to induce OPC proliferation, whereas PDGF can act alone [94,104]. Knockout models of NT-3 and TrkC show severe depletion in PDGFRα+ OPCs in both the brain and spinal cord, although the distribution of OPCs in the CNS was similar to wild type, indicating NT-3 does not influence migration or distribution of OPCs [105]. In addition to acting as a mitogen during development, NT-3 is also a potent survival factor, promoting OPC survival in the absence of other trophic support [104].

2.3. Differentiation

The transition from progenitor cell to differentiated OLs involves multiple signals, including intracellular transcription factors and non-coding RNAs and extracellular molecules such as neurotransmitters, growth factors and extracellular matrix components (for an excellent recent review, see [5]). Changes in intracellular redox state may also be involved [57,106]. An additional molecular mechanism believed to underlie the switch in cell fate involves cyclin-dependent kinase-2 (Cdk2), which controls OPC cell cycle progression as it regulates the transition of cells from G1 to S phase [107,108]. To stop cell division, p27 binds to Cdk2 and promotes cell cycle arrest [109]. As OPCs proliferate, p27 slowly accumulates and regulates the timing of differentiation. If p27 is overexpressed, OPCs become unresponsive to mitogens resulting in significantly more mature OLs. Therefore, as time progresses, p27 levels reach a tipping point after which sufficient levels of Cdk2 are inhibited and cell proliferation is halted, in correlation with reduced PDGF and increased thyroid hormone (T3). Collectively, these experiments indicate OPC differentiation is regulated through multiple signaling mechanisms that ensure proper timing of OL maturation. Here, we will mainly focus on developmental factors that have also been examined in the injured CNS.

2.3.1. Hormones

Thyroid hormone is an important regulator of OPC differentiation. In the absence of T3 in culture, OPCs fail to differentiate and instead proliferate continuously [110–113]. Levels of T3 peak at birth and remain elevated for two weeks, coinciding with post-natal OL differentiation and myelination [114]. Once secreted, T3 binds to two receptors: T3α on OPCs and T3β on mature OLs [115,116]. During myelination, T3 binds to T3β receptors and drives myelin basic protein (MBP) expression through direct interaction with the MBP promoter [117–119]. Mature OLs exposed to T3 also have increased branching, a morphology beneficial to myelination [118]. The diverse roles of T3 on OL development are likely due to distinct receptors, as T3 modulates OPC survival and OL differentiation through T3α receptor and promotes myelination after cells upregulate T3β receptor.

In vitro about 80% of OPCs differentiate into OLs in the presence of IGF-1, whereas only 30% differentiate without it [84,85]. Conditional IGF-1 knockout mice show severely reduced brain size due to fewer OLs and axons, leading to an overall reduction in white matter [120,121], whereas excess IGF-1 inhibits OL apoptosis and promotes OL survival [122]. The higher number of mature OLs leads to increased MBP and proteolipid protein (PLP) expression, and a higher percentage of myelinated axons with thicker myelin [122–124]. Manipulating IGF-1 expression in vivo in either direction reveals the importance of IGF-1 in later stages, but due to its multiple roles throughout OL development, a model focused on OL maturation is more beneficial. Luzi et al. developed a transgenic mouse that overexpresses IGF-1 through the MBP promoter, thereby driving its overexpression only after myelination begins, around P10 [125]. The result was extensive myelination on axons due to more myelin produced per OL [125].

2.3.2. Neurotrophic Factors

Ciliary neurotrophic factor (CNTF) was originally identified for its role in neuronal support and survival [126], but since then, its importance in regulating OL development has become clear. CNTF is synthesized by astrocytes during the first postnatal week when OL generation peaks, and is continually expressed throughout early stages of oligodendrogenesis [127]. While CNTF does enhance the rate of OPC proliferation [128], it is more extensively involved in differentiation, maturation, and survival of OLs [129,130]. Spinal cord and cortical OPCs cultured in media supplemented with CNTF show increased differentiation, which is amplified when T3 is added [129,131]. Further in vitro studies uncovered a role for CNTF in myelination. When added to cultures, CNTF increased myelin production and the number of myelin internodes by upregulating MBP and myelin oligodendrocyte glycoprotein (MOG) expression [130,132]. Overexpressing CNTF in vivo is also correlated with increased MOG expression, while CNTF-deficient mice have higher rates of OL apoptosis and fewer myelinated axons [133,134]. Despite CNTF being a survival factor, the increased myelin gene expression is not due to increased OLs, but instead to more MBP and MOG expressed per OL [130].

Neurotrophin-3 plays a vital role in OL development. It is widely accepted that NT-3 promotes myelination and acts as a support factor in both the peripheral and central nervous system. It is highly expressed in the late prenatal period, peaks shortly after birth, then remains high 1–2 weeks postnatally before rapidly declining [135]. This expression pattern coincides with OPC differentiation and ultimately promotes axon myelination. Without NT-3, fewer OPCs differentiate, and those that do appear immature with short, stubby processes [105,136]. Overexpression of NT-3 in OPCs co-cultured with hippocampal neurons results in a 10-fold increase in MBP expression with a higher percent of axons becoming myelinated [137]. Thus, NT-3 is one of many influential signaling molecules in proper axon myelination.

Like NT-3, BDNF promotes myelin protein production in the peripheral nervous system (PNS) and CNS. In the PNS, BDNF activates p75NTR, while in the CNS it binds to TrkB, stimulating MAPK to upregulate MBP, PLP, and myelin-associated glycoprotein in OLs [102,138–140]. The need for BDNF developmentally is seen in BDNF null and heterozygous mice, which display hypomyelinated white matter due to reduced myelin gene expression [139,141–143]. This reduced myelin is not due to fewer myelinated axons, but instead thinner myelin per axon. Moreover, the number of differentiated OLs is comparable to controls, suggesting BDNF does not influence OL-axon contact, but may be necessary for establishing proper myelin thickness [144,145].

Neuregulin-1 (Nrg-1) is an extrinsic growth factor expressed by neurons in the brain and spinal cord that signals through ErbB receptor tyrosine kinases [146]. Initially, Nrg-1 was studied for its role in stimulating OPC proliferation; however, Nrg-1 is secreted throughout development and influences all stages of OL lineage cells, from proliferation through myelination [147–150]. Similar to PDGF, Nrg-1 stimulates OPC proliferation through the PI3K-Akt pathway [33,151,152]. Neuregulin works cooperatively with integrin signaling as ErbB2 associates with $\alpha_v\beta_3$ on OPCs to stimulate proliferation via the PI3K-Akt pathway. This co-association is mediated by the Src family kinase (SFK) Lyn, a group of kinases that integrate external signals by regulating integrin and growth factor behaviors. As development progresses, OLs contact laminins which activate an integrin-regulated switch from proliferation to pro-differentiation and myelination. This switch reverses Nrg-1 inhibition of differentiation when Fyn, an SFK, binds integrin $\alpha_6\beta_1$ to change Nrg-1 signaling from PI3K-Akt to the

MAPK pathway, thereby promoting myelination [151,152]. Blocking Erb signaling developmentally reduces differentiated OL number, and OLs that do differentiate fail to ensheath axons [153–155]. Together, these experiments suggest Nrg-1 signals through ErbB receptors and integrins to enhance OPC proliferation, differentiation, and OL myelination of axons.

CNS development is a sequential process that requires communication between secreted factors and their receptors (Figure 1), input from transcription factors (see reviews [5,156,157]), and cross talk between cell types. Oligodendrocyte progenitors migrate from the pMN domain of the neural tube, proliferate, differentiate into OLs, and then mature OLs myelinate axons. OPCs continue to proliferate and differentiate throughout adulthood, and OLs continuously generate new myelin to either replace myelin lost to aging or to accommodate new myelin in support of learning new tasks [55]. Myelination, a process tightly regulated during development, is disrupted after injury to the brain or spinal cord, altering the tissue milieu and complicating neural–glia interactions.

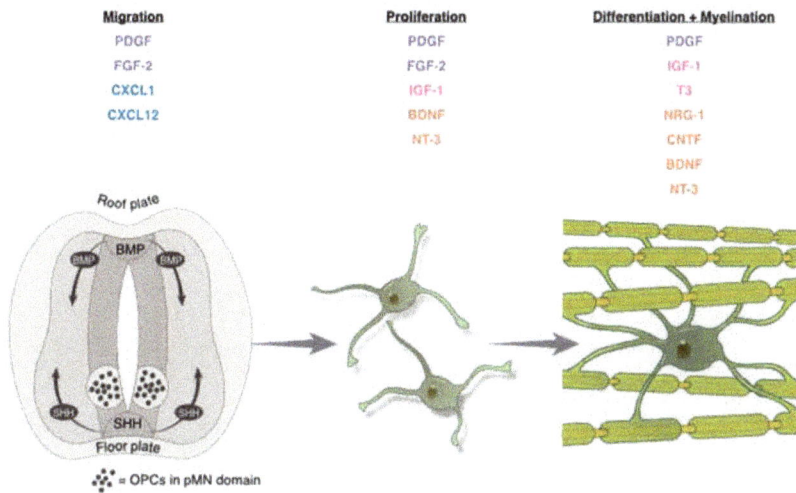

Migration	**Proliferation**	**Differentiation + Myelination**
PDGF	PDGF	PDGF
FGF-2	FGF-2	IGF-1
CXCL1	IGF-1	T3
CXCL12	BDNF	NRG-1
	NT-3	CNTF
		BDNF
		NT-3

Root plate

BMP

BMP

BMP

SHH

SHH

SHH

Floor plate

= OPCs in pMN domain

Figure 1. Environmental stimuli that influence the various stages of oligodendrocyte (OL) development. Oligodendrocyte progenitor cells (OPCs) originate in the neural tube, migrate dorsally and ventrally throughout the brain and spinal cord, proliferate, then differentiate into myelinating OLs. Environmental cues are grouped based category: growth factors (purple), chemokines (blue), hormones (pink), neurotrophic factors (orange). PDGF: platelet-derived growth factor; FGF-2: fibroblast growth factor-2; IGF-1: insulin-like growth factor-1; BDNF: brain-derived neurotrophic factor; NT-3: neurotrophin-3; T3: thyroid hormone; NRG-1: Neuregulin-1; CNTF: ciliary neurotrophic factor.

3. Central Nervous System Trauma

Brain and spinal cord trauma is characterized by a transient primary injury induced by a mechanical impact followed by protracted secondary injury processes. The hemorrhage, hypoxia, and extensive loss of neurons, glia, and axon tracts during the secondary injury phase is a large contributor to the cognitive, motor, and sensory dysfunction observed in human trauma patients and in pre-clinical models of central nervous system (CNS) trauma. In rodent models of spinal cord injury (SCI), there is a significant acute loss of OLs within 15 min at the injury epicenter that continues for at least 3 weeks post-injury (wpi) [158–161]. Traumatic brain injury (TBI) studies in rodents also show OLs within and proximal to the lesion are most susceptible to caspase-3-mediated apoptosis [162].

Myelinating OLs are terminally differentiated; thus, the primary source of post-injury myelin biogenesis is adult OPCs. Trauma to the CNS induces a robust oligodendrogenic response in which adult NG2+ OPCs proliferate in and around the injury epicenter and regenerate OLs that remyelinate spared axons [161,163–167]. Central canal ependymal cells can also proliferate and regenerate OLs, but this is specific to some models of SCI and has not been reproduced in other models of CNS insult [167–170]. Ultrastructural observations of axons in the injured cat spinal cord were among the first demonstrations of axon remyelination following CNS trauma [171,172]. Remyelinated axons are typically characterized by thinner myelin and shorter internodes, although myelin as thin as 3% of normal may still allow action potential conduction, revealing that thin myelin is likely preferable to no myelin [173,174]. Despite robust oligodendrogenesis persisting for at least 3 months post-injury (mpi) [164], spared axons experience a chronic increase in conduction block and their myelin displays a concurrent decrease in MBP messenger RNA (mRNA) expression [175], suggesting that endogenous remyelination of spared axons is suboptimal. Indeed, persistent myelin pathology has been detected for at least 10 wpi in a pre-clinical rat SCI model [164,176] and up to a decade after injury in some human SCI patients [177], making efforts to promote spontaneous myelin repair a promising therapeutic endeavor.

While necrosis and apoptosis are widely recognized as significant contributors to acute OL death after CNS injury [158,162,178], the mechanisms behind chronic demyelination remain unknown. As in development, OL lineage cells are exquisitely sensitive to their environment. The factors, mitogens, and signaling cues that drive healthy development of OLs are largely dysregulated after CNS trauma, creating an environment in which functional myelin regeneration is potentially deterred. While the successful response of OL lineage cells to chemically induced focal demyelination has been well characterized, their response to the multiple biochemical cascades that define an injury microenvironment remains largely unknown. The following outlines primary components of the traumatically injured CNS milieu that are permissive or inhibitory for functional myelin repair (Figure 2). To develop effective therapeutics that provide meaningful recovery for CNS trauma patients, it is essential that we understand the impact of the injury microenvironment on spontaneous myelin repair and how the injury milieu changes over time.

3.1. Growth Factors, Neurotrophic Factors, and Hormones Modulate Myelin Regeneration

3.1.1. Growth Factors

The role of BMP proteins in adult myelin regeneration is not fully understood. Spinal cord injury induces BMP expression similar to other models of CNS injury [164,165,179,180]. While both BMP2 and BMP4 inhibit the early stages of OPC differentiation during development, BMP4 is the primary BMP member to inhibit OL lineage cell differentiation after CNS trauma [181–183]. Indeed, inhibiting BMP4 signaling promotes OL regeneration and axon remyelination and decreases glial scarring in models of CNS trauma and chemically induced demyelination [179,182,184].

During development, exposure to PDGF promotes OPC proliferation by activating Wnt-β-catenin signaling [53]. The pattern of expression of Wnt signaling is modulated by SCI [53,185,186]. Moreover, genetic deletion of β-catenin from PDGFRα-expressing cells suppressed OPC proliferation and accumulation around the SCI epicenter [187]. Thus, increased exposure to PDGFA could potentially stimulate Wnt/β-catenin activation and promote OPC proliferation following SCI.

OPC differentiation and remyelination of spared axons are also modulated post-injury by PDGF-A, which primarily upregulates *Olig2* [61,188]. Evidence suggests that PDGF-A positively modulates OL lineage cells via synergistic effects with components of the extracellular matrix and other pro-proliferation growth factors, such as FGF-2 and IGF-1, which are upregulated for weeks after SCI [68,164,189–191]. After experimental rat SCI, intraspinal transplantation of Schwann cells promotes host OPC proliferation and recruitment to the lesion via secretion of FGF-2 and PDGF-A, a treatment that promoted remyelination of spared axons and enhanced recovery of function [188]. Further studies evaluating the synergistic effects of these protective, pro-OL lineage growth factors could provide novel therapeutic avenues that robustly promote OPC proliferation and differentiation.

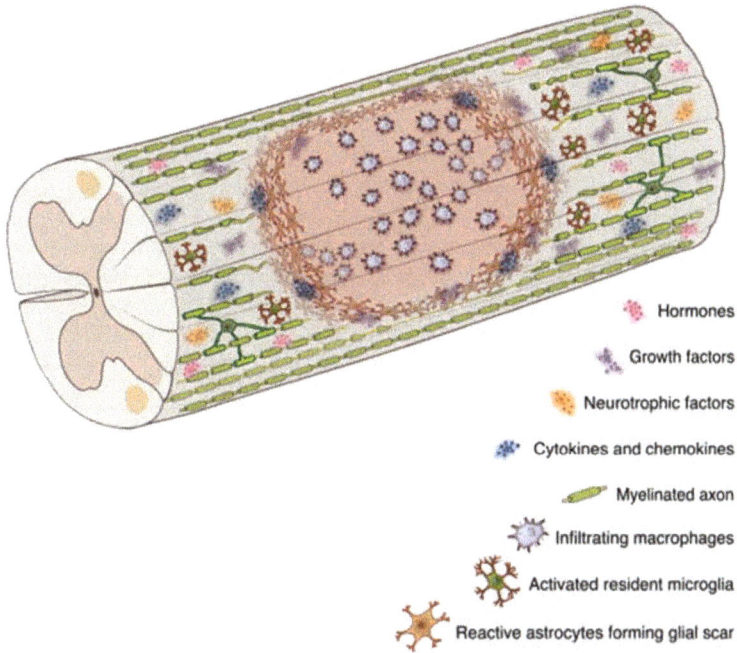

Figure 2. Primary factors that define a central nervous system (CNS) injury milieu. The injury microenvironment impacts the ability for OL lineage cells to effectively remyelinate all spared axons. Hormones (pink), growth factors (purple) and neurotrophic factors (orange) that promote myelination during development are dysregulated after spinal cord injury. Reactive astrocytes and immune cells (macrophages and microglia) secrete pro-reparative and pro-inflammatory cytokines and chemokines that differentially affect OL lineage cells.

3.1.2. Neurotrophic Factors

Ciliary neurotrophic factor is a pro-reparative protein that protects OPCs from TNFα-induced apoptosis and promotes proliferation during development and after CNS injury [94,192]. Following TBI and SCI in adult rat models, both CNTF and FGF-2 are upregulated acutely and remain elevated chronically, particularly within the glial scar and in regions of increased OPC proliferation [164,191,193,194] suggesting that CNTF is a somewhat "permanent" component of a microenvironment permissive to OL lineage cells. Indeed, transplanting OPCs overexpressing CNTF into the injured adult rat cord not only promotes OPC survival and axon remyelination, but also significantly restores signal conduction of demyelinated axons and improves recovery of hindlimb motor function [195]. Thus, CNTF's pro-proliferative and pro-survival role in development is maintained after CNS injury, making it a promising therapeutic factor in promoting myelin regeneration.

The developmental role of NT-3 in promoting OPC survival and maturation is potentiated after injury. Neurotrophin-3 can promote the in vitro survival of OLs at a higher rate than CNTF, and stimulates OPC proliferation and axon remyelination in vivo [94,196]. The effect of NT-3 on OL lineage cells becomes increasingly neuroprotective in synergy with other intrinsic and extrinsic factors both during development and after trauma. For example, the effect of NT-3 on developmental OL survival is potentiated in the presence of PDGF [94]. Similarly, co-expression of NT-3 and BDNF in the injured adult rat spinal cord not only promotes regeneration of propriospinal axons but also stimulates OL lineage cell proliferation and axon remyelination [104,196,197]. Moreover, co-expression of NT-3 and Shh increases Olig2+ cell number and enhances remyelination after injury to the adult mouse spinal cord [198]. Transplanting fibrin scaffolds loaded with purified neural progenitor cells, NT-3, and PDGF-AA into the acutely injured mouse spinal cord establishes a pro-reparative microenvironment in which tissue sparing is promoted and OL differentiation and axon remyelination is increased [199].

After rat spinal contusion, neurons and glia upregulate BDNF acutely, suggesting it is in position to play a neuroprotective role during the secondary injury processes [200–202]. BDNF treatment increases MBP expression in spared white matter of the spinal cord, promotes long-term OL survival and axon remyelination, and increases functional recovery [196,203,204]. Brain-derived neurotrophic factor and IGF-1 synergistically attenuate expression of nitric oxide synthase, a mediator of OL death in several demyelinating conditions, including SCI [205–207]. Moreover, intrathecal administration of BDNF promotes OL survival by preventing downregulation of Cu/Zn superoxide dismutase (CuZnSOD), an antioxidant that limits cell death by attenuating the formation of reactive oxygen species (ROS). Brain-derived neurotrophic factor also promotes myelin regeneration after CNS injury by positively modulating pro-myelinating transcription factors, such as Olig2, as well as promoting expression of PLP, a major myelin protein [208–210]. While the primary developmental role of BDNF is to modulate myelin thickness, BDNF becomes a potent extrinsic regulator of OPC differentiation and OL survival after CNS injury and may have significant potential in translational clinical applications.

The developmental role of Nrg-1 in stimulating OPC proliferation, survival, and differentiation is conserved after adult CNS injury. Intrathecal administration of Nrg-1 enhances OPC differentiation, promotes survival of existing OPCs, and stimulates remyelination by newly generated OLs and infiltrating Schwann cells [148,211,212]. Additionally, selectively ablating Nrg-1 prevents CNS OL lineage cells from differentiating into peripheral-like Schwann cells that remyelinate spared axons [212]. As Nrg-1 levels significantly drop acutely after injury and remain profoundly low chronically [148], perhaps Nrg-1 deregulation, which impacts signaling cascades integral for proliferation and cell survival, contributes to impaired OPC proliferation and maturation. Dysregulated levels of Nrg-1 in the spinal cord have recently been suggested to underlie myelin thinning on remyelinated axons [211]. Neuregulin-1 is also suggested to modulate the reparative and pro-inflammatory response of glial cells to CNS trauma. The immediate administration of Nrg-1 after rat-compressive SCI deceases pro-inflammatory components (e.g., interleukin (IL)-1β, TNFα, nitric oxide) and harmful matrix metalloproteinases. It also increases factors characteristic of a pro-reparative permissive environment, such as IL-10 and arginase-1 [148,213]. The effects of Nrg-1 on OL lineage cells, as well as its ability to modulate the inflammatory response to trauma, make Nrg-1 therapy a promising direction in CNS injury research.

3.1.3. Hormones

Thyroid hormone, a potent regulator of the timing of developmental OL differentiation, is also modulated by CNS trauma. Thyroid hormone levels are significantly lower in SCI patients, both acutely and chronically, compared to non-injured individuals [214,215]. In vitro studies demonstrate that compared to BDNF and NT-3, T3 is more potent in stimulating OL differentiation [216]. Moreover, local delivery of T3 directly to the spinal cord significantly accelerates oligodendrogenesis and axon myelination following cervical contusion injury [216]. While the beneficial effects of T3 have been extensively studied in multiple sclerosis (MS) and other demyelinating conditions, further work is needed in models of CNS trauma to fully elucidate its potential in myelin repair.

A key player in both CNS and PNS reparative processes, IGF-1 is secreted by astrocytes, microglia, and macrophages after CNS injury [217–219]. It stimulates OPC proliferation and differentiation, increases myelin related gene expression, and decreases astrogliosis after CNS injury [220–223]. Moreover, IGF-1 robustly promotes OPC survival and OL maturation via synergistic effects with other growth factors, including BDNF, PDGF, and NT-3 [205,224]. Systemic administration of IGF-1 reverses TBI-induced reductions in NT-3 and BDNF, inhibits OL apoptosis, and improves injury outcome [224]. Neurological outcome after traumatic brain and spinal cord injury in humans has been linked to

IGF-1 levels in peripheral blood serum. Patients with elevated serum IGF-1 levels demonstrate greater neurological improvement chronically compared to those with lower serum IGF-1 [225,226]. Levels of IGF-1 may be elevated in response to prolonged injury-associated inflammation, and exogenous IGF-1 treatment could potentially supplement the neuroprotective role of IGF-1 and serve as a potent therapeutic target.

Progesterone (P4) is an endogenous hormone and steroid from the progestogens family and has emerged as a neuroprotective strategy to promote endogenous repair. Daily progesterone treatments between three to five days following SCI in rats reduces the lesion size, stimulates OPC proliferation, and increases mRNA expression of Olig2 and Nkx2.2, a major OPC specification protein [227–229]. Continued administration of P4 for 21 days in a complete SCI rat model increases newly differentiated OLs and stimulates Olig1 expression, a transcription factor that promotes myelin regeneration [228,230]. Systemic progesterone treatment following TBI in rats also significantly attenuates secondary pathology and improves behavioral function, but its ability to restore white matter integrity has yet to be evaluated in these models [231,232].

3.2. Components of the Injury-Induced Glial Scar Affect OL Lineage Cells

Central nervous system trauma promotes the formation of a glial scar whose primary astrocytic component secretes chondroitin sulfate proteoglycans (CSPGs) [233]. These CSPGs negatively regulate OL lineage cells both in vitro and in vivo [234,235]. Macrophage-secreted transforming growth factor (TGF)β can also induce CSPG upregulation via PI3K–Akt–mTOR signaling [236–238]. Evidence suggests there is a relationship between the concentrations of CSPG and the degree of remyelination of spared axons [233,239]. Not only do CSPGs deter axon regeneration, but they also signal through PTPσ receptors to inhibit OL process outgrowth and axon myelination [235]. Several studies have targeted CSPGs and while these have proven effective in reducing tissue damage and promoting axon growth, only CSPG degradation using chondroitinase ABC (ChABC) treatment, or ChABC combined with a cocktail of growth factors (FGF, PDGF) has successfully promoted OL differentiation after SCI [169,235,240,241].

Macrophage and glial-scar-derived Endothelin-1, LRR and Ig domain-containing, Nogo Receptor-interacting protein (LINGO-1), TNFα, and IL-1β also suppress OPC differentiation and OL maturation [242–244]. It is important to note, however, that both TNFα and IL-1β also positively modulate OL lineage cells. Mice lacking TNFα and its associated receptor, TNFR2, have a significant delay in remyelination after toxin-induced demyelination [245]. Interleukin-1β can also induce OPC differentiation and promote OL survival; however, in the presence of PDGF and FGF in vitro, it arrests OPC proliferation [246]. These lines of evidence suggest that further research is needed to elucidate the interactions of astrocyte- and macrophage-derived cytokines with OL lineage cells and the ways in which their response to demyelination and trauma may change over time.

Astrocytes can positively modulate remyelination by their ability to produce CNTF and take up significant amounts of iron, maintaining the homeostasis that is necessary for the proliferation, maturation, and survival of OL lineage cells [164,247,248]. Notably, prior work from our lab demonstrated the SCI-induced glial scar is an area of robust OPC proliferation and accumulation as well as OL differentiation and myelination [164,249]. This area contains high levels of pro-oligogenic factors CNTF, FGF-2, and peroxisome proliferator-activated receptor delta (PPAR-δ), an intracellular nuclear receptor that promotes OL differentiation [164,191,250]. Notably, when proliferating NG2+ OPCs (and pericytes) were ablated after SCI, the astrocytic glial scar was significantly less dense and more axons spontaneously grew into the lesions, revealing OPCs not only respond to their environment but also affect the response of other post-injury parenchymal elements [251]. Astrocyte–oligodendrocyte crosstalk drives developmental myelin formation, trauma-induced myelin damage, and spontaneous axon remyelination. Thus, clarifying the complex mechanisms behind astrocyte–OL lineage crosstalk could potentially lead to novel therapeutics in which the beneficial effects of astrocytes and OPCs are harnessed and the detrimental effects are attenuated.

3.3. The Neuroimmune Axis

In the homeostatic CNS, the balance of genes expressed by adult OPCs are similar to OLs [252]. However, in response to toxin-induced demyelination, OPCs revert to a neonatal transcriptome and increase expression of IL-1β and CCL2, immune cues that promote progenitor cell migration [252,253]. On the other hand, several chemokines and cytokines can inhibit OPC differentiation and axon remyelination [213,246,254] suggesting that a neuroimmune axis exists that may dynamically modulate OL lineage cells and myelin repair after CNS trauma [255].

3.3.1. Cytokines and Microglia/Macrophage Signaling

Activated macrophages, a population composed of resident microglia and infiltrating monocytes, play divergent pro-inflammatory and pro-reparative roles in response to CNS trauma. Pro-inflammatory M1 polarized macrophages secrete toxic cytokines, chemokines, reactive oxygen species, and promote excitotoxicity—all of which engender a microenvironment inhibitory for OL regeneration [253].

Pro-reparative M2 macrophages not only facilitate the clearance of myelin debris that can inhibit OL differentiation but also secrete factors that stimulate OL differentiation and remyelination, such as IL-10, leukemia inhibitory factor (LIF), CNTF, and, TGFβ [256–258]. Experimental strategies in SCI models where LIF is administered arrests OL death, enhances OL differentiation, and promotes OL survival by activating the Janus kinase—signal transducers and activators of transcription (JAK-STAT) and Akt pathways [259–261]. However, evidence from a mouse model of MS suggests that while LIF administration promotes axon remyelination, it fails to increase the thickness of regenerated myelin [262]. Transforming growth factor-β is suggested to potently regulate the initiation and resolution of inflammation [263]. Indeed, following spinal contusion, TGFβ mRNA levels are significantly elevated, particularly in regions of dense microglia and macrophages [264]. Attenuation of TGFβ following SCI decreases fibrotic scar formation, and promotes axon regeneration through lesion [265,266]; remyelination, however, was not evaluated in that study.

The mechanism of microglia and macrophage activation also has consequences for OL lineage cells (for a recent review, see [267]). For instance, in vivo activation of the Toll-like receptor 2 (TLR2) on microglia and macrophages results in death of all OPCs and OLs (and astrocytes) in the region [268]. However, intraspinal activation of the receptor TLR4 causes initial demyelination and loss of OPCs and OLs, followed by subsequent and robust OPC proliferation and migration into the area of activated macrophages, after which a significant portion of OPCs differentiate into new OLs [268,269]. Notably, this oligodendrogenic response depended on sufficient iron levels and we showed that macrophages can transfer iron-containing ferritin to OPCs in vivo [270,271]. This may be an intriguing mechanism of OL genesis after SCI since TLR4 is activated on microglia and macrophages after SCI and this signaling pathway induces iron uptake by macrophages [272,273]. The SCI site is rich in iron due to intraspinal hemorrhage and cell death, and iron-laden macrophages accumulate acutely and are sustained chronically in the injured spinal cord [274–276]. Notably, in the absence of TLR4 signaling after SCI, OPC accumulation and OL production are significantly reduced [273]. Microglia play a central role in CNS development and myelin biogenesis; thus, the ways in which activated microglia and macrophages influence OL lineage cells after CNS trauma needs further study as it could provide important insight into how the neuroimmune axis can be harnessed to promote myelin repair.

3.3.2. Cytokine Signaling Regulators

Suppressors of cytokine signaling (SOCS) proteins are key components of the innate and adaptive immune system (extensively reviewed in [277]). Cytokines and interleukins induce SOCS expression via JAK/STAT signaling. SOCS, in turn, inhibits the JAK/STAT pathway and negatively regulates cytokine signaling [278–280]. Of the SOCS protein family, SOCS1 and SOCS3 have been best characterized in their response to CNS trauma and their differential influence on endogenous myelin repair. SOCS1 proteins positively modulate pro-reparative M2 macrophage polarization and attenuate pro-inflammatory M1 macrophages [281]. Enhanced expression of SOCS1 in a mouse model of contusive SCI is linked to improved sensory and locomotor function, decreased demyelination, and reduced pro-inflammatory cytokine expression [282]. On the other hand, SOCS3 expression is upregulated by M1 polarized macrophages within pro-inflammatory environments [283]. Inhibition of SOCS3 activity in rodents attenuates demyelination, enhances NG2+ cell proliferation, and promotes OL survival after SCI [279,284,285]. Understanding the expression and function of SOCS proteins in CNS trauma may hold promise for immunomodulatory therapeutics that suppress a hostile trauma microenvironment and promote myelin repair.

3.3.3. Chemokines

Several chemokines and cytokines in the C-X-C family have been implicated in the response of OL lineage cells to CNS trauma.

Following mid-thoracic SCI in adult mice, there is a significant and persistent upregulation of CX3CR1 expression, a microglia-specific receptor for fractalkine [286]. Genetic deletion of CX3CR1 modulates macrophages towards a pro-reparative phenotype, enhances NG2 responses to injury, and increases myelin and axon sparing at the lesion epicenter [286,287].

CXCL12 and its receptor, CXCR4, are expressed by PDGFRα+ OPCs and positively modulate OPC proliferation, survival, migration, and differentiation after CNS trauma [50,51,288,289]. Reactive astrocytes in regions of demyelination upregulate CXCL12, which has been proposed to serve as a potent chemoattractant to guide migrating oligodendrocyte precursor cells to the injury site and promote their differentiation [290].

Both CXCL1 and its receptor, CXCR2, are upregulated after CNS injury [289]. During development, CXCL1 primarily promotes OPC proliferation; however, after injury, CXCL1 signaling promotes OPC survival by restricting interferon (IFN)-γ- and CXCL10-induced apoptosis [44,291]. Evidence from the experimental allergic encephalomyelitis (EAE) model demonstrates that CXCL1 overexpression can rescue OPCs from apoptosis and significantly reduce the severity of myelin pathology [292], though this has yet to be shown in SCI. The CXCR2 receptor is expressed on human OLs [293], and CXCL1 ligand has been detected on human-activated microglia and reactive astrocytes [294,295] making this chemokine and its modulation of OL lineage cells a potentially translatable focus of study that should be explored further within the pathology of brain and spinal cord injury.

4. Summary and Conclusions

Myelination is an evolutionarily advantageous specialization that enables rapid communication between neurons in the CNS. Oligodendrocyte lineage cells are incredibly sensitive to their environment. A healthy microenvironment is integral for myelin biogenesis during development as well myelin maintenance in adults and repair following CNS trauma. Mechanisms regulating OL progression during development are well studied; however, the individual and synergistic roles of these regulatory factors after CNS trauma are not fully understood. Overwhelming evidence demonstrates the ways in which downregulating beneficial factors combined with the poor resolution of pro-inflammatory factors hinders endogenous axon remyelination. Thus, manipulating various components of the injury milieu is a promising strategy to promote spontaneous myelin repair. For instance, understanding the synergistic effects of pro-myelination growth factors and hormones could inform the development of treatments that harness their synergistic neuroprotective effects. Importantly, future work aimed at promoting myelin repair should also focus on elucidating the effects of glial cross talk on endogenous remyelination. While the physiology and pathophysiology of individual glial cells in a trauma microenvironment is incompletely understood [243], clarifying how OL lineage cells are influenced by astrocytes and microglia/macrophages could not only provide insight into the importance of glial cross talk during development but also provide novel avenues through which those signaling pathways can be harnessed to promote myelin repair.

With the rising field of tissue engineering and the significant strides made in stem cell biology, several of the beneficial and toxic factors that comprise post-injury milieu can be manipulated to promote CNS injury repair [296]. Additionally, the prevalent and validated use of transgenic mice with inducible gene expression has allowed for the evaluation of pro-myelination developmental factors within the post-injury microenvironment. For instance, myelin regulatory factor (MYRF), a factor critical for myelination during development, is expressed by newly generated OLs in response to induced focal demyelination and is required for new OL genesis [297]. The recent use of mice in which OPC-specific MYRF can be deleted or inducibly expressed is promising for research aimed towards promoting myelin repair after CNS trauma. To develop novel therapeutics geared to promote myelin regeneration after CNS injury, it is vital that the factors driving healthy myelin development are manipulated after injury to support OL lineage progression. Harnessing these pathways to improve myelin repair may promote meaningful functional recovery for patients.

Author Contributions: N.P. and R.Y., contributed the original draft preparation; D.M.M., N.P., and R.Y., reviewed and edited the paper.

Acknowledgments: We would like to thank Anthony Baker of the Ohio State University Neurological Institute for the manuscript illustrations.

Conflicts of Interest: The authors declare no conflict of interest.

References

1. Boullerne, A.I. The history of myelin. *Exp. Neurol.* **2016**, *283*, 431–445. [CrossRef] [PubMed]
2. Rasband, M.N.; Peles, E. The Nodes of Ranvier: Molecular Assembly and Maintenance. *Cold Spring Harb. Perspect. Biol.* **2015**, *8*, a020495. [CrossRef] [PubMed]
3. Pan, S.; Chan, J.R. Regulation and dysregulation of axon infrastructure by myelinating glia. *J. Cell Biol.* **2017**, *216*, 3903–3916. [CrossRef] [PubMed]
4. Zalc, B. The acquisition of myelin: An evolutionary perspective. *Brain Res.* **2016**, *1641*, 4–10. [CrossRef] [PubMed]
5. Santos, A.K.; Vieira, M.S.; Vasconcellos, R.; Goulart, V.A.M.; Kihara, A.H.; Resende, R.R. Decoding cell signalling and regulation of oligodendrocyte differentiation. *Semin. Cell Dev. Biol.* **2018**. [CrossRef] [PubMed]
6. Nishiyama, A.; Boshans, L.; Goncalves, C.M.; Wegrzyn, J.; Patel, K.D. Lineage, fate, and fate potential of NG2-glia. *Brain Res.* **2016**, *1638*, 116–128. [CrossRef] [PubMed]
7. Nishiyama, A.; Komitova, M.; Suzuki, R.; Zhu, X. Polydendrocytes (NG2 cells): multifunctional cells with lineage plasticity. *Nat. Rev. Neurosci.* **2009**, *10*, 9–22. [CrossRef] [PubMed]
8. Watanabe, M.; Toyama, Y.; Nishiyama, A. Differentiation of proliferated NG2-positive glial progenitor cells in a remyelinating lesion. *J. Neurosci. Res.* **2002**, *69*, 826–836. [CrossRef] [PubMed]
9. Gans, C.; Northcutt, R.G. Neural crest and the origin of vertebrates: a new head. *Science* **1983**, *220*, 268–273. [CrossRef] [PubMed]
10. Noll, E.; Miller, R.H. Oligodendrocyte precursors originate at the ventral ventricular zone dorsal to the ventral midline region in the embryonic rat spinal cord. *Development* **1993**, *118*, 563–573. [PubMed]
11. Rowitch, D.H. Glial specification in the vertebrate neural tube. *Nat. Rev. Neurosci.* **2004**, *5*, 409–419. [CrossRef] [PubMed]
12. Richardson, W.D.; Kessaris, N.; Pringle, N. Oligodendrocyte wars. *Nat. Rev. Neurosci.* **2006**, *7*, 11–18. [CrossRef] [PubMed]
13. Tripathi, R.B.; Clarke, L.E.; Burzomato, V.; Kessaris, N.; Anderson, P.N.; Attwell, D.; Richardson, W.D. Dorsally and ventrally derived oligodendrocytes have similar electrical properties but myelinate preferred tracts. *J. Neurosci.* **2011**, *31*, 6809–6819. [CrossRef] [PubMed]
14. Levison, S.W.; Goldman, J.E. Both oligodendrocytes and astrocytes develop from progenitors in the subventricular zone of postnatal rat forebrain. *Neuron* **1993**, *10*, 201–212. [CrossRef]
15. Lachapelle, F.; Gumpel, M.; Baulac, M.; Jacque, C.; Duc, P.; Baumann, N. Transplantation of CNS Fragments into the Brain of Shiverer Mutant Mice: Extensive Myelination by Implanted Oligodendrocytes. *Dev. Neurosci.* **1983**, *6*, 325–334. [CrossRef] [PubMed]

16. Cai, J.; Qi, Y.; Hu, X.; Tan, M.; Liu, Z.; Zhang, J.; Li, Q.; Sander, M.; Qiu, M. Generation of Oligodendrocyte Precursor Cells from Mouse Dorsal Spinal Cord Independent of Nkx6 Regulation and Shh Signaling. *Neuron* **2005**, *45*, 41–53. [CrossRef] [PubMed]

17. Jessell, T.M. Neuronal specification in the spinal cord: inductive signals and transcriptional codes. *Nat. Rev. Genet.* **2000**, *1*, 20–29. [CrossRef] [PubMed]

18. Mekki-Dauriac, S.; Agius, E.; Kan, P.; Cochard, P. Bone morphogenetic proteins negatively control oligodendrocyte precursor specification in the chick spinal cord. *Development* **2002**, *129*, 5117–5130. [PubMed]

19. Bond, A.M.; Bhalala, O.G.; Kessler, J.A. The dynamic role of bone morphogenetic proteins in neural stem cell fate and maturation. *Dev. Neurobiol.* **2012**, *72*, 1068–1084. [CrossRef] [PubMed]

20. Kessaris, N.; Fogarty, M.; Iannarelli, P.; Grist, M.; Wegner, M.; Richardson, W.D. Competing waves of oligodendrocytes in the forebrain and postnatal elimination of an embryonic lineage. *Nat. Neurosci.* **2006**, *9*, 173–179. [CrossRef] [PubMed]

21. Hughes, E.G.; Kang, S.H.; Fukaya, M.; Bergles, D.E. Oligodendrocyte progenitors balance growth with self-repulsion to achieve homeostasis in the adult brain. *Nat. Neurosci.* **2013**, *16*, 668–676. [CrossRef] [PubMed]

22. Kirby, B.B.; Takada, N.; Latimer, A.J.; Shin, J.; Carney, T.J.; Kelsh, R.N.; Appel, B. In vivo time-lapse imaging shows dynamic oligodendrocyte progenitor behavior during zebrafish development. *Nat. Neurosci.* **2006**, *9*, 1506–1511. [CrossRef] [PubMed]

23. Chong, S.Y.C.; Rosenberg, S.S.; Fancy, S.P.J.; Zhao, C.; Shen, Y.-A.A.; Hahn, A.T.; McGee, A.W.; Xu, X.; Zheng, B.; Zhang, L.I.; et al. Neurite outgrowth inhibitor Nogo-A establishes spatial segregation and extent of oligodendrocyte myelination. *Proc. Natl. Acad. Sci. USA* **2012**, *109*, 1299–1304. [CrossRef] [PubMed]

24. Richardson, W.D.; Pringle, N.; Mosley, M.J.; Westermark, B.; Dubois-Dalcqt, M. A Role for Platelet-Derived Growth Factor in Normal Gliogenesis in the Central Nervous System. *Cell* **1988**, *53*, 309–319. [CrossRef]

25. Pringle, N.P.; Mudhar, H.S.; Collarini, E.J.; Richardson, W.D. PDGF receptors in the rat CNS: during late neurogenesis, PDGF alpha- receptor expression appears to be restricted to glial cells of the oligodendrocyte lineage. *Development* **1992**, *115*, 535–551. [PubMed]

26. Frost, E.E.; Zhou, Z.; Krasnesky, K.; Armstrong, R.C. Initiation of oligodendrocyte progenitor cell migration by a PDGF-A activated extracellular regulated kinase (ERK) signaling pathway. *Neurochem. Res.* **2009**, *34*, 169–181. [CrossRef] [PubMed]

27. Kennedy, T.E.; Serafini, T.; de la Torre, J.; Tessier-Lavigne, M. Netrins are diffusible chemotropic factors for commissural axons in the embryonic spinal cord. *Cell* **1994**, *78*, 425–435. [CrossRef]

28. Jarjour, A.A.; Manitt, C.; Moore, S.W.; Thompson, K.M.; Yuh, S.-J.; Kennedy, T.E. Netrin-1 is a chemorepellent for oligodendrocyte precursor cells in the embryonic spinal cord. *J. Neurosci.* **2003**, *23*, 3735–3744. [CrossRef] [PubMed]

29. Hart, I.K.; Richardson, W.D.; Heldin, C.-H.; Westermark, B.; Raff, M.C. PDGF receptors on cells of the oligodendrocyte-type-2 astrocyte (O-2A) cell lineage. *Development* **1989**, *105*, 595–603. [PubMed]

30. Tsai, H.-H.; Tessier-Lavigne, M.; Miller, R.H. Netrin 1 mediates spinal cord oligodendrocyte precursor dispersal. *Development* **2003**, *130*, 2095–2105. [CrossRef] [PubMed]

31. Tsai, H.-H.; Macklin, W.B.; Miller, R.H. Netrin-1 is required for the normal development of spinal cord oligodendrocytes. *J. Neurosci.* **2006**, *26*, 1913–1922. [CrossRef] [PubMed]

32. Leferink, P.S.; Breeuwsma, N.; Bugiani, M.; van der Knaap, M.S.; Heine, V.M. Affected astrocytes in the spinal cord of the leukodystrophy vanishing white matter. *Glia* **2018**, *66*, 862–873. [CrossRef] [PubMed]

33. Baron, W.; Shattil, S.J.; ffrench-Constant, C. The oligodendrocyte precursor mitogen PDGF stimulates proliferation by activation of alpha(v)beta3 integrins. *EMBO J.* **2002**, *21*, 1957–1966. [CrossRef] [PubMed]

34. Ferrara, N.; Ousley, F.; Gospodarowicz, D. Bovine brain astrocytes express basic fibroblast growth factor, a neurotropic and angiogenic mitogen. *Brain Res.* **1988**, *462*, 223–232. [CrossRef]

35. Wolswijk, G.; Noble, M. Cooperation Between PDGF and FGF Converts Slowly Dividing O-2A adutt Progenitor Cells to Rapidly Dividing Cells with Characteristics of O_2A perinatal Progenitor Cells. *J. Cell Biol.* **1992**, *118*, 889–900. [CrossRef] [PubMed]

36. Milner, R.; Anderson, H.J.; Rippon, R.F.; McKay, J.S.; Franklin, R.J.M.; Marchionni, M.A.; Reynolds, R.; Ffrench-Constant, C. Contrasting effects of mitogenic growth factors on oligodendrocyte precursor cell migration. *Glia* **1997**, *19*, 85–90. [CrossRef]

37. Vora, P.; Pillai, P.P.; Zhu, W.; Mustapha, J.; Namaka, M.P.; Frost, E.E. Differential effects of growth factors on oligodendrocyte progenitor migration. *Eur. J. Cell Biol.* **2011**, *90*, 649–656. [CrossRef] [PubMed]

38. Chen, Y.-J.; Zhang, J.-X.; Shen, L.; Qi, Q.; Cheng, X.-X.; Zhong, Z.-R.; Jiang, Z.-Q.; Wang, R.; Lü, H.-Z.; Hu, J.-G. Schwann cells induce Proliferation and Migration of Oligodendrocyte Precursor Cells Through Secretion of PDGF-AA and FGF-2. *J. Mol. Neurosci.* **2015**, *56*, 999–1008. [CrossRef] [PubMed]

39. Murcia-Belmonte, V.; Medina-Rodríguez, E.M.; Bribián, A.; de Castro, F.; Esteban, P.F. ERK1/2 signaling is essential for the chemoattraction exerted by human FGF2 and human anosmin-1 on newborn rat and mouse OPCs via FGFR1. *Glia* **2014**, *62*, 374–386. [CrossRef] [PubMed]

40. Osterhout, D.J.; Ebner, S.; Xu, J.; Ornitz, D.M.; Zazanis, G.A.; McKinnon, R.D. Transplanted oligodendrocyte progenitor cells expressing a dominant-negative FGF receptor transgene fail to migrate in vivo. *J. Neurosci.* **1997**, *17*, 9122–9132. [CrossRef] [PubMed]

41. Robinson, S.; Tani, M.; Strieter, R.M.; Ransohoff, R.M.; Miller, R.H. The chemokine growth-regulated oncogene-alpha promotes spinal cord oligodendrocyte precursor proliferation. *J. Neurosci.* **1998**, *18*, 10457–10463. [CrossRef] [PubMed]

42. Nguyen, D.; Stangel, M. Expression of the chemokine receptors CXCR1 and CXCR2 in rat oligodendroglial cells. *Brain Res. Dev. Brain Res.* **2001**, *128*, 77–81. [CrossRef]

43. Padovani-Claudio, D.A.; Liu, L.; Ransohoff, R.M.; Miller, R.H. Alterations in the oligodendrocyte lineage, myelin, and white matter in adult mice lacking the chemokine receptor CXCR2. *Glia* **2006**, *54*, 471–483. [CrossRef] [PubMed]

44. Tirotta, E.; Ransohoff, R.M.; Lane, T.E. CXCR2 signaling protects oligodendrocyte progenitor cells from IFN-γ/CXCL10-mediated apoptosis. *Glia* **2011**, *59*, 1518–1528. [CrossRef] [PubMed]

45. Tsai, H.-H.; Frost, E.; To, V.; Robinson, S.; ffrench-Constant, C.; Geertman, R.; Ransohoff, R.M.; Miller, R.H. The Chemokine Receptor CXCR2 Controls Positioning of Oligodendrocyte Precursors in Developing Spinal Cord by Arresting Their Migration. *Cell* **2002**, *110*, 373–383. [CrossRef]

46. Li, M.; Ransohoff, R.M. Multiple roles of chemokine CXCL12 in the central nervous system: a migration from immunology to neurobiology. *Prog. Neurobiol.* **2008**, *84*, 116–131. [CrossRef] [PubMed]

47. Lavi, E.; Strizki, J.M.; Ulrich, A.M.; Zhang, W.; Fu, L.; Wang, Q.; O'Connor, M.; Hoxie, J.A.; González-Scarano, F. CXCR-4 (Fusin), a co-receptor for the type 1 human immunodeficiency virus (HIV-1), is expressed in the human brain in a variety of cell types, including microglia and neurons. *Am. J. Pathol.* **1997**, *151*, 1035–1042. [PubMed]

48. McGrath, K.E.; Koniski, A.D.; Maltby, K.M.; McGann, J.K.; Palis, J. Embryonic Expression and Function of the Chemokine SDF-1 and Its Receptor, CXCR4. *Dev. Biol.* **1999**, *213*, 442–456. [CrossRef] [PubMed]

49. Ma, Q.; Jones, D.; Borghesani, P.R.; Segal, R.A.; Nagasawa, T.; Kishimoto, T.; Bronson, R.T.; Springer, T.A. Impaired B-lymphopoiesis, myelopoiesis, and derailed cerebellar neuron migration in CXCR4- and SDF-1-deficient mice. *Proc. Natl. Acad. Sci. USA* **1998**, *95*, 9448–9453. [CrossRef] [PubMed]

50. Dziembowska, M.; Tham, T.N.; Lau, P.; Vitry, S.; Lazarini, F.; Dubois-Dalcq, M.; Lau, P. A Role for CXCR4 Signaling in Survival and Migration of Neural and Oligodendrocyte Precursors. *Glia* **2005**, *50*, 258–269. [CrossRef] [PubMed]

51. Kadi, L.; Selvaraju, R.; de Lys, P.; Proudfoot, A.E.I.; Wells, T.N.C.; Boschert, U. Differential effects of chemokines on oligodendrocyte precursor proliferation and myelin formation in vitro. *J. Neuroimmunol.* **2006**, *174*, 133–146. [CrossRef] [PubMed]

52. Miller, R.H.; David, S.; Patel, R.; Abney, E.R.; Raff, M.C. A quantitative immunohistochemical study of macroglial cell development in the rat optic nerve: in vivo evidence for two distinct astrocyte lineages. *Dev. Biol.* **1985**, *111*, 35–41. [CrossRef]

53. Hill, R.A.; Patel, K.D.; Medved, J.; Reiss, A.M.; Nishiyama, A. NG2 cells in white matter but not gray matter proliferate in response to PDGF. *J. Neurosci.* **2013**, *33*, 14558–14566. [CrossRef] [PubMed]

54. Young, K.M.; Psachoulia, K.; Tripathi, R.B.; Dunn, S.-J.; Cossell, L.; Attwell, D.; Tohyama, K.; Richardson, W.D. Oligodendrocyte dynamics in the healthy adult CNS: evidence for myelin remodeling. *Neuron* **2013**, *77*, 873–885. [CrossRef] [PubMed]

55. Rivers, L.E.; Young, K.M.; Rizzi, M.; Jamen, F.; Psachoulia, K.; Wade, A.; Kessaris, N.; Richardson, W.D. PDGFRA/NG2 glia generate myelinating oligodendrocytes and piriform projection neurons in adult mice. *Nat. Neurosci.* **2008**, *11*, 1392–1401. [CrossRef] [PubMed]

56. Accetta, R.; Damiano, S.; Morano, A.; Mondola, P.; Paternò, R.; Avvedimento, E.V.; Santillo, M. Reactive Oxygen Species Derived from NOX3 and NOX5 Drive Differentiation of Human Oligodendrocytes. *Front. Cell. Neurosci.* **2016**, *10*, 146. [CrossRef] [PubMed]

57. Noble, M.; Smith, J.; Ladi, E.; Mayer-Proschel, M. Redox state is a central modulator of the balance between self-renewal and differentiation in a dividing glial precursor cell. *Proc. Natl. Acad. Sci. USA* **2000**, *97*, 10032–10037. [CrossRef]

58. Clarke, L.E.; Young, K.M.; Hamilton, N.B.; Li, H.; Richardson, W.D.; Attwell, D. Properties and fate of oligodendrocyte progenitor cells in the corpus callosum, motor cortex, and piriform cortex of the mouse. *J. Neurosci.* **2012**, *32*, 8173–8185. [CrossRef] [PubMed]

59. Noble, M.; Murray, K. Purified astrocytes promote the in vitro division of a bipotential glial progenitor cell. *EMBO J.* **1984**, *3*, 2243–2247. [PubMed]

60. Raff, M.C.; Lillien, L.E.; Richardson, W.D.; Burne, J.F.; Noble, M.D. Platelet-derived growth factor from astrocytes drives the clock that times oligodendrocyte development in culture. *Nature* **1988**, *333*, 562–565. [CrossRef] [PubMed]

61. Hu, J.-G.; Fu, S.-L.; Wang, Y.-X.; Li, Y.; Jiang, X.-Y.; Wang, X.-F.; Qiu, M.-S.; Lu, P.-H.; Xu, X.-M. Platelet-derived growth factor-AA mediates oligodendrocyte lineage differentiation through activation of extracellular signal-regulated kinase signaling pathway. *Neuroscience* **2008**, *151*, 138–147. [CrossRef] [PubMed]

62. Barateiro, A.; Fernandes, A. Temporal oligodendrocyte lineage progression: In vitro models of proliferation, differentiation and myelination. *Biochim. Biophys. Acta - Mol. Cell Res.* **2014**, *1843*, 1917–1929. [CrossRef] [PubMed]

63. McKinnon, R.D.; Matsui, T.; Dubois-Dalcq, M.; Aaronson, S.A. FGF modulates the PDGF-driven pathway of oligodendrocyte development. *Neuron* **1990**, *5*, 603–614. [CrossRef]

64. Raff, M.C.; Miller, R.H.; Noble, M. A glial progenitor cell that develops in vitro into an astrocyte or an oligodendrocyte depending on culture medium. *Nature* **1983**, *303*, 390–396. [CrossRef] [PubMed]

65. Soriano, P. The PDGF alpha receptor is required for neural crest cell development and for normal patterning of the somites. *Development* **1997**, *124*, 2691–2700. [PubMed]

66. Fruttiger, M.; Karlsson, L.; Hall, A.C.; Abramsson, A.; Calver, A.R.; Bostrom, H.; Willetts, K.; Bertold, C.H.; Heath, J.K.; Betsholtz, C.; et al. Defective oligodendrocyte development and severe hypomyelination in PDGF-A knockout mice. *Development* **1999**, *126*, 457–467. [PubMed]

67. Calver, A.R.; Hall, A.C.; Yu, W.-P.; Walsh, F.S.; Heath, J.K.; Betsholtz, C.; Richardson, W.D. Oligodendrocyte Population Dynamics and the Role of PDGF In Vivo. *Neuron* **1998**, *20*, 869–882. [CrossRef]

68. Hu, J.-G.; Wang, X.-F.; Deng, L.-X.; Liu, N.-K.; Gao, X.; Chen, J.; Zhou, F.C.; Xu, X.-M. Cotransplantation of Glial Restricted Precursor Cells and Schwann Cells Promotes Functional Recovery after Spinal Cord Injury. *Cell Transplant.* **2013**, *22*, 2219–2236. [CrossRef] [PubMed]

69. McKinnon, R.D.; Matsui, T.; Aranda, M.; Dubois-Dalcq, M. A Role for Fibroblast Growth Factor in Oligodendrocyte Development. *Ann. N. Y. Acad. Sci.* **1991**, *638*, 378–386. [CrossRef] [PubMed]

70. Gard, A.L.; Pfeiffer, S.E. Glial Cell Mitogens bFGF and PDGF Differentially Regulate Development of O4+GalC- Oligodendrocyte Progenitors. *Dev. Biol.* **1993**, *159*, 618–630. [CrossRef] [PubMed]

71. Bögler, O.; Wren, D.; Barnett, S.C.; Land, H.; Noble, M. Cooperation between two growth factors promotes extended self-renewal and inhibits differentiation of oligodendrocyte-type-2 astrocyte (O-2A) progenitor cells. *Proc. Natl. Acad. Sci. USA* **1990**, *87*, 6368–6372. [CrossRef] [PubMed]

72. Eccleston, P.A.; Silberberg, D.H. Fibroblast growth factor is a mitogen for oligodendrocytes in vitro. *Brain Res.* **1985**, *353*, 315–318. [CrossRef]

73. Vaccarino, F.M.; Schwartz, M.L.; Raballo, R.; Nilsen, J.; Rhee, J.; Zhou, M.; Doetschman, T.; Coffin, J.D.; Wyland, J.J.; Hung, Y.-T.E. Erratum: Changes in cerebral cortex size are governed by fibroblast growth factor during embryogenesis. *Nat. Neurosci.* **1999**, *2*, 246–253. [CrossRef] [PubMed]

74. Murtie, J.C.; Zhou, Y.-X.; Le, T.Q.; Armstrong, R.C. In vivo analysis of oligodendrocyte lineage development in postnatal FGF2 null mice. *Glia* **2005**, *49*, 542–554. [CrossRef] [PubMed]

75. Bansal, R.; Kumar, M.; Murray, K.; Morrison, R.S.; Pfeiffer, S.E. Regulation of FGF Receptors in the Oligodendrocyte Lineage. *Mol. Cell. Neurosci.* **1996**, *7*, 263–275. [CrossRef] [PubMed]

76. Fortin, D.; Rom, E.; Sun, H.; Yayon, A.; Bansal, R. Distinct Fibroblast Growth Factor (FGF)/FGF Receptor Signaling Pairs Initiate Diverse Cellular Responses in the Oligodendrocyte Lineage. *J. Neurosci.* **2005**, *25*, 7470–7479. [CrossRef] [PubMed]

77. Zhou, Y.-X.; Flint, N.C.; Murtie, J.C.; Le, T.Q.; Armstrong, R.C. Retroviral lineage analysis of fibroblast growth factor receptor signaling in FGF2 inhibition of oligodendrocyte progenitor differentiation. *Glia* **2006**, *54*, 578–590. [CrossRef] [PubMed]

78. Goddard, D.R.; Berry, M.; Kirvell, S.L.; Butt, A.M. Fibroblast Growth Factor-2 Inhibits Myelin Production by Oligodendrocytes in Vivo. *Mol. Cell. Neurosci.* **2001**, *18*, 557–569. [CrossRef] [PubMed]

79. Fressinaud, C.; Vallat, J.M.; Labourdette, G. Basic fibroblast growth factor down-regulates myelin basic protein gene expression and alters myelin compaction of mature oligodendrocytes in vitro. *J. Neurosci. Res.* **1995**, *40*, 285–293. [CrossRef] [PubMed]

80. Wang, Z.; Colognato, H.; ffrench-Constant, C. Contrasting effects of mitogenic growth factors on myelination in neuron–oligodendrocyte co-cultures. *Glia* **2007**, *55*, 537–545. [CrossRef] [PubMed]

81. Jiang, F.; Frederick, T.J.; Wood, T.L. IGF-I Synergizes with FGF-2 to Stimulate Oligodendrocyte Progenitor Entry into the Cell Cycle. *Dev. Biol.* **2001**, *232*, 414–423. [CrossRef] [PubMed]

82. Shemer, J.; Raizada, M.K.; Masters, B.A.; Ota, A.; Leroith, D. Insulin-like Growth Factor I Receptors in Neuronal and Glial Cells CHARACTERIZATION AND BIOLOGICAL EFFECTS IN PRIMARY CULTURE*. *J. Biol. Chem.* **1987**, *262*, 7693–7699. [PubMed]

83. Jones, J.I.; Clemmons, D.R. Insulin-Like Growth Factors and Their Binding Proteins: Biological Actions*. *Endocr. Rev.* **1995**, *16*, 3–34. [CrossRef] [PubMed]

84. McMorris, F.A.; Smith, T.M.; DeSalvo, S.; Furlanetto, R.W. Insulin-like growth factor I/somatomedin C: a potent inducer of oligodendrocyte development. *Proc. Natl. Acad. Sci. USA* **1986**, *83*, 822–826. [CrossRef] [PubMed]

85. McMorris, F.A.; Dubois-Dalcq, M. Insulin-like growth factor I promotes cell proliferation and oligodendroglial commitment in rat glial progenitor cells developing in vitro. *J. Neurosci. Res.* **1988**, *21*, 199–209. [CrossRef] [PubMed]

86. Popken, G.J.; Hodge, R.D.; Ye, P.; Zhang, J.; Ng, W.; O'Kusky, J.R.; D'Ercole, A.J. In vivo effects of insulin-like growth factor-I (IGF-I) on prenatal and early postnatal development of the central nervous system. *Eur. J. Neurosci.* **2004**, *19*, 2056–2068. [CrossRef] [PubMed]

87. Hodge, R.D.; D'Ercole, A.J.; O'Kusky, J.R. Insulin-like growth factor-I accelerates the cell cycle by decreasing G1 phase length and increases cell cycle reentry in the embryonic cerebral cortex. *J. Neurosci.* **2004**, *24*, 10201–10210. [CrossRef] [PubMed]

88. Frederick, T.J.; Min, J.; Altieri, S.C.; Mitchell, N.E.; Wood, T.L. Synergistic induction of cyclin D1 in oligodendrocyte progenitor cells by IGF-I and FGF-2 requires differential stimulation of multiple signaling pathways. *Glia* **2007**, *55*, 1011–1022. [CrossRef] [PubMed]

89. Cui, Q.-L.; Almazan, G. IGF-I-induced oligodendrocyte progenitor proliferation requires PI3K/Akt, MEK/ERK, and Src-like tyrosine kinases. *J. Neurochem.* **2007**, *100*, 1480–1493. [CrossRef] [PubMed]

90. Palacios, N.; Sanchez-Franco, F.; Fernandez, M.; Sanchez, I.; Cacicedo, L. Intracellular events mediating insulin-like growth factor I-induced oligodendrocyte development: modulation by cyclic AMP. *J. Neurochem.* **2005**, *95*, 1091–1107. [CrossRef] [PubMed]

91. Frederick, T.J.; Wood, T.L. IGF-I and FGF-2 coordinately enhance cyclin D1 and cyclin E-cdk2 association and activity to promote G1 progression in oligodendrocyte progenitor cells. *Mol. Cell. Neurosci.* **2004**, *25*, 480–492. [CrossRef] [PubMed]

92. Mairet-Coello, G.; Tury, A.; DiCicco-Bloom, E. Insulin-like growth factor-1 promotes G(1)/S cell cycle progression through bidirectional regulation of cyclins and cyclin-dependent kinase inhibitors via the phosphatidylinositol 3-kinase/Akt pathway in developing rat cerebral cortex. *J. Neurosci.* **2009**, *29*, 775–788. [CrossRef] [PubMed]

93. Barres, B.A.; Hart, I.K.; Coles, H.S.R.; Burne, J.F.; Voyvodic, J.T.; Richardson, W.D.; Raff, M.C. Cell death in the oligodendrocyte lineage. *J. Neurobiol.* **1992**, *23*, 1221–1230. [CrossRef] [PubMed]

94. Barres, B.A.; Schmid, R.; Sendtner, M.; Raff, M.C. Multiple extracellular signals are required for long-term oligodendrocyte survival. *Development* **1993**, *118*, 283–295. [PubMed]

95. Pang, Y.; Zheng, B.; Fan, L.-W.; Rhodes, P.G.; Cai, Z. IGF-1 protects oligodendrocyte progenitors against TNFα-induced damage by activation of PI3K/Akt and interruption of the mitochondrial apoptotic pathway. *Glia* **2007**, *55*, 1099–1107. [CrossRef] [PubMed]

96. Chao, M.V. The p75 neurotrophin receptor. *J. Neurobiol.* **1994**, *25*, 1373–1385. [CrossRef] [PubMed]

97. Huang, E.J.; Reichardt, L.F. Trk Receptors: Roles in Neuronal Signal Transduction. *Annu. Rev. Biochem.* **2003**, *72*, 609–642. [CrossRef] [PubMed]
98. Xiao, J.; Kilpatrick, T.J.; Murray, S.S. The Role of Neurotrophins in the Regulation of Myelin Development. *Neurosignals* **2009**, *17*, 265–276. [CrossRef] [PubMed]
99. Barbacid, M. Neurotrophic factors and their receptors. *Curr. Opin. Cell Biol.* **1995**, *7*, 148–155. [CrossRef]
100. Chao, M.V.; Hempstead, B.L. p75 and Trk: a two-receptor system. *Trends Neurosci.* **1995**, *18*, 321–326. [CrossRef]
101. Van't Veer, A.; Du, Y.; Fischer, T.Z.; Boetig, D.R.; Wood, M.R.; Dreyfus, C.F. Brain-derived neurotrophic factor effects on oligodendrocyte progenitors of the basal forebrain are mediated through trkB and the MAP kinase pathway. *J. Neurosci. Res.* **2009**, *87*, 69–78. [CrossRef] [PubMed]
102. Du, Y.; Fischer, T.Z.; Clinton-Luke, P.; Lercher, L.D.; Dreyfus, C.F. Distinct effects of p75 in mediating actions of neurotrophins on basal forebrain oligodendrocytes. *Mol. Cell. Neurosci.* **2006**, *31*, 366–375. [CrossRef] [PubMed]
103. Johnson, J.R.; Chu, A.K.; Sato-Bigbee, C. Possible role of CREB in the stimulation of oligodendrocyte precursor cell proliferation by neurotrophin-3. *J. Neurochem.* **2000**, *74*, 1409–1417. [CrossRef] [PubMed]
104. Barres, B.A.; Raff, M.C.; Gaese, F.; Bartke, I.; Dechant, G.; Barde, Y.-A. A crucial role for neurotrophin-3 in oligodendrocyte development. *Nature* **1994**, *367*, 371–375. [CrossRef] [PubMed]
105. Kahn, M.A.; Kumar, S.; Liebl, D.; Chang, R.; Parada, L.F.; De Vellis, J. Mice lacking NT-3, and its receptor TrkC, exhibit profound deficiencies in CNS glial cells. *Glia* **1999**, *26*, 153–165. [CrossRef]
106. Olguín-Albuerne, M.; Morán, J. Redox Signaling Mechanisms in Nervous System Development. *Antioxid. Redox Signal.* **2018**, *28*, 1603–1625. [CrossRef] [PubMed]
107. Caillava, C.; Baron-Van Evercooren, A. Differential requirement of cyclin-dependent kinase 2 for oligodendrocyte progenitor cell proliferation and differentiation. *Cell Div.* **2012**, *7*, 14. [CrossRef] [PubMed]
108. Belachew, S.; Aguirre, A.A.; Wang, H.; Vautier, F.; Yuan, X.; Anderson, S.; Kirby, M.; Gallo, V. Cyclin-dependent kinase-2 controls oligodendrocyte progenitor cell cycle progression and is downregulated in adult oligodendrocyte progenitors. *J. Neurosci.* **2002**, *22*, 8553–8562. [CrossRef] [PubMed]
109. Sherr, C.J.; Roberts, J.M. Inhibitors of mammalian G1 cyclin-dependent kinases. *Genes Dev.* **1995**, *9*, 1149–1163. [CrossRef] [PubMed]
110. Jones, S.A.; Jolson, D.M.; Cuta, K.K.; Mariash, C.N.; Anderson, G.W. Triiodothyronine is a survival factor for developing oligodendrocytes. *Mol. Cell. Endocrinol.* **2003**, *199*, 49–60. [CrossRef]
111. Ahlgren, S.C.; Wallace, H.; Bishop, J.; Neophytou, C.; Raff, M.C. Effects of Thyroid Hormone on Embryonic Oligodendrocyte Precursor Cell Development in Vivo and in Vitro. *Mol. Cell. Neurosci.* **1997**, *9*, 420–432. [CrossRef] [PubMed]
112. Gao, F.-B.; Apperly, J.; Raff, M. Cell-Intrinsic Timers and Thyroid Hormone Regulate the Probability of Cell-Cycle Withdrawal and Differentiation of Oligodendrocyte Precursor Cells. *Dev. Biol.* **1998**, *197*, 54–66. [CrossRef] [PubMed]
113. Barres, B.A.; Lazar, M.A.; Raff, M.C. A novel role for thyroid hormone, glucocorticoids and retinoic acid in timing oligodendrocyte development. *Development* **1994**, *120*, 1097–1108. [PubMed]
114. Sarliève, L.L.; Rodríguez-Peña, A.; Langley, K. Expression of Thyroid Hormone Receptor Isoforms in the Oligodendrocyte Lineage. *Neurochem. Res.* **2003**, *29*, 903–922. [CrossRef]
115. Baas, D.; Fressinaud, C.; Ittel, M.E.; Reeber, A.; Dalençon, D.; Puymirat, J.; Sarliève, L.L. Expression of thyroid hormone receptor isoforms in rat oligodendrocyte cultures. Effect of 3,5,3′-triiodo-l-thyronine. *Neurosci. Lett.* **1994**, *176*, 47–51. [CrossRef]
116. Carré, J.-L.; Demerens, C.; Rodríguez-Peñ, A.; Floch, H.H.; Vincendon, G.; Sarliève, L.L. Thyroid Hormone Receptor Isoforms Are Sequentially Expressed in Oligodendrocyte Lineage Cells During Rat Cerebral Development. *J. Neurosci. Res* **1998**, *54*, 584–594. [CrossRef]
117. Almazan, G.; Honegger, P.; Matthieu, J.M. Triiodothyronine stimulation of oligodendroglial differentiation and myelination. A developmental study. *Dev. Neurosci.* **1985**, *7*, 45–54. [CrossRef] [PubMed]
118. Baas, D.; Bourbeau, D.; Sarli Ve, L.L.; Ittel, M.-E.; Dussault, J.H.; Puymirat, J. Oligodendrocyte Maturation and Progenitor Cell Proliferation Are Independently Regulated by Thyroid Hormone. *Glia* **1997**, *19*, 324–332. [CrossRef]
119. Almeida, R.; Lyons, D. Oligodendrocyte Development in the Absence of Their Target Axons In Vivo. *PLoS ONE* **2016**, *11*, e0164432. [CrossRef] [PubMed]

120. Beck, K.D.; Powell-Braxton, L.; Widmer, H.R.; Valverde, J.; Hefti, F. Igf1 gene disruption results in reduced brain size, CNS hypomyelination, and loss of hippocampal granule and striatal parvalbumin-containing neurons. *Neuron* **1995**, *14*, 717–730. [CrossRef]

121. Zeger, M.; Popken, G.; Zhang, J.; Xuan, S.; Lu, Q.R.; Schwab, M.H.; Nave, K.-A.; Rowitch, D.; D'Ercole, A.J.; Ye, P. Insulin-like growth factor type 1 receptor signaling in the cells of oligodendrocyte lineage is required for normalin vivo oligodendrocyte development and myelination. *Glia* **2007**, *55*, 400–411. [CrossRef] [PubMed]

122. Carson, M.J.; Behringer, R.R.; Brinster, R.L.; McMorris, F.A. Insulin-like growth factor I increases brain growth and central nervous system myelination in transgenic mice. *Neuron* **1993**, *10*, 729–740. [CrossRef]

123. Ye, P.; Carson, J.; D'Ercole, A.J. In vivo actions of insulin-like growth factor-I (IGF-I) on brain myelination: studies of IGF-I and IGF binding protein-1 (IGFBP-1) transgenic mice. *J. Neurosci.* **1995**, *15*, 7344–7356. [CrossRef] [PubMed]

124. Mozell, R.L.; McMorris, F.A. Insulin-like growth factor I stimulates oligodendrocyte development and myelination in rat brain aggregate cultures. *J. Neurosci. Res.* **1991**, *30*, 382–390. [CrossRef] [PubMed]

125. Luzi, P.; Zaka, M.; Rao, H.Z.; Curtis, M.; Rafi, M.A.; Wenger, D.A. Generation of transgenic mice expressing insulin-like growth factor-1 under the control of the myelin basic protein promoter: increased myelination and potential for studies on the effects of increased IGF-1 on experimentally and genetically induced demyelination. *Neurochem. Res.* **2004**, *29*, 881–889. [PubMed]

126. Adler, R.; Landa, K.B.; Manthorpe, M.; Varon, S. Cholinergic neuronotrophic factors: intraocular distribution of trophic activity for ciliary neurons. *Science* **1979**, *204*, 1434–1436. [CrossRef] [PubMed]

127. Stöckli, K.A.; Lillien, L.E.; Näher-Noé, M.; Breitfeld, G.; Hughes, R.A.; Raff, M.C.; Thoenen, H.; Sendtner, M. Regional Distribution, Developmental Changes, and Cellular Localization of CNTF-mRNA and Protein in the Rat Brain. *J. Cell Biol.* **1991**, *115*, 447–459. [CrossRef] [PubMed]

128. Barres, B.A.; Burne, J.F.; Holtmann, B.; Thoenen, H.; Sendtner, M.; Raff, M.C. Ciliary Neurotrophic Factor Enhances the Rate of Oligodendrocyte Generation. *Mol. Cell. Neurosci.* **1996**, *8*, 146–156. [CrossRef] [PubMed]

129. Marmur, R.; Kessler, J.A.; Zhu, G.; Gokhan, S.; Mehler, M.F. Differentiation of oligodendroglial progenitors derived from cortical multipotent cells requires extrinsic signals including activation of gp130/LIFbeta receptors. *J. Neurosci.* **1998**, *18*, 9800–9811. [CrossRef] [PubMed]

130. Stankoff, B.; Aigrot, M.-S.; Noël, F.; Wattilliaux, A.; Zalc, B.; Lubetzki, C. Ciliary neurotrophic factor (CNTF) enhances myelin formation: A novel role for CNTF and CNTF-related molecules. *J. Neurosci.* **2002**, *22*, 9221–9227. [CrossRef] [PubMed]

131. Ibarrola, N.; Mayer-Pröschel, M.; Rodriguez-Peña, A.; Noble, M. Evidence for the Existence of at Least Two Timing Mechanisms That Contribute to Oligodendrocyte Generationin Vitro. *Dev. Biol.* **1996**, *180*, 1–21. [CrossRef] [PubMed]

132. Mayer, M.; Bhakoo, K.; Noble, M. Ciliary neurotrophic factor and leukemia inhibitory factor promote the generation, maturation and survival of oligodendrocytes in vitro. *Development* **1994**, *120*, 143–153. [PubMed]

133. Salehi, Z.; Hadiyan, S.P.; Navidi, R. Ciliary Neurotrophic Factor Role in Myelin Oligodendrocyte Glycoprotein Expression in Cuprizone-Induced Multiple Sclerosis Mice. *Cell. Mol. Neurobiol.* **2013**, *33*, 531–535. [CrossRef] [PubMed]

134. Linker, R.A.; Mäurer, M.; Gaupp, S.; Martini, R.; Holtmann, B.; Giess, R.; Rieckmann, P.; Lassmann, H.; Toyka, K.V.; Sendtner, M.; et al. CNTF is a major protective factor in demyelinating CNS disease: A neurotrophic cytokine as modulator in neuroinflammation. *Nat. Med.* **2002**, *8*, 620–624. [CrossRef] [PubMed]

135. Ernfors, P.; Ibáñez, C.F.; Ebendal, T.; Olson, L.; Persson, H. Molecular cloning and neurotrophic activities of a protein with structural similarities to nerve growth factor: developmental and topographical expression in the brain. *Proc. Natl. Acad. Sci. USA* **1990**, *87*, 5454–5458. [CrossRef] [PubMed]

136. Heinrich, M.; Gorath, M.; Richter-Landsberg, C. Neurotrophin-3 (NT-3) Modulates Early Differentiation of Oligodendrocytes in Rat Brain Cortical Cultures. *Glia* **1999**, *28*, 244–255. [CrossRef]

137. Rubio, N.; Rodriguez, R.; Arevalo, M.A. In vitro myelination by oligodendrocyte precursor cells transfected with the neurotrophin-3 gene. *Glia* **2004**, *47*, 78–87. [CrossRef] [PubMed]

138. Du, Y.; Lercher, L.D.; Zhou, R.; Dreyfus, C.F. Mitogen-activated protein kinase pathway mediates effects of brain-derived neurotrophic factor on differentiation of basal forebrain oligodendrocytes. *J. Neurosci. Res.* **2006**, *84*, 1692–1702. [CrossRef] [PubMed]

139. Xiao, J.; Wong, A.W.; Willingham, M.M.; van den Buuse, M.; Kilpatrick, T.J.; Murray, S.S. Brain-Derived Neurotrophic Factor Promotes Central Nervous System Myelination via a Direct Effect upon Oligodendrocytes. *Neurosignals* **2010**, *18*, 186–202. [CrossRef] [PubMed]

140. Cosgaya, J.M.; Chan, J.R.; Shooter, E.M. The Neurotrophin Receptor p75NTR as a Positive Modulator of Myelination. *Science* **2002**, *298*, 1245–1248. [CrossRef] [PubMed]

141. Cellerino, A.; Carroll, P.; Thoenen, H.; Barde, Y.-A. Reduced Size of Retinal Ganglion Cell Axons and Hypomyelination in Mice Lacking Brain-Derived Neurotrophic Factor. *Mol. Cell. Neurosci.* **1997**, *9*, 397–408. [CrossRef] [PubMed]

142. Djalali, S.; Holtje, M.; Grosse, G.; Rothe, T.; Stroh, T.; Grosse, J.; Deng, D.R.; Hellweg, R.; Grantyn, R.; Hortnagl, H.; et al. Effects of brain-derived neurotrophic factor (BDNF) on glial cells and serotonergic neurones during development. *J. Neurochem.* **2005**, *92*, 616–627. [CrossRef] [PubMed]

143. Vondran, M.W.; Clinton-Luke, P.; Honeywell, J.Z.; Dreyfus, C.F. BDNF+/- mice exhibit deficits in oligodendrocyte lineage cells of the basal forebrain. *Glia* **2010**, *58*, 848–856. [CrossRef] [PubMed]

144. Wong, A.W.; Xiao, J.; Kemper, D.; Kilpatrick, T.J.; Murray, S.S. Oligodendroglial expression of TrkB independently regulates myelination and progenitor cell proliferation. *J. Neurosci.* **2013**, *33*, 4947–4957. [CrossRef] [PubMed]

145. Du, Y.; Fischer, T.Z.; Lee, L.N.; Lercher, L.D.; Dreyfus, C.F. Regionally Specific Effects of BDNF on Oligodendrocytes. *Dev. Neurosci.* **2003**, *25*, 116–126. [CrossRef] [PubMed]

146. Mei, L.; Nave, K.-A. Neuregulin-ERBB signaling in the nervous system and neuropsychiatric diseases. *Neuron* **2014**, *83*, 27–49. [CrossRef] [PubMed]

147. Canoll, P.D.; Kraemer, R.; Teng, K.K.; Marchionni, M.A.; Salzer, J.L. GGF/Neuregulin Induces a Phenotypic Reversion of Oligodendrocytes. *Mol. Cell. Neurosci.* **1999**, *13*, 79–94. [CrossRef] [PubMed]

148. Gauthier, M.-K.; Kosciuczyk, K.; Tapley, L.; Karimi-Abdolrezaee, S. Dysregulation of the neuregulin-1-ErbB network modulates endogenous oligodendrocyte differentiation and preservation after spinal cord injury. *Eur. J. Neurosci.* **2013**, *38*, 2693–2715. [CrossRef] [PubMed]

149. Flores, A.I.; Mallon, B.S.; Matsui, T.; Ogawa, W.; Rosenzweig, A.; Okamoto, T.; Macklin, W.B. Akt-mediated survival of oligodendrocytes induced by neuregulins. *J. Neurosci.* **2000**, *20*, 7622–7630. [CrossRef] [PubMed]

150. Fernandez, P.A.; Tang, D.G.; Cheng, L.; Prochiantz, A.; Mudge, A.W.; Raff, M.C. Evidence that axon-derived neuregulin promotes oligodendrocyte survival in the developing rat optic nerve. *Neuron* **2000**, *28*, 81–90. [CrossRef]

151. Colognato, H.; Baron, W.; Avellana-Adalid, V.; Relvas, J.B.; Evercooren, A.B.-V.; Georges-Labouesse, E.; ffrench-Constant, C. CNS integrins switch growth factor signalling to promote target-dependent survival. *Nat. Cell Biol.* **2002**, *4*, 833–841. [CrossRef] [PubMed]

152. Colognato, H.; Ramachandrappa, S.; Olsen, I.M.; ffrench-Constant, C. Integrins direct Src family kinases to regulate distinct phases of oligodendrocyte development. *J. Cell Biol.* **2004**, *167*, 365–375. [CrossRef] [PubMed]

153. Kim, J.Y.; Sun, Q.; Oglesbee, M.; Yoon, S.O. The role of ErbB2 signaling in the onset of terminal differentiation of oligodendrocytes in vivo. *J. Neurosci.* **2003**, *23*, 5561–5571. [CrossRef] [PubMed]

154. Roy, K.; Murtie, J.C.; El-Khodor, B.F.; Edgar, N.; Sardi, S.P.; Hooks, B.M.; Benoit-Marand, M.; Chen, C.; Moore, H.; O'Donnell, P.; Brunner, D.; Corfas, G. Loss of erbB signaling in oligodendrocytes alters myelin and dopaminergic function, a potential mechanism for neuropsychiatric disorders. *Proc. Natl. Acad. Sci. USA* **2007**, *104*, 8131–8136. [CrossRef] [PubMed]

155. Park, S.K.; Miller, R.; Krane, I.; Vartanian, T. The erbB2 gene is required for the development of terminally differentiated spinal cord oligodendrocytes. *J. Cell Biol.* **2001**, *154*, 1245–1258. [CrossRef] [PubMed]

156. Küspert, M.; Wegner, M. SomethiNG 2 talk about—Transcriptional regulation in embryonic and adult oligodendrocyte precursors. *Brain Res.* **2016**, *1638*, 167–182. [CrossRef] [PubMed]

157. Traiffort, E.; Zakaria, M.; Laouarem, Y.; Ferent, J. Hedgehog: A Key Signaling in the Development of the Oligodendrocyte Lineage. *J. Dev. Biol.* **2016**, *4*, 28. [CrossRef] [PubMed]

158. Crowe, M.J.; Bresnahan, J.C.; Shuman, S.L.; Masters, J.N.; Crowe, M.S. Apoptosis and delayed degeneration after spinal cord injury in rats and monkeys. *Nat. Med.* **1997**, *3*, 73–76. [CrossRef] [PubMed]

159. Lytle, J.M.; Vicini, S.; Wrathall, J.R. Phenotypic changes in NG2+ cells after spinal cord injury. *J. Neurotrauma* **2006**, *23*, 1726–1738. [CrossRef] [PubMed]

160. Grossman, S.D.; Rosenberg, L.J.; Wrathall, J.R. Temporal-spatial pattern of acute neuronal and glial loss after spinal cord contusion. *Exp. Neurol.* **2001**. [CrossRef] [PubMed]

161. McTigue, D.M.; Wei, P.; Stokes, B.T. Proliferation of NG2-positive cells and altered oligodendrocyte numbers in the contused rat spinal cord. *J. Neurosci.* **2001**, *21*, 3392–3400. [CrossRef] [PubMed]

162. Lotocki, G.; de Rivero Vaccari, J.; Alonso, O.; Molano, J.S.; Nixon, R.; Dietrich, W.D.; Bramlett, H.M. Oligodendrocyte Vulnerability Following Traumatic Brain Injury in Rats: Effect of Moderate Hypothermia. *Ther. Hypothermia Temp. Manag.* **2011**, *1*, 43–51. [CrossRef] [PubMed]

163. Gensert, J.M.; Goldman, J.E. Endogenous progenitors remyelinate demyelinated axons in the adult CNS. *Neuron* **1997**, *19*, 197–203. [CrossRef]

164. Hesp, Z.C.; Goldstein, E.Z.; Goldstein, E.A.; Miranda, C.J.; Kaspar, B.K.; Kaspar, B.K.; McTigue, D.M. Chronic oligodendrogenesis and remyelination after spinal cord injury in mice and rats. *J. Neurosci.* **2015**, *35*, 1274–1290. [CrossRef] [PubMed]

165. Sellers, D.L.; Maris, D.O.; Horner, P.J. Postinjury Niches Induce Temporal Shifts in Progenitor Fates to Direct Lesion Repair after Spinal Cord Injury. *J. Neurosci.* **2009**, *29*, 6722–6733. [CrossRef] [PubMed]

166. Zai, L.J.; Wrathall, J.R. Cell proliferation and replacement following contusive spinal cord injury. *Glia* **2005**, *50*, 247–257. [CrossRef] [PubMed]

167. Barnabé-Heider, F.; Göritz, C.; Sabelström, H.; Takebayashi, H.; Pfrieger, F.W.; Meletis, K.; Frisén, J. Origin of New Glial Cells in Intact and Injured Adult Spinal Cord. *Cell Stem Cell* **2010**, *7*, 470–482. [CrossRef] [PubMed]

168. Meletis, K.; Barnabé-Heider, F.; Carlén, M.; Evergren, E.; Tomilin, N.; Shupliakov, O.; Frisén, J. Spinal cord injury reveals multilineage differentiation of ependymal cells. *PLoS Biol.* **2008**, *6*, e182. [CrossRef] [PubMed]

169. Karimi-Abdolrezaee, S.; Billakanti, R. Reactive Astrogliosis after Spinal Cord Injury—Beneficial and Detrimental Effects. *Mol. Neurobiol.* **2012**, *46*, 251–264. [CrossRef] [PubMed]

170. Lacroix, S.; Hamilton, L.K.; Vaugeois, A.; Beaudoin, S.; Breault-Dugas, C.; Pineau, I.; Lévesque, S.A.; Grégoire, C.-A.; Fernandes, K.J.L. Central Canal Ependymal Cells Proliferate Extensively in Response to Traumatic Spinal Cord Injury but Not Demyelinating Lesions. *PLoS ONE* **2014**, *9*, e85916. [CrossRef] [PubMed]

171. BUNGE, M.B.; BUNGE, R.P.; RIS, H. Ultrastructural study of remyelination in an experimental lesion in adult cat spinal cord. *J. Biophys. Biochem. Cytol.* **1961**, *10*, 67–94. [CrossRef] [PubMed]

172. Gledhill, R.F.; Harrison, B.M.; McDonald, W.I. Demyelination and Remyelination after Acute Spinal Cord Compression. *Exp. Neurol.* **1973**, *38*, 472–487. [CrossRef]

173. Rasminsky, M.; Sears, T.A. Internodal conduction in undissected demyelinated nerve fibres. *J. Physiol.* **1972**, *227*, 323–350. [CrossRef] [PubMed]

174. Mcdonald, W.I. Pathophysiology in multiple sclerosis. *Brain* **1974**, *97*, 179–196. [CrossRef] [PubMed]

175. Wrathall, J.R.; Li, W.; Hudson, L.D. Myelin gene expression after experimental contusive spinal cord injury. *J. Neurosci.* **1998**, *18*, 8780–8793. [CrossRef] [PubMed]

176. Totoiu, M.O.; Keirstead, H.S. Spinal cord injury is accompanied by chronic progressive demyelination. *J. Comp. Neurol.* **2005**, *486*, 373–383. [CrossRef] [PubMed]

177. Guest, J.D.; Hiester, E.D.; Bunge, R.P. Demyelination and Schwann cell responses adjacent to injury epicenter cavities following chronic human spinal cord injury. *Exp. Neurol.* **2005**, *192*, 384–393. [CrossRef] [PubMed]

178. Blight, A.R. Delayed Demyelination and Macrophage Invasion: A Candidate for Secondary Cell Damage in Spinal Cord Injury. *Cent. Nerv. Syst. Trauma* **1985**, *2*, 299–315. [CrossRef] [PubMed]

179. Park, Y.M.; Lee, W.T.; Bokara, K.K.; Seo, S.K.; Park, S.H.; Kim, J.H.; Yenari, M.A.; Park, K.A.; Lee, J.E. The Multifaceted Effects of Agmatine on Functional Recovery after Spinal Cord Injury through Modulations of BMP-2/4/7 Expressions in Neurons and Glial Cells. *PLoS ONE* **2013**, *8*, e53911. [CrossRef] [PubMed]

180. Setoguchi, T.; Yone, K.; Matsuoka, E.; Takenouchi, H.; Nakashima, K.; Sakou, T.; Komiya, S.; Izumo, S. Traumatic injury-induced BMP7 expression in the adult rat spinal cord. *Brain Res.* **2001**, *921*, 219–225. [CrossRef]

181. Grinspan, J.B.; Edell, E.; Carpio, D.F.; Beesley, J.S.; Lavy, L.; Pleasure, D.; Golden, J.A. Stage-specific effects of bone morphogenetic proteins on the oligodendrocyte lineage. *J. Neurobiol.* **2000**, *43*, 1–17. [CrossRef]

182. Sabo, J.K.; Aumann, T.D.; Merlo, D.; Kilpatrick, T.J.; Cate, H.S. Remyelination Is Altered by Bone Morphogenic Protein Signaling in Demyelinated Lesions. *J. Neurosci.* **2011**, *31*, 4504–4510. [CrossRef] [PubMed]

183. See, J.; Zhang, X.; Eraydin, N.; Golden, J.A.; Grinspan, J.B. Oligodendrocyte maturation is inhibited by bone morphogenetic protein. *Mol. Cell. Neurosci.* **2004**, *26*, 481–492. [CrossRef] [PubMed]

184. Cate, H.S.; Sabo, J.K.; Merlo, D.; Kemper, D.; Aumann, T.D.; Robinson, J.; Merson, T.D.; Emery, B.; Perreau, V.M.; Kilpatrick, T.J. Modulation of bone morphogenic protein signalling alters numbers of astrocytes and oligodendroglia in the subventricular zone during cuprizone-induced demyelination. *J. Neurochem.* **2010**, *115*, 11–22. [CrossRef] [PubMed]

185. González-Fernández, C.; Fernández-Martos, C.M.; Shields, S.D.; Arenas, E.; Javier Rodríguez, F. Wnts are expressed in the spinal cord of adult mice and are differentially induced after injury. *J. Neurotrauma* **2014**, *31*, 565–581. [CrossRef] [PubMed]

186. Fernández-Martos, C.M.; González-Fernández, C.; González, P.; Maqueda, A.; Arenas, E.; Rodríguez, F.J. Differential expression of Wnts after spinal cord contusion injury in adult rats. *PLoS ONE* **2011**, *6*, e27000. [CrossRef] [PubMed]

187. Rodriguez, J.P.; Coulter, M.; Miotke, J.; Meyer, R.L.; Takemaru, K.-I.; Levine, J.M. Abrogation of β-catenin signaling in oligodendrocyte precursor cells reduces glial scarring and promotes axon regeneration after CNS injury. *J. Neurosci.* **2014**, *34*, 10285–10297. [CrossRef] [PubMed]

188. Yao, Z.-F.; Wang, Y.; Lin, Y.-H.; Wu, Y.; Zhu, A.-Y.; Wang, R.; Shen, L.; Xi, J.; Qi, Q.; Jiang, Z.-Q.; Lü, H.-Z.; Hu, J.-G. Transplantation of PDGF-AA-Overexpressing Oligodendrocyte Precursor Cells Promotes Recovery in Rat Following Spinal Cord Injury. *Front. Cell. Neurosci.* **2017**, *11*, 79. [CrossRef] [PubMed]

189. Tripathi, A.; Parikh, Z.S.; Vora, P.; Frost, E.E.; Pillai, P.P. pERK1/2 Peripheral Recruitment and Filopodia Protrusion Augment Oligodendrocyte Progenitor Cell Migration: Combined Effects of PDGF-A and Fibronectin. *Cell. Mol. Neurobiol.* **2017**, *37*, 183–194. [CrossRef] [PubMed]

190. Yang, J.; Cheng, X.; Qi, J.; Xie, B.; Zhao, X.; Zheng, K.; Zhang, Z.; Qiu, M. EGF Enhances Oligodendrogenesis from Glial Progenitor Cells. *Front. Mol. Neurosci.* **2017**, *10*, 106. [CrossRef] [PubMed]

191. Tripathi, R.B.; McTigue, D.M. Chronically increased ciliary neurotrophic factor and fibroblast growth factor-2 expression after spinal contusion in rats. *J. Comp. Neurol.* **2008**. [CrossRef] [PubMed]

192. Louis, J.C.; Magal, E.; Takayama, S.; Varon, S. CNTF protection of oligodendrocytes against natural and tumor necrosis factor-induced death. *Science* **1993**, *259*, 689–692. [CrossRef] [PubMed]

193. Oyesiku, N.M.; Wilcox, J.N.; Wigston, D.J. Changes in expression of ciliary neurotrophic factor (CNTF) and CNTF-receptor alpha after spinal cord injury. *J. Neurobiol.* **1997**, *32*, 251–261. [CrossRef]

194. Oyesiku, N.M.; Evans, C.-O.; Houston, S.; Darrell, R.S.; Smith, J.S.; Fulop, Z.L.; Dixon, C.E.; Stein, D.G. Regional changes in the expression of neurotrophic factors and their receptors following acute traumatic brain injury in the adult rat brain. *Brain Res.* **1999**, *833*, 161–172. [CrossRef]

195. Cao, Q.; He, Q.; Wang, Y.; Cheng, X.; Howard, R.M.; Zhang, Y.; DeVries, W.H.; Shields, C.B.; Magnuson, D.S.K.; Xu, X.-M.; et al. Transplantation of ciliary neurotrophic factor-expressing adult oligodendrocyte precursor cells promotes remyelination and functional recovery after spinal cord injury. *J. Neurosci.* **2010**, *30*, 2989–3001. [CrossRef] [PubMed]

196. McTigue, D.M.; Horner, P.J.; Stokes, B.T.; Gage, F.H. Neurotrophin-3 and brain-derived neurotrophic factor induce oligodendrocyte proliferation and myelination of regenerating axons in the contused adult rat spinal cord. *J. Neurosci.* **1998**, *18*, 5354–5365. [CrossRef] [PubMed]

197. Xu, X.M.; Guénard, V.; Kleitman, N.; Aebischer, P.; Bunge, M.B. A Combination of BDNF and NT-3 Promotes Supraspinal Axonal Regeneration into Schwann Cell Grafts in Adult Rat Thoracic Spinal Cord. *Exp. Neurol.* **1995**, *134*, 261–272. [CrossRef] [PubMed]

198. Thomas, A.M.; Seidlits, S.K.; Goodman, A.G.; Kukushliev, T.V.; Hassani, D.M.; Cummings, B.J.; Anderson, A.J.; Shea, L.D. Sonic hedgehog and neurotrophin-3 increase oligodendrocyte numbers and myelination after spinal cord injury. *Integr. Biol. (Camb).* **2014**, *6*, 694–705. [CrossRef] [PubMed]

199. McCreedy, D.A.; Wilems, T.S.; Xu, H.; Butts, J.C.; Brown, C.R.; Smith, A.W.; Sakiyama-Elbert, S.E. Survival, Differentiation, and Migration of High-Purity Mouse Embryonic Stem Cell-derived Progenitor Motor Neurons in Fibrin Scaffolds after Sub-Acute Spinal Cord Injury. *Biomater. Sci.* **2014**, *2*, 1672–1682. [CrossRef] [PubMed]

200. Bartholdi, D.; Schwab, M.E. Oligodendroglial reaction following spinal cord injury in rat: transient upregulation of MBP mRNA. *Glia* **1998**, *23*, 278–284. [CrossRef]

201. Dougherty, K.D.; Dreyfus, C.F.; Black, I.B. Brain-Derived Neurotrophic Factor in Astrocytes, Oligodendrocytes, and Microglia/Macrophages after Spinal Cord Injury. *Neurobiol. Dis.* **2000**, *7*, 574–585. [CrossRef] [PubMed]

202. Ikeda, O.; Murakami, M.; Ino, H.; Yamazaki, M.; Nemoto, T.; Koda, M.; Nakayama, C.; Moriya, H. Acute up-regulation of brain-derived neurotrophic factor expression resulting from experimentally induced injury in the rat spinal cord. *Acta Neuropathol.* **2001**, *102*, 239–245. [CrossRef] [PubMed]

203. Ikeda, O.; Murakami, M.; Ino, H.; Yamazaki, M.; Koda, M.; Nakayama, C.; Moriya, H. Effects of Brain-Derived Neurotrophic Factor (BDNF) on Compression-Induced Spinal Cord Injury: BDNF Attenuates Down-Regulation of Superoxide Dismutase Expression and Promotes Up-Regulation of Myelin Basic Protein Expression. *J. Neuropathol. Exp. Neurol.* **2002**, *61*, 142–153. [CrossRef] [PubMed]

204. Zhao, J.; Sun, W.; Cho, H.M.; Ouyang, H.; Li, W.; Lin, Y.; Do, J.; Zhang, L.; Ding, S.; Liu, Y.; et al. Integration and long distance axonal regeneration in the central nervous system from transplanted primitive neural stem cells. *J. Biol. Chem.* **2013**, *288*, 164–168. [CrossRef] [PubMed]

205. Sharma, H.S.; Nyberg, F.; Westman, J.; Alm, P.; Gordh, T.; Lindholm, D. Brain derived neurotrophic factor and insulin like growth factor-1 attenuate upregulation of nitric oxide synthase and cell injury following trauma to the spinal cord. *Amino Acids* **1998**, *14*, 121–129. [CrossRef] [PubMed]

206. Kwak, E.K.; Kim, J.W.; Kang, K.S.; Lee, Y.H.; Hua, Q.H.; Park, T.I.; Park, J.Y.; Sohn, Y.K. The Role of Inducible Nitric Oxide Synthase Following Spinal Cord Injury in Rat. *J. Korean Med. Sci.* **2005**, *20*, 663. [CrossRef] [PubMed]

207. Thorburne, S.K.; Juurlink, B.H. Low glutathione and high iron govern the susceptibility of oligodendroglial precursors to oxidative stress. *J. Neurochem.* **1996**, *67*, 1014–1022. [CrossRef] [PubMed]

208. Li, L.; Xu, Q.; Wu, Y.; Hu, W.; Gu, P.; Fu, Z. Combined therapy of methylprednisolone and brain-derived neurotrophic factor promotes axonal regeneration and functional recovery after spinal cord injury in rats. *Chin. Med. J. (Engl.)* **2003**, *116*, 414–418. [PubMed]

209. Hu, J.-G.; Shen, L.; Wang, R.; Wang, Q.-Y.; Zhang, C.; Xi, J.; Ma, S.-F.; Zhou, J.-S.; Lü, H.-Z. Effects of Olig2-overexpressing neural stem cells and myelin basic protein-activated T cells on recovery from spinal cord injury. *Neurotherapeutics* **2012**, *9*, 422–445. [CrossRef] [PubMed]

210. Ramos-Cejudo, J.; Gutierrez-Fernandez, M.; Otero-Ortega, L.; Rodriguez-Frutos, B.; Fuentes, B.; Vallejo-Cremades, M.T.; Hernanz, T.N.; Cerdan, S.; Diez-Tejedor, E. Brain-Derived Neurotrophic Factor Administration Mediated Oligodendrocyte Differentiation and Myelin Formation in Subcortical Ischemic Stroke. *Stroke* **2015**, *46*, 221–228. [CrossRef] [PubMed]

211. Kataria, H.; Alizadeh, A.; Shahriary, G.M.; Saboktakin Rizi, S.; Henrie, R.; Santhosh, K.T.; Thliveris, J.A.; Karimi-Abdolrezaee, S. Neuregulin-1 promotes remyelination and fosters a pro-regenerative inflammatory response in focal demyelinating lesions of the spinal cord. *Glia* **2018**, *66*, 538–561. [CrossRef] [PubMed]

212. Bartus, K.; Galino, J.; James, N.D.; Hernandez-Miranda, L.R.; Dawes, J.M.; Fricker, F.R.; Garratt, A.N.; McMahon, S.B.; Ramer, M.S.; Birchmeier, C.; et al. Neuregulin-1 controls an endogenous repair mechanism after spinal cord injury. *Brain* **2016**, *139*, 1394–1416. [CrossRef] [PubMed]

213. Alizadeh, A.; Karimi-Abdolrezaee, S. Microenvironmental regulation of oligodendrocyte replacement and remyelination in spinal cord injury. *J. Physiol.* **2016**, *594*, 3539–3552. [CrossRef] [PubMed]

214. Cheville, A.L.; Kirshblum, S.C. Thyroid hormone changes in chronic spinal cord injury. *J. Spinal Cord Med.* **1995**, *18*, 227–232. [CrossRef] [PubMed]

215. Bugaresti, J.M.; Tator, C.H.; Silverberg, J.D.; Szalai, J.P.; Malkin, D.G.; Malkin, A.; Tay, S.K. Changes in thyroid hormones, thyroid stimulating hormone and cortisol in acute spinal cord injury. *Spinal Cord* **1992**, *30*, 401–409. [CrossRef] [PubMed]

216. Shultz, R.B.; Wang, Z.; Nong, J.; Zhang, Z.; Zhong, Y. Local delivery of thyroid hormone enhances oligodendrogenesis and myelination after spinal cord injury. *J. Neural Eng.* **2017**, *14*, 36014. [CrossRef] [PubMed]

217. Annunziata, M.; Granata, R.; Ghigo, E. The IGF system. *Acta Diabetol.* **2011**, *48*, 1–9. [CrossRef] [PubMed]

218. Garcia-Estrada, J.; Garcia-Segura, L.M.; Torres-Aleman, I. Expression of insulin-like growth factor I by astrocytes in response to injury. *Brain Res.* **1992**, *592*, 343–347. [CrossRef]

219. O'Donnell, S.L.; Frederick, T.J.; Krady, J.K.; Vannucci, S.J.; Wood, T.L. IGF-I and microglia/macrophage proliferation in the ischemic mouse brain. *Glia* **2002**, *39*, 85–97. [CrossRef] [PubMed]

220. Latov, N.; Nilaver, G.; Zimmerman, E.A.; Johnson, W.G.; Silverman, A.J.; Defendini, R.; Cote, L. Fibrillary astrocytes proliferate in response to brain injury: a study combining immunoperoxidase technique for glial fibrillary acidic protein and radioautography of tritiated thymidine. *Dev. Biol.* **1979**, *72*, 381–384. [CrossRef]
221. Dusart, I.; Schwab, M.E. Secondary cell death and the inflammatory reaction after dorsal hemisection of the rat spinal cord. *Eur. J. Neurosci.* **1994**, *6*, 712–724. [CrossRef] [PubMed]
222. Hinks, G.L.; Franklin, R.J.M. Distinctive Patterns of PDGF-A, FGF-2, IGF-I, and TGF-β1 Gene Expression during Remyelination of Experimentally-Induced Spinal Cord Demyelination. *Mol. Cell. Neurosci.* **1999**, *14*, 153–168. [CrossRef] [PubMed]
223. Yao, D.-L.; West, N.R.; Bondy, C.A.; Brenner, M.; Hudson, L.D.; Zhou, J.; Collins, G.H.; Webster, H.D. Cryogenic spinal cord injury induces astrocytic gene expression of insulin-like growth factor I and insulin-like growth factor binding protein 2 during myelin regeneration. *J. Neurosci. Res.* **1995**, *40*, 647–659. [CrossRef] [PubMed]
224. Kazanis, I.; Giannakopoulou, M.; Philippidis, H.; Stylianopoulou, F. Alterations in IGF-I, BDNF and NT-3 levels following experimental brain trauma and the effect of IGF-I administration. *Exp. Neurol.* **2004**, *186*, 221–234. [CrossRef] [PubMed]
225. Moghaddam, A.; Sperl, A.; Heller, R.; Kunzmann, K.; Graeser, V.; Akbar, M.; Gerner, H.J.; Biglari, B. Elevated Serum Insulin-Like Growth Factor 1 Levels in Patients with Neurological Remission after Traumatic Spinal Cord Injury. *PLoS ONE* **2016**, *11*, e0159764. [CrossRef] [PubMed]
226. Feeney, C.; Sharp, D.J.; Hellyer, P.J.; Jolly, A.E.; Cole, J.H.; Scott, G.; Baxter, D.; Jilka, S.; Ross, E.; Ham, T.E.; et al. Serum insulin-like growth factor-I levels are associated with improved white matter recovery after traumatic brain injury. *Ann. Neurol.* **2017**, *82*, 30–43. [CrossRef] [PubMed]
227. Thomas, A.J.; Nockels, R.P.; Pan, H.Q.; Shaffrey, C.I.; Chopp, M. Progesterone is Neuroprotective After Acute Experimental Spinal Cord Trauma in Rats. *Spine (Phila. Pa. 1976).* **1999**, *24*, 2134. [CrossRef]
228. Labombarda, F.; González, S.L.; Lima, A.; Roig, P.; Guennoun, R.; Schumacher, M.; de Nicola, A.F. Effects of progesterone on oligodendrocyte progenitors, oligodendrocyte transcription factors, and myelin proteins following spinal cord injury. *Glia* **2009**, *57*, 884–897. [CrossRef] [PubMed]
229. Zhou, Q.; Choi, G.; Anderson, D.J. The bHLH transcription factor Olig2 promotes oligodendrocyte differentiation in collaboration with Nkx2.2. *Neuron* **2001**, *31*, 791–807. [CrossRef]
230. Arnett, H.A.; Fancy, S.P.J.; Alberta, J.A.; Zhao, C.; Plant, S.R.; Kaing, S.; Raine, C.S.; Rowitch, D.H.; Franklin, R.J.M.; Stiles, C.D. bHLH Transcription Factor Olig1 Is Required to Repair Demyelinated Lesions in the CNS. *Science* **2004**, *306*, 2111–2115. [CrossRef] [PubMed]
231. Galani, R.; Hoffman, S.W.; Stein, D.G. Effects of the duration of progesterone treatment on the resolution of cerebral edema induced by cortical contusions in rats. *Restor. Neurol. Neurosci.* **2001**, *18*, 161–166. [PubMed]
232. Cutler, S.M.; Cekic, M.; Miller, D.M.; Wali, B.; VanLandingham, J.W.; Stein, D.G. Progesterone Improves Acute Recovery after Traumatic Brain Injury in the Aged Rat. *J. Neurotrauma* **2007**, *24*, 1475–1486. [CrossRef] [PubMed]
233. Fawcett, J.W.; Asher, R.A. The glial scar and central nervous system repair. *Brain Res. Bull.* **1999**, *49*, 377–391. [CrossRef]
234. Siebert, J.R.; Osterhout, D.J. The inhibitory effects of chondroitin sulfate proteoglycans on oligodendrocytes. *J. Neurochem.* **2011**, *119*, 176–188. [CrossRef] [PubMed]
235. Pendleton, J.C.; Shamblott, M.J.; Gary, D.S.; Belegu, V.; Hurtado, A.; Malone, M.L.; McDonald, J.W. Chondroitin sulfate proteoglycans inhibit oligodendrocyte myelination through PTPσ. *Exp. Neurol.* **2013**, *247*, 113–121. [CrossRef] [PubMed]
236. Jahan, N.; Hannila, S.S. Transforming growth factor β-induced expression of chondroitin sulfate proteoglycans is mediated through non-Smad signaling pathways. *Exp. Neurol.* **2015**, *263*, 372–384. [CrossRef] [PubMed]
237. Schachtrup, C.; Ryu, J.K.; Helmrick, M.J.; Vagena, E.; Galanakis, D.K.; Degen, J.L.; Margolis, R.U.; Akassoglou, K. Fibrinogen triggers astrocyte scar formation by promoting the availability of active TGF-beta after vascular damage. *J. Neurosci.* **2010**, *30*, 5843–5854. [CrossRef] [PubMed]
238. Susarla, B.T.S.; Laing, E.D.; Yu, P.; Katagiri, Y.; Geller, H.M.; Symes, A.J. Smad proteins differentially regulate transforming growth factor-β-mediated induction of chondroitin sulfate proteoglycans. *J. Neurochem.* **2011**, *119*, 868–878. [CrossRef] [PubMed]

239. Lau, L.W.; Keough, M.B.; Haylock-Jacobs, S.; Cua, R.; Döring, A.; Sloka, S.; Stirling, D.P.; Rivest, S.; Yong, V.W. Chondroitin sulfate proteoglycans in demyelinated lesions impair remyelination. *Ann. Neurol.* **2012**, *72*, 419–432. [CrossRef] [PubMed]

240. Karimi-Abdolrezaee, S.; Eftekharpour, E.; Wang, J.; Schut, D.; Fehlings, M.G. Synergistic Effects of Transplanted Adult Neural Stem/Progenitor Cells, Chondroitinase, and Growth Factors Promote Functional Repair and Plasticity of the Chronically Injured Spinal Cord. *J. Neurosci.* **2010**, *30*, 1657–1676. [CrossRef] [PubMed]

241. Siebert, J.R.; Stelzner, D.J.; Osterhout, D.J. Chondroitinase treatment following spinal contusion injury increases migration of oligodendrocyte progenitor cells. *Exp. Neurol.* **2011**, *231*, 19–29. [CrossRef] [PubMed]

242. Hammond, T.R.; Gadea, A.; Dupree, J.; Kerninon, C.; Nait-Oumesmar, B.; Aguirre, A.; Gallo, V. Astrocyte-Derived Endothelin-1 Inhibits Remyelination through Notch Activation. *Neuron* **2014**, *81*, 588–602. [CrossRef] [PubMed]

243. Domingues, H.S.; Portugal, C.C.; Socodato, R.; Relvas, J.B. Oligodendrocyte, Astrocyte, and Microglia Crosstalk in Myelin Development, Damage, and Repair. *Front. cell Dev. Biol.* **2016**, *4*, 71. [CrossRef] [PubMed]

244. Wang, H.-F.; Liu, X.-K.; Li, R.; Zhang, P.; Chu, Z.; Wang, C.-L.; Liu, H.-R.; Qi, J.; Lv, G.-Y.; Wang, G.-Y.; et al. Effect of glial cells on remyelination after spinal cord injury. *Neural Regen. Res.* **2017**, *12*, 1724–1732. [CrossRef] [PubMed]

245. Arnett, H.A.; Mason, J.; Marino, M.; Suzuki, K.; Matsushima, G.K.; Ting, J.P.-Y. TNFα promotes proliferation of oligodendrocyte progenitors and remyelination. *Nat. Neurosci.* **2001**, *4*, 1116–1122. [CrossRef] [PubMed]

246. Vela, J.M.; Molina-Holgado, E.; Arévalo-Martín, Á.; Almazán, G.; Guaza, C. Interleukin-1 Regulates Proliferation and Differentiation of Oligodendrocyte Progenitor Cells. *Mol. Cell. Neurosci.* **2002**, *20*, 489–502. [CrossRef] [PubMed]

247. Schulz, K.; Kroner, A.; David, S. Iron efflux from astrocytes plays a role in remyelination. *J. Neurosci.* **2012**, *32*, 4841–4847. [CrossRef] [PubMed]

248. Kıray, H.; Lindsay, S.L.; Hosseinzadeh, S.; Barnett, S.C. The multifaceted role of astrocytes in regulating myelination. *Exp. Neurol.* **2016**, *283*, 541–549. [CrossRef]

249. Tripathi, R.; McTigue, D.M. Prominent oligodendrocyte genesis along the border of spinal contusion lesions. *Glia* **2007**. [CrossRef] [PubMed]

250. Almad, A.; McTigue, D.M. Chronic expression of PPAR-δ by oligodendrocyte lineage cells in the injured rat spinal cord. *J. Comp. Neurol.* **2010**, *518*, 785–799. [CrossRef] [PubMed]

251. Hesp, Z.C.; Yoseph, R.Y.; Suzuki, R.; Jukkola, P.; Wilson, C.; Nishiyama, A.; McTigue, D.M. Proliferating NG2-Cell-Dependent Angiogenesis and Scar Formation Alter Axon Growth and Functional Recovery After Spinal Cord Injury in Mice. *J. Neurosci.* **2018**, *38*, 1366–1382. [CrossRef] [PubMed]

252. Moyon, S.; Dubessy, A.L.; Aigrot, M.S.; Trotter, M.; Huang, J.K.; Dauphinot, L.; Potier, M.C.; Kerninon, C.; Melik Parsadaniantz, S.; Franklin, R.J.M.; et al. Demyelination Causes Adult CNS Progenitors to Revert to an Immature State and Express Immune Cues That Support Their Migration. *J. Neurosci.* **2015**, *35*, 4–20. [CrossRef] [PubMed]

253. Gensel, J.C.; Zhang, B. Macrophage activation and its role in repair and pathology after spinal cord injury. *Brain Res.* **2015**, *1619*, 1–11. [CrossRef] [PubMed]

254. Levine, J. The reactions and role of NG2 glia in spinal cord injury. *Brain Res.* **2016**, *1638*, 199–208. [CrossRef] [PubMed]

255. Goldstein, E.Z.; Church, J.S.; Hesp, Z.C.; Popovich, P.G.; McTigue, D.M. A silver lining of neuroinflammation: Beneficial effects on myelination. *Exp. Neurol.* 2016. [CrossRef] [PubMed]

256. Setzu, A.; Lathia, J.D.; Zhao, C.; Wells, K.; Rao, M.S.; Ffrench-Constant, C.; Franklin, R.J.M. Inflammation stimulates myelination by transplanted oligodendrocyte precursor cells. *Glia* **2006**, *54*, 297–303. [CrossRef] [PubMed]

257. Miron, V.E.; Boyd, A.; Zhao, J.-W.; Yuen, T.J.; Ruckh, J.M.; Shadrach, J.L.; van Wijngaarden, P.; Wagers, A.J.; Williams, A.; Franklin, R.J.M.; et al. M2 microglia and macrophages drive oligodendrocyte differentiation during CNS remyelination. *Nat. Neurosci.* **2013**, *16*, 1211–1218. [CrossRef] [PubMed]

258. Kigerl, K.A.; Gensel, J.C.; Ankeny, D.P.; Alexander, J.K.; Donnelly, D.J.; Popovich, P.G. Identification of two distinct macrophage subsets with divergent effects causing either neurotoxicity or regeneration in the injured mouse spinal cord. *J. Neurosci.* **2009**, *29*, 13435–13444. [CrossRef] [PubMed]

259. Azari, M.F.; Profyris, C.; Karnezis, T.; Bernard, C.C.; Small, D.H.; Cheema, S.S.; Ozturk, E.; Hatzinisiriou, I.; Petratos, S. Leukemia Inhibitory Factor Arrests Oligodendrocyte Death and Demyelination in Spinal Cord Injury. *J. Neuropathol. Exp. Neurol.* **2006**, *65*, 914–929. [CrossRef] [PubMed]

260. Kerr, B.J.; Patterson, P.H. Leukemia inhibitory factor promotes oligodendrocyte survival after spinal cord injury. *Glia* **2005**, *51*, 73–79. [CrossRef] [PubMed]

261. Zang, D.W.; Cheema, S.S. Leukemia Inhibitory Factor Promotes Recovery of Locomotor Function following Spinal Cord Injury in the Mouse. *J. Neurotrauma* **2003**, *20*, 1215–1222. [CrossRef] [PubMed]

262. Rittchen, S.; Boyd, A.; Burns, A.; Park, J.; Fahmy, T.M.; Metcalfe, S.; Williams, A. Myelin repair in vivo is increased by targeting oligodendrocyte precursor cells with nanoparticles encapsulating leukaemia inhibitory factor (LIF). *Biomaterials* **2015**, *56*, 78–85. [CrossRef] [PubMed]

263. Letterio, J.J.; Roberts, A.B. REGULATION OF IMMUNE RESPONSES BY TGF-β. *Annu. Rev. Immunol.* **1998**, *16*, 137–161. [CrossRef] [PubMed]

264. McTigue, D.M.; Popovich, P.G.; Morgan, T.E.; Stokes, B.T. Localization of Transforming Growth Factor-β1 and Receptor mRNA after Experimental Spinal Cord Injury. *Exp. Neurol.* **2000**, *163*, 220–230. [CrossRef] [PubMed]

265. Hellal, F.; Hurtado, A.; Ruschel, J.; Flynn, K.C.; Laskowski, C.J.; Umlauf, M.; Kapitein, L.C.; Strikis, D.; Lemmon, V.; Bixby, J.; et al. Microtubule stabilization reduces scarring and causes axon regeneration after spinal cord injury. *Science* **2011**, *331*, 928–931. [CrossRef] [PubMed]

266. Kohta, M.; Kohmura, E.; Yamashita, T. Inhibition of TGF-β1 promotes functional recovery after spinal cord injury. *Neurosci. Res.* **2009**, *65*, 393–401. [CrossRef] [PubMed]

267. Miron, V.E. Microglia-driven regulation of oligodendrocyte lineage cells, myelination, and remyelination. *J. Leukoc. Biol.* **2017**, *101*, 1103–1108. [CrossRef] [PubMed]

268. Schonberg, D.L.; Popovich, P.G.; McTigue, D.M. Oligodendrocyte Generation Is Differentially Influenced by Toll-Like Receptor (TLR) 2 and TLR4-Mediated Intraspinal Macrophage Activation. *J. Neuropathol. Exp. Neurol.* **2007**, *66*, 1124–1135. [CrossRef] [PubMed]

269. Goldstein, E.Z.; Church, J.S.; Pukos, N.; Gottipati, M.K.; Popovich, P.G.; McTigue, D.M. Intraspinal TLR4 activation promotes iron storage but does not protect neurons or oligodendrocytes from progressive iron-mediated damage. *Exp. Neurol.* **2017**, *298*, 42–56. [CrossRef] [PubMed]

270. Schonberg, D.L.; McTigue, D.M. Iron is essential for oligodendrocyte genesis following intraspinal macrophage activation. *Exp. Neurol.* **2009**. [CrossRef] [PubMed]

271. Schonberg, D.L.; Goldstein, E.Z.; Sahinkaya, F.R.; Wei, P.; Popovich, P.G.; McTigue, D.M. Ferritin Stimulates Oligodendrocyte Genesis in the Adult Spinal Cord and Can Be Transferred from Macrophages to NG2 Cells In Vivo. *J. Neurosci.* **2012**, *32*, 5374–5384. [CrossRef] [PubMed]

272. Kigerl, K.A.; Lai, W.; Rivest, S.; Hart, R.P.; Satoskar, A.R.; Popovich, P.G. Toll-like receptor (TLR)-2 and TLR-4 regulate inflammation, gliosis, and myelin sparing after spinal cord injury. *J. Neurochem.* **2007**, *102*, 37–50. [CrossRef] [PubMed]

273. Church, J.S.; Kigerl, K.A.; Lerch, J.K.; Popovich, P.G.; McTigue, D.M. TLR4 Deficiency Impairs Oligodendrocyte Formation in the Injured Spinal Cord. *J. Neurosci.* **2016**, *36*, 6352–6364. [CrossRef] [PubMed]

274. Sauerbeck, A.; Schonberg, D.L.; Laws, J.L.; McTigue, D.M. Systemic iron chelation results in limited functional and histological recovery after traumatic spinal cord injury in rats. *Exp. Neurol.* **2013**. [CrossRef] [PubMed]

275. Sahinkaya, F.R.; Milich, L.M.; McTigue, D.M. Changes in NG2 cells and oligodendrocytes in a new model of intraspinal hemorrhage. *Exp. Neurol.* **2014**. [CrossRef] [PubMed]

276. Rathore, K.I.; Kerr, B.J.; Redensek, A.; López-Vales, R.; Jeong, S.Y.; Ponka, P.; David, S. Ceruloplasmin protects injured spinal cord from iron-mediated oxidative damage. *J. Neurosci.* **2008**, *28*, 12736–12747. [CrossRef] [PubMed]

277. Yoshimura, A.; Naka, T.; Kubo, M. SOCS proteins, cytokine signalling and immune regulation. *Nat. Rev. Immunol.* **2007**, *7*, 454–465. [CrossRef] [PubMed]

278. Schmitz, J.; Weissenbach, M.; Haan, S.; Heinrich, P.C.; Schaper, F. SOCS3 exerts its inhibitory function on interleukin-6 signal transduction through the SHP2 recruitment site of gp130. *J. Biol. Chem.* **2000**, *275*, 12848–12856. [CrossRef] [PubMed]

279. Park, K.W.; Lin, C.-Y.; Li, K.; Lee, Y.-S. Effects of Reducing Suppressors of Cytokine Signaling-3 (SOCS3) Expression on Dendritic Outgrowth and Demyelination after Spinal Cord Injury. *PLoS ONE* **2015**, *10*, e0138301. [CrossRef] [PubMed]

280. Yoshimura, A.; Suzuki, M.; Sakaguchi, R.; Hanada, T.; Yasukawa, H. SOCS, Inflammation, and Autoimmunity. *Front. Immunol.* **2012**, *3*, 20. [CrossRef] [PubMed]
281. Whyte, C.S.; Bishop, E.T.; Rückerl, D.; Gaspar-Pereira, S.; Barker, R.N.; Allen, J.E.; Rees, A.J.; Wilson, H.M. Suppressor of cytokine signaling (SOCS) 1 is a key determinant of differential macrophage activation and function. *J. Leukoc. Biol* **2011**, *90*, 845–854. [CrossRef] [PubMed]
282. Kerr, B.J.; Girolami, E.I.; Ghasemlou, N.; Jeong, S.Y.; David, S. The protective effects of 15-deoxy-Δ-12,14-prostaglandin J2 in spinal cord injury. *Glia* **2008**, *56*, 436–448. [CrossRef] [PubMed]
283. Arnold, C.E.; Whyte, C.S.; Gordon, P.; Barker, R.N.; Rees, A.J.; Wilson, H.M. A critical role for suppressor of cytokine signalling 3 in promoting M1 macrophage activation and function in vitro and in vivo. *Immunology* **2014**, *141*, 96–110. [CrossRef] [PubMed]
284. Okada, S.; Nakamura, M.; Katoh, H.; Miyao, T.; Shimazaki, T.; Ishii, K.; Yamane, J.; Yoshimura, A.; Iwamoto, Y.; Toyama, Y.; et al. Conditional ablation of Stat3 or Socs3 discloses a dual role for reactive astrocytes after spinal cord injury. *Nat. Med.* **2006**, *12*, 829–834. [CrossRef] [PubMed]
285. Hackett, A.R.; Lee, J.K. Understanding the NG2 Glial Scar after Spinal Cord Injury. *Front. Neurol.* **2016**, *7*, 199. [CrossRef] [PubMed]
286. Donnelly, D.J.; Longbrake, E.E.; Shawler, T.M.; Kigerl, K.A.; Lai, W.; Tovar, C.A.; Ransohoff, R.M.; Popovich, P.G. Deficient CX3CR1 signaling promotes recovery after mouse spinal cord injury by limiting the recruitment and activation of Ly6Clo/iNOS+ macrophages. *J. Neurosci.* **2011**, *31*, 9910–9922. [CrossRef] [PubMed]
287. Freria, C.M.; Hall, J.C.E.; Wei, P.; Guan, Z.; McTigue, D.M.; Popovich, P.G. Deletion of the Fractalkine Receptor, CX3CR1, Improves Endogenous Repair, Axon Sprouting, and Synaptogenesis after Spinal Cord Injury in Mice. *J. Neurosci.* **2017**, *37*, 3568–3587. [CrossRef] [PubMed]
288. Patel, J.R.; McCandless, E.E.; Dorsey, D.; Klein, R.S. CXCR4 promotes differentiation of oligodendrocyte progenitors and remyelination. *Proc. Natl. Acad. Sci. USA* **2010**, *107*, 11062–11067. [CrossRef] [PubMed]
289. Jaerve, A.; Müller, H.W. Chemokines in CNS injury and repair. *Cell Tissue Res.* **2012**, *349*, 229–248. [CrossRef] [PubMed]
290. Patel, J.R.; Williams, J.L.; Muccigrosso, M.M.; Liu, L.; Sun, T.; Rubin, J.B.; Klein, R.S. Astrocyte TNFR2 is required for CXCL12-mediated regulation of oligodendrocyte progenitor proliferation and differentiation within the adult CNS. *Acta Neuropathol.* **2012**, *124*, 847–860. [CrossRef] [PubMed]
291. Tirotta, E.; Kirby, L.A.; Hatch, M.N.; Lane, T.E. IFN-γ-induced apoptosis of human embryonic stem cell derived oligodendrocyte progenitor cells is restricted by CXCR2 signaling. *Stem Cell Res.* **2012**, *9*, 208–217. [CrossRef] [PubMed]
292. Omari, K.M.; Lutz, S.E.; Santambrogio, L.; Lira, S.A.; Raine, C.S. Neuroprotection and Remyelination after Autoimmune Demyelination in Mice that Inducibly Overexpress CXCL1. *Am. J. Pathol.* **2009**, *174*, 164–176. [CrossRef] [PubMed]
293. Filipovic, R.; Zecevic, N. The effect of CXCL1 on human fetal oligodendrocyte progenitor cells. *Glia* **2008**, *56*, 1–15. [CrossRef] [PubMed]
294. Omari, K.M.; John, G.R.; Sealfon, S.C.; Raine, C.S. CXC chemokine receptors on human oligodendrocytes: implications for multiple sclerosis. *Brain* **2005**, *128*, 1003–1015. [CrossRef] [PubMed]
295. Omari, K.M.; John, G.; Lango, R.; Raine, C.S. Role for CXCR2 and CXCL1 on glia in multiple sclerosis. *Glia* **2006**, *53*, 24–31. [CrossRef] [PubMed]
296. Niu, W.; Zeng, X. The Application of Stem Cell Based Tissue Engineering in Spinal Cord Injury Repair. *J. Tissue Sci. Eng.* **2015**, *6*. [CrossRef]
297. Duncan, G.J.; Plemel, J.R.; Assinck, P.; Manesh, S.B.; Muir, F.G.W.; Hirata, R.; Berson, M.; Liu, J.; Wegner, M.; Emery, B.; et al. Myelin regulatory factor drives remyelination in multiple sclerosis. *Acta Neuropathol.* **2017**, *134*, 403–422. [CrossRef] [PubMed]

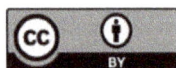

neuroglia

MDPI

Article

Sequential Contribution of Parenchymal and Neural Stem Cell-Derived Oligodendrocyte Precursor Cells toward Remyelination

David R. Serwanski [1], Andrew L. Rasmussen [1], Christopher B. Brunquell [1], Scott S. Perkins [1] and Akiko Nishiyama [1,2,3,*]

[1]   Department of Physiology and Neurobiology, University of Connecticut, 75 North Eagleville Road, Storrs, CT 06269-3156, USA; drsbeek@gmail.com (D.R.S.); andy.l.rasmussen@gmail.com (A.L.R.); christopherbrunquell@gmail.com (C.B.B.); scoperk11@gmail.com (S.S.P.)
[2]   Institute for Systems Genomics, University of Connecticut, Storrs, CT 06269, USA
[3]   Institute for Brain and Cognitive Science, University of Connecticut, Storrs, CT 06269, USA
*   Correspondence: akiko.nishiyama@uconn.edu

Received: 1 May 2018; Accepted: 4 June 2018; Published: 12 June 2018

Abstract: In the adult mammalian forebrain, oligodendrocyte precursor cells (OPCs), also known as NG2 glia are distributed ubiquitously throughout the gray and white matter. They remain proliferative and continuously generate myelinating oligodendrocytes throughout life. In response to a demyelinating insult, OPCs proliferate rapidly and differentiate into oligodendrocytes which contribute to myelin repair. In addition to OPCs, neural stem cells (NSCs) in the subventricular zone (SVZ) also contribute to remyelinating oligodendrocytes, particularly in demyelinated lesions in the vicinity of the SVZ, such as the corpus callosum. To determine the relative contribution of local OPCs and NSC-derived cells toward myelin repair, we performed genetic fate mapping of OPCs and NSCs and compared their ability to generate oligodendrocytes after acute demyelination in the corpus callosum created by local injection of α-lysophosphatidylcholine (LPC). We have found that local OPCs responded rapidly to acute demyelination, expanded in the lesion within seven days, and produced oligodendrocytes by two weeks after lesioning. By contrast, NSC-derived NG2 cells did not significantly increase in the lesion until four weeks after demyelination and generated fewer oligodendrocytes than parenchymal OPCs. These observations suggest that local OPCs could function as the primary responders to repair acutely demyelinated lesion, and that NSCs in the SVZ contribute to repopulating OPCs following their depletion due to oligodendrocyte differentiation.

Keywords: demyelination; oligodendrocyte precursor; myelin; subventricular zone; NG2; neural stem cell

---

1. Introduction

In the mammalian central nervous system (CNS), oligodendrocyte precursor cells (OPCs), also known as NG2 glia or polydendrocytes, represent a fourth major glial cell population that persists in the adult and continue to proliferate and generate myelinating oligodendrocytes throughout life, even after developmental myelination is largely completed (reviewed in [1,2]). Studies in the adult rat spinal cord have shown that OPCs proliferate in response to acute demyelination, and that the proliferated cells differentiate into oligodendrocytes [3–5]. Oligodendrocyte precursor cells in the telencephalon also contribute to remyelination of acute and chronic demyelinated lesions [3,6,7]. Genetic fate mapping has allowed more precise determination of the fate of OPCs under normal conditions [8–11] and established that the postnatal fate of OPCs is restricted to oligodendrocytes. This approach was also used to confirm that OPCs are an important source of remyelinating oligodendrocytes that repair demyelinated lesions [12,13].

In addition to local proliferating NG2 glia, the adult brain also contains neural stem cells (NSCs) that reside in the subventricular zone (SVZ). Neural stem cells in the adult SVZ pass through a transit-amplifying progenitor stage as they differentiate into neuroblasts that migrate through the rostral migratory stream (RMS) into the olfactory bulb, and their multipotential ability to generate astrocytes as well as neurons has been well characterized [14,15]. When demyelination occurs in the vicinity of the SVZ, cells in the SVZ become mobilized and may contribute to remyelination [16–18]. The availability of genetic fate mapping tools to identify the fate of OPCs and NSCs have allowed a direct comparison of the contribution of local OPCs and SVZ-derived cells toward myelin repair, and several studies were published recently with varying results. While two studies suggest a robust ability of NSCs to generate remyelinating oligodendrocytes [19,20], another recent study suggests that although SVZ cells proliferate in response to acute demyelination, they are unable to produce oligodendrocytes that contribute to myelin repair [21]. We have used Tg(Cspg4-creER^{TM}) and Tg(Nes-creER^{T2}) transgenic mice crossed to a reporter line and have compared the ability of local OPCs and nestin+ NSCs to generate oligodendrocytes in response to acute demyelination caused by α-lysophosphatidylcholine (LPC) injection into the adult corpus callosum. We show that local OPCs generate oligodendrocytes more rapidly than NSCs, whereas NSCs contribute to repopulating OPCs in the corpus callosum after myelin repair.

2. Materials and Methods

2.1. Animals

A bacterial artificial chromosome (BAC) transgenic mouse line expressing tamoxifen-inducible Cre in OPCs (Tg(Cspg4-creER^{TM}) [9]; Jackson Laboratory stock #008538, Bar Harbor, ME, USA) was crossed to the cre reporter gt(ROSA)26Sor$^{tm1(EYFP)}$ (YFP) [22] (Jackson Laboratory stock #006148) and maintained as double homozygotes. Tg(Nes-creER^{T2}) mice were obtained from Dr. Amelia Eisch (University of Pennsylvania, Philadelphia, PA, USA) [23] and also crossed to YFP mice. Cre was induced by four consecutive days of intraperitoneal injection of 1 mg of 4-hydroxytamoxifen (4OHT, Sigma H-7904, St. Louis, MO, USA) every 12 h, as previously described [9].

To create acute demyelinating lesions, 1 μL of 2% LPC in phosphate-buffered saline (PBS) was stereotaxically injected into the right rostral corpus callosum using a Hamilton syringe at the coordinates (−1.3 mm from the bregma, 1 mm lateral, and 1.7 mm from the surface of the skull). Mice were sacrificed at 7, 14, and 28 days after LPC injection (7, 14, and 28 dpl) by intracardiac perfusion of 4% paraformaldehyde in 0.1 M sodium phosphate buffer, pH 7.4, containing 0.1 M L-lysine and 0.01 M sodium metaperiodate. Brains were isolated and post-fixed in the same fixative for 2 h at 4 °C. For NG2creER;YFP mice, LPC injection was performed three days after the last 4OHT injection. For Tg(Nes-creER^{T2}):gt(ROSA)26Sor$^{tm1(EYFP)}$ mice, LPC injection was performed 28 days after 4OHT injection to allow for greater accumulation of YFP+ cells in the SVZ.

All animal procedures were approved by the Institutional Animal Care and Usage Committee in a protocol A16-018 "NG2 cells in the neural network" from June 24, 2016 through June 23, 2019.

2.2. Tissue Processing and Immunohistochemistry

Serial 50 μm coronal sections were cut on a vibratome (Leica VTS1000, Leica Biosystems Inc., Buffalo Grove, IL, USA) and stored at −20 °C in 98-well plates in cryostorage solution consisting of 10 g of polyvinylpyrolidone, 500 mL 0.2 M sodium phosphate buffer, pH 7.4, 300 g sucrose, and 300 mL ethylene glycol in 1 L. Sections were processed for immunohistochemistry as previously described [9]. The primary antibodies used are listed in Table 1. Secondary antibodies were Alexa 488-labeled anti-chick antibody (1:1000), Cy3-labeled anti-mouse, rabbit, or goat (1:200), and Cy5- (1:100) or Alexa 647-labeled (1:200) anti-mouse, rabbit, or goat antibodies from Jackson ImmunoResearch (West Grove, PA, USA). Five or six sections from each mouse that were 600 μm apart were labeled with the antibodies and mounted with Vectashield containing 4′,6-diamidino-2-phenylindole dihydrochloride

(DAPI, Vector Labs, Burlingame, CA, USA). Stained sections were analyzed on Leica TCS SP2 or SP8 confocal microscope and Zeiss Axiovert 200 M with ORCA ER camera and apotome (Carl Zeiss Microscopy, Jena, Germany).

Table 1. Primary antibodies used.

Antibody	Host Species	Source	Dilution
Dcx	Rabbit	Cell Signaling Technology (Danvers, MA, USA)	1:300
NG2	Rabbit	EMD Millipore (Burlington, MA, USA)	1:500
Pdgfra	Goat	R&D Systems (Minneapolis, MN, USA)	1:1000
CC1 (Quaking 7)	Mouse	EMD Millipore (Burlington, MA, USA)	1:100
MBP, smi99 antibody	Mouse	Covance (Princeton, NJ, USA)	1:3000
Smi32	Mouse	Covance (Princeton, NJ, USA)	1:1000
GFP	Chick	Aves Labs (Tigard, OR, USA)	1:1000
Olig2	Mouse	EMD Millipore (Burlington, MA, USA)	1:1000
Olig2	Rabbit	Novus Biologicals (Littleton, CO, USA)	1:1000
PSA-NCAM, 12E3 antibody	Mouse	Dr. Tatsunori Seki (Tokyo Medical University, Tokyo, Japan)	1:1000
GFAP	Rabbit	DAKO-Agilent (Santa Clara, CA, USA)	1:2000

Dcx: Doublecortin; Pdgfra: Platelet-derived growth factor receptor α; MBP: Myelin basic protein; Smi32: Non-phosphorylated neurofilaments; GFP: Green fluorescent protein; Olig2: Oligodendrocyte transcription factor 2; PSA-NCAM: Polysialic acid-neural cell adhesion molecule; GFAP: Glial fibrillary acidic protein.

2.3. Cell Quantification

Demyelinated lesions were assessed by a combination of immunolabeling for myelin basic protein (MBP) and non-phosphorylated neurofilaments. For quantification, a series of tiled confocal z-stack images were collected over a z-distance of 20–30 μm, encompassing the lesion from at least two sections for each animal. Cell numbers were estimated by scoring each YFP+ cell for the expression of specific antigens within a defined area for each section. The area for quantification was defined as the area that lacked MBP immunofluorescence in adjacent sections for the early time points. For later time points, the lesioned and repaired areas were defined as areas that contained dense reactive NG2 glia and astrocytes. To obtain the density of the cells, the area from which cell numbers were obtained was calculated using ImageJ [24] and multiplied by the thickness of the z-stack.

2.4. Statistical Analysis

Quantification results are expressed as mean ± standard deviation. Statistical analyses were performed using two-way analysis of variance (ANOVA) with uncorrected Fisher's least significant difference (LSD) test for the quantification of % YFP+ cells that were NG2+ or CC1+ and the density of YFP+ NG2+ and YFP+ CC1+ cells. Student's t-test (two-way, unpaired) was used for the quantification of the percentage of CC1+ cells derived from NG2+ or nestin+ precursor cells over 14 days. Sample sizes ranged from three to four.

3. Results

3.1. Evolution of LPC-Induced Demyelinated Lesion

In the normal adult mouse corpus callosum, MBP was robustly detected in the corpus callosum, and there was little detectable non-phosphorylated neurofilaments, with the exception of axons in the cingulate cortex (Figure 1A–C). Injection of LPC into the corpus callosum resulted in focal demyelination, characterized by a well demarcated loss of MBP immunoreactivity at 7 days after lesioning (dpl) (Figure 1D–F, arrowheads in D), accompanied by increased immunoreactivity for non-phosphorylated neurofilaments, which have been shown to increase in demyelinated axons [25]. By 14 dpl, the area of demyelinated lesion had decreased, and a substantial amount of myelin had been regenerated, while non-phosphorylated neurofilaments were still present. By 28 dpl, the lesion was indistinguishable from the surrounding myelinated region in the majority of the animals. The evolution of the lesion was consistent with previously published reports (for example, [26]).

3.2. Contribution of Local OPCs to Remyelinating Oligodendrocytes

To investigate the extent to which local OPCs contribute to remyelination, we used Tg(Cspg4-creER^{TM};gt(ROSA)26Sor$^{tm1(EYFP)}$ (NG2-YFP) double transgenic mice. The fate of local OPCs was followed during the course of demyelination and remyelination by activating cre-mediated recombination and YFP expression in OPCs 3–4 days prior to LPC injection (Figure 2A). One day after the last tamoxifen injection, 40–50% of OPCs in the corpus callosum were YFP+ [9]. We induced cre before LPC injection to avoid activating YFP expression in macrophages that could also express NG2 [27]. This regimen also minimized labeling of SVZ progenitor cells that were mobilized and upregulated NG2 expression after demyelination.

To determine the dynamics of oligodendrocyte differentiation from parenchymal OPCs, we determined the percentage of YFP+ cells that were NG2+ oligodendrocyte precursor cells or CC1+ differentiated oligodendrocytes at 7, 14, and 28 dpl. At 7 dpl, when there was a well-defined demyelinated lesion characterized by a lack of MBP reactivity, clusters of YFP+ cells were seen in and around the lesion suggestive of local proliferation (Figure 2B,C). Among the YFP+ cells, 80% were NG2+, while only 10% were CC1+ oligodendrocytes (Figure 2E,K,L). By 14 dpl, the proportion of YFP+ cells that were NG2+ decreased to 62%, while the proportion of YFP+ cells that were CC1+ increased to 44% (Figure 2D,E,K,L), and clusters of YFP+ CC1+ cells were found inside the lesion (Figure 2F,G). Some YFP+ cells expressed both NG2 and CC1, which suggests that OPCs were rapidly differentiating into CC1+ oligodendrocytes. Outside the lesion, both YFP+ NG2+ cells and YFP+ CC1+ oligodendrocytes were detected as well (Figure 2H). The proportion of YFP+ cells that were CC1+ in and around the lesion at 14 dpl was more than 4-fold greater than that at 7 dpl, suggesting that OPCs that were recruited to the lesion were undergoing oligodendrocyte differentiation. At 28 dpl, the proportion of YFP+ cells that were NG2+ remained at 63%, while the proportion of YFP+ cells that were CC1+ decreased slightly to 30% (Figure 2I–L).

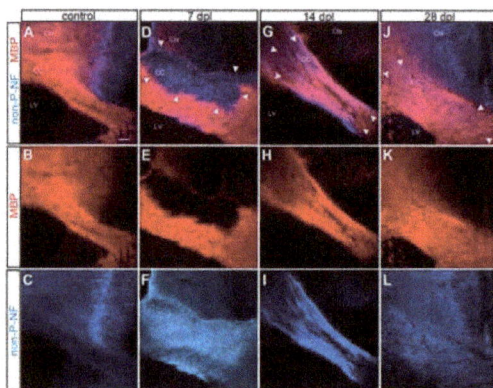

Figure 1. Evolution of α-lysophosphatidylcholine (LPC)-induced demyelinated lesion. Immunofluorescence labeling for myelin basic protein (MBP) and non-phosphorylated neurofilaments. (**A–C**) Control unlesioned brain. Intact MBP+ myelin in the corpus callosum. Non-phosphorylated neurofilaments are restricted to the neurons in the cingulate cortex. Ctx: cortex, CC: corpus callosum, LV: lateral ventricle. (**D–F**) Demyelinated corpus callosum at 7 days post lesioning (dpl) showing a well-defined lesion lacking MBP and upregulated non-phosphorylated neurofilaments. Boundary of the lesion is indicated by arrowheads. (**G–I**) Demyelinated corpus callosum at 14 dpl showing partial remyelination, characterized by uneven MBP labeling and persistent presence non-phosphorylated neurofilaments. (**J–L**) Remyelinated corpus callosum at 28 dpl showing uniform MBP labeling and reduced levels of non-phosphorylated neurofilaments, though they are higher than unlesioned corpus callosum. Scale bar: 100 μm.

When we examined the density of total YFP+ cells and YFP+ NG2+ cells, there was no significant difference between 7 and 14 dpl, but a 3-fold increase at 28 dpl (Figures 2J and 3P,Q). By contrast, the density of YFP+ CC1+ cells continued to rise from 7 to 28 dpl (Figure 3R). This suggests that after demyelination local OPCs already proliferated by 7 dpl and actively generated oligodendrocytes over the course of four weeks. The increase in the density of YFP+ NG2+ cells at 28 dpl likely reflects continued proliferation of local OPCs that existed prior to demyelination, as well as migration of OPCs from the surrounding areas into the lesion and the surrounding corpus callosum.

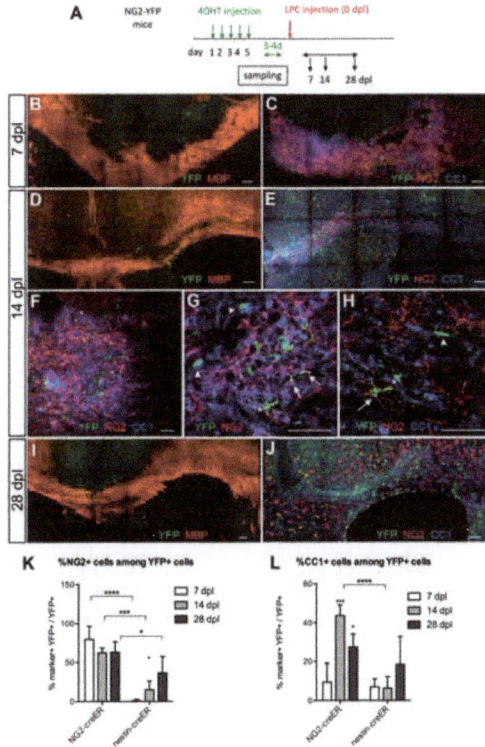

Figure 2. Response of local oligodendrocyte precursor cells (OPCs) to LPC-induced demyelination in the corpus callosum. (**A**) Scheme showing the experimental outline. (**B,C**) Lesion at 7 dpl. Low magnification images of immunolabeling for MBP and yellow fluorescent protein (YFP) showing an area of demyelination (**B**) and immunolabeling for YFP, NG2, and CC1 showing scattered YFP+NG2+ cells in the lesion (**C**). (**D–H**) Lesion at 14 dpl. Low magnification images of immunolabeling for MBP and YFP showing partially remyelinated lesion (**D**), characterized by uneven MBP staining, and immunolabeling for YFP, NG2, and CC1 showing increased number of YFP+ cells in the lesion (**E,F**). Higher magnification shows a significant proportion of YFP+ cells express CC1 (arrowheads), while other YFP+ cells are NG2+ (arrows). Some YFP+ cells express both NG2 and CC1 (asterisks) at varying ratios. (**G**) is a higher magnification of the lesion. (**H**) is from a site further away from the lesion. (**I,J**) Lesion at 28 dpl. Immunolabeling for MBP and YFP shows largely repaired lesion (**I**) and a cluster of YFP+CC1+ cells in the center of the repaired lesion while YFP+ NG2+ cells are seen at the periphery (**J**). Scale bars: 100 μm for (**B–F**) and (**I,J**); 50 μm for (**F–H**). (**K,L**) The proportion of YFP+ cells that were NG2+ (**K**) or CC1+ (**L**) in Tg(Cspg4-creER^{TM};gt(ROSA)26Sor$^{tm1(EYFP)}$ (NG2-YFP) and Tg(Nes-creER^{T2});gt(ROSA)26Sor$^{tm1(EYFP)}$ (nestin-YFP) mice. * $p < 0.05$, *** $p < 0.001$, **** $p < 0.0001$. $n = 3$, two-way ANOVA, uncorrected Fisher's least significant difference (LSD) test.

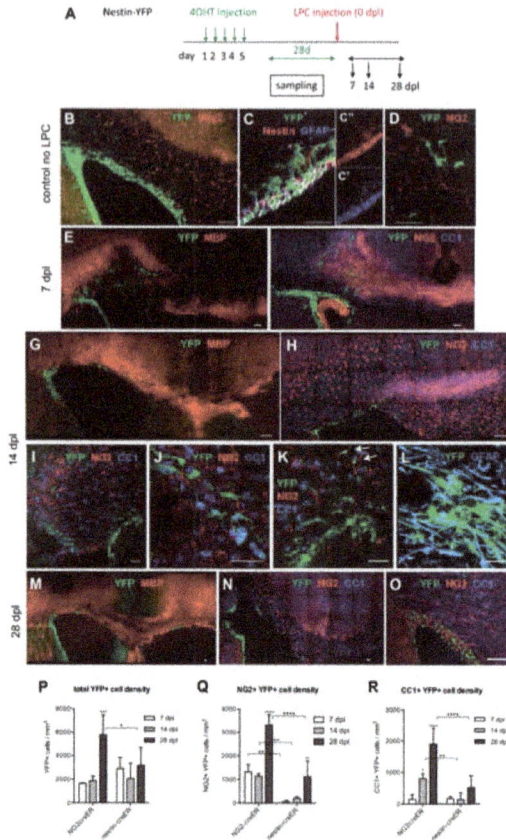

Figure 3. Response of subventricular zone (SVZ) cells to LPC-induced demyelination in the corpus callosum. (**A**) Scheme showing the experimental outline. (**B–D**) The distribution and phenotype of YFP+ cells prior to LPC injection. The majority of the YFP+ cells are found in the SVZ (**B**) and very few of the YFP+ cells expressed Olig2. The majority of the YFP+ cells expressed nestin and GFAP (**C**) but not NG2 (**D**). (**E,F**) Lesion at 7 dpl. Low magnification images of MBP and YFP immunolabeling showing an area of demyelination with YFP+ cells mostly above the lateral ventricle (**E**) and immunolabeling for YFP, NG2, and CC1 showing that most of the YFP+ cells are neither NG2+ nor CC1+. There is strongly upregulated NG2 immunoreactivity throughout the lesion. Note that YFP+ cells line the SVZ. Some YFP+ cells appear to be migrating toward the needle track (arrows). (**G–L**) Lesion at 14 dpl. Low magnification of immunolabeling for MBP and YFP showing partially remyelinated lesion (**G**) and immunolabeling for YFP, NG2, and CC1 showing a slightly increased number of YFP+ cells in the lesion (**H**). Higher magnification shows that most of the YFP+ cells were confined to the lesion border (**I**). Higher magnification of **I** shows that most of the YFP+ cells did not express NG2 or CC1. (**J**) A region from the periphery of the lesion above the lateral angle of SVZ showing two YFP+ NG2+ cells (arrowheads). Some of the large, YFP+ cells were glial fibrillary acidic protein (GFAP)+ (**L**). (**M–O**) Lesion at 28 dpl. YFP and MBP labeling show remyelinated lesion with increased YFP+ cells in the lesion (**M**) and that the majority of the YFP+ cells were NG2+ (**N**). (**O**) Control mouse injected with PBS and stained for YFP, NG2, and CC1 at 28 dpl, showing that the majority of the YFP+ cells are confined to the SVZ and few YFP+ cells were detectable in the corpus callosum. Scale bar: 50 μm. (**P–R**) The density of YFP+ cells (**P**), YFP+ NG2+ cells (**Q**), and YFP+ CC1+ cells at 7, 14, and 28 dpl in NG2-YFP and nestin-YFP mice. * $p < 0.05$, ** $p < 0.01$, *** $p < 0.001$, **** $p < 0.0001$. n = 3–4, two-way ANOVA, uncorrected Fisher's LSD.

3.3. Contribution of SVZ-Derived Cells to Remyelinating Oligodendrocytes

Distribution and Phenotype of YFP+ Cells in Tg(Nes-creER^{T2});gt(ROSA)26Sor$^{tm1(EYFP)}$ Mice

To assess the contribution of SVZ progenitor cells to remyelination, we performed a similar experiment in Tg(Nes-creER^{T2});gt(ROSA)26Sor$^{tm1(EYFP)}$ (nestin-YFP) mice. We induced YFP in nestin+ progenitor cells in the SVZ 28 days prior to LPC injection, as the YFP labeling efficiency was too low immediately after tamoxifen injection (Figure 3A). At 28 days after tamoxifen injection, YFP expression was detected in 30–50% of nestin+ cells in dorsal and dorsolateral SVZ, as well as in medial and latera SVZ and the rostral migratory stream (RMS). Thus, the YFP labeling efficiency among nestin+ NSCs with this induction protocol was comparable to the efficiency among OPCs in NG2cre-YFP mice. In this study, we focused on YFP+ cells in the dorsal and dorsolateral SVZ and the corpus callosum of nestin-YFP mice. Almost 90% of the YFP+ cells resided in the SVZ, where they expressed nestin and glial fibrillary acidic protein (GFAP), two proteins known to be expressed by NSCs in the SVZ (Doetsch et al., 1999) (Figure 3B,C). A small fraction of YFP+ cells in the SVZ expressed the oligodendrocyte transcription factor Olig2, and most of the Olig2+ YFP+ cells were located in the outer layers of the SVZ. Of the YFP+ cells, 11.7% were in the corpus callosum, mostly above the dorsolateral angle of the SVZ (Figure 3B, upper left). Among the YFP+ cells in the corpus callosum, 64% were GFAP+, 47% were nestin+, and 77% were positive for the polysialylated form of neural cell adhesion molecule (PSA-NCAM), which is known to be expressed by neuroblasts and neural progenitor cells in the neurogenic niches of the SVZ and dentate subgranular zone [28,29], as well as on growing axons that are defasciculating at the target [30,31]. Among the YFP+ cells in the corpus callosum, 7.5% expressed NG2 (Figure 3D), and only 0.8% of the total YFP+ cells in the corpus callosum and in the dorsal and dorsolateral SVZ expressed NG2 prior to LPC injection.

3.4. Response of Nestin+ SVZ Cells to Acute Demyelination

To examine whether nestin+ SVZ progenitor cells generated OPCs that were recruited to acutely demyelinated lesions in the corpus callosum, we examined the changes in YFP+ NG2+ and YFP+ CC1+ cells in nestin-YFP mice over the course of four weeks after LPC injection. At the time of peak demyelination at 7 dpl, we saw an infiltration of YFP+ cells in the demyelinated corpus callosum (Figure 3E). In addition to scattered YFP+ cells in the demyelinated corpus callosum, there was a line of YFP+ cells that extended into the injection site in the more rostral sections that had the needle track (e.g., Figure 3F, arrowheads). Fewer than 3% of the YFP+ cells were NG2+ (Figures 2K and 3F), in stark contrast to NG2-YFP mice in which 80% of the YFP+ cells were NG2+ (Figure 2K).

By 14 dpl, 18% of the YFP+ cells had become NG2+, but the density of YFP+ NG2+ cells remained less than one-fourth of that in NG2-YFP mice (Figure 3G,H,Q). Many of the YFP+ cells, including those found in the lesion, had large polygonal cell bodies that were morphologically distinct from oligodendrocyte lineage cells, and some expressed GFAP (Figure 3J–L). Some YFP+ NG2+ cells with typical polydendrocyte morphology were found at the border of the lesion (Figure 3K, upper right). The percentage of YFP+ CC1+ oligodendrocytes in nestin-YFP mice did not increase from 7 dpl to 14 dpl (Figure 2L). Neither did the density of YFP+ CC1+ cells increase from 7 to 14 dpl (Figure 3R) and remained 5.7-fold lower than that in NG2-YFP mice.

At 28 dpl, the most notable change was that the density of YFP+ NG2+ cells in nestin-YFP mice increased 5.3-fold over that at 14 dpl (Figure 3Q). The average density of YFP+ CC1+ oligodendrocytes in these mice at 28 dpl was three-fold higher than at 14 dpl but did not reach statistical significance ($p = 0.0876$) and remained 3.6-fold lower than the density of YFP+ CC1+ cells in NG2-YFP mice at 28 dpl. Thus, between 14 and 28 dpl, NSC-derived cells seemed to be most actively generating OPCs, while the parenchymal OPCs were actively producing oligodendrocytes between 7 and 14 dpl, having expanded the precursor population earlier, by 7 dpl. The density of NSC-derived OPCs in the lesion at 28 dpl reached a comparable level to that of OPCs derived from the local population seen at 7 and 14 dpl. These observations indicate that after acute demyelination, local parenchymal OPCs initially responded more rapidly and robustly than SVZ-derived cells to produce oligodendrocytes, and the response of NSCs lagged behind by 2–3 weeks.

To further evaluate the contribution of parenchymal OPCs and NSC-derived cells in the supply of oligodendrocytes to the lesion, we estimated the proportion of total CC1+ oligodendrocytes in the dorsal aspect of the corpus callosum that were generated from parenchymal OPCs or NSCs at 14 dpl, as previously estimated in the normal adult corpus callosum [9,11]. We obtained the percentage of CC1+ oligodendrocytes that were YFP+ in NG2-YFP and nestin-YFP mice at 14 dpl and adjusted for the recombination efficiency in the respective mice. We found that 0.222% and 0.060% of CC1+ oligodendrocytes were generated from local OPCs and nestin+ NSCs, respectively, during the two weeks after demyelination. Thus, NG2-YFP mice had generated 4.3 times more CC1+ oligodendrocytes than nestin-YFP mice ($p = 0.0188$). This corroborates the other quantifications and indicates that after acute demyelination, local OPCs were more likely to contribute to remyelinating oligodendrocytes than SVZ-derived oligodendrocyte lineage cells.

The density of total YFP+ cells and YFP+ NG2+ cells in nestin-YFP mice was more than two-fold greater at 28 dpl than at 14 dpl. In contrast to clusters of YFP+ cells found at 7 and 14 dpl, many YFP+ NG2+ cells at 28 dpl were distributed more uniformly throughout the remyelinated and neighboring corpus callosum (Figure 3M,N). In PBS-injected mice, very few YFP+ cells were detected in the corpus callosum, similar to uninjured mice prior to LPC injection (Figure 3O). This suggests that demyelination triggered SVZ cells to generate oligodendrocyte lineage cells, and that the SVZ-derived cells were likely to be contributing to the replenishment of the OPC population that had been depleted due to their differentiation into remyelinating oligodendrocytes.

3.5. Transient Migration of NSC-Derived Neuroblasts into Corpus Callosum after Demyelination

We noticed that the dorsal SVZ was thicker in LPC-injected mice than in control PBS-injected mice. When we measured the height of the dorsal SVZ at 28 dpl, it was approximately two-fold greater in LPC-injected mice compared to PBS-injected control mice (Figure 4A,B), suggesting that there was sustained proliferative activity in the SVZ after remyelination had occurred. We examined the cellular composition in the dorsal SVZ that was expanded after demyelination. Previous studies had described PSA-NCAM+ and doublecortin (Dcx)+cells that emerged from the SVZ into acutely demyelinated corpus callosum [16,18,32]. In the SVZ at 14 dpl, we also found large clusters of PSA-NCAM+ and Dcx+ cells, many of which co-expressed the two antigens and had small, round, or oval cell bodies and long slender processes (Figure 4C,D). Some of them were also YFP+ in nestin-YFP mice. These YFP+ cells had a distinct morphology from flat polygonal NSCs that were YFP+ nestin+, suggesting that they were progeny of the NSCs.

In the corpus callosum of control PBS-injected mice, there were very few PSA-NCAM+ Dcx+ cells at 14 dpl (Figure 4E). In LPC-injected mice, a larger number of PSA-NCAM+ Dcx+ cells were seen migrating into the corpus callosum, mostly from the dorsolateral angle of the SVZ (Figure 4F–H). Their processes were oriented parallel to the axons in the corpus callosum, and many had the typical unipolar tadpole shape, as previously described [16,18], consistent with their neuroblast identity (see Figure 4H, top left cell that is also YFP+).

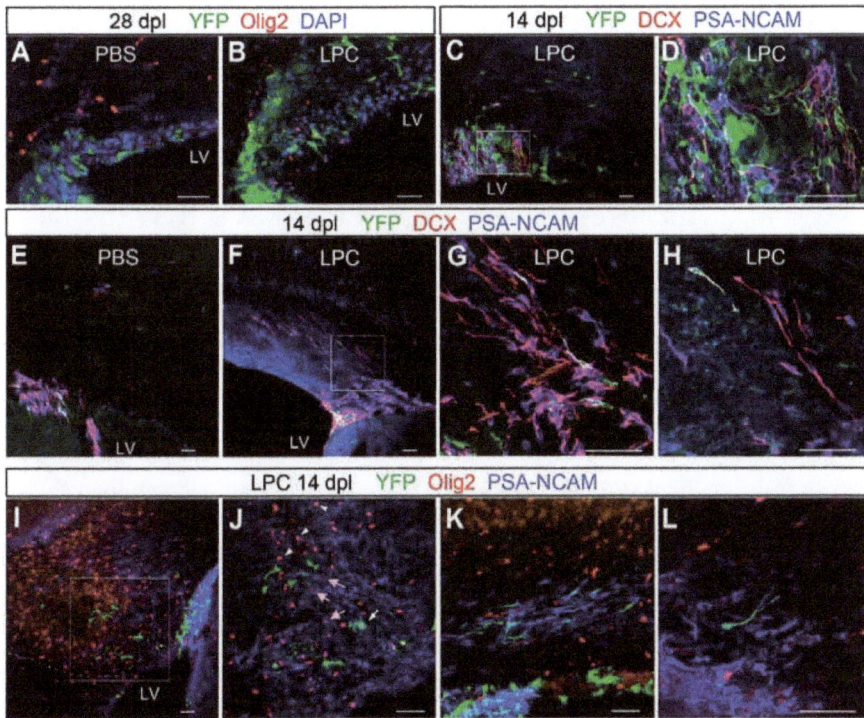

Figure 4. Changes in subventricular zone (SVZ) cells after LPC-induced demyelination. (**A,B**) Immunolabeling for YFP, Olig2, and DAPI showing increased thickness of the dorsal SVZ 28 days after LPC injection (**B**) compared with PBS-injected control (**A**). Very few Olig2+ cells are found in the control SVZ after PBS injection, whereas several Olig2+ cells are detected in the thickened SVZ after LPC injection. (**C,D**) Immunolabeling for doublecortin (Dcx) and PSA-NCAM showing that many of the YFP+ cells co-express Dcx and PSA-NCAM. (**D**) represents a higher magnification of the boxed area in C. (**E–H**) Immunolabeling for YFP, Dcx, and (PSA-NCAM) showing that most of the Dcx/PSA-NCAM+ cells are confined to the SVZ in control (**E**), whereas LPC-injected animals show a greater number of Dcx+ PSA-NCAM+ cells migrating dorsally into the SVZ (**F–H**). (**H**) is a higher magnification image of the boxed area in (**F**). (**I,J**) Immunolabeling for YFP, Olig2, and PSA-NCAM near the lesion (dotted line) at 14 dpl. There is a dense cluster of PSA-NCAM+ cells in the lateral angle of the SVZ (right side in I). Higher magnification of the boxed area in (**I**), showing a YFP+ cell that is also PSA-NCAM+ (**J**, white arrow). There is a cluster of strongly Olig2+ cells inside the lesion (arrowheads in (**J**)), and weakly Olig2+ PSA-NCAM+ cells are detected at the lesion border (pink arrows in (**J**)). (**K,L**) PSA-NCAM+ cells, some of which are YFP+, appear to be migrating in the corpus callosum in clusters (**K**), and many of them have a tadpole-shaped unipolar morphology (**L**). Scale bar: 50 µm.

To examine whether PSA-NCAM+ or Dcx+ cells contributed to the repair of the demyelinated lesion, we examined the phenotype and distribution of YFP+ PSA-NCAM+ cells in nestin-YFP mice after demyelination. At 14 dpl, many PSA-NCAM+ cells were found at the periphery of the lesion, while very few were seen in the core of the lesion where there was a high density of Olig2+ cells (Figure 4I,J). While the majority of the cells inside the lesion that were strongly positive for Olig2 did not express PSA-NCAM (Figure 4J, arrowheads), a few weakly Olig2+ cells around the lesion also expressed PSA-NCAM (Figure 4J, arrows). Most of the PSA-NCAM+ cells around the lesion were YFP-negative in nestin-YFP mice, suggesting that they had been generated from cells that were already neuroblasts or transit amplifying cells by the time of LPC injection. There were occasional clusters of PSA-NCAM+ cells oriented parallel to each other but not necessarily in the direction of the demyelinated lesion (Figure 4K,L). Some of the PSA-NCAM+ cells had the typical tadpole morphology, with their leading edge pointing away from the SVZ, suggestive of emigration from the SVZ into the corpus callosum. At 28 dpl, fewer than 2% of the PSA-NCAM+ cells expressed Olig2, and the majority of PSA-NCAM+ cells appeared to remain as migrating neuroblasts. These findings suggest that acute demyelination triggered emigration of PSA-NCAM+ Dcx+ neuroblasts from the SVZ. However, during the four weeks after demyelination, we did not detect a significant contribution of YFP+ PSA-NCAM+ cells into the lesion, even at 28 dpl when we saw a significant number of YFP+ NG2+ cells in the corpus callosum. This makes it more likely that many of the NSC-derived OPCs that populated the corpus callosum after remyelination had directly differentiated into oligodendrocyte lineage cells from NSCs, rather than having passed through an intermediate stage of PSA-NCAM+ Dcx+ neuroblasts.

4. Discussion

We have shown that after chemically induced acute demyelination in the adult corpus callosum, local OPCs were rapidly recruited to the demyelinated lesion where they generated oligodendrocytes by 14 dpl. By contrast, nestin+ SVZ cells expanded and migrated into the lesion but did so after a delay of two weeks and continued to generate OPCs in the corpus callosum through 28 dpl when remyelination had already occurred. These observations suggest that local OPCs provide the major source of myelin repair after acute demyelination, while NSCs in the SVZ are an important source of repopulating the OPC population following their loss due to their differentiation into remyelinating oligodendrocytes.

4.1. Oligodendroglial Fate of Local Parenchymal OPCs and NSCs in the SVZ

It is well established that parenchymal OPCs that reside in the corpus callosum proliferate and generate remyelinating cells after an acute demyelinating injury created by local LPC injection [6], reviewed in [1,33]. There is also evidence that PSA-NCAM+ and/or Dcx+ neuroblasts in the SVZ migrate toward an acutely demyelinated lesion in the corpus callosum, although it has remained uncertain as to whether they generate remyelinating cells [16,18,34], see below).

The cuprizone-induced demyelinating model is another commonly used demyelination model with a more protracted time course. In mice fed on a cuprizone diet, demyelination occurs over five to six weeks, and remyelination ensues over the two to six weeks after the mice are returned to normal diet [35,36]. Moreover, if mice are continued on the cuprizone diet for 12 weeks, persistent demyelination occurs with poor remyelination [7]. Two recent studies used Tg(Nes-creER^{T2}) mice and Tg(Pdgfra-creER^{T2}) mice crossed to the ROSA-YFP reporter mice to compare the fate of NSCs and parenchymal OPCs, respectively, during the remyelination phase of cuprizone-induced demyelination [19,20]. In both studies, the progeny of NSCs, particularly those in rostral corpus callosum, robustly generated remyelinating oligodendrocytes to a greater extent than local OPCs. Furthermore, in regions above the SVZ, NSC-derived oligodendrocytes produced thicker myelin than local NG2 cell-derived oligodendrocytes [19].

On the contrary, another recent study used Tg(GFAP-creER^{T2}) crossed to the YFP reporter to examine the fate of GFAP+ NSCs in the SVZ following LPC-induced acute demyelination [21]. Despite a robust proliferative response in the SVZ in both the young and old mice, NSC-derived cells generated only a very small fraction of oligodendrocyte lineage cells, and the vast majority of oligodendrocyte lineage cells in the remyelinated lesion were generated from parenchymal cells [21], consistent with an earlier imaging study [37]. In our LPC-induced demyelination model, our observations were similar to the Kazanis study in that we found a greater contribution of local OPCs to oligodendrocyte regeneration but differed in that we saw a more significant influx of SVZ-derived OPCs by 28 dpl.

4.2. Temporal and Regional Determinants of Mobilizing Local OPCs and SVZ Cells

The difference between our findings and those from the cuprizone studies may be partly attributed to the temporal difference in the evolution of myelin damage and repair in the cuprizone and LPC models. The more robust remyelination, mediated by the progeny of NSCs in the cuprizone model, could be because the SVZ has had time to expand during the prolonged two to six weeks of demyelination stage, and that two to seven days of demyelination in the LPC lesion was too short for these responses to occur in the SVZ. The increased density of NSC-derived OPCs in the lesioned corpus callosum that we observed at 28 dpl is consistent with this, as is the observation that oligodendrocyte production from NSCs does not occur during the first four weeks [19]. Other studies that examined the response of more differentiated progeny of neural stem cells such as PSA-NCAM+ or Dcx+ neuroblasts in the SVZ have observed a more rapid response [16,18,32].

In the two cuprizone studies described above, the progeny of NSCs contribute significantly more to remyelination in the rostral corpus callosum, whereas local OPCs contribute more toward remyelination in the caudal corpus callosum. This could reflect the normal physiological dynamics of SVZ cells in rostral and caudal corpus callosum [38] and may reflect a greater abundance of oligodendrogliogenic progenitor cells in the caudal SVZ. In our experiments, LPC was injected into the rostral corpus callosum, and in most mice, demyelination spread laterally and caudally, so that the center of the demyelinated lesion typically occurred more than 500 μm caudal from the injection site. Thus, our observation that local OPCs generated oligodendrocytes before NSC-derived cells did reflect the location of the demyelinated lesion. In addition to the rostro-caudal difference, there is medio-lateral heterogeneity among NSCs, those with oligodendroglial fate potential being more abundant along the dorsal SVZ than in the dorsolateral angle, where neurogenic NSCs reside [39].

4.3. Plasticity of Neuronal and Oligodendrocyte Lineages in the SVZ

The SVZ constitutes one of the two neurogenic niches in the mammalian CNS where neural stem cells reside and continue to generate new neurons and glia in the adult. Cells isolated from the adult mouse SVZ undergo self-renewal and can be induced to generate astrocytes, neurons, and a few oligodendrocytes [14,39,40]. Under normal physiological conditions, oligodendrocytes are a minor fate among the cells of the SVZ [41]. The adult mouse SVZ consists of nestin+ GFAP+ neural stem cells, PSA-NCAM+ Dcx+ neuroblasts that migrate through the RMS to the olfactory bulb, and rapidly amplify type C cells, which express Distal-less homeobox 2 (Dlx2) and give rise to neuroblasts [15,42]. In the SVZ, committed oligodendrocyte lineage cells are sparse, and importantly, OPCs are distinct from GFAP+ neural stem cells, rapidly proliferating type C cells, and Dcx+ neuroblasts [43].

After acute demyelination in the corpus callosum, PSA-NCAM+/Dcx+ progeny of NSCs, likely to be neuroblasts, extensively proliferate and migrate out of the SVZ toward the demyelinated lesion [16,18]. In response to an inflammatory lesion, the number of oligodendrocyte lineage cells increase in the SVZ at the expense of neurons in the olfactory bulb, resulting in impaired olfactory memory, suggesting plasticity of neuronal and glial fates of SVZ stem cells [17]. However, because oligodendrocyte lineage cells, particularly OPCs, actively transcribe low levels of neuronally expressed genes such as Dcx, Dlx2, and glutamic acid decarboxylase 67 (Gad1) [2], it has been a challenge to study the fate of neuroblasts or type C cells [18,43]. Thus, it still remains unclear whether demyelination triggers reprogramming of normally neuronally committed NSCs or their progeny or amplifies oligodendrocyte-fated NSC cell clones.

4.4. Mechanisms that Could Affect Oligodendrogliogenesis from the SVZ

Local OPCs in the corpus callosum are capable of sensing a change in the degree of myelination or oligodendrocyte density and rapidly expand to repair the deficit [6,44]. Nestin+ NSCs, on the other hand, require two to three weeks to initiate the program to produce oligodendrocyte lineage cells, but given the necessary time, they can migrate and generate OPCs. How might a demyelinating lesion in the corpus callosum signal to the SVZ? Some proposed mechanisms include soluble factors such as netrin-1 [45] and epidermal growth factor [46] that promote emigration of cells out of the SVZ, and factors such as chordin [18], and Wnt7 [39] that promote oligodendroglial fate of NSCs. Besides these positive signals, negative regulators of oligodendrogliogenesis such as Gli1 [47], neurofibromin 1 [48], and Drosha [49] are beginning to be uncovered. How these mechanisms are coordinately regulated in response to demyelination remains to be elucidated.

5. Conclusions

In summary, we have shown that after acute demyelination in the corpus callosum, local OPCs rapidly expand and differentiate into remyelinating oligodendrocytes within the first two weeks. By contrast, NSCs in the SVZ begin their oligodendrogliogenic program with a temporal delay of two weeks, resulting in an increased population of SVZ-derived OPCs by four weeks after demyelination. The SVZ may be a limited source for repopulating OPCs, as it becomes depleted after sustained or repeated demyelination [20], which often occurs in chronic cases of multiple sclerosis (MS). Furthermore, the potential of SVZ-derived supply of OPCs in MS would be limited to lesions near the SVZ. Interestingly, NG2 cell density declines after remyelination of acutely demyelinated lesion in the spinal cord [3], while OPCs in the corpus callosum maintain their ability to self-renew even after prolonged cuprizone treatment for 12 weeks [20]. Further elucidation of the differences in the cellular properties of newly generated OPCs and those that have been residing in the white matter for an extended period of time could lead to new strategies to harness the ubiquitous population of local OPCs with enhanced ability for myelin repair.

Author Contributions: The study was conceived and developed by D.R.S. and A.N. D.R.S., S.S.P. and A.N. performed the experiments. A.L.R., S.S.P., C.C.B. and A.N. analyzed the data and performed the quantification. A.N. and D.R.S. wrote the manuscript.

Funding: The work was supported by grants from the National Institutes of Health (NIH) (R01NS049267, R01NS074870, and R01 NS073425 to AN), the National Multiple Sclerosis Society (RG4579A5/1 to AN), and Connecticut Stem Cell Program (06SCB03 to AN). The Leica SP8 confocal microscope was purchased using NIH Shared Instrumentation Grant S10OD016435 (PI, AN) and is maintained by Chris O'Connell, Director of Advanced Microscopy Facility.

Acknowledgments: We thank Youfen Sun for maintaining the mouse colony. We thank Amelia Eisch (University of Pennsylvania, Philadelphia, PA, USA) for the Tg(Nes-creER^{T2}) mice and Tatsunori Seki (Tokyo Medical University) for the monoclonal 12E3 antibody to PSA-NCAM. We thank William Wood (University of Connecticut, Physiology and Neurobiology) for discussions and critical reading of the manuscript.

Conflicts of Interest: The authors declare no conflicts of interest.

References

1. Nishiyama, A.; Komitova, M.; Suzuki, R.; Zhu, X. Polydendrocytes (NG2 cells): Multifunctional cells with lineage plasticity. *Nat. Rev. Neurosci.* **2009**, *10*, 9–22. [CrossRef] [PubMed]
2. Nishiyama, A.; Boshans, L.; Goncalves, C.M.; Wegrzyn, J.; Patel, K.D. Lineage, fate, and fate potential of NG2-glia. *Brain Res.* **2016**, *1638 (Pt B)*, 116–128. [CrossRef] [PubMed]
3. Keirstead, H.S.; Levine, J.M.; Blakemore, W.F. Response of the oligodendrocyte progenitor cell population (defined by NG2 labelling) to demyelination of the adult spinal cord. *Glia* **1998**, *22*, 161–170. [CrossRef]
4. Di Bello, C.I.; Dawson, M.R.; Levine, J.M.; Reynolds, R. Generation of oligodendroglial progenitors in acute inflammatory demyelinating lesions of the rat brain stem is associated with demyelination rather than inflammation. *J. Neurocytol.* **1999**, *28*, 365–381. [CrossRef] [PubMed]
5. Watanabe, M.; Toyama, Y.; Nishiyama, A. Differentiation of proliferated NG2-positive glial progenitor cells in a remyelinating lesion. *J. Neurosci. Res.* **2002**, *69*, 826–836. [CrossRef] [PubMed]
6. Gensert, J.M.; Goldman, J.E. Endogenous progenitors remyelinate demyelinated axons in the adult CNS. *Neuron* **1997**, *19*, 197–203. [CrossRef]

7. Mason, J.L.; Toews, A.; Hostettler, J.D.; Morell, P.; Suzuki, K.; Goldman, J.E.; Matsushima, G.K. Oligodendrocytes and progenitors become progressively depleted within chronically demyelinated lesions. *Am. J. Pathol.* **2004**, *164*, 1673–1682. [CrossRef]

8. Dimou, L.; Simon, C.; Kirchhoff, F.; Takebayashi, H.; Gotz, M. Progeny of Olig2-expressing progenitors in the gray and white matter of the adult mouse cerebral cortex. *J. Neurosci.* **2008**, *28*, 10434–10442. [CrossRef] [PubMed]

9. Zhu, X.; Hill, R.A.; Dietrich, D.; Komitova, M.; Suzuki, R.; Nishiyama, A. Age-dependent fate and lineage restriction of single NG2 cells. *Development* **2011**, *138*, 745–753. [CrossRef] [PubMed]

10. Kang, S.H.; Fukaya, M.; Yang, J.K.; Rothstein, J.D.; Bergles, D.E. NG2+ CNS glial progenitors remain committed to the oligodendrocyte lineage in postnatal life and following neurodegeneration. *Neuron* **2010**, *68*, 668–681. [CrossRef] [PubMed]

11. Young, K.M.; Psachoulia, K.; Tripathi, R.B.; Dunn, S.J.; Cossell, L.; Attwell, D.; Tohyama, K.; Richardson, W.D. Oligodendrocyte dynamics in the healthy adult CNS: Evidence for myelin remodeling. *Neuron* **2013**, *77*, 873–885. [CrossRef] [PubMed]

12. Tripathi, R.B.; Rivers, L.E.; Young, K.M.; Jamen, F.; Richardson, W.D. NG2 glia generate new oligodendrocytes but few astrocytes in a murine experimental autoimmune encephalomyelitis model of demyelinating disease. *J. Neurosci.* **2010**, *30*, 16383–16390. [CrossRef] [PubMed]

13. Zawadzka, M.; Rivers, L.E.; Fancy, S.P.; Zhao, C.; Tripathi, R.; Jamen, F.; Young, K.; Goncharevich, A.; Pohl, H.; Rizzi, M.; et al. CNS-resident glial progenitor/stem cells produce Schwann cells as well as oligodendrocytes during repair of CNS demyelination. *Cell Stem Cell* **2010**, *6*, 578–590. [CrossRef] [PubMed]

14. Reynolds, B.A.; Weiss, S. Generation of neurons and astrocytes from isolated cells of the adult mammalian central nervous system. *Science* **1992**, *255*, 1707–1710. [CrossRef] [PubMed]

15. Doetsch, F.; Caille, I.; Lim, D.A.; Garcia-Verdugo, J.M.; Alvarez-Buylla, A. Subventricular zone astrocytes are neural stem cells in the adult mammalian brain. *Cell* **1999**, *97*, 703–716. [CrossRef]

16. Nait-Oumesmar, B.; Decker, L.; Lachapelle, F.; Avellana-Adalid, V.; Bachelin, C.; Van Evercooren, A.B. Progenitor cells of the adult mouse subventricular zone proliferate, migrate and differentiate into oligodendrocytes after demyelination. *Eur. J. Neurosci.* **1999**, *11*, 4357–4366. [CrossRef] [PubMed]

17. Tepavcevic, V.; Lazarini, F.; Alfaro-Cervello, C.; Kerninon, C.; Yoshikawa, K.; Garcia-Verdugo, J.M.; Lledo, P.M.; Nait-Oumesmar, B.; Baron-Van Evercooren, A. Inflammation-induced subventricular zone dysfunction leads to olfactory deficits in a targeted mouse model of multiple sclerosis. *J. Clin. Investig.* **2011**, *121*, 4722–4734. [CrossRef] [PubMed]

18. Jablonska, B.; Aguirre, A.; Raymond, M.; Szabo, G.; Kitabatake, Y.; Sailor, K.A.; Ming, G.L.; Song, H.; Gallo, V. Chordin-induced lineage plasticity of adult SVZ neuroblasts after demyelination. *Nat. Neurosci.* **2010**, *13*, 541–550. [CrossRef] [PubMed]

19. Xing, Y.L.; Roth, P.T.; Stratton, J.A.; Chuang, B.H.; Danne, J.; Ellis, S.L.; Ng, S.W.; Kilpatrick, T.J.; Merson, T.D. Adult neural precursor cells from the subventricular zone contribute significantly to oligodendrocyte regeneration and remyelination. *J. Neurosci.* **2014**, *34*, 14128–14146. [CrossRef] [PubMed]

20. Brousse, B.; Magalon, K.; Durbec, P.; Cayre, M. Region and dynamic specificities of adult neural stem cells and oligodendrocyte precursors in myelin regeneration in the mouse brain. *Biol. Open* **2015**, *4*, 980–992. [CrossRef] [PubMed]

21. Kazanis, I.; Evans, K.A.; Andreopoulou, E.; Dimitriou, C.; Koutsakis, C.; Karadottir, R.T.; Franklin, R.J.M. Subependymal zone-derived oligodendroblasts respond to focal demyelination but fail to generate myelin in young and aged mice. *Stem Cell Reports* **2017**, *8*, 685–700. [CrossRef] [PubMed]

22. Srinivas, S.; Watanabe, T.; Lin, C.S.; William, C.M.; Tanabe, Y.; Jessell, T.M.; Costantini, F. Cre reporter strains produced by targeted insertion of EYFP and ECFP into the ROSA26 locus. *BMC Dev. Biol.* **2001**, *1*, 4. [CrossRef]

23. Lagace, D.C.; Whitman, M.C.; Noonan, M.A.; Ables, J.L.; DeCarolis, N.A.; Arguello, A.A.; Donovan, M.H.; Fischer, S.J.; Farnbauch, L.A.; Beech, R.D.; et al. Dynamic contribution of nestin-expressing stem cells to adult neurogenesis. *J. Neurosci.* **2007**, *27*, 12623–12629. [CrossRef] [PubMed]

24. Schneider, C.A.; Rasband, W.S.; Eliceiri, K.W. NIH Image to ImageJ: 25 years of image analysis. *Nat. Methods* **2012**, *9*, 671–675. [CrossRef] [PubMed]

25. Trapp, B.D.; Peterson, J.; Ransohoff, R.M.; Rudick, R.; Mork, S.; Bo, L. Axonal transection in the lesions of multiple sclerosis. *N. Engl. J. Med.* **1998**, *338*, 278–285. [CrossRef] [PubMed]

26. Miron, V.E.; Boyd, A.; Zhao, J.W.; Yuen, T.J.; Ruckh, J.M.; Shadrach, J.L.; van Wijngaarden, P.; Wagers, A.J.; Williams, A.; Franklin, R.J.; et al. M2 microglia and macrophages drive oligodendrocyte differentiation during CNS remyelination. *Nat. Neurosci.* **2013**, *16*, 1211–1218. [CrossRef] [PubMed]

27. Kucharova, K.; Stallcup, W.B. Distinct NG2 proteoglycan-dependent roles of resident microglia and bone marrow-derived macrophages during myelin damage and repair. *PLoS ONE* **2017**, *12*, e0187530. [CrossRef] [PubMed]

28. Seki, T.; Arai, Y. Highly polysialylated neural cell adhesion molecule (NCAM-H) is expressed by newly generated granule cells in the dentate gyrus of the adult rat. *J. Neurosci.* **1993**, *13*, 2351–2358. [CrossRef] [PubMed]

29. Doetsch, F.; Garcia-Verdugo, J.M.; Alvarez-Buylla, A. Cellular composition and three-dimensional organization of the subventricular germinal zone in the adult mammalian brain. *J. Neurosci.* **1997**, *17*, 5046–5061. [CrossRef] [PubMed]

30. Rutishauser, U.; Landmesser, L. Polysialic acid on the surface of axons regulates patterns of normal and activity-dependent innervation. *Trends Neurosci.* **1991**, *14*, 528–532. [CrossRef]

31. Rutishauser, U.; Landmesser, L. Polysialic acid in the vertebrate nervous system: A promoter of plasticity in cell-cell interactions. *Trends Neurosci.* **1996**, *19*, 422–427. [CrossRef]

32. Picard-Riera, N.; Decker, L.; Delarasse, C.; Goude, K.; Nait-Oumesmar, B.; Liblau, R.; Pham-Dinh, D.; Baron-Van Evercooren, A. Experimental autoimmune encephalomyelitis mobilizes neural progenitors from the subventricular zone to undergo oligodendrogenesis in adult mice. *Proc. Natl. Acad. Sci. USA* **2002**, *99*, 13211–13216. [CrossRef] [PubMed]

33. Franklin, R.J.; Ffrench-Constant, C. Remyelination in the CNS: From biology to therapy. *Nat. Rev. Neurosci.* **2008**, *9*, 839–855. [CrossRef] [PubMed]

34. Menn, B.; Garcia-Verdugo, J.M.; Yaschine, C.; Gonzalez-Perez, O.; Rowitch, D.; Alvarez-Buylla, A. Origin of oligodendrocytes in the subventricular zone of the adult brain. *J. Neurosci.* **2006**, *26*, 7907–7918. [CrossRef] [PubMed]

35. Blakemore, W.F. Observations on oligodendrocyte degeneration, the resolution of status spongiosus and remyelination in cuprizone intoxication in mice. *J. Neurocytol.* **1972**, *1*, 413–426. [CrossRef] [PubMed]

36. Ludwin, S.K. Central nervous system demyelination and remyelination in the mouse. *Lab. Investig.* **1978**, *39*, 597–612. [PubMed]

37. Guglielmetti, C.; Praet, J.; Rangarajan, J.R.; Vreys, R.; De Vocht, N.; Maes, F.; Verhoye, M.; Ponsaerts, P.; Van der Linden, A. Multimodal imaging of subventricular zone neural stem/progenitor cells in the cuprizone mouse model reveals increased neurogenic potential for the olfactory bulb pathway, but no contribution to remyelination of the corpus callosum. *Neuroimage* **2014**, *86*, 99–110. [CrossRef] [PubMed]

38. Luskin, M.B. Restricted proliferation and migration of postnatally generated neurons derived from the forebrain subventricular zone. *Neuron* **1993**, *11*, 173–189. [CrossRef]

39. Ortega, F.; Gascon, S.; Masserdotti, G.; Deshpande, A.; Simon, C.; Fischer, J.; Dimou, L.; Chichung Lie, D.; Schroeder, T.; Berninger, B. Oligodendrogliogenic and neurogenic adult subependymal zone neural stem cells constitute distinct lineages and exhibit differential responsiveness to Wnt signalling. *Nat. Cell Biol.* **2013**, *15*, 602–613. [CrossRef] [PubMed]

40. Gonzalez-Perez, O.; Alvarez-Buylla, A. Oligodendrogenesis in the subventricular zone and the role of epidermal growth factor. *Brain Res. Rev.* **2011**, *67*, 147–156. [CrossRef] [PubMed]

41. Maki, T.; Liang, A.C.; Miyamoto, N.; Lo, E.H.; Arai, K. Mechanisms of oligodendrocyte regeneration from ventricular-subventricular zone-derived progenitor cells in white matter diseases. *Front Cell Neurosci.* **2013**, *7*, 275. [CrossRef] [PubMed]

42. Komitova, M.; Zhu, X.; Serwanski, D.R.; Nishiyama, A. NG2 cells are distinct from neurogenic cells in the postnatal mouse subventricular zone. *J. Comp. Neurol.* **2009**, *512*, 702–716. [CrossRef] [PubMed]

43. Dayer, A.G.; Cleaver, K.M.; Abouantoun, T.; Cameron, H.A. New GABAergic interneurons in the adult neocortex and striatum are generated from different precursors. *J. Cell Biol.* **2005**, *168*, 415–427. [CrossRef] [PubMed]

44. Bu, J.; Banki, A.; Wu, Q.; Nishiyama, A. Increased NG2(+) glial cell proliferation and oligodendrocyte generation in the hypomyelinating mutant shiverer. *Glia* **2004**, *48*, 51–63. [CrossRef] [PubMed]

45. Cayre, M.; Courtes, S.; Martineau, F.; Giordano, M.; Arnaud, K.; Zamaron, A.; Durbec, P. Netrin 1 contributes to vascular remodeling in the subventricular zone and promotes progenitor emigration after demyelination. *Development* **2013**, *140*, 3107–3117. [CrossRef] [PubMed]

46. Aguirre, A.; Dupree, J.L.; Mangin, J.M.; Gallo, V. A functional role for EGFR signaling in myelination and remyelination. *Nat. Neurosci.* **2007**, *10*, 990–1002. [CrossRef] [PubMed]

47. Samanta, J.; Grund, E.M.; Silva, H.M.; Lafaille, J.J.; Fishell, G.; Salzer, J.L. Inhibition of Gli1 mobilizes endogenous neural stem cells for remyelination. *Nature* **2015**, *526*, 448–452. [CrossRef] [PubMed]

48. Sun, G.J.; Zhou, Y.; Ito, S.; Bonaguidi, M.A.; Stein-O'Brien, G.; Kawasaki, N.K.; Modak, N.; Zhu, Y.; Ming, G.L.; Song, H. Latent tri-lineage potential of adult hippocampal neural stem cells revealed by Nf1 inactivation. *Nat. Neurosci.* **2015**, *18*, 1722–1724. [CrossRef] [PubMed]

49. Rolando, C.; Erni, A.; Grison, A.; Beattie, R.; Engler, A.; Gokhale, P.J.; Milo, M.; Wegleiter, T.; Jessberger, S.; Taylor, V. Multipotency of adult hippocampal NSCs in vivo is restricted by Drosha/NFIB. *Cell Stem Cell* **2016**, *19*, 653–662. [CrossRef] [PubMed]

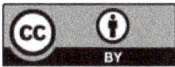

neuroglia

MDPI

Article

Action Potential Firing Induces Sodium Transients in Macroglial Cells of the Mouse *Corpus Callosum*

Behrouz Moshrefi-Ravasdjani, Daniel Ziemens, Nils Pape, Marcel Färfers and Christine R. Rose *

Institute of Neurobiology, Faculty of Mathematics and Natural Sciences, Heinrich Heine University Düsseldorf, Universitätsstrasse 1, D-40225 Düsseldorf, Germany; Behrouz.Moshrefi-Ravasdjani@hhu.de (B.M.-R.); Daniel.Ziemens@hhu.de (D.Z.); nipap101@uni-duesseldorf.de (N.P.); Marcel.Faerfers@hhu.de (M.F.)
* Correspondence: rose@hhu.de; Tel.: +49-211-81-13416

Received: 14 June 2018; Accepted: 27 June 2018; Published: 3 July 2018

Abstract: Recent work has established that glutamatergic synaptic activity induces transient sodium elevations in grey matter astrocytes by stimulating glutamate transporter 1 (GLT-1) and glutamate-aspartate transporter (GLAST). Glial sodium transients have diverse functional consequences but are largely unexplored in white matter. Here, we employed ratiometric imaging to analyse sodium signalling in macroglial cells of mouse *corpus callosum*. Electrical stimulation resulted in robust sodium transients in astrocytes, oligodendrocytes and NG2 glia, which were blocked by tetrodotoxin, demonstrating their dependence on axonal action potentials (APs). Action potential-induced sodium increases were strongly reduced by combined inhibition of ionotropic glutamate receptors and glutamate transporters, indicating that they are related to release of glutamate. While AMPA receptors were involved in sodium influx into all cell types, oligodendrocytes and NG2 glia showed an additional contribution of NMDA receptors. The transporter subtypes GLT-1 and GLAST were detected at the protein level and contributed to glutamate-induced glial sodium signals, indicating that both are functionally relevant for glutamate clearance in *corpus callosum*. In summary, our results demonstrate that white matter macroglial cells experience sodium influx through ionotropic glutamate receptors and glutamate uptake upon AP generation. Activity-induced glial sodium signalling may thus contribute to the communication between active axons and macroglial cells.

Keywords: astrocyte; oligodendrocyte; NG2 cell; SBFI; glutamate; GLT-1; GLAST

1. Introduction

In the grey matter of the vertebrate brain, astrocytes can be subject to transient activity-related increases in their sodium concentration, which can either be local or global depending on neuronal activity patterns [1,2]. A major pathway for the generation of these astrocyte sodium transients is the activation of sodium-dependent glutamate uptake in response to synaptic release of glutamate [3–7]. Glutamate uptake by grey matter astrocytes is realized by two transporter subtypes, namely glutamate transporter 1 (GLT-1) and glutamate-aspartate transporter (GLAST) [8,9].

Activity-related astrocyte sodium transients have been suggested to serve important functional roles in the interaction between neurons and astrocytes. Sodium increases caused by glutamate transport activate the astrocytic Na^+/K^+-ATPase, leading to the consumption of cellular ATP and thereby stimulating glial metabolism and lactate production, a key step in the so-called astrocyte-neuron lactate shuttle [10,11]. Moreover, sodium influx into astrocytes changes the driving force for sodium-dependent secondary active transporters. For example, this may result in the reversal of the plasma membrane Na^+/Ca^{2+}-exchanger (NCX), which then switches from a calcium exporter to an importer for calcium, contributing to intracellular calcium increases under both physiological and pathophysiological conditions [12–15].

In contrast to grey matter, the properties of sodium signalling in white matter glia are largely unexplored. While white matter tracts do not feature classical chemical synapses between neurons, axons can release glutamate in an activity-dependent manner (e.g., [16–19]). It is also established that white matter macroglia express sodium-dependent glutamate transporters, which are especially important to protect the tissue from glutamate-induced excitotoxicity [20–24]. In line with this, we could recently demonstrate that application of glutamate results in sodium transients in astrocytes and cells of the oligodendroglial lineage (representing mature oligodendrocytes as well as NG2 cells) in tissue slices of *corpus callosum* of the mouse, which were strongly dampened upon pharmacological inhibition of glutamate uptake in both groups [25]. Furthermore, we found that sodium not only propagated intercellularly between gap-junction coupled astrocytes, but also from astrocytes to oligodendrocytes and NG2 cells. This indicates that the different macroglia cell types in this white matter area are directly functionally coupled [25].

In addition to glutamate transporters, white matter macroglia express a large repertoire of receptors for different transmitters [26,27]. Their activation upon action potential (AP) propagation triggers calcium signals in astrocytes in the optic nerve and *corpus callosum*, involving both glutamate and purine receptors [19,28–30]. Axonal AP propagation and glutamate release moreover activate α-amino-3-hydroxy-5-methyl-4-isoxazolepropionic acid (AMPA) and N-methyl-D-aspartate (NMDA) receptors expressed on the myelin sheath, inducing intracellular calcium signals in the myelin compartment and stimulating oligodendrocyte glycolysis [27]. In NG2 cells, calcium signals are generated upon opening of AMPA receptors [17,19,31–33].

While it is thus established that glial cells in white matter can undergo calcium signalling in response to axonal AP firing [26,27], it is not known, if axonal activity does induce detectable increases in the sodium concentration of surrounding macroglial cells. In the present study, we addressed this question by performing quantitative ratiometric imaging with the fluorescent sodium indicator sodium-binding benzofurane isophthalate (SBFI) in acute tissue slices of the juvenile mouse *corpus callosum*. Using pharmacological tools, different genetically-modified mice, immunohistochemistry, and immunoblotting, we investigated the cellular pathways of sodium influx into the main macroglial cell types, namely astrocytes, oligodendrocytes, and NG2 glia.

2. Materials and Methods

2.1. Animals, Tissue Preparation, and Salines

The present study was carried out in strict accordance with the institutional guidelines of the Heinrich Heine University Düsseldorf and the European Community Council Directive (86/609/EEC). All experiments were communicated to and approved by the Animal Welfare Office at the Animal Care and Use Facility of the Heinrich Heine University Düsseldorf (institutional act number: O50/05) in accordance with the recommendations of the European Commission [34]. In accordance with the German Animal Welfare Act (Tierschutzgesetz, Articles 4 and 7), no formal additional approval for the post-mortem removal of brain tissue was necessary.

Coronal tissue slices (250 µm) were prepared from mouse *corpus callosum* (*Mus musculus*, Balb/C; postnatal days (P) 15-20; both sexes). Moreover, the following transgenic animals were used (P15-20; both sexes): NG2/EYFP knock-in mice, in which enhanced yellow fluorescent protein (EYFP) is expressed under the control of the NG2 promoter [35]; connexin knock-out (Cx-k.o.) mice that display astrocyte-directed conditional deletion of *connexin43* as well as additional, unrestricted deletion of *connexin30* [36]; and GLAST-k.o. mice that feature inactivation of the gene for GLAST [37]. In accordance with the recommendations of the European Commission (published in "Euthanasia of experimental animals," Luxembourg: Office for Official Publications of the European Communities, 1997; ISBN 92-827-9694-9), mice were anaesthetized with CO_2 before the animals were quickly decapitated for slice preparation.

For imaging experiments, *corpus callosum* slices were prepared in ice-cold saline composed of (in mM): 125 NaCl, 2.5 KCl, 2 CaCl$_2$, 1 MgCl$_2$, 1.25 NaH$_2$PO$_4$, 26 NaHCO$_3$, and 20 glucose, bubbled with 95% O$_2$ and 5% CO$_2$, resulting in a pH of 7.4. After slice preparation, the tissue was kept at 34 °C for 20 min in saline containing 0.5–1 μM sulforhodamine 101 (SR101) for specific labelling of astrocytes [38]. Afterwards, slices were incubated in SR101-free saline and kept at room temperature (20–22 °C). Experiments were performed at room temperature as well.

2.2. Sodium Imaging and Electrophysiology

For intracellular sodium imaging, sodium-binding benzofuran isophthalate-acetoxymethyl ester (SBFI-AM) (TEFLabs Inc., Austin, TX, USA), the membrane-permeant form of SBFI, was injected into the *corpus callosum*, following a procedure reported before [39]. Ratiometric wide-field sodium imaging was performed as described earlier in detail [4] using a variable scan digital imaging system (Nikon NIS-Elements v4.3, Nikon GmbH Europe, Düsseldorf, Germany) attached to an upright microscope (Nikon Eclipse FN-PT, Nikon GmbH Europe, Düsseldorf, Germany) equipped with 40×/N.A. 0.8 LUMPlanFI water immersion objective (Olympus Deutschland GmbH, Hamburg, Germany) and an orca FLASH V2 camera (Hamamatsu Photonics Deutschland GmbH, Herrsching, Germany).

Excitation light was generated by a PolychromeV monochromator (TILL Photonics, Martinsried, Germany). SBFI was alternately excited at 340 and 380 nm at 5 Hz and resulting emission was collected >440 nm. Fluorescence was evaluated in regions of interest (ROI) positioned around SBFI-labelled cell bodies. Signals were background-corrected as described before [4,40] and analysed using OriginPro Software (OriginLab Corporation, Northampton, MA, USA). The fluorescence ratio was calculated from the emission at single wavelengths (F_{340}/F_{380}). SBFI fluorescence was calibrated in situ as described earlier [4,39].

Corpus callosum axons were electrically stimulated using a saline-filled glass pipette with a tip diameter of around 1 μM connected to an isolated stimulator (A-M systems, Model 2100, Sequim, WA, USA). A train of rectangular electrical pulses (250 μsec/50–80 V) was delivered at 50 Hz for 0.5 s to evoke APs. Local field potentials were recorded using a glass electrode (1-3 MΩ resistance) connected to a HEKA EPC10 patch amplifier and analysed with Patchmaster software (HEKA electronics, Lambrecht, Germany).

In several sets of experiments, glutamate (1 mM) was focally ejected into the *corpus callosum* through a fine glass micropipette attached to a pressure application device (PDES-02D, NPI Electronic GmbH, Tamm, Germany). All other substances were applied with the bath perfusion. The following blockers were used: tetrodotoxin, TTX (Biotrend, Köln, Germany); (3S)-3-[[3-[[4-(Trifluoromethyl)benzoyl] amino]phenyl]methoxy]-L-aspartic acid, TFB-TBOA (Tocris, Bristol, UK), 2-amino-5-phosphonopentanoic acid, AP5 (Cayman chemical, Hamburg, Germany); 2,3-Dihydroxy-6-nitro-7-sulfamoyl-benzo(F) quinoxaline, NBQX (Biotrend, Köln, Germany); dihydrokainate, DHK (Tocris, Bristol, UK).

2.3. Immunohistochemistry

Balb/C mouse brains of both sexes (P15-17) were fixed in 0.1 M PBS (phosphate buffered saline) containing 4% PFA (paraformaldehyde) at 4 °C for 24 h. Then, 30 μm coronal slices of the *corpus callosum* were prepared with a vibratome. For indirect immunostainings, sections were first incubated in blocking solution comprised of normal goat serum (Gibco/Life Technologies, Darmstadt, Germany; 5% in PBS, 1 h) and TritonX-100 (Sigma-Aldrich Chemical, Munich, Germany, 0.4%). Afterwards, sections were incubated in blocking solution (overnight, 4 °C) containing primary antibodies guinea pig anti-GLT1 (Merck Millipore, Darmstadt, Germany, 1:1000), mouse anti-GLAST (Miltenyi, Bergisch Gladbach, Germany, 1:100), rabbit anti-GLAST (Tocris, Bristol, UK, 1:1000), rabbit anti-glial fibrillary acidic protein (GFAP) (DAKO, Santa Clara, CA, USA, 1:1000), and mouse anti-CC1 (GeneTex, Irvine, CA, USA, 1:250). Mouse anti-NG2 (Merck Millipore, Darmstadt, Germany, 1:100) was incubated for 19 h at room temperature.

Finally, sections were incubated in secondary antibody solution (PBS with 0.4% TritonX-100, 1 h) containing goat anti-mouse Alexa 488 or 594 (1:500), goat anti-rabbit Alexa 488 or 594 (1:500) and goat anti-guinea pig Alexa 488 (1:500). In control sections, the primary antibodies were omitted from the protocol. The sections were coverslipped in Mowiol (Calbiochem, Fluka, distributed by Sigma-Aldrich Chemical, Munich, Germany).

Image z-stacks (10–20 optical sections, 0.3–0.5 µm each) were captured using a motorized confocal laser scanning microscope (Nikon Eclipse C1, Nikon Instruments, Düsseldorf, Germany), equipped with a Nikon 60×/1.4 oil objective. Adequate excitation was realized through argon (488 nm) and helium-neon (543 nm) and 407 nm lasers. The parameters of image acquisition and processing were identical for all stacks.

2.4. SDS-PAGE and Western Blot

For Western blotting, parts of the *corpus callosum* were excised from mouse brains of different postnatal stages (P5, P10, P15, P25) and homogenized in radioimmunoprecipitation assay (RIPA) buffer (pH 7.4) containing 1% deoxycholic acid (NP-40), 0.25% sodium deoxycholate, protease inhibitors (CompleteMini, Roche, Germany), 150 mM NaCl and 50 mM Tris-HCL. The homogenate was centrifuged at 13,200 g at 4 °C for 30 min and the supernatant was supplemented with 4× Laemmli sample buffer (5% sodium dodecyl sulfate (SDS), 43.5% glycerol, 100 mM DL-dithiothreitol (DTT), 0.002% bromphenol blue, 20% 2-mercaptoethanol, 125 mM Tris-HCl). Proteins were then separated on 5% (stacking) and 10% (separation) gels by sodium dodecyl sulfate polyacrylamide gel electrophoresis (SDS-PAGE), with a voltage of 60 V for 45 min and 120 V for 90 min, respectively. Proteins were then transferred to polyvinylidenfluorid (PVDF)-membranes (Roth830.1, pore size 0.45 µm) for 70 min using the semi-dry western blot procedure [41,42] with a constant current of 54 mA (one gel) or 108 mA (two gels).

Membranes were then incubated in a blocking solution comprised of PBS, 0.1% (v/v) tween and 5% (w/v) milk powder for 1 h. Blocking solution containing primary antibodies guinea pig anti-GLT1 (Merck Millipore, Darmstadt, Germany, 1:5000), rabbit anti-GLAST (Abcam, Cambridge, UK, 1:1000) and rabbit anti-actin (Sigma-Aldrich Chemical, Munich, Germany, 1:2000) was added overnight at 4 °C. Afterwards, membranes were incubated with a solution containing horseradish peroxidase (HRP)-conjugated secondary antibodies goat anti-rabbit (Invitrogen, Carlsbad, CA, USA, 1:5000) and rabbit anti-guinea pig (Sigma-Aldrich Chemical, Munich, Germany, 1:5000) for 30 min at room temperature.

Immunoreactive protein bands were visualized using the enhanced chemiluminescence technique (ECL-kit, Amersham, Germany). Densitometric analysis was performed at a luminescent image analyser ImageQuant LAS-4000 (Fujifilm Europe, Düsseldorf, Germany). Background corrected grey values of the respective proteins were divided by the grey values of α-actin and normalized to the P25 bands of the separate blots.

2.5. Data Analysis and Presentation

Unless differently specified, data are presented as mean values ± standard error of mean (SEM) and, depending on the experimental setup, analysed by Wilcoxon paired test or student's *t*-test. p represents error probability, * $0.01 \leq p < 0.05$, ** $0.001 \leq p < 0.01$, *** $p < 0.001$. "*n*" represents the number of individual cells analysed, while "*N*" represents the number of individual experiments/slice preparations. Each set of experiments was obtained from slices of at least three different animals. Images were edited in ImageJ (NIH Image, Bethesda, MD, USA), and figures were prepared using Adobe Illustrator (Adobe Systems Incorporated, San Jose, CA, USA).

3. Results

3.1. Action Potentials Evoke Sodium Transients in Macroglial Cells of the Corpus Callosum

For imaging activity-related glial sodium transients in the *corpus callosum*, we first stained tissue slices with the vital fluorescence marker SR101 to identify astrocytes (Figure 1A). Upon additional bolus-loading of the membrane-permeant form of the sodium indicator SBFI, cell bodies of (SR101-positive) astrocytes and SR101-negative cells could be distinguished (Figure 1A). In a recent study [25], we found that SBFI-AM stains virtually the entire macroglial cell population, confirming that microglia do not take up the dye [30]. SR101-negative, SBFI-loaded cells thus most likely represent oligodendrocytes and NG2 cells. No obvious differences in the baseline ratio levels were observed between the different types of macroglial cells, indicating that their resting sodium concentrations are similar.

To evoke AP's, a glass electrode was positioned in the fibre tract and axons were electrically stimulated for 0.5 s at 50 Hz. The electrical stimulation induced a transient increase in the sodium concentration of astrocytes and SR101-negative cells ($N = 19$) (Figure 1B). The average peak amplitude of these sodium transients was similar in both cell types, amounting to 1.2 ± 0.1 mM in astrocytes ($n = 94$) and to 1.4 ± 0.1 mM in SR101-negative cells ($n = 171$) (Figure 1C). Notably, recovery from sodium transients was rather slow, and full recovery typically took several minutes (Figure 1B,C). Sodium transients evoked by electrical stimulation were completely suppressed after perfusion of slices with 0.5 µM TTX ($n = 34$ astrocytes and $n = 66$ SR101-negative cells; $N = 5$) (Figure 1C), indicating that they were indeed related to axonal AP generation.

To test if AP-related sodium transients could be evoked repetitively, we performed experiments, in which the electrical stimulation was repeated after 20 min ($N = 4$). Figure 1D illustrates that sodium signals in astrocytes ($n = 12$) and SR101-negative cells ($n = 29$) exhibited similar amplitudes and kinetics with four consecutive stimulations. Similarly, extracellular compound APs (CAPs) were stable with three subsequent stimulations ($N = 5$; not shown). Perfusion with 0.5 µM TTX completely suppressed CAPs ($N = 3$, not shown).

Taken together, our data show that electrical stimulation results in well-detectable transient sodium increases in astrocytes as well as SR101-negative glial cells of the *corpus callosum*. These increases are completely blocked during perfusion with TTX, showing that they are dependent on the opening of voltage-gated sodium channels and the generation of APs, respectively.

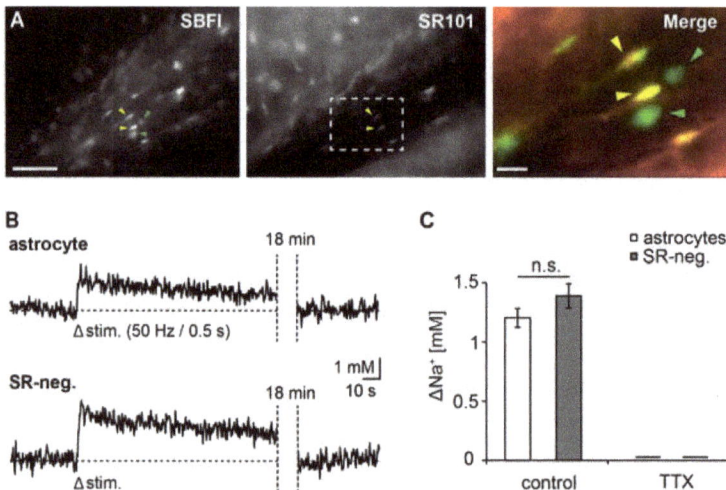

Figure 1. *Cont.*

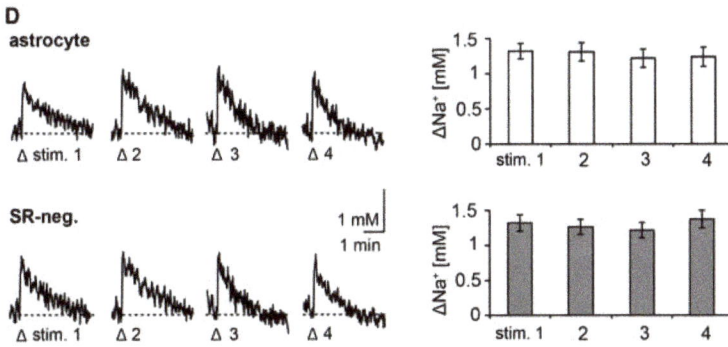

Figure 1. Action potential-induced sodium signals in macroglial cells of the *corpus callosum*. (**A**) Images of sodium-binding benzofurane isophthalate (SBFI) fluorescence (left) and sulforhodamine 101 (SR101) fluorescence (centre) of a tissue slice. The dotted box indicates the region depicted in the merged image on the right. Yellow arrowheads point to SBFI-loaded, SR101-positive cells (astrocytes), green arrowheads show SBFI-loaded, SR101-negative cells (cells of the oligodendrocyte lineage). Scale bars: 50 µm (left and centre) and 10 µm (right). (**B**) Sodium transients evoked by electrical stimulation (arrowheads) in an astrocyte and a SR101-negative cell. The measurement was interrupted for 18 min; note that cells fully recovered to baseline sodium within this time. (**C**) Histogram showing average peak amplitudes ± standard error of mean (SEM) of action potential (AP)-induced sodium signals in astrocytes and SR101-negative cells in control and after perfusion with tetrodotoxin (TTX). n.s.: not significant. (**D**) Transient AP-induced sodium changes in an astrocyte and a SR101-negative cell with four consecutive stimulations (arrowheads). Right: Histograms showing average peak amplitudes ± S.E.M. of AP-induced sodium signals in astrocytes and SR101-negative cells with four consecutive stimulations.

3.2. Pharmacology of Action Potential-Induced Sodium Transients in Macroglial Cells

In grey matter astrocytes of the mouse hippocampus, activity-related sodium transients are mainly due to activation of glutamate transport [4], while in cerebellar Bergman glial cells, an additional contribution of AMPA receptors was described [6]. To study the relevance of glutamate transporter versus glutamate receptor-mediated sodium influx into macroglial cells of the *corpus callosum*, we performed experiments in which axons were stimulated repetitively while different blockers were added successively ($N = 12$).

Addition of NBQX (10 µM) to block AMPA receptors reduced the peak amplitude of sodium transients significantly to $70.8 \pm 5.3\%$ of control stimulation in astrocytes ($n = 29$) and to $66.8 \pm 4.3\%$ in SR101-negative cells ($n = 43$) (Figure 2A,B). Subsequent addition of AP5 (50 µM) to additionally block NMDA receptors did not alter the amplitude of sodium signals in astrocytes, while significantly reducing them in SR101-negative cells to $47 \pm 4.1\%$ of control. Finally, addition of TFB-TBOA (1 µM), which blocks high-affinity glutamate transporters, significantly reduced amplitudes to $32.1 \pm 6.8\%$ in astrocytes and to $21.3 \pm 4.2\%$ in SR101-negative cells (Figure 2A,B).

SBFI-loaded, SR101-negative cells in *corpus callosum* slices mainly represent oligodendrocytes and NG2 cells [25]. To further distinguish between these two cell types, we used tissue slices from transgenic NG2/EYFP-reporter mice [35], in which NG2 cells can be identified based on their expression of EYFP (and absence of SR101-staining), while oligodendrocytes are both SR101 and EYFP-negative (Figure 3A).

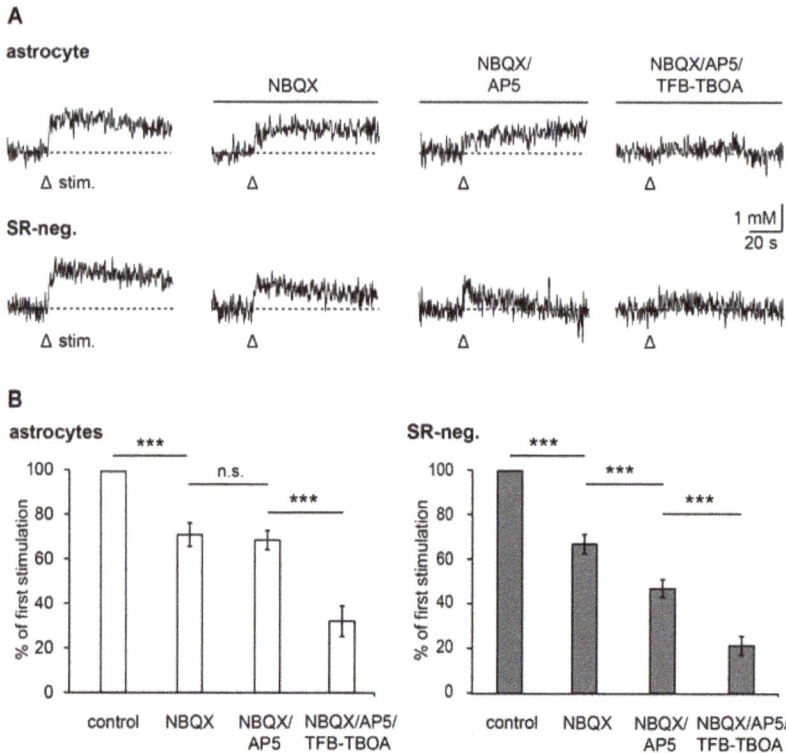

Figure 2. Pharmacology of AP-induced sodium transients. (**A**) Action potential-induced (arrowheads) changes in sodium in an astrocyte and a SR101-negative cell with four consecutive stimulations under control conditions and after addition of different blockers as indicated by the bars (for abbreviations see text). (**B**) Histograms showing peak amplitudes $\pm$ SEM of AP-induced sodium signals in astrocytes and SR101-negative cells in control and after perfusion with different blockers as indicated, normalized to the respective controls. *** $p < 0.001$; n.s.: not significant.

Electrical fibre stimulation triggered intracellular sodium transients in both NG2 cells and oligodendrocytes ($N = 7$) (Figure 3B). The peak amplitude of these sodium transients was not significantly different between the two cell types (NG2-cells: 1.7 ± 0.2 mM, $n = 37$; oligodendrocytes: 1.5 ± 0.1 mM, $n = 68$; not shown). Moreover, the pharmacological profiles were similar in both cell types, essentially recapitulating the results obtained before with "SR101-negative" cells (see Figure 2). As compared to controls in the absence of blockers, NBQX reduced peak amplitudes to $57.4 \pm 5.3\%$ in NG2 cells ($n = 37$) and to $63.2 \pm 6.1\%$ in oligodendrocytes ($n = 68$). AP5 additionally reduced amplitudes to $45.6 \pm 5.4\%$ (NG2 cells) and $41.3 \pm 4.4\%$ (oligodendrocytes), while TFB-TBOA caused a reduction to $22.1 \pm 4.8\%$ (NG2 cells) and $20 \pm 2.5\%$ (oligodendrocytes) (Figure 3C).

In summary, these experiments show that axonal AP generation induces transient sodium signals in all three classes of macroglial cells of the *corpus callosum*, namely astrocytes, oligodendrocytes, and NG2 glia. Action potential-induced sodium increases are strongly reduced by combined inhibition of glutamate receptors and glutamate transport, indicating that they are largely related to axonal release of glutamate. The exact pharmacological profile, however, slightly differs between the different cell types. While high-affinity glutamate transport and opening of AMPA receptors contribute to AP-related sodium influx into all three macroglia cell types, only oligodendrocytes and NG2 glia (but not astrocytes) show an additional contribution of NMDA receptors.

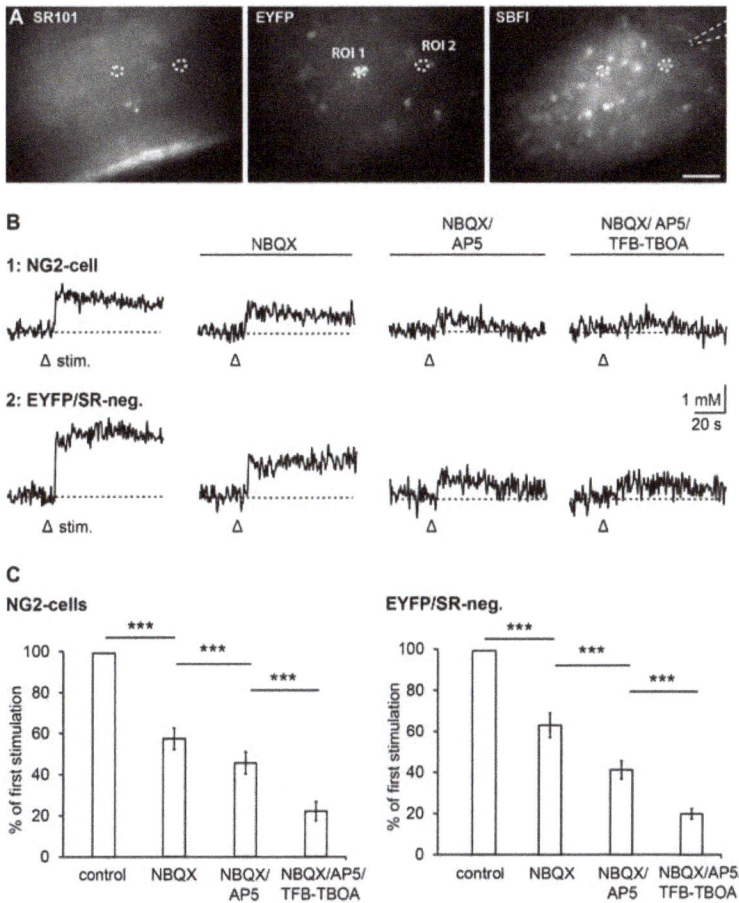

Figure 3. Pharmacology of AP-induced sodium transients in NG2 cells and oligodendrocytes. (**A**) Images of SR101 (left), EYFP (middle), and SBFI fluorescence (right) of a tissue slice prepared from a NG2/EYFP transgenic mouse. The pipette for electrical stimulation is indicated in the right image. Areas encircled by dotted lines represent regions of interest in which sodium signals were measured as depicted in (**B**) (regions of interest (ROI) 1: NG2-cell; ROI2: oligodendrocyte). Scale bar: 50 μm. (**B**) AP-induced (arrowheads) changes in sodium in an NG2 cell and an oligodendrocyte with four consecutive stimulations under control conditions and after addition of different blockers as indicated by the bars (for abbreviations see text). (**C**) Histograms showing peak amplitudes ± SEM of AP-induced sodium signals in NG2 cells and (EYFP/SR101-negative) oligodendrocytes in control and after perfusion with blockers as indicated, normalized to the respective controls. ***: $p < 0.001$.

3.3. Relevance of Gap Junctional Coupling

The results presented so far show that electrical stimulation of axons and AP generation are accompanied by transient elevations in the sodium concentration of astrocytes, oligodendrocytes, as well as NG2 cells of the *corpus callosum* and that these signals are largely related to activation of glutamate receptors and transporters. We have reported previously that sodium signals can spread through gap junctions among astrocytes and from astrocytes to oligodendrocytes and NG2 cells in the *corpus callosum* [25], suggesting that glutamate may not act directly on all macroglial cells. To analyse the involvement of sodium spread through gap junctions in the generation of glutamate-related sodium transients, we prepared tissue slices from animals, which exhibit a conditional (cre-recombinase-dependent) deletion of *connexin43* in astrocytes as well as an unrestricted deletion of connexin30 [36] ("Cx-k.o. mice"). Cre-recombinase-negative mice, featuring undisturbed gap junctional coupling, were used as controls.

Focal pressure application of glutamate (1 mM/250 ms) induced sodium transients in the majority of astrocytes and SR101-negative cells in the field of view in control animals as well as in Cx-k.o. mice ($N = 5$) (Figure 4A). In control, these amounted to 2.0 ± 0.1 mM in astrocytes ($n = 51$) and to 1.2 ± 0.1 mM in SR101-negative cells ($n = 54$) (Figure 4B). In Cx-k.o. mice, glutamate-evoked sodium increases were significantly larger as compared to controls in both astrocytes (2.8 ± 0.4 mM; $n = 40$) and SR101-negative cells (1.7 ± 0.2 mM; $n = 64$) (Figure 4A,B).

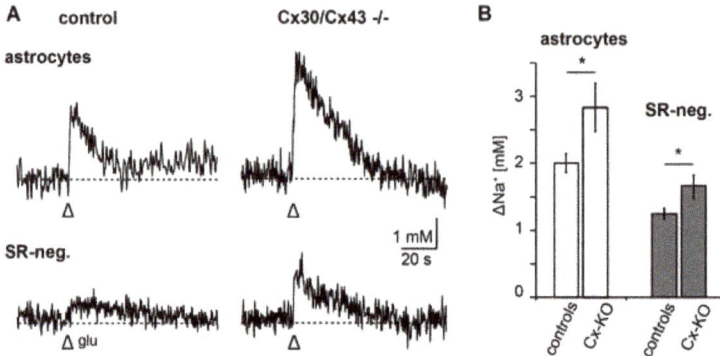

Figure 4. Relevance of gap junctional coupling for glutamate-induced sodium transients. (**A**) Sodium increases evoked by pressure application of glutamate (1 mM/250 ms; arrowheads) in astrocytes (upper traces) and SR101-negative cells (lower traces) in slices obtained from control mice (left) and Cx-k.o. mice (right). (**B**) Histogram showing peak amplitudes $\pm$ SEM of glutamate-induced sodium signals in astrocytes and SR101-negative cells in control and Cx-k.o. mice. *: $0.01 \leq p < 0.05$.

These experiments thus show that sodium signals induced by direct application of glutamate in astrocytes and SR101-negative cells are augmented in animals lacking connexins 30 and 43 in astrocytes. This indicates that sodium signals in the latter group are caused by direct action of glutamate onto individual cells and not primarily caused by an intercellular spread of sodium from astrocytes to SR101-negative cells through gap junctions.

3.4. Relevance of Different Glutamate Transporter Subtypes

Grey matter astrocytes express two different subtypes of sodium-dependent glutamate transporters, GLT-1 and GLAST, with the former being dominant after the first postnatal week [8,9,43]. To address the specific involvement of GLAST and GLT-1 in the generation of sodium signals in macroglia of the *corpus callosum*, we studied the effect of different pharmacological blockers on sodium transients evoked by puff application of glutamate (1 mM/250 ms). Under control conditions ($N = 15$), this caused transient increase in sodium by 4.5 ± 0.3 mM in astrocytes ($n = 71$) and by 1.8 ± 0.1 mM in SR101-negative cells ($n = 66$) (Figure 5A–C).

We first applied the non-transported, competitive inhibitor TFB-TBOA (1 µM), which blocks both transporter subtypes [44]. In the presence of this blocker, the amplitude of glutamate-induced sodium transients in astrocytes was reduced to $24.1 \pm 4.7\%$ ($n = 14$, $N = 4$) as compared to control (Figure 5A,D). In SR101-negative cells, TFB-TBOA reduced the amplitude of sodium signals to $42.3 \pm 9.2\%$ ($n = 16$, $N = 4$) relative to control (Figure 5A,D). In another set of experiments, dihydrokainate (DHK, 100 µM), a GLT1-specific antagonist, was applied ($N = 7$). Dihydrokainate reduced the peak amplitude of sodium transients in astrocytes to $81.1 \pm 8.1\%$ ($n = 30$) of respective control. In SR101-negative cells, sodium transients were reduced to $76.4 \pm 6.2\%$ ($n = 28$) of control (Figure 5B,D).

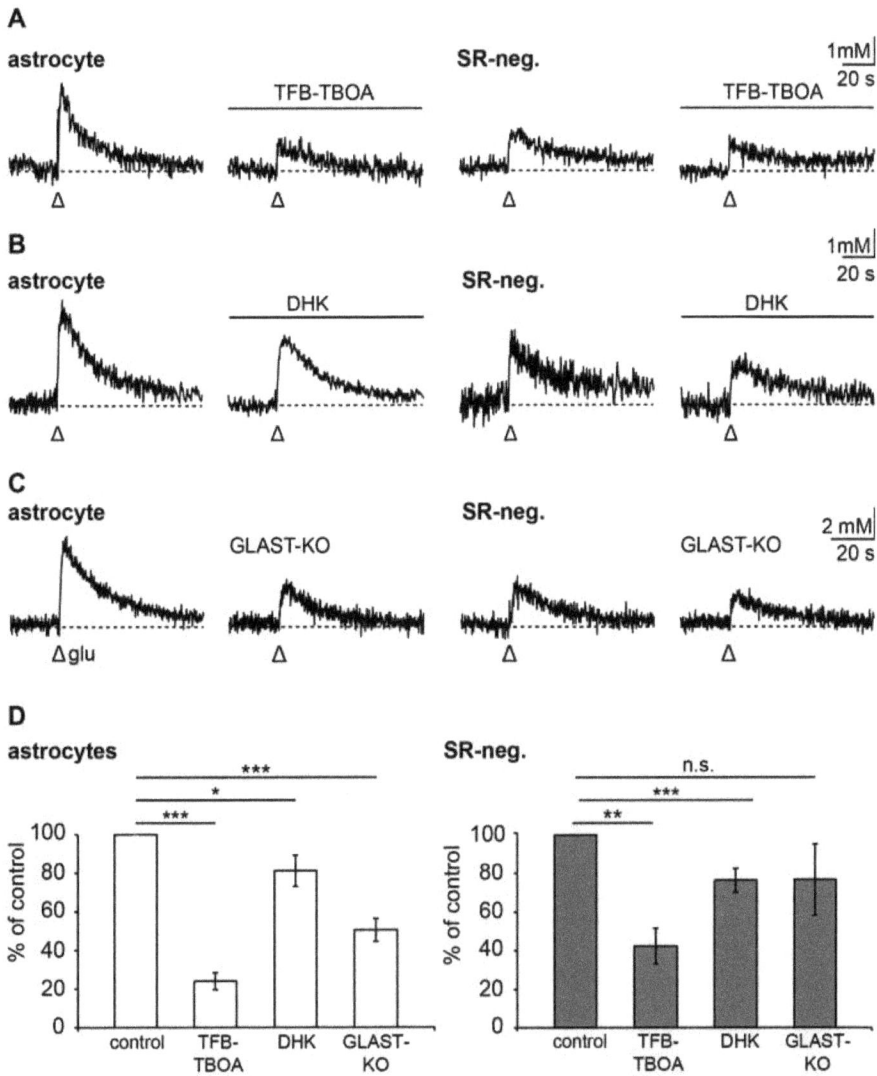

Figure 5. Involvement of glutamate-aspartate-transporter (GLAST) and glutamate transporter 1 (GLT-1) in the generation of sodium signals. (**A**) Sodium increase evoked by pressure application of glutamate (1 mM/250 ms; arrowheads) in an astrocyte (left) and a SR101-negative cell (right) in control and after application of (3*S*)-3-[[3-[[4-(Trifluoromethyl)benzoyl]amino]phenyl]methoxy]-L-aspartic acid (TFB-TBOA). (**B**) Same as in (**A**), but with application of dihydrokainate (DHK). (**C**) Sodium increase evoked by pressure application of glutamate (1 mM/250 ms; arrowheads) in a representative wild type astrocyte and SR101-negative cell (left traces) and in cells from a GLAST-k.o. animal (right traces). (**D**) Histograms showing peak amplitudes ± S.E.M. of glutamate-induced sodium signals in astrocytes and SR101-negative cells in control and after perfusion with different blockers as well as in GLAST-k.o. animals, normalized to the respective controls. n.s.: not significant, *: $0.01 \leq p < 0.05$, **: $0.001 \leq p < 0.01$, ***: $p < 0.001$.

In addition, we performed experiments in brain slices taken from GLAST-k.o. animals [37] ($N = 6$). Here, glutamate application induced sodium increases by 2.3 ± 0.3 mM in astrocytes ($n = 20$) and by 1.4 ± 0.3 mM ($n = 33$) in SR101-negative cells (Figure 5C,D). Compared to the mean peak amplitude of control experiments performed in wild type astrocytes as presented above, amplitudes were thus significantly reduced to $50.5 \pm 6\%$. In SR101-negative cells, peak amplitudes were not significantly different between wild type controls and GLAST-k.o. animals (Figure 5D).

Taken together, these results show that sodium-dependent glutamate transport is a major pathway involved in the generation of glutamate-induced sodium signals in astrocytes as well as SR101-negative macroglial cells of the *corpus callosum*. Moreover, our data suggest that both glial transporter subtypes, GLT-1 and GLAST, contribute to glutamate-induced sodium influx.

3.5. Spatial and Developmental Expression Profile of Glutamate-Aspartate-Transporter and Glutamate Transporter-1 in Corpus Callosum

Our results indicated that activation of the glutamate transporter subtypes GLT-1 and GLAST is involved in sodium influx in response to AP generation in macroglial cells. To study GLT-1 and GLAST expression at the protein level, we performed immunohistochemical stainings and immunoblotting of *corpus callosum* tissue.

For immunohistochemistry, tissue slices of *corpus callosum*, taken from mice at postnatal day 15–17, were labelled with antibodies targeting the astrocyte intermediate filament GFAP. Figure 6A,B illustrate the typical staining pattern of GFAP in white matter tracts, consisting of elongated fibres presumably running in parallel to axonal tracts. CC-1 antibodies were used to visualize the oligodendrocytic protein adenomatous polyposis coli (APC). CC-1 immunoreactivity showed the typical labelling of oligodendrocyte somata without labelling myelin (Figure 6C,D). Antibodies for NG2 proteoglycan were used to label NG2 glia. NG2 immunoreactivity resulted in plasma membrane labelling as shown in Figure 6E,F. Double labelling for GLT-1 (Figure 6A,C,E) or GLAST (Figure 6B,D,F) resulted in punctate labelling patterns for both transporters, which partially co-localized with GFAP, CC-1, and NG2-positive structures.

In addition, we performed SDS-PAGE and Western blots of tissue dissected from *corpus callosum* of animals at different postnatal stages (P5, 10, 15, 25). For both GLT-1 and GLAST several distinct bands (60, 130, 180 kd and 55, 130, 150, 190 kd, respectively) were detected in all age groups most likely due to monomeric and multimeric fractions of the transporters (Figure 7A), confirming earlier studies indicating that both exist as homomultimers [45,46]. Numerical analysis of GLT-1 expression (60, 130, 180 kDa) revealed a steady increase in relative protein content during postnatal development ($N = 4$ per age group) as shown before for mouse hippocampus [43]. At the neonatal stage (P5), GLT-1 expression was low (10.4%) compared to P25 (100%). Its expression increased significantly at P10 (40.7%) and again at P15 (52.7%). In contrast, relative GLAST expression (55, 130, 150, 190 kDa) at P5 was already about half (51.5%) that of P25. While the GLAST protein expression level significantly rose from P5 to P10 (87.6%), there was no further significant increase at P15 (74.0%) as compared to P25 ($N = 3$ per age group) (Figure 7B). Again, this general expression profile was similar to that reported from early postnatal hippocampus [43].

These experiments clearly indicate that both GLT-1 and GLAST are expressed at the protein levels in the *corpus callosum* of mice during the first three weeks after birth. Both transporters show an increase in relative protein content between P5 and P25 that is similar to what was reported from hippocampus. However, the upregulation of GLT-1 expression appears to be slightly delayed when compared to GLAST, which already shows high expression levels in the neonatal *corpus callosum*.

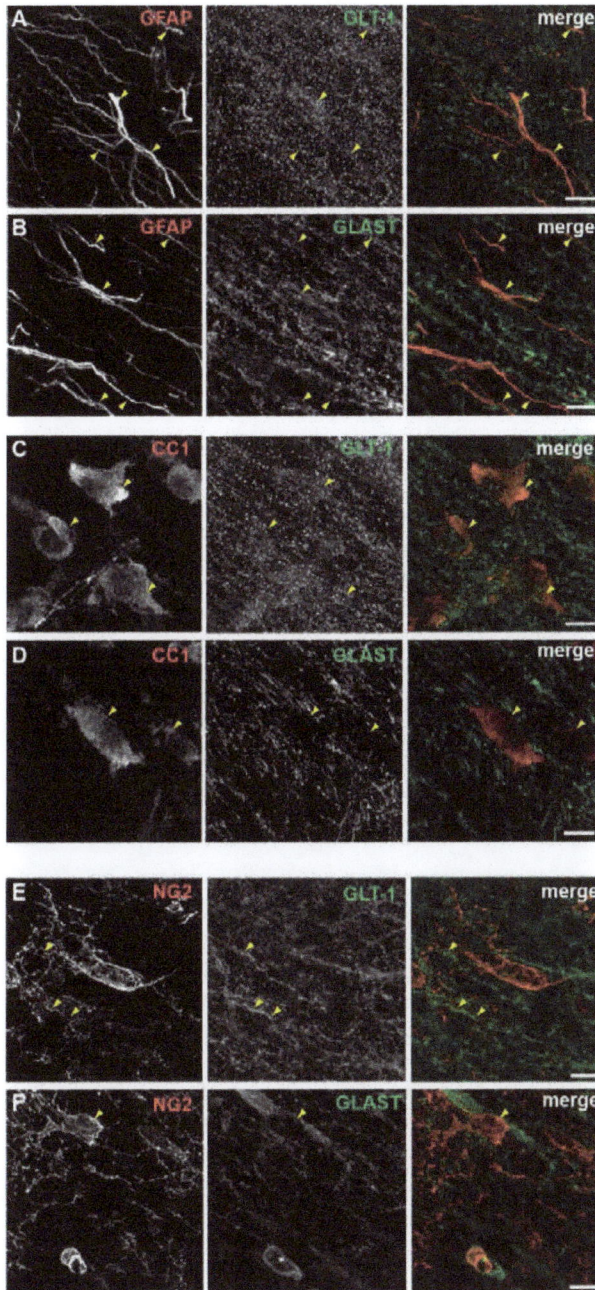

Figure 6. Immunohistochemical analysis of glutamate transporter expression in macroglia of *corpus callosum* at P15-17. (**A**) GFAP and GLT-1 immunoreactivity and merge. (**B**) GFAP and GLAST immunoreactivity and merge. (**C**) CC-1 and GLT-1 immunoreactivity and merge. (**D**) CC-1 and GLAST immunoreactivity and merge. (**E**) NG2 and GLT-1 immunoreactivity and merge. (**F**) NG2 and GLAST immunoreactivity and merge. Yellow arrowheads point to structures with apparent co-labelling. Scale bar: 5 μm.

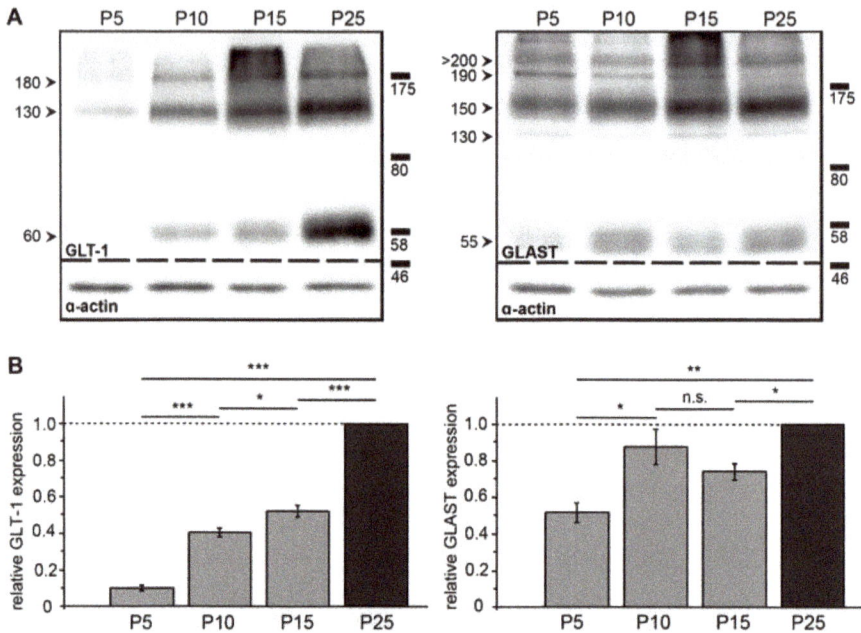

Figure 7. Quantitative analysis of glutamate transporter expression. (**A**) Western blots incubated with anti-GLT-1/GLAST and α-actin from *corpus callosum* preparations taken from mice aged P5, P10, P15 and P25. (**B**) Mean relative intensities of GLT-1 and GLAST bands normalized to P25. n.s.: not significant, *: $0.01 \leq p < 0.05$, **: $0.001 \leq p < 0.01$, ***: $p < 0.001$.

4. Discussion

4.1. Action Potentials Induce Sodium Transients in White Matter Glial Cells That Are Related to Glutamate

In this study, we analysed activity-related intracellular sodium transients in mouse *corpus callosum* after injection of the chemical sodium indicator SBFI-AM into acutely isolated tissue slices. According to our previous work, this results in selective loading of the dye into macroglia, excluding microglial cells [25,30]. To separate between different subtypes of macroglia, astrocytes were additionally stained with the vital dye SR101 [38,47]. The population of SBFI-labelled SR101-negative cells, representing cells of the oligodendrocyte lineage, was further distinguished employing NG2 reporter mice [35], in which NG2 cells and mature oligodendrocytes of *corpus callosum* slices can be identified based on EYFP fluorescence [25]. Using these tools, we could demonstrate that the generation of APs is accompanied by sodium transients in all three main classes of macroglial cells, namely astrocytes, oligodendrocytes as well as NG2 glia in the *corpus callosum*.

Activity-related sodium transients are well described from astrocytes of different grey matter regions, including hippocampus, neocortex, cerebellar cortex and Calyx of Held [4–7,48,49]. They are mainly caused by activation of sodium-dependent glutamate transporters in response to presynaptic release of glutamate [10,12,50]. Knowledge on sodium signalling of cells of the oligodendrocyte lineage is sparse. Studies performed on cultured oligodendrocytes reported that application of glutamate or AMPA increases intracellular sodium [51,52]. In cultured NG2 cells, γ-aminobutyric acid (GABA) induced an elevation of intracellular sodium probably by opening non-inactivating sodium channels in response to GABA-mediated depolarization [53]. In addition, we recently described glutamate-induced sodium increases in *corpus callosum* oligodendrocytes and NG2 glia [25].

In our earlier study [25], we also showed that sodium can easily spread from astrocytes to both oligodendrocytes and NG2 cells and that this panglial spread of sodium depends on the presence of gap junctions composed of connexins 30 and 43. In the present study, application of glutamate in slices obtained from animals lacking connexins 30 and 43 in astrocytes induced prominent sodium transients in astrocytes and also in SR101-negative cells. This strongly suggests that glutamate directly acted on both cell types, namely on astrocytes and cells of the oligodendrocyte lineage. Glutamate-induced sodium signalling thus seems to be a widespread property of different macroglial cells of grey as well as of white matter.

As mentioned above, activity-induced sodium transients, resulting from synaptic release of glutamate and subsequent transporter-mediated uptake into glial cells, are well known from grey matter. Our data now show that macroglial cells also undergo activity-related sodium transients in the *corpus callosum*, that is in the absence of classical chemical synapses and presynaptic glutamate release. In this context it is worth mentioning that our stimulation protocol was relatively moderate, comprising only 25 pulses within 0.5 s. We thus assume that the stimulation resulted in a maximum of 25 APs fired at 50 Hz. Action potential-induced sodium increases in *corpus callosum* macroglial cells were strongly reduced by combined inhibition of glutamate receptors and glutamate transport, indicating that they are largely related to release of glutamate. This is in line with numerous earlier reports suggesting that active axons release glutamate into the periaxonal space (e.g., [16–19,26]). In addition, there is evidence that glutamate is also released by astrocytes [19].

Interestingly, while AP-induced sodium signals were of similar amplitude in astrocytes and in SR101-negative cells, sodium transients induced by direct pressure application of glutamate were significantly larger in astrocytes as compared to SR101-negative macroglia. The latter observation confirms data obtained in our earlier study [25]. A likely reason for this disparity is the different spatial relationship between the sources of glutamate (axonal versus external pipette) and the distribution of glutamate receptors/transporters on macroglial cells. Axonal glutamate release will most likely reach receptors/transporters on the innermost layer of myelin facing the axonal membrane directly and may less efficiently escape at nodes of Ranvier to activate receptors on nearby astrocytes. Applying glutamate by a pipette will probably activate receptors/transporters on astrocytes efficiently, whereas it may not fully reach those underneath the myelin sheath.

While our measurements enabled detection of activity-related sodium transients in white matter astrocytes, oligodendrocytes as well as NG2 cells, axonal fibres were not visible with the experimental approach employed. Action potential generation in axons obviously depends on the opening of voltage-gated sodium channels and it was indeed shown that this results in prominent transient elevation in intra-axonal sodium concentrations in different central neurons [54–57]. It is therefore probably safe to assume that AP generation also caused sodium transients in axonal fibres of *corpus callosum*. Finally, sodium influx into neuronal and glial compartments will most likely be accompanied by a transient decrease in extracellular sodium as shown e.g., for cortex [58].

4.2. Relevance of Different Sodium Influx Pathways

In the present study, perfusing slices with NBQX reduced the peak amplitude of AP-induced sodium transients by 30–40% in astrocytes, oligodendrocytes and NG2 cells. This indicates that activation of AMPA receptors in response to AP-related release of glutamate provides a prominent pathway for sodium influx into all three types of macroglial cells in *corpus callosum*. Moreover, sodium influx into oligodendrocytes and NG2 glia was significantly reduced upon additional pharmacological inhibition of NMDA receptors. This in in line with earlier reports describing expression of ionotropic glutamate receptors in white matter glia [26,27]. White matter astrocytes, in addition to ionotropic glutamate receptors, express a wide variety of different other transmitter receptors, most notably ionotropic P2X$_7$ purinoceptors [28,29]. The latter, activated by axonal release of ATP, might represent a further influx pathway for sodium into astrocytes [28].

Like astrocytes in white matter, cells of the oligodendrocytic lineage express different glutamate receptors, including ionotropic AMPA and NMDA receptors, which are activated in response to AP firing [59–63]. For example, it was shown that glutamate released by axons is sensed by AMPA receptors on oligodendrocyte precursor (NG2) cells, which influences their proliferation and differentiation [17,19,32,64–66]. There is also firm evidence that glutamate derived from active axons is sensed by AMPA and NMDA receptors expressed on the surrounding myelin sheath, resulting in calcium signals proposed to play a central role in coupling axonal activity and integrity with oligodendrocyte metabolism and driving formation of myelin [67–72]. Metabolic support of axons was moreover suggested to be provided by astrocytes, which break down glycogen and release lactate into the extracellular space that can then be taken up by axons during periods of high energy demand [73,74].

Our data in addition demonstrate a significant contribution of high-affinity glutamate uptake to AP-related sodium signals in astrocytes, oligodendrocytes as well as NG2 cells, suggesting that glutamate transporters are activated upon AP propagation in the *corpus callosum*. These results are thus in line with earlier reports showing expression of different subtypes of glutamate transporters in white matter [21–24,75,76]. To address the involvement of glutamate transporter subtypes GLT-1 and GLAST, we performed immunohistochemical stainings and immunoblotting, demonstrating expression of both transporters at the protein level during the first three weeks after birth in *corpus callosum*. Their expression levels increased between P5 and P25, which is similar to hippocampus and neocortex [43,77].

We also tested the effect of DHK, a selective pharmacological inhibitor of GLT-1, on glutamate-induced sodium signals. DHK resulted in a significant reduction of sodium increases in both astrocytes and cells of the oligodendrocyte lineage, indicating that this subtype is functionally relevant for both groups. Moreover, in GLAST-k.o. animals, glutamate-induced sodium signals were significantly altered in astrocytes as compared to wild type controls. In contrast, sodium signals were unaltered in cells of the oligodendrocyte lineage in animals lacking GLAST, suggesting that GLAST is not ultimately required for efficient uptake of glutamate in SR101-negative cells. This in in agreement with studies demonstrating that glutamate uptake in white matter oligodendrocytes additionally involves excitatory amino acid carrier 1 (EAAC1) [24,76].

5. Conclusions

Our study establishes that the propagation of APs in the *corpus callosum*, a major white matter tract, generates transient sodium elevations in macroglial cells. While many studies have demonstrated the existence of glial calcium signalling in white matter [26,27], activity-related sodium signalling has, to the best of our knowledge, not been reported so far. Interestingly, sodium transients in astrocytes and cells of the oligodendrocyte lineage shared many characteristics. Their amplitudes and time courses were rather similar, and the majority of sodium influx was mediated by glutamate-related pathways, namely ionotropic receptors and high-affinity glutamate transport. The only essential differences found were the apparent involvement of GLAST in astrocytes, but not in cells of the oligodendrocyte lineage, and the contribution of NMDA receptors to sodium signals of the latter, but not the former group of cells. Along with these considerations, it is important to keep in mind that measurements in the present study were taken from somata and that signal properties as well as sodium influx pathways might be different in cellular processes and in myelin compartments.

At present, we can only speculate about the possible functional relevance of macroglial sodium signals in white matter. In general, it is of note that glial calcium and sodium signals share a common influx pathway, namely inotropic glutamate receptors, emphasizing the involvement of the latter in the communication between axons and surrounding glia. Sodium elevations are additionally augmented by high-affinity glutamate uptake, which is not directly involved in the generation of calcium signalling. In grey matter, activity-related sodium signals induced upon activation of glutamate transport were suggested to stimulate astrocyte glycolysis and lactate release, thereby representing important mediators of metabolic interaction between neurons and glial cells [10,11]. In analogy, they might also drive lactate production in white matter oligodendrocytes and astrocytes and thereby be involved in metabolic support of axons by both cell types [74,78,79].

Several studies have correlated sodium elevations with migration, proliferation and differentiation of oligodendrocyte precursor cells. Direct modulation of K^+ channels by sodium influx resulting from activation of AMPA receptors was shown to inhibit proliferation of oligodendrocyte precursor cells [64,80–82]. In rat oligodendrocytes in culture, stimulating sodium-dependent glutamate uptake was associated with intracellular calcium signals most likely based on reverse mode NCX activity, which promoted their morphological differentiation [83]. Increased sodium and resulting reverse NCX activity were also found to promote synthesis of myelin basic protein in mouse oligodendrocyte precursor cells in culture [84]. Finally, NCX-mediated calcium signalling promoted by a persistent sodium current was involved in the migration of NG2 cells during early brain development [53].

Sodium transients induced in astrocytes and cells of the oligodendrocyte lineage by propagating APs along axonal fibre tracts might thus exert a role in the metabolic support of axons. In addition, they might promote the establishment of a compact myelin sheath. Activity-related sodium signalling in white matter macroglia is therefore likely to represent an essential component in the communication between axons and surrounding glia.

Author Contributions: Conceptualization and supervision of experimental work: C.R.R.; Experimental work and primary data analysis, B.M.-R., D.Z., N.P., M.F.; Figure preparation, B.M.-R., D.Z., N.P., M.F., C.R.R.; Writing of original text version, B.M.-R., C.R.R.; Writing of final text version: C.R.R., Final editing and approval of text, B.M.-R., D.Z., N.P., M.F., C.R.R., Project administration: C.R.R., Funding acquisition: C.R.R.

Funding: This research was funded by the Deutsche Forschungsgemeinschaft (DFG), Special Priority Programme 1757 ("glial heterogeneity"), grant number Ro2327/8-2.

Acknowledgments: We thank the following colleagues for providing transgenic animals: Gerald Seifert and Christian Steinhäuser, University of Bonn, Germany (Cx-k.o.), Nikolaj Klöcker, Heinrich Heine University Düsseldorf, Germany (NG2-EYFP), and Christoph Fahlke and Verena Untiet, Forschungszentrum Jülich, Germany (GLAST-k.o). We thank Ulrich Rüther, Heinrich Heine University Düsseldorf, Germany, for support in the densitometric analysis of immunoblots.

Conflicts of Interest: The authors declare no conflict of interest.

References

1. Rose, C.R.; Verkhratsky, A. Principles of sodium homeostasis and sodium signalling in astroglia. *Glia* **2016**, *64*, 1611–1627. [CrossRef] [PubMed]

2. Kirischuk, S.; Heja, L.; Kardos, J.; Billups, B. Astrocyte sodium signaling and the regulation of neurotransmission. *Glia* **2016**, *64*, 1655–1666. [CrossRef] [PubMed]

3. Chatton, J.Y.; Marquet, P.; Magistretti, P.J. A quantitative analysis of L-glutamate-regulated Na^+ dynamics in mouse cortical astrocytes: Implications for cellular bioenergetics. *Eur. J. Neurosci.* **2000**, *12*, 3843–3853. [CrossRef] [PubMed]

4. Langer, J.; Rose, C.R. Synaptically induced sodium signals in hippocampal astrocytes in situ. *J. Physiol.* **2009**, *587*, 5859–5877. [CrossRef] [PubMed]

5. Kirischuk, S.; Kettenmann, H.; Verkhratsky, A. Membrane currents and cytoplasmic sodium transients generated by glutamate transport in bergmann glial cells. *Pflugers Arch.* **2007**, *454*, 245–252. [CrossRef] [PubMed]

6. Bennay, M.; Langer, J.; Meier, S.D.; Kafitz, K.W.; Rose, C.R. Sodium signals in cerebellar Purkinje neurons and Bergmann glial cells evoked by glutamatergic synaptic transmission. *Glia* **2008**, *56*, 1138–1149. [CrossRef] [PubMed]

7. Karus, C.; Mondragao, M.A.; Ziemens, D.; Rose, C.R. Astrocytes restrict discharge duration and neuronal sodium loads during recurrent network activity. *Glia* **2015**, *63*, 936–957. [CrossRef] [PubMed]

8. Danbolt, N.C. Glutamate uptake. *Prog. Neurobiol.* **2001**, *65*, 1–105. [CrossRef]

9. Rose, C.R.; Ziemens, D.; Untiet, V.; Fahlke, C. Molecular and cellular physiology of sodium-dependent glutamate transporters. *Brain Res. Bull.* **2018**, *136*, 13–16. [CrossRef] [PubMed]

10. Chatton, J.Y.; Magistretti, P.J.; Barros, L.F. Sodium signaling and astrocyte energy metabolism. *Glia* **2016**, *64*, 1667–1676. [CrossRef] [PubMed]

11. Magistretti, P.J.; Allaman, I. Lactate in the brain: From metabolic end-product to signalling molecule. *Nat. Rev. Neurosci.* **2018**, *19*, 235–249. [CrossRef] [PubMed]

12. Kirischuk, S.; Parpura, V.; Verkhratsky, A. Sodium dynamics: Another key to astroglial excitability? *Trends Neurosci.* **2012**, *35*, 497–506. [CrossRef] [PubMed]

13. Parpura, V.; Sekler, I.; Fern, R. Plasmalemmal and mitochondrial Na^+-Ca^{2+} exchange in neuroglia. *Glia* **2016**, *64*, 1646–1654. [CrossRef] [PubMed]

14. Jackson, J.G.; O'Donnell, J.C.; Takano, H.; Coulter, D.A.; Robinson, M.B. Neuronal activity and glutamate uptake decrease mitochondrial mobility in astrocytes and position mitochondria near glutamate transporters. *J. Neurosci.* **2014**, *34*, 1613–1624. [CrossRef] [PubMed]

15. Gerkau, N.J.; Rakers, C.; Durry, S.; Petzold, G.; Rose, C.R. Reverse NCX attenuates cellular sodium loading in metabolically compromised cortex. *Cereb. Cortex* **2017**, 1–7. [CrossRef] [PubMed]

16. Kukley, M.; Capetillo-Zarate, E.; Dietrich, D. Vesicular glutamate release from axons in white matter. *Nat. Neurosci.* **2007**, *10*, 311–320. [CrossRef] [PubMed]

17. Ziskin, J.L.; Nishiyama, A.; Rubio, M.; Fukaya, M.; Bergles, D.E. Vesicular release of glutamate from unmyelinated axons in white matter. *Nat. Neurosci.* **2007**, *10*, 321–330. [CrossRef] [PubMed]

18. Fruhbeis, C.; Frohlich, D.; Kuo, W.P.; Amphornrat, J.; Thilemann, S.; Saab, A.S.; Kirchhoff, F.; Mobius, W.; Goebbels, S.; Nave, K.A.; et al. Neurotransmitter-triggered transfer of exosomes mediates oligodendrocyte-neuron communication. *PLoS Biol.* **2013**, *11*, e1001604. [CrossRef] [PubMed]

19. Hamilton, N.; Vayro, S.; Wigley, R.; Butt, A.M. Axons and astrocytes release ATP and glutamate to evoke calcium signals in NG2-glia. *Glia* **2010**, *58*, 66–79. [CrossRef] [PubMed]

20. Fern, R.F.; Matute, C.; Stys, P.K. White matter injury: Ischemic and nonischemic. *Glia* **2014**, *62*, 1780–1789. [CrossRef] [PubMed]

21. Domercq, M.; Matute, C. Expression of glutamate transporters in the adult bovine *corpus callosum*. *Brain Res. Mol. Brain Res.* **1999**, *67*, 296–302. [CrossRef]

22. Goursaud, S.; Kozlova, E.N.; Maloteaux, J.M.; Hermans, E. Cultured astrocytes derived from *corpus callosum* or cortical grey matter show distinct glutamate handling properties. *J. Neurochem.* **2009**, *108*, 1442–1452. [CrossRef] [PubMed]

23. Lundgaard, I.; Osorio, M.J.; Kress, B.T.; Sanggaard, S.; Nedergaard, M. White matter astrocytes in health and disease. *Neuroscience* **2014**, *276*, 161–173. [CrossRef] [PubMed]

24. Arranz, A.M.; Hussein, A.; Alix, J.J.; Perez-Cerda, F.; Allcock, N.; Matute, C.; Fern, R. Functional glutamate transport in rodent optic nerve axons and glia. *Glia* **2008**, *56*, 1353–1367. [CrossRef] [PubMed]

25. Moshrefi-Ravasdjani, B.; Hammel, E.L.; Kafitz, K.W.; Rose, C.R. Astrocyte sodium signalling and panglial spread of sodium signals in brain white matter. *Neurochem. Res.* **2017**, *42*, 2505–2518. [CrossRef] [PubMed]

26. Butt, A.M.; Fern, R.F.; Matute, C. Neurotransmitter signaling in white matter. *Glia* **2014**, *62*, 1762–1779. [CrossRef] [PubMed]

27. Micu, I.; Plemel, J.R.; Caprariello, A.V.; Nave, K.A.; Stys, P.K. Axo-myelinic neurotransmission: A novel mode of cell signalling in the central nervous system. *Nat. Rev. Neurosci.* **2018**, *19*, 49–58. [CrossRef] [PubMed]

28. Hamilton, N.; Vayro, S.; Kirchhoff, F.; Verkhratsky, A.; Robbins, J.; Gorecki, D.C.; Butt, A.M. Mechanisms of ATP- and glutamate-mediated calcium signaling in white matter astrocytes. *Glia* **2008**, *56*, 734–749. [CrossRef] [PubMed]

29. Bernstein, M.; Lyons, S.A.; Moller, T.; Kettenmann, H. Receptor-mediated calcium signalling in glial cells from mouse *corpus callosum* slices. *J. Neurosci. Res.* **1996**, *46*, 152–163. [CrossRef]

30. Schipke, C.G.; Boucsein, C.; Ohlemeyer, C.; Kirchhoff, F.; Kettenmann, H. Astrocyte Ca^{2+} waves trigger responses in microglial cells in brain slices. *FASEB J.* **2002**, *16*, 255–257. [CrossRef] [PubMed]

31. Hamilton, N.; Hubbard, P.S.; Butt, A.M. Effects of glutamate receptor activation on NG2-glia in the rat optic nerve. *J. Anat.* **2009**, *214*, 208–218. [CrossRef] [PubMed]

32. Bergles, D.E.; Jabs, R.; Steinhäuser, C. Neuron-glia synapses in the brain. *Brain Res. Rev.* **2010**, *63*, 130–137. [CrossRef] [PubMed]

33. Dimou, L.; Gallo, V. NG2-glia and their functions in the central nervous system. *Glia* **2015**, *63*, 1429–1451. [CrossRef] [PubMed]

34. Close, B.; Banister, K.; Baumans, V.; Bernoth, E.M.; Bromage, N.; Bunyan, J.; Erhardt, W.; Flecknell, P.; Gregory, N.; Hackbarth, H.; et al. Recommendations for euthanasia of experimental animals: Part 2. DGXT of the european commission. *Lab. Anim.* **1997**, *31*, 1–32. [CrossRef] [PubMed]

35. Karram, K.; Goebbels, S.; Schwab, M.; Jennissen, K.; Seifert, G.; Steinhauser, C.; Nave, K.A.; Trotter, J. NG2-expressing cells in the nervous system revealed by the NG2-EYFP-knockin mouse. *Genesis* **2008**, *46*, 743–757. [CrossRef] [PubMed]

36. Wallraff, A.; Kohling, R.; Heinemann, U.; Theis, M.; Willecke, K.; Steinhauser, C. The impact of astrocytic gap junctional coupling on potassium buffering in the hippocampus. *J. Neurosci.* **2006**, *26*, 5438–5447. [CrossRef] [PubMed]

37. Watase, K.; Hashimoto, K.; Kano, M.; Yamada, K.; Watanabe, M.; Inoue, Y.; Okuyama, S.; Sakagawa, T.; Ogawa, S.-i.; Kawashima, N.; et al. Motor discoordination and increased susceptibility to cerebellar injury in glast mutant mice. *Eur. J. Neurosci.* **1998**, *10*, 976–988. [CrossRef] [PubMed]

38. Kafitz, K.W.; Meier, S.D.; Stephan, J.; Rose, C.R. Developmental profile and properties of sulforhodamine 101-labeled glial cells in acute brain slices of rat hippocampus. *J. Neurosci. Methods* **2008**, *169*, 84–92. [CrossRef] [PubMed]

39. Meier, S.D.; Kovalchuk, Y.; Rose, C.R. Properties of the new fluorescent Na^+ indicator corona green: Comparison with SBFI and confocal Na^+ imaging. *J. Neurosci. Methods* **2006**, *155*, 251–259. [CrossRef] [PubMed]

40. Langer, J.; Stephan, J.; Theis, M.; Rose, C.R. Gap junctions mediate intercellular spread of sodium between hippocampal astrocytes in situ. *Glia* **2012**, *60*, 239–252. [CrossRef] [PubMed]

41. Towbin, H.; Staehelin, T.; Gordon, J. Electrophoretic transfer of proteins from polyacrylamide gels to nitrocellulose sheets: Procedure and some applications. *Proc. Natl. Acad. Sci. USA* **1979**, *76*, 4350–4354. [CrossRef] [PubMed]

42. Burnette, W.N. "Western blotting": Electrophoretic transfer of proteins from sodium dodecyl sulfate—Polyacrylamide gels to unmodified nitrocellulose and radiographic detection with antibody and radioiodinated protein a. *Anal. Biochem.* **1981**, *112*, 195–203. [CrossRef]

43. Schreiner, A.E.; Durry, S.; Aida, T.; Stock, M.C.; Rüther, U.; Tanaka, K.; Rose, C.R.; Kafitz, K.W. Laminar and subcellular heterogeneity of GLAST and GLT-1 immunoreactivity in the developing postnatal mouse hippocampus. *J. Comp. Neurol.* **2014**, *522*, 204–224. [CrossRef] [PubMed]

44. Tsukada, S.; Iino, M.; Takayasu, Y.; Shimamoto, K.; Ozawa, S. Effects of a novel glutamate transporter blocker, (2s, 3s)-3-[3-[4-(trifluoromethyl)benzoylamino]benzyloxy]aspartate (TFB-TBOA), on activities of hippocampal neurons. *Neuropharmacology* **2005**, *48*, 479–491. [CrossRef] [PubMed]

45. Haugeto, O.; Ullensvang, K.; Levy, L.M.; Chaudhry, F.A.; Honore, T.; Nielsen, M.; Lehre, K.P.; Danbolt, N.C. Brain glutamate transporter proteins form homomultimers. *J. Biol. Chem.* **1996**, *271*, 27715–27722. [CrossRef] [PubMed]

46. Peacey, E.; Miller, C.C.; Dunlop, J.; Rattray, M. The four major N- and C-terminal splice variants of the excitatory amino acid transporter GLT-1 form cell surface homomeric and heteromeric assemblies. *Mol. Pharmacol.* **2009**, *75*, 1062–1073. [CrossRef] [PubMed]

47. Nimmerjahn, A.; Kirchhoff, F.; Kerr, J.N.; Helmchen, F. Sulforhodamine 101 as a specific marker of astroglia in the neocortex in vivo. *Nat. Methods* **2004**, *1*, 31–37. [CrossRef] [PubMed]

48. Uwechue, N.M.; Marx, M.C.; Chevy, Q.; Billups, B. Activation of glutamate transport evokes rapid glutamine release from perisynaptic astrocytes. *J. Physiol.* **2012**, *590*, 2317–2331. [CrossRef] [PubMed]

49. Lamy, C.M.; Chatton, J.Y. Optical probing of sodium dynamics in neurons and astrocytes. *Neuroimage* **2011**, *58*, 572–578. [CrossRef] [PubMed]

50. Rose, C.R.; Chatton, J.Y. Astrocyte sodium signaling and neuro-metabolic coupling in the brain. *Neuroscience* **2016**, *323*, 121–134. [CrossRef] [PubMed]

51. Ballanyi, K.; Kettenmann, H. Intracellular Na^+ activity in cultured mouse oligodendrocytes. *J. Neurosci. Res.* **1990**, *26*, 455–460. [CrossRef] [PubMed]

52. Chen, H.; Kintner, D.B.; Jones, M.; Matsuda, T.; Baba, A.; Kiedrowski, L.; Sun, D. Ampa-mediated excitotoxicity in oligodendrocytes: Role for Na^+-K^+-Cl^- co-transport and reversal of Na^+/Ca^{2+} exchanger. *J. Neurochem.* **2007**, *102*, 1783–1795. [CrossRef] [PubMed]

53. Tong, X.P.; Li, X.Y.; Zhou, B.; Shen, W.; Zhang, Z.J.; Xu, T.L.; Duan, S. Ca^{2+} signaling evoked by activation of Na^+ channels and Na^+/Ca^{2+} exchangers is required for GABA-induced NG2 cell migration. *J. Cell Biol.* **2009**, *186*, 113–128. [CrossRef] [PubMed]

54. Baranauskas, G.; David, Y.; Fleidervish, I.A. Spatial mismatch between the Na^+ flux and spike initiation in axon initial segment. *Proc. Natl. Acad. Sci. USA* **2013**, *110*, 4051–4056. [CrossRef] [PubMed]

55. Miyazaki, K.; Ross, W.N. Simultaneous sodium and calcium imaging from dendrites and axons. *eNeuro* **2015**, *2*. [CrossRef] [PubMed]

56. Ona-Jodar, T.; Gerkau, N.J.; Sara Aghvami, S.; Rose, C.R.; Egger, V. Two-photon Na$^+$ imaging reports somatically evoked action potentials in rat olfactory bulb mitral and granule cell neurites. *Front. Cell. Neurosci.* **2017**, *11*, 50. [CrossRef] [PubMed]

57. Kole, M.H.; Ilschner, S.U.; Kampa, B.M.; Williams, S.R.; Ruben, P.C.; Stuart, G.J. Action potential generation requires a high sodium channel density in the axon initial segment. *Nat. Neurosci.* **2008**, *11*, 178–186. [CrossRef] [PubMed]

58. Dietzel, I.; Heinemann, U.; Hofmeier, G.; Lux, H.D. Stimulus-induced changes in extracellular Na$^+$ and Cl$^-$ concentration in relation to changes in the size of the extracellular space. *Exp. Brain Res.* **1982**, *46*, 73–84. [CrossRef] [PubMed]

59. Deng, W.; Rosenberg, P.A.; Volpe, J.J.; Jensen, F.E. Calcium-permeable AMPA/kainate receptors mediate toxicity and preconditioning by oxygen-glucose deprivation in oligodendrocyte precursors. *Proc. Natl. Acad. Sci. USA* **2003**, *100*, 6801–6806. [CrossRef] [PubMed]

60. Karadottir, R.; Cavelier, P.; Bergersen, L.H.; Attwell, D. NMDA receptors are expressed in oligodendrocytes and activated in ischaemia. *Nature* **2005**, *438*, 1162–1166. [CrossRef] [PubMed]

61. Salter, M.G.; Fern, R. Nmda receptors are expressed in developing oligodendrocyte processes and mediate injury. *Nature* **2005**, *438*, 1167–1171. [CrossRef] [PubMed]

62. Matute, C.; Alberdi, E.; Domercq, M.; Sanchez-Gomez, M.V.; Perez-Samartin, A.; Rodriguez-Antiguedad, A.; Perez-Cerda, F. Excitotoxic damage to white matter. *J. Anat.* **2007**, *210*, 693–702. [CrossRef] [PubMed]

63. Micu, I.; Ridsdale, A.; Zhang, L.; Woulfe, J.; McClintock, J.; Brantner, C.A.; Andrews, S.B.; Stys, P.K. Real-time measurement of free Ca^{2+} changes in CNS myelin by two-photon microscopy. *Nat. Med.* **2007**, *13*, 874–879. [CrossRef] [PubMed]

64. Gallo, V.; Zhou, J.M.; McBain, C.J.; Wright, P.; Knutson, P.L.; Armstrong, R.C. Oligodendrocyte progenitor cell proliferation and lineage progression are regulated by glutamate receptor-mediated k$^+$ channel block. *J. Neurosci.* **1996**, *16*, 2659–2670. [CrossRef] [PubMed]

65. Yuan, X.; Eisen, A.M.; McBain, C.J.; Gallo, V. A role for glutamate and its receptors in the regulation of oligodendrocyte development in cerebellar tissue slices. *Development* **1998**, *125*, 2901–2914. [PubMed]

66. Nagy, B.; Hovhannisyan, A.; Barzan, R.; Chen, T.J.; Kukley, M. Different patterns of neuronal activity trigger distinct responses of oligodendrocyte precursor cells in the *corpus callosum*. *PLoS Biol.* **2017**, *15*, e2001993. [CrossRef] [PubMed]

67. Funfschilling, U.; Supplie, L.M.; Mahad, D.; Boretius, S.; Saab, A.S.; Edgar, J.; Brinkmann, B.G.; Kassmann, C.M.; Tzvetanova, I.D.; Mobius, W.; et al. Glycolytic oligodendrocytes maintain myelin and long-term axonal integrity. *Nature* **2012**, *485*, 517–521. [CrossRef] [PubMed]

68. Saab, A.S.; Tzvetavona, I.D.; Trevisiol, A.; Baltan, S.; Dibaj, P.; Kusch, K.; Mobius, W.; Goetze, B.; Jahn, H.M.; Huang, W.; et al. Oligodendroglial NMDA receptors regulate glucose import and axonal energy metabolism. *Neuron* **2016**, *91*, 119–132. [CrossRef] [PubMed]

69. Meyer, N.; Richter, N.; Fan, Z.; Siemonsmeier, G.; Pivneva, T.; Jordan, P.; Steinhauser, C.; Semtner, M.; Nolte, C.; Kettenmann, H. Oligodendrocytes in the mouse *corpus callosum* maintain axonal function by delivery of glucose. *Cell Rep.* **2018**, *22*, 2383–2394. [CrossRef] [PubMed]

70. Lee, Y.; Morrison, B.M.; Li, Y.; Lengacher, S.; Farah, M.H.; Hoffman, P.N.; Liu, Y.; Tsingalia, A.; Jin, L.; Zhang, P.W.; et al. Oligodendroglia metabolically support axons and contribute to neurodegeneration. *Nature* **2012**, *487*, 443–448. [CrossRef] [PubMed]

71. Baraban, M.; Koudelka, S.; Lyons, D.A. Ca^{2+} activity signatures of myelin sheath formation and growth in vivo. *Nat. Neurosci.* **2018**, *21*, 19–23. [CrossRef] [PubMed]

72. Krasnow, A.M.; Ford, M.C.; Valdivia, L.E.; Wilson, S.W.; Attwell, D. Regulation of developing myelin sheath elongation by oligodendrocyte calcium transients in vivo. *Nat. Neurosci.* **2018**, *21*, 24–28. [CrossRef] [PubMed]

73. Brown, A.M.; Sickmann, H.M.; Fosgerau, K.; Lund, T.M.; Schousboe, A.; Waagepetersen, H.S.; Ransom, B.R. Astrocyte glycogen metabolism is required for neural activity during aglycemia or intense stimulation in mouse white matter. *J. Neurosci. Res.* **2005**, *79*, 74–80. [CrossRef] [PubMed]

74. Brown, A.M.; Ransom, B.R. Astrocyte glycogen and brain energy metabolism. *Glia* **2007**, *55*, 1263–1271. [CrossRef] [PubMed]

75. Regan, M.R.; Huang, Y.H.; Kim, Y.S.; Dykes-Hoberg, M.I.; Jin, L.; Watkins, A.M.; Bergles, D.E.; Rothstein, J.D. Variations in promoter activity reveal a differential expression and physiology of glutamate transporters by glia in the developing and mature CNS. *J. Neurosci.* **2007**, *27*, 6607–6619. [CrossRef] [PubMed]

76. DeSilva, T.M.; Kabakov, A.Y.; Goldhoff, P.E.; Volpe, J.J.; Rosenberg, P.A. Regulation of glutamate transport in developing rat oligodendrocytes. *J. Neurosci.* **2009**, *29*, 7898–7908. [CrossRef] [PubMed]

77. Hanson, E.; Armbruster, M.; Cantu, D.; Andresen, L.; Taylor, A.; Danbolt, N.C.; Dulla, C.G. Astrocytic glutamate uptake is slow and does not limit neuronal nmda receptor activation in the neonatal neocortex. *Glia* **2015**, *63*, 1784–1796. [CrossRef] [PubMed]

78. Morrison, B.M.; Lee, Y.; Rothstein, J.D. Oligodendroglia: Metabolic supporters of axons. *Trends Cell Biol.* **2013**, *23*, 644–651. [CrossRef] [PubMed]

79. Hirrlinger, J.; Nave, K.A. Adapting brain metabolism to myelination and long-range signal transduction. *Glia* **2014**, *62*, 1749–1761. [CrossRef] [PubMed]

80. Borges, K.; Kettenmann, H. Blockade of K^+ channels induced by AMPA/kainate receptor activation in mouse oligodendrocyte precursor cells is mediated by Na^+ entry. *J. Neurosci. Res.* **1995**, *42*, 579–593. [CrossRef] [PubMed]

81. Knutson, P.; Ghiani, C.A.; Zhou, J.M.; Gallo, V.; McBain, C.J. K^+ channel expression and cell proliferation are regulated by intracellular sodium and membrane depolarization in oligodendrocyte progenitor cells. *J. Neurosci.* **1997**, *17*, 2669–2682. [CrossRef] [PubMed]

82. Schroder, W.; Seifert, G.; Huttmann, K.; Hinterkeuser, S.; Steinhauser, C. AMPA receptor-mediated modulation of inward rectifier K^+ channels in astrocytes of mouse hippocampus. *Mol. Cell. Neurosci.* **2002**, *19*, 447–458. [CrossRef] [PubMed]

83. Martinez-Lozada, Z.; Waggener, C.T.; Kim, K.; Zou, S.; Knapp, P.E.; Hayashi, Y.; Ortega, A.; Fuss, B. Activation of sodium-dependent glutamate transporters regulates the morphological aspects of oligodendrocyte maturation via signaling through calcium/calmodulin-dependent kinase IIβ's actin-binding/-stabilizing domain. *Glia* **2014**, *62*, 1543–1558. [CrossRef] [PubMed]

84. Friess, M.; Hammann, J.; Unichenko, P.; Luhmann, H.J.; White, R.; Kirischuk, S. Intracellular ion signaling influences myelin basic protein synthesis in oligodendrocyte precursor cells. *Cell Calcium* **2016**, *60*, 322–330. [CrossRef] [PubMed]

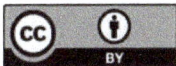

neuroglia

MDPI

Review

Astrogliopathy in Tauopathies

Isidro Ferrer [1,2,3,4]

1   Department of Pathology and Experimental Therapeutics, University of Barcelona, Feixa Llarga sn, 08907 Hospitalet de Llobregat, Spain; 8082ifa@gmail.com
2   IDIBELL (Bellvitge Biomedical Research Centre), Bellvitge University Hospital, 08907 Hospitalet de Llobregat, Spain; Tel.: +34-93-403-5808
3   CIBERNED (Network Centre of Biomedical Research of Neurodegenerative Diseases), Institute of Health Carlos III, Ministry of Economy, Industry and Competitiveness, 08907 Hospitalet de Llobregat, Spain
4   Institute of Neurosciences, University of Barcelona, 08907 Hospitalet de Llobregat, Spain

Received: 24 June 2018; Accepted: 29 June 2018; Published: 4 July 2018

Abstract: Astrocytes are involved in many diseases of the central nervous system, not only as reactive cells to neuronal damage but also as primary actors in the pathological process. Astrogliopathy is a term used to designate the involvement of astrocytes as key elements in the pathogenesis and pathology of diseases and injuries of the central nervous system. Astrocytopathy is utilized to name non-reactive astrogliosis covering hypertrophy, atrophy and astroglial degeneration with loss of function in astrocytes and pathological remodeling, as well as senescent changes. Astrogliopathy and astrocytopathy are hallmarks of tauopathies—neurodegenerative diseases with abnormal hyper-phosphorylated tau aggregates in neurons and glial cells. The involvement of astrocytes covers different disease-specific types such as tufted astrocytes, astrocytic plaques, thorn-shaped astrocytes, granular/fuzzy astrocytes, ramified astrocytes and astrocytes with globular inclusions, as well as others which are unnamed but not uncommon in familial frontotemporal degeneration linked to mutations in the tau gene. Knowledge of molecular differences among tau-containing astrocytes is only beginning, and their distinct functional implications remain rather poorly understood. However, tau-containing astrocytes in certain conditions have deleterious effects on neuronal function and nervous system integrity. Moreover, recent studies have shown that tau-containing astrocytes obtained from human brain tauopathies have a capacity for abnormal tau seeding and spreading in wild type mice. Inclusive conceptions include a complex scenario involving neurons, glial cells and local environmental factors that potentiate each other and promote disease progression in tauopathies.

Keywords: astrocytes; tau; seeding; spreading; tauopathies; progressive supranuclear palsy; corticobasal degeneration; Pick's disease; aging-related tau astrogliopathy; primary age-related tauopathy; frontotemporal degeneration-tau; astrocytopathy

1. Introduction

Tauopathies are adult-age clinically, biochemically and anatomically heterogeneous neurodegenerative diseases, defined by the depositing of excessively phosphorylated tau protein, which is abnormally folded and eventually forms aggregates in nerve cells. Tau deposits in nerve cells form neurofibrillary tangles (NFT, neurofibrillary degeneration) and pre-tangle deposits, aggregates in neuronal and glial cell processes form neuropil threads, inclusions in astrocytes give rise to different morphological types, and inclusions in oligodendrocytes mainly form coiled bodies and, rarely, globular inclusions. Certain regions of the brain, and certain cell populations, are vulnerable to the pathology of tau, although the mechanisms of regional vulnerability and selective cellular vulnerability in tauopathies are poorly understood. Tau proteins are encoded by the microtubule-associated protein tau gene *MAPT*, the transcription of which, by alternative splicing, produces six isoforms in the brain. Some tauopathies are identified as 4R-tauopathies (4Rtau) and others as 3R-tauopathies (3Rtau) depending on the axon 10 splicing.

2. Human Tauopathies

The clinical and pathological phenotype of human tauopathies is, in part, determined by (a) the types of tau deposits (3Rtau or 4Rtau); (b) the specific regional and cellular vulnerability to each tauopathy; (c) the involvement of neurons and/or glial cells (astrocytes and oligodendrocytes); (d) the type of mutation in *MAPT* in familial tauopathy; and (e) the accompanying presence of extracellular amyloids, as in Alzheimer's disease (AD) (in which the tauopathy is associated with extracellular deposits of amyloid β (Aβ) giving rise to β-amyloid plaques), but also in British familial dementia (FBD) and Danish familial dementia (FDD) linked to distinct mutations in *BRI2* (or *ITMM2B)* and producing amyloids ABri and ADan, respectively. Certain families with Gerstmann–Sträussler–Scheinker syndrome (GSS) linked to mutations in *PRNP* (which encodes the prion protein) are associated with prionopathy and tauopathy.

The most frequent human sporadic tauopathy, in addition to sporadic AD, are primary age-related tauopathy (PART), a neuronal 4Rtau + 3Rtau similar to AD but without the Aβ component; aging-related tau astrogliopathy (ARTAG), a selective astrocyte 4Rtau; argyrophilic grain disease (AGD), a 4Rtau with predominant pre-tangles in neurons, protrusions in dendrites (grains) and inclusions in astrocytes and oligodendrocytes; Pick's disease (PiD), a 3Rtau with mainly neuronal involvement (Pick bodies) but also with tau deposits in astrocytes and oligodendrocytes; progressive supranuclear palsy (PSP) and corticobasal degeneration (CBD), both 4R-tauopathies with the involvement of neurons and oligodendrocytes, and with disease-specific tau deposits in astrocytes; and globular glial tauopathy (GGT), a 4Rtau with neuronal involvement and unique tau inclusions in astrocytes and globular tau deposits in oligodendrocytes [1–29].

The most common pure hereditary tauopathy is frontotemporal lobar degeneration linked to *MAPT* mutations (FTLD-tau). Clinically, FTLD-tau is manifested by frontal dementia (FTD) and parkinsonism; tau deposits are composed of 4Rtau, 3Rtau or 4Rtau + 3Rtau depending on the site of the mutation [30–34]. Globular glial tauopathy is mostly sporadic but certain tauopathies linked to *MAPT* mutations show variable amounts of globular inclusions in oligodendrocytes and bizarre astrocytic inclusions resembling sporadic GGT [35–38].

The most frequent combined tauopathy and amyloidopathy is familial AD linked to mutations in amyloid β precursor protein (APP)-related genes: *APP*, presenilin1 (*PSEN1*), or presenilin 2 (*PSEN2*). British familial dementia, FDD and GSS with tauopathy are extremely rare [21,39–41]. Other tauopathies can be reviewed elsewhere [25].

A combination of different tauopathies is not rare in old-age individuals [28,42,43]. The combination of AD, AGD and ARTAG is frequent in old-age individuals. The association of PSP or CBD and ARTAG and AGD is usual.

3. Non-Human Primate Tauopathies in Old Age

Tauopathy also occurs in aged non-human primates. Major research is focused on AD-related changes (Aβ deposits and tau deposits) in old-age animals. Interestingly, AD-like pathology is not rare in non-human primates, although there are marked species differences.

In cynomologous monkey (*Macaca fascicularis*), intraneuronal and oligodendroglial tau accumulation is found in the temporal cortex and hippocampus before the age of 20 years and before the presence of amyloid deposits; at advanced ages, NFTs and tau accumulate in dystrophic neurites [44]. An age-related increase of Aβ deposits in the form of plaques and around blood vessels is frequent, with gender differences, in the neocortex and hippocampus of western lowland gorilla (*Gorilla gorilla gorilla*), housed in American zoos and aquarium-accredited facilities. Neurons stained for the tau marker Alz50 are found in the neocortex and hippocampus of gorillas at all ages. Occasional Alz50-, MC1- and AT8-immunoreactive astrocyte and oligodendrocyte coiled bodies and neuritic clusters are seen in the neocortex and hippocampus of the oldest gorillas [45]. Aged wild mountain gorillas (*Gorilla beringei beringei*) which spent their entire lives in their natural habitat also display an age-related increase in APP and/or Aβ-immunoreactive blood vessels and plaques, but very limited tau pathology, in the frontal cortex [46]. In contrast, old-age baboons (*Papio hamadryas*) show NFTs in the hippocampus and limbic system, and tau-positive inclusions in astrocytes located in subependymal, subpial and perivascular locations, as well as in oligodendrocytes [47]. The first description of AD-like neuropathology in an aged chimpanzee (*Pan troglodytes*) included tau deposits in neurons, neuropil threads and plaque-like clusters throughout the neocortex with moderate Aβ deposition in blood vessels and rarely in plaques [48]. Subsequent studies in a larger series of chimpanzees revealed Aβ plaques, Aβ-angiopathy, and neurons with pre-tangles, NFTs and neuritic clusters [49].

Cerebral Aβ deposition is found in aged cotton-top tamarins (*Saguinus oedipus*), lemurs (*Lemuroidae*), marmosets, cynomologous monkeys, rhesus monkeys (*Macaca mulatta*), vervets (*Chlorocebus pygerythrus*), squirrel monkeys (*Saimiri* sp.), baboons, orangutans (*Pongo* sp.), gorillas and chimpanzees [50]. The amyloid precursor protein and its shorter fragment, Aβ, are homologous in humans and non-human primates. However, *MAPT* sequence varies among primates, with differences being minimal between human and chimpanzees. This may account for differences between humans and non-human primates regarding tau pathology in old-age and related tauopathies [51]. Further studies are needed to elucidate possibly overlooked tau deposition in glial cells, and additional abnormal tau-containing deposits such as grains in aged non-human primates.

4. Main Types of Tau-Containing Astrocytes

Astrocytes containing hyper-phosphorylated tau have disease-specific traits in the majority of tauopathies: tufted astrocytes in PSP, astrocytic plaques in CBD, thorn-shaped astrocytes (TSAs) and granular/fuzzy astrocytes (GFAs) in ARTAG, ramified astrocytes in PiD and astrocytes with globular inclusions in GGT [4,17,18,20,24,25,52–66]. (Figures 1–3).

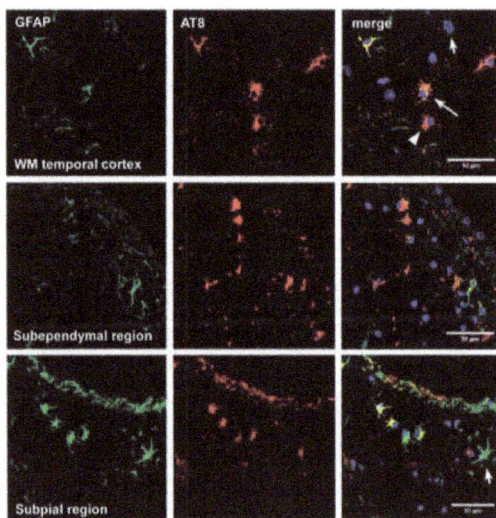

Figure 1. Double-labeling immunofluorescence to glial fibrillary acidic protein (GFAP) (green) and phospho-tau AT8 (red) showing the morphology of thorn-shaped astrocytes in the white matter of the temporal cortex, subependymal region and subpial region. Long arrow: cells with double staining; short arrow: cells only stained green; arrowhead: cells only stained red. Hyper-phosphorylated tau-containing astrocytes have reduced GFAP immunoreactivity. Paraffin sections; nuclei (blue) are stained with DRAQ5 (Biostatus, Leicestershire, UK); WM: withe matter; bar = 50 μm.

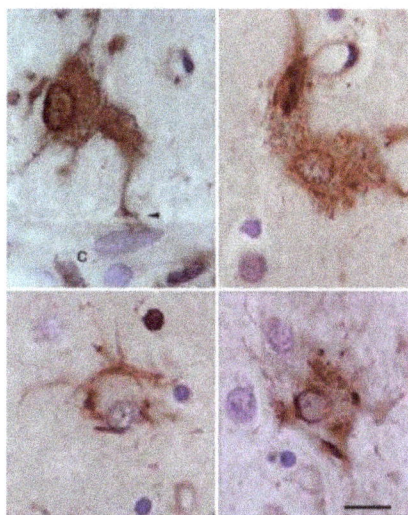

Figure 2. Tau-containing astrocytes in progressive supernuclear palsy (PSP). Typical tufted astrocytes are seen in the lower row. A perivascular astrocyte with a podocyte (arrowhead) in the vicinity of a capillary (C), and a reactive astrocyte also contain hyper-phosphorylated tau (upper row). Paraffin section, AT8 immunohistochemistry, slightly counterstained with hematoxylin, bar = 10 µm.

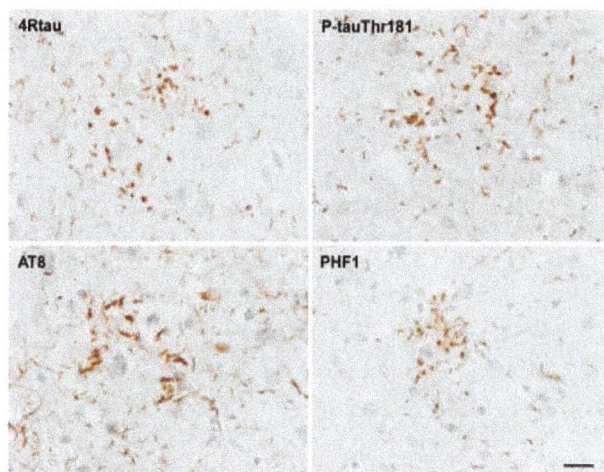

Figure 3. Astrocytic plaques in corticobasal degeneration (CBD), stained with 4Rtau, P-tauThr181, AT8 (P-tau Ser202-Thr205) and antibody PHF1 (P-tauSer396-Ser404). Paraffin sections slightly counterstained with hematoxilin, bar = 25 µm.

However, some tau-containing astrocytes are found in different tauopathies—for example, TSAs occur in aging, AGD, AD, PSP and CBD [14,19,67–72], and in traumatic chronic encephalopathy [73]. Granular/fuzzy astrocytes are seen in the elderly and ARTAG [26,70], but also in other tauopathies such as in PSP [37].

Interestingly, tau-containing astrocytes are early lesions in PSP, CBD and FTLD-tau [28,74–76].

Various types of astrocytic inclusions are generated in familial FTLD-tau linked to mutations in exons 1 and 10 and in introns following exons 9 and 10, the morphology of which largely depends on the *MAPT* mutation. Intracytoplasmic tau-immunoreactive inclusions in FTLD-tau are represented by tufted-like astrocytes, astrocytic plaques, ramified astrocytes, TSAs, astrocytes with globular inclusions and other types with no specific names [17,33,34,36,37,66,77–86]. Tufted astrocytes and astrocytic plaques practically do not co-exist in PSP and CBD [57], but these lesions appear in combination in FTLD-tau [29] (Figure 4).

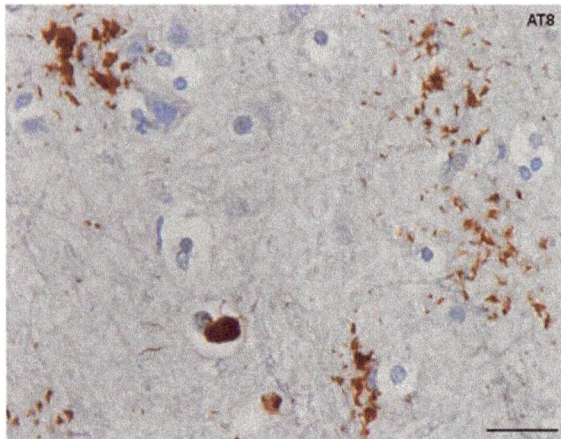

Figure 4. Frontotemporal lobar degeneration linked to *MAPT* mutations (FTLD-tau) K317M stained with antibody AT8 showing tufted-like astrocytes (reminiscent of tau-containing astrocytes in globular glial tauopathy (GGT)), astrocytic plaques and globular inclusion in an oligodendrocyte. Paraffin sections, slightly counterstained with hematoxylin, bar = 25 µm.

Extensive astrocyte-predominant tauopathy involving brain astrocytes and Bergmann glia has been reported in familial behavioral variant frontotemporal dementia associated with astrocyte-predominant tauopathy; the morphology of abnormal astrocytes, including deposits in Bergmann glia, differs from all other tauopathies [87].

The localization of tau-containing astrocytes does not always match that of tau-containing neurons in tauopathies [14,19,28,76,88–92]. Curiously, tufted astrocytes and astrocytic plaques are often located near the blood vessels [93], and perivascular distribution is overwhelming in a rare familial behavioral variant frontotemporal dementia associated with astrocyte-predominant tauopathy [87]. Regarding ARTAG, TSAs are found in regions proximal to the CSF and blood vessels [72].

Hyper-phosphorylated tau intracytoplasmic filamentous inclusions are common in transgenic mouse models of tauopathies both in animals over-expressing human tau and those bearing different tau mutations which are causative of human familial FTLD-tau. Tau pathology in glial cells has been generated in transgenic mice over-expressing human tau in neurons and glial cells. In these animals, a tau pathology resembling astrocytic plaques and coiled bodies in oligodendrocytes is found in old mice; these changes are associated with glial and axonal degeneration [94].

Transgenic mice bearing P301L tau develop cytoplasmic neuronal inclusions, and oligodendroglial and astrocytic filamentous inclusions composed of abnormal hyper-phosphorylated tau aggregates [95]. Similar neuronal and glial tau-immunoreactive inclusions occur in the P301S transgenic mouse (Figure 5).

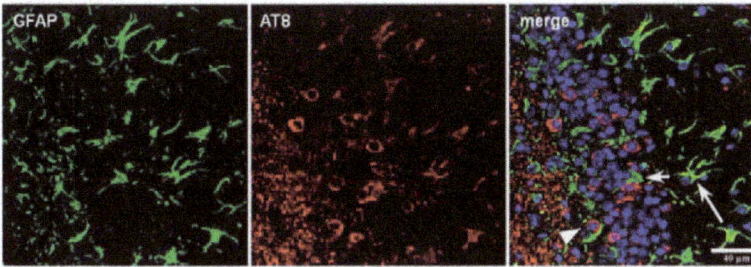

Figure 5. P301S transgenic mice aged 10 months. Double-labeling immunofluorescence to GFAP (green) and AT8 (red) showing cells with double staining (long arrow), cells only stained green (short arrow) and cells only stained red (arrowhead). Some astrocytes contain hyper-phosphorylated tau deposits. Paraffin sections; nuclei stained with DRAQ5 (Biostatus) (blue); bar = 40 μm.

5. Post-Translational Tau Modifications and Tau Kinases in Tau-Containing Astrocytes in Tauopathies

Tau in astrocytes is hyper-phosphorylated at different sites including Thr181, Ser199, Thr231, Ser262, Ser422, Ser202-Thr205 (antibody AT8), Ser396-Ser404 (antibody PHF1) and Thr212/Ser214 (tau-100), and it has an altered conformation as revealed with the antibodies Alz50 (amino acids 5–15) and MC-1 (amino acids 312–322) [37]. All these astrocytic inclusions in sporadic tauopathies are composed of 4Rtau isoforms, but certain astrocytes in PiD and PSP contain 3Rtau [37]. Astrocytic inclusions in FTLD-tau depend on the mutation, but they are largely composed of 4Rtau [33,37,66].

Astrocytes containing hyper-phosphorylated tau inclusions co-express phosphorylated tau kinases: mitogen-activated protein kinase/extracellular signal-regulated kinase (MAPK/ERK), p-38 kinase, stress-activated kinase/c-Jun N-terminal kinase (SAPK/JNK) and glycogen synthase kinase-3 [14,82,96–100]. Co-expression in astrocytes suggests active phosphorylation of tau by specific kinases; such co-localization also occurs in neurons with pre-tangles and tangles in the same tauopathies.

The presence of truncated forms of tau in tau-containing astrocytes is not documented in detail. Most tau-containing astrocytes in tauopathies are not stained with the antibody tau-C3 which recognizes tau truncated at aspartic acid 421 [37]. Only small tau-C3 immunoreactive dots are occasionally seen in TSAs [71]. Exceptions are astrocytes with globular inclusions in GGT, astrocytes in certain FTLD-tau (as in the familial tauopathy linked to *MAPT* K317M), and astrocytes in familial behavioral variant frontotemporal dementia associated with astrocyte-predominant tauopathy [37,87]. In such cases, tau-containing astrocytes are always ubiquitinated [37]. In contrast, tufted astrocytes, astrocytic plaques, TSAs and ramified astrocytes only very rarely contain ubiquitin-immunoreactive deposits [37] (Figure 6).

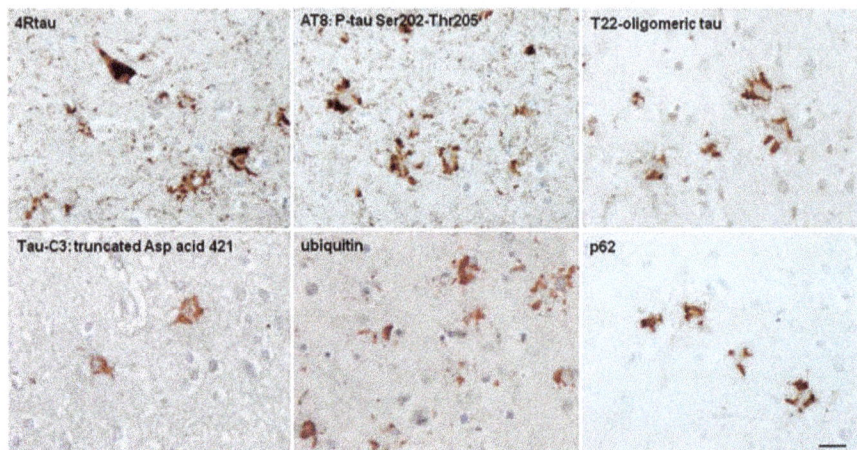

Figure 6. Globular glial tauopathy (GGT) showing abnormal tau-containing astrocytes with distinctive features stained with antibodies against 4Rtau, clone AT8 (directed against P-tau Ser202-Thr205), tau22 (anti-oligomeric tau), tau-C3 (against tau truncation at aspartic acid 421), ubiquitin and p62. One neuron is also observed in the section stained with anti-4Rtau. Paraffin sections slightly counterstained with hematoxylin, bar = 25 μm.

Tau phosphorylation, conformation and truncation in astrocytes have characteristics similar to their neuronal counterparts in tauopathies with equivalents to pre-tangles and tangle stages [37]. However, this must be interpreted with caution as knowledge is still limited. For example, a lack of epitopes derived from alternatively spliced exon 2 and 3 has been reported in glial tau when compared with neuronal tau in certain tauopathies [56,101]. Tau acetylation is rarer in astrocytes when compared to neurons in tauopathies [102]. Tau is acetylated in glial inclusions in FTLD-tau [102] but apparently not in AGD [103]. This is an important point, as tau acetylation inhibits tau function and promotes tau aggregation [104,105].

Finally, tau truncation may occur at different sites of tau; western blots of total brain homogenates show bands of low molecular weight in most tauopathies, but the method does not discriminate between neurons and glial cells. Immunohistochemistry utilizing tau antibodies directed against specific amino acids of tau (amino-terminal, carboxyl-terminal, middle segments) can be useful to uncover possible sites of tau truncation in astrocytes in tauopathies in addition to the characteristic truncation at aspartic acid 421 in astrocytes in minority tauopathies. Thorn-shaped astrocytes (TSAs) are stained with antibody 394 (amino acids 394–398, corresponding to the carboxyl-terminal); antibody 229 (against amino acids 229–233, middle region) and antibody 499 (directed against amino acids 14–26, amino-terminal) [106]. Tau-containing astrocytes in FTLD-tau 301T are stained with antibodies tau 7 (directed against amino acids 426–441), 394, 229 and 499 (Figure 7A). However, tufted astrocytes in PSP and astrocytic plaques in CBD are decorated with antibodies tau 7, 229 and 394 but barely or not at all with antibody 499, thus suggesting the reduction or absence of tau species containing the amino terminal of tau protein in tufted astrocytes and astrocytic plaques (Figure 7B,C).

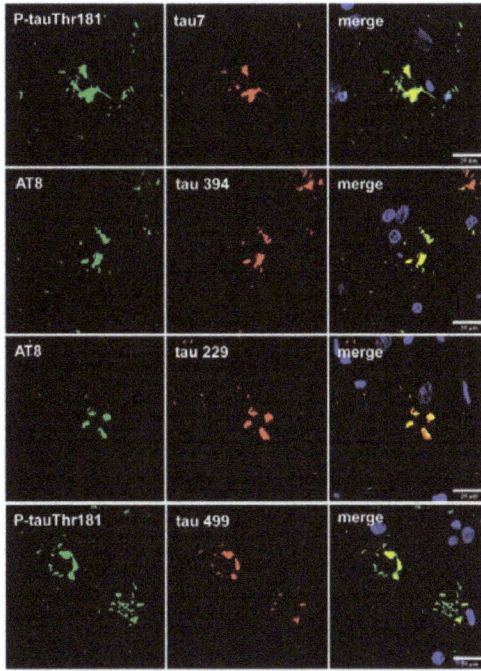

(A)

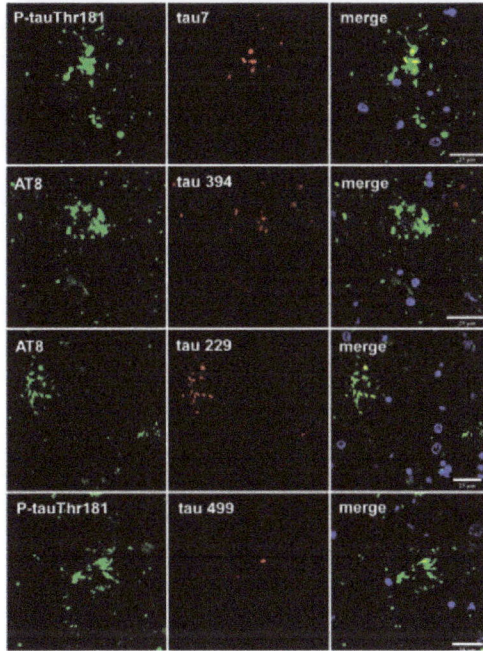

(B)

Figure 7. *Cont.*

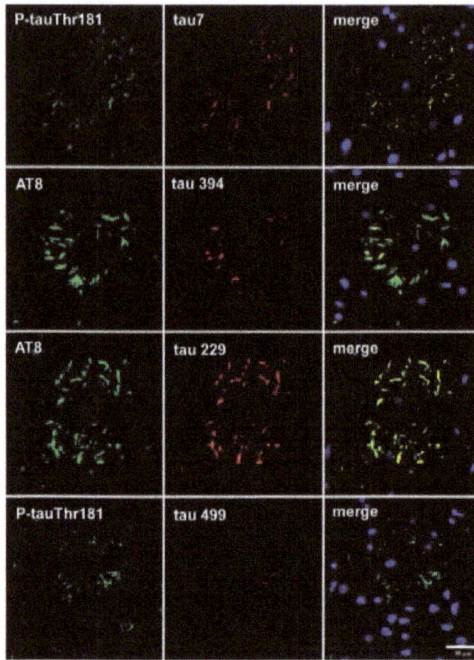

(C)

Figure 7. Double-labeling immunofluorescence and confocal microscopy using antibodies tau 7 (directed against amino acids 426–441), 394 (amino acids 394–398, corresponding to the carboxyl terminal), 229 (against amino acids 229–233, middle region), and 499 (directed against amino acids 14–26, amino terminal) (green); and P-tauThr181 or AT8 (depending on the mouse or rabbit origin of the first anti-tau antibodies) (red) in FTLD-tau linked to 301T mutation (**A**); PSP (**B**) and CBD (**C**). Tau 7, 229 and 394 co-localize with phospho-tau deposits in astrocytes in FTLD-tau 301T, tufted astrocytes and astrocytic plaques; antibody 499 also co-localizes with phospho-tau in FTLD-tau 301T, but tufted astrocytes and astrocytic plaques almost lack 499 tau immunostaining, thus suggesting tau amino terminal truncation. Paraffin sections; nuclei (blue) are stained with DRAQ5 (Biostatus); A, bar= 20 μm; B, bar = 25 μm C; bar = 30 μm.

6. Cytoarchitectonic Changes Linked to Tau Deposits in Astrocytes

Not all astrocytes are immunoreactive to glial fibrillary acidic protein (GFAP) [107–110]. However, GFAP is currently used as a marker of astrocytes, mainly for reactive astrocytes.

Even considering these limitations, double-labeling immunofluorescence and confocal microscopy have been used to learn about cytoskeletal anomalies in astrocytes containing hyper-phosphorylated tau. Glial fibrillary acidic protein has been reported to be absent in tufted astrocytes in PSP [58,111]. However, small amounts of GFAP are commonly redistributed around the nucleus in tufted astrocytes in PSP and FTLD-tau. GFAP is disrupted by short segments or dots of hyper-phosphorylated tau throughout the astrocytic processes in astrocytic plaques in CBD, and in astrocytes with proximal granular inclusions in FTLD-tau/P301L. Glial fibrillary acidic protein immunoreactivity is also displaced by hyper-phosphorylated tau deposits in ramified astrocytes in PiD, TSAs in ARTAG, tau-containing astrocytes in GGT, and astrocytes in familial behavioral variant frontotemporal dementia associated with astrocyte-predominant tauopathy [37,87,92] (Figure 8).

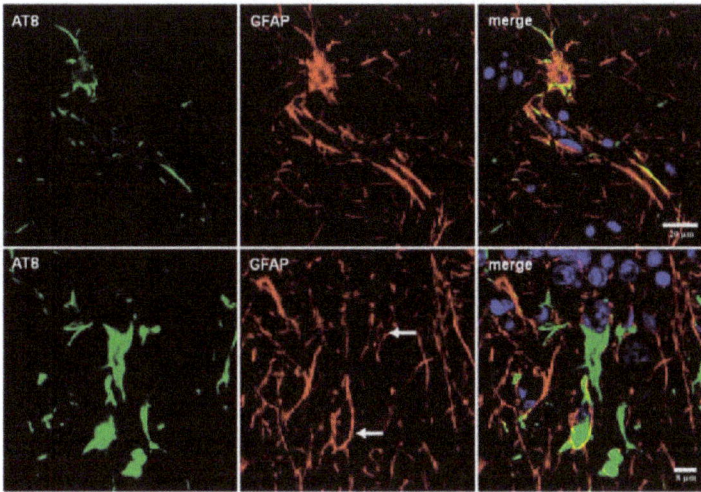

Figure 8. Double-labeling immunofluorescence and confocal microscopy to phospho-tau clone AT8 (green) and glial fibrillary acidic protein (red) in the cerebral cortex (upper row) and cerebellum (lower row) in familial behavioral variant frontotemporal dementia associated with astrocyte-predominant tauopathy. Variable distortion of the glial cytoskeleton is found mainly in Bergmann glia. Nuclei are stained with DRAQ5 (Biostatus) (blue). Upper row, bar = 20 μm; lower row, bar = 8 μm.

7. Astrogliopathy

This term refers to alterations of astrocytes occurring in diseases of the nervous system, implying the involvement of astrocytes as key elements in the pathogenesis and pathology of diseases and in injuries of the central nervous system [112–122].

Reactive astrogliosis is a reaction secondary to neuronal damage in various injuries such as trauma and ischemia, external toxins, metabolic disorders and neurodegenerative diseases. The term astrocytopathy is used for non-reactive astrogliosis including hypertrophy, atrophy and astroglial degeneration with loss of function manifested by variable and distinct molecular changes in astrocytes, and pathological remodeling [112,117]. Senescent astrocytes are a particular form of astrocytophathy linked to old age which is manifested by modifications in the morphology of the nucleus and cytoplasm, cytoskeletal changes, oxidative damage, reduced energy production and secretory phenotype including production of inflammatory cytokines [92].

8. Reactive Astrogliosis

Reactive astrogliosis is common to all tauopathies and its distribution correlates with the degree of regional vulnerability to neuronal degeneration and neuronal loss [17,123,124]. However, tau-containing astrocytes do not match reactive astrocytes and they represent different although occasionally co-existent lesions [17,18,92,124].

Reactive astrogliosis also occurs in transgenic mouse models; the hippocampus is mainly affected in mice bearing the P301S mutation [125].

The expression of small heat shock proteins (HSP25/27 and αB-crystallin) is a characteristic response of reactive astrocytes in most tauopathies. However, HSPs are rarely co-expressed in astrocytes containing hyper-phosphorylated tau [126–129] (Figure 9). This suggests that generalized stress, rather than the restricted response in glial cells with abnormal protein aggregates, induces HSP expression [129]. Alternatively, it may be postulated that stress responses are directed to correcting protein misfolding, and that they succeed to a certain extent, in that aggregates are not formed in many glial cells [92].

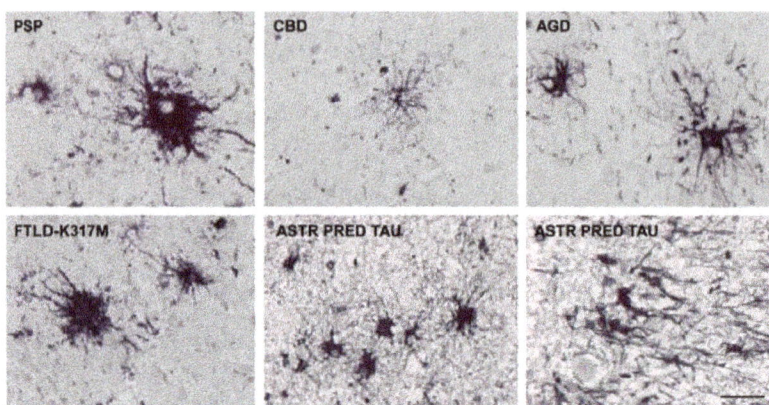

Figure 9. αB-crystallin-immunoreactive astrocytes in PSP, CBD, argyrophilic gain disease (AGD), FTLD-tau K317M and familial behavioral variant frontotemporal dementia associated with astrocyte-predominant tauopathy. Paraffin sections visualized with diaminobenzidine, NH_4NiSO_4 and H_2O_2 without hematoxylin counterstaining; bar = 50 μm.

Additionally, it has been reported that intraneuronal accumulation of misfolded tau protein induces over-expression of Hsp27 in activated astrocytes [130].

9. Astrocytopathy

In spite of the evident astrocytopathy characterized by disease-dependent stereotyped tau deposits, little is known about the functional effects of hyper-phosphorylated tau in tau-containing astrocytes in tauopathies [131]. This is due to several factors: the diversity of astrocytes, diversity of functions and gene expression profiles under various conditions and regions, as well as the lack of studies considering these variables in tauopathies.

Astrocytes are not homogeneous cells. They can be classified into protoplasmic astrocytes of the grey matter, interlaminar astrocytes of the cerebral cortex, subpial astrocytes of the cerebral cortex, fibrous astrocytes of the white matter, perivascular astrocytes, Bergmann glia, stem astrocytes of subventricular zones, radial glia of the developing brain, tanycytes of the hypothalamus, pituicytes and Müller glia of the retina [116]. Moreover, they are heterogeneous with respect to their coverage domains, ion channels, calcium responses, glutamate transporters and expression of neurotransmitter receptors [92,132].

Gene expression studies of neurons and glial cells have contributed to our understanding of the variety of gene expression profiles that advance distinct functions in different cell types [133–140]. Microarray analyses of isolated astrocytes have identified particular transcription profiles in AD and related animal models [141,142].

Unfortunately, this approach has not been utilized in human tauopathies, and we are still in the dark concerning gene expression differences among TSAs, tufted astrocytes, astrocytic plaques and astrocytes with globular inclusions, to name just some examples.

Moreover, we do not know about similarities and differences among tau-containing astrocytes in the same disease but located in different regions; for example, subependymal, subpial, clusters in the frontal and temporal white matter, basal forebrain and perivascular TSAs in ARTAG.

These aspects are important in the present context as we do not know whether different tau inclusions affect different astrocyte types with particular vulnerability to tau species, or even if different tau species modify the morphology and function of the same type of astrocyte.

The over-expression of tau in cultured astrocytes produces degeneration of the cytoskeleton and Golgi complex, eventually leading to cell death [143]. Altered nuclear function and DNA transcription has also been posited for tau-containing neurons in tauopathies and fly models [144–147].

The expression of solute carrier family 1 member 2 (SLC1A2 or GLT-1) is markedly reduced in most astrocytes bearing hyper-phosphorylated tau in familial behavioral variant frontotemporal dementia associated with astrocyte-predominant tauopathy [87]. Decreased expression of GLT-1 and solute carrier family 1 member 3 (SLC1A3 or GLAST) also occurs in transgenic mice selectively expressing hyper-phosphorylated tau in astrocytes [148,149].

Whether tau-containing astrocytes have deleterious effects on neurons is an important question, as decreased GLT-1 expression alters glutamate metabolism and enhances excitotxicity. Hyper-phosphorylated tau deposits also have effects on the redistribution of organelles and reactive responses, but their functional effects are not known (Figure 10).

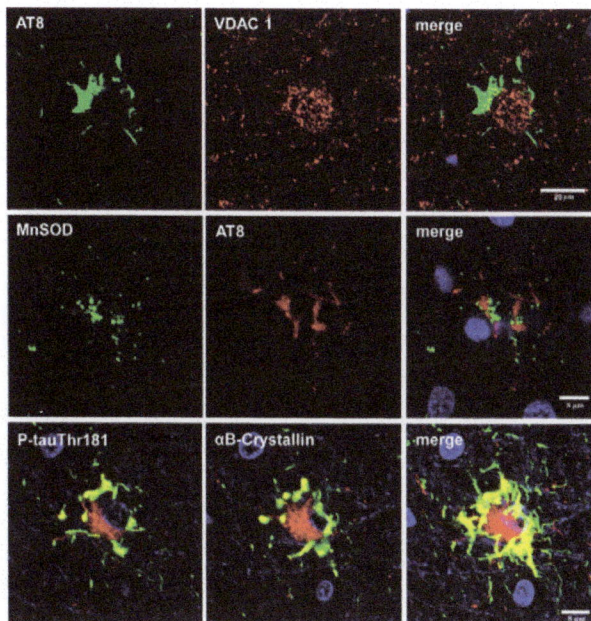

Figure 10. Double-labeling immunofluorescence and confocal microscopy of tufted astrocytes in PSP to AT8 and voltage-dependent anion-selective channel 1: VDAC1 (upper row), AT8 and superoxide dismutase 2: MnSOD, SOD2 (middle row), and serial sections of P-tauThr181 and αB-crystallin (lower row). VDAC1 is concentrated at the center of the cell due to the displacement of peripheral tau whereas SOD2 immunoreactivity is intermingled with phospho-tau deposits. αB-crystallin is found around the nucleus and surrounded by hyper-phosphorylated tufts. Paraffin sections; nuclei (blue) are stained with DRAQ5 (Biostatus); upper row, bar =20 μm; middle and lower row, bar =8μm.

Moreover, extracellular tau oligomers rapidly accumulate in astrocytes and reduce the release of gliotransmitters, thus impairing neuronal function [150].

Furthermore, FTLD-N279K *MAPT* astrocytes derived from neural stem cells increase oxidative stress and produce marked modifications in the genomic expression of co-cultured healthy neurons [151]. Finally, P301S-derived astrocytes significantly decrease pre-synaptic and post-synaptic protein expression in cortical neuron cultures, whereas normal astrocytes enhance these markers, thereby suggesting that mutant astrocytes have reduced neuroprotective capacities [152].

10. Disease Progression: Seeding and Spreading; Role of Astrocytes

Tauopathies are progressive biological processes with a preclinical phase, prodromal phases and phases with clinical manifestations. The stages of NFT progression (stages I–VI of Braak) in AD are well known [153,154]. The stages of NFT pathology in PART are the same as those proposed for AD; whether PART is part of AD is a matter of discussion [155,156]. The majority of cases formerly classified as early stages of sporadic AD lack Aβ plaques [157,158] and are now considered PART, whereas the majority of cases with advanced Braak NFT stages are considered AD because of the presence of abundant Aβ deposits. Whatever the name, early stages of NFT are very common in old people as they occur in about 85% of individuals aged 65 years [157,159].

Different stages have also been proposed to categorize disease progression in AGD [14,160]. In contrast, only short series of incidental and early stages of PSP and CBD are available [74–76,161,162] to permit a validation of the several proposed sequences of events in disease progression.

The progression of AD and tauopathies is thought to occur by trans-cellular and trans-regional propagation of the abnormal protein in a similar way to what happens in prion diseases [163]. The exact mechanism of transmission is not known. Release and trans-synaptic transmission of tau [164,165], tau uptake via exosomes [166–168] or nanotubules [169] and free uptake of fibrillar proteins [170,171] have all been suggested as putative mechanisms using cultured neurons. Although astrocyte-to-neuron intercellular transfer mediated by cell-to-cell contact has been postulated for prions [172], no information is available concerning astrocyte-to-neuron transfer in tauopathies.

Transgenic mice with human tau over-expression or with tau mutations have been used to facilitate the mechanism of seeding and progression. Seeding and spreading of abnormal tau occurs after inoculation of brain homogenates from AD and other tauopathies into the brain of transgenic mice over-expressing human tau or mutated tau [163,173–175]. The type of deposits in the inoculated animals seems to be disease-dependent in the few tauopathies so far studied, which suggests the occurrence of different species or strains of tau depending on the disease [176–178]. However, these models have a natural substrate of abnormal tau production that makes it difficult to separate the propagation itself from what is induced.

Seeding of human tau from homogenates of AD and tauopathies with neuronal and glial components is also observed after inoculation into the brain of wild-type mice [178,179].

Additionally, the inoculation effect of recombinant tau is different from the effects using human brain homogenates enriched with tau fibrils from brains with tauopathy [178]. This suggests that different species ('strains') of tau have different properties and produce different effects. Another difference between the inoculation of recombinant tau fibrils and inoculation of tau from human brain homogenates is the accompanying inoculation, in the latter, of a number of associated proteins and enzymes which represents a probably disease-specific environment with unexplored properties.

All these experiments have been performed using brain samples of tauopathies with tau pathology only in neurons or with tau pathology in neurons and in glial cells. Abnormal tau in these paradigms can spread to resident neurons, astrocytes and oligodendroglia [176–178]. In other words, certain tau prion strains have the capacity to induce tauopathy not only in neurons but also in glial cells [180] (Figure 11).

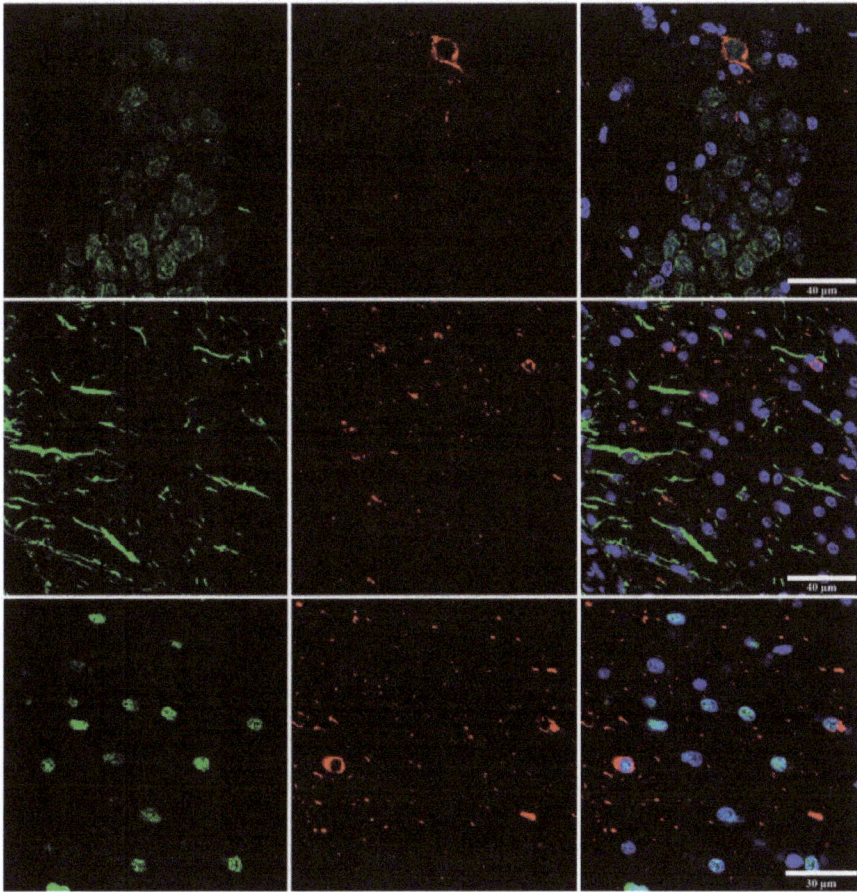

Figure 11. Wild-type (WT) mice inoculated with primary age-related tauopathy (PART) in the hippocampus at the age of 7 months and killed at the age of 10 months. Double-labeling immunofluorescence to neuronal nuclear protein (NeuN), GFAP and Olig-2 (green) and P-tauThr181 or clone AT8 (red). Subpopulations of neurons, astrocytes and oligodendrocytes contain hyper-phosphorylated tau (arrows). Paraffin sections, nuclei stained with DRAQ5 (Biostatus) (blue), bar, upper and middle row, bar = 30 μm; lower row, bar = 40 μm.

Whether astrocytic tau alone is able to induce tauopathy has recently been assessed. Tau-enriched fractions of brain homogenates from pure ARTAG (with no associated tauopathy) inoculated into the hippocampus (dentate gyrus and *cornu ammonis* (CA1) of wild-type mice generate intracytoplasmic hyper-phosphorylated tau inclusions in astrocytes, oligodendrocytes and neurons near the site of injection, and in nerve fiber tracts in the fimbria and *corpus callosum* [106] (Figure 12). These observations indicate that astrocytes containing hyper-phosphorylated tau have the capability of seeding tau to neurons and glial cells, thus highlighting the putatively cardinal role of astrocytopathy in the pathogenesis of tauopathies [106]. Moreover, inoculation of ARTAG, containing 4Rtau astrocytes, produces 3Rtau seeding in neurons and glial cells in addition to 4Rtau deposition [106]. This also points to the likely involvement of astrocytes in the development of tau-containing neuronal processes in the aged brain [181].

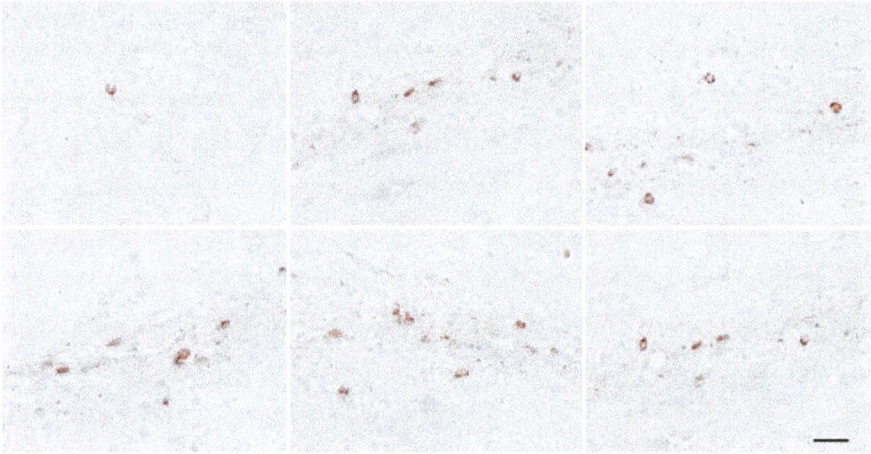

Figure 12. Wild-type mice inoculated with aging-related tau astrogliopathy (ARTAG) in the hippocampus at the age of 12 months and killed at the age of 19 months. The upper row corresponds to one mouse in which a hyper-phosphorylated tau-containing neuron is seen in CA1 region of the hippocampus (left) and several glial cells and fibers in the *corpus callosum* radiation of the ipsilateral side (middle) and contralateral side of injection (right). The lower row corresponds to another mouse showing hyper-phosphorylated tau fibers and glial cells in the *corpus callosum* radiation of the ipsilateral side (left), middle region of the *corpus callosum* (middle) and contralateral radiation of the *corpus callosum* (right). Paraffin sections immunostained with the AT8 antibody and slightly counterstained with hematoxylin, bar = 25 μm.

The fact that a neuronal tauopathy such as PART (only containing NFTs and threads) or pure forms of ARTAG (only containing TSAs) can produce seeding in neurons, astrocytes and oligodendrocytes in WT mice is an unexpected observation. This may be in part because different murine tau isoforms can be distinguished by the carboxyl terminal domains, and murine tau differs from human tau in a number of ways, including the absence of residues which are involved in tubulin binding [182].

Finally, environmental factors may influence tau pathology and seeding in astrocytes (and other cell types). Phosphoproteomics using bi-dimensional gel electrophoresis and mass spectrometry have shown a large number of phosphorylated proteins in addition to tau and related molecules in AD [183–185]. Other studies have identified GFAP phosphorylation in AD and in many other tauopathies [186,187]. More precise methods in several regions and different stages of disease have demonstrated the occurrence of very large numbers of phosphorylated proteins including kinases and synaptic proteins in areas with no relationship to β-amyloid deposits and NFTs [188]. Similar studies have recognized a number of phosphorylated proteins including phospho-kinases, neurofilaments, and synaptic and other neuronal proteins, in addition to phospho-GFAP and phosphorylated aquaporine-4 in the white matter in pure cases of ARTAG [106]. Although similar studies are not available in other tauopathies, these observations suggest that tau pathology in astrocytes should be interpreted not as an isolated process but in the context of a very particular environment which is hospitable to tau phosphorylation.

Funding: This study was funded by Ministry of Economy, Industry and Competitiveness, Institute of Health Carlos III (ISCIII–ERDF, a way to build Europe) PI17/00809, and co-financed by ERDF under the program Interreg Poctefa: RedPrion 148/16.

Acknowledgments: I wish to thank M. Carmona and B. Torrejón-Escribano for the preparation of figures and T. Yohannan for editorial help.

Conflicts of Interest: The author declares no conflict of interest.

References

1. Tolnay, M.; Spillantini, M.G.; Goedert, M.; Ulrich, J.; Langui, D.; Probst, A. Argyrophilic grain disease: Widespread hyperphosphorylation of tau protein in limbic neurons. *Acta Neuropathol.* **1997**, *93*, 477–484. [CrossRef] [PubMed]
2. Molina, J.A.; Probst, A.; Villanueva, C.; Jimenez-Jimenez, F.J.; Madero, S.; Torres, N.; Bermejo, F. Primary progressive aphasia with glial cytoplasmic inclusions. *Eur. Neurol.* **1998**, *40*, 71–77. [CrossRef] [PubMed]
3. Jellinger, K.A. Dementia with grains (argyrophilic grain disease). *Brain Pathol.* **1998**, *8*, 377–386. [CrossRef] [PubMed]
4. Bigio, E.H.; Lipton, A.M.; Yen, S.H.; Hutton, M.L.; Baker, M.; Nacharaju, P.; White, C.L., 3rd; Davies, P.; Lin, W.; Dickson, D.W. Frontal lobe dementia with novel tauopathy: Sporadic multiple system tauopathy with dementia. *J. Neuropathol. Exp. Neurol.* **2001**, *60*, 328–341. [CrossRef] [PubMed]
5. Berry, R.W.; Quinn, B.; Johnson, N.; Cochran, E.J.; Ghoshal, N.; Binder, L.I. Pathological glial tau accumulations in neurodegenerative disease: Review and case report. *Neurochem. Int.* **2001**, *39*, 469–479. [CrossRef]
6. Ferrer, I.; Hernandez, I.; Boada, M.; Llorente, A.; Rey, M.J.; Cardozo, A.; Ezquerra, M.; Puig, B. Primary progressive aphasia as the initial manifestation of corticobasal degeneration and unusual tauopathies. *Acta Neuropathol.* **2003**, *106*, 419–435. [CrossRef] [PubMed]
7. Powers, J.M.; Byrne, N.P.; Ito, M.; Takao, M.; Yankopoulou, D.; Spillantini, M.G.; Ghetti, B. A novel leukoencephalopathy associated with tau deposits primarily in white matter glia. *Acta Neuropathol.* **2003**, *106*, 181–187. [CrossRef] [PubMed]
8. Clark, C.N.; Lashley, T.; Mahoney, C.J.; Warren, J.D.; Revesz, T.; Rohrer, J.D. Temporal Variant Frontotemporal dementia is associated with globular glial tauopathy. *Cogn. Behav. Neurol.* **2015**, *28*, 92–97. [CrossRef] [PubMed]
9. Piao, Y.S.; Tan, C.F.; Iwanaga, K.; Kakita, A.; Takano, H.; Nishizawa, M.; Lashley, T.; Revesz, T.; Lees, A.; de Silva, R.; et al. Sporadic four-repeat tauopathy with frontotemporal degeneration, parkinsonism and motor neuron disease. *Acta Neuropathol.* **2005**, *110*, 600–609. [CrossRef] [PubMed]
10. Josephs, K.A.; Katsuse, O.; Beccano-Kelly, D.A.; Lin, W.L.; Uitti, R.J.; Fujino, Y.; Boeve, B.F.; Hutton, M.L.; Baker, M.C.; Dickson, D.W. Atypical progressive supranuclear palsy with corticospinal tract degeneration. *J. Neuropathol. Exp. Neurol.* **2006**, *65*, 396–405. [CrossRef] [PubMed]
11. Williams, D.R. Tauopathies: Classification and clinical update on neurodegenerative diseases associated with microtubule-associated protein tau. *Intern. Med. J.* **2006**, *36*, 652–660. [CrossRef] [PubMed]
12. Kovacs, G.G.; Majtenyi, K.; Spina, S.; Murrell, J.R.; Gelpi, E.; Hoftberger, R.; Fraser, G.; Crowther, R.A.; Goedert, M.; Budka, H.; et al. White matter tauopathy with globular glial inclusions: A distinct sporadic frontotemporal lobar degeneration. *J. Neuropathol. Exp. Neurol.* **2008**, *67*, 963–975. [CrossRef] [PubMed]
13. Giaccone, G.; Marcon, G.; Mangieri, M.; Morbin, M.; Rossi, G.; Fetoni, V.; Patriarca, C.; Catania, M.; Di Fede, G.; Tagliavini, F.; et al. Atypical tauopathy with massive involvement of the white matter. *Neuropathol. Appl. Neurobiol.* **2008**, *34*, 468–472. [PubMed]
14. Ferrer, I.; Santpere, G.; van Leeuwen, F.W. Argyrophilic grain disease. *Brain* **2008**, *146*, 1640–1651. [CrossRef] [PubMed]
15. Fu, Y.J.; Nishihira, Y.; Kuroda, S.; Toyoshima, Y.; Ishihara, T.; Shinozaki, M.; Miyashita, A.; Piao, Y.S.; Tan, C.F.; Tani, T.; et al. Sporadic four-repeat tauopathy with frontotemporal lobar degeneration, parkinsonism, and motor neuron disease: A distinct clinicopathological and biochemical disease entity. *Acta Neuropathol.* **2010**, *120*, 21–32. [CrossRef] [PubMed]
16. Ahmed, Z.; Doherty, K.M.; Silveira-Moriyama, L.; Bandopadhyay, R.; Lashley, T.; Mamais, A.; Hondhamuni, G.; Wray, S.; Newcombe, J.; O'Sullivan, S.S.; et al. Globular glial tauopathies (GGT) presenting with motor neuron disease or frontotemporal dementia: An emerging group of 4-repeat tauopathies. *Acta Neuropathol.* **2011**, *122*, 415–428. [CrossRef] [PubMed]
17. Dickson, D.W.; Hauw, J.J.; Agid, Y.; Litvan, I. Progressive supranuclear palsy and corticobasal degeneration. In *Neurodegeneration: The Molecular Pathology of Dementia and Movement Disorders*, 2nd ed.; Dickson, D.W., Weller, R.O., Eds.; Willey-Blackwell: Chichester, UK, 2011; pp. 135–155.
18. Muñoz, D.G.; Morris, H.R.; Rossor, M. Pick's disease. In *Neurodegeneration: The Molecular Pathology of Dementia and Movement Disorders*, 2nd ed.; Dickson, D.W., Weller, R.O., Eds.; Willey-Blackwell: Chichester, UK, 2011; pp. 156–164.

19. Tolnay, M.; Braak, H. Argyrophilic grain disease. In *Neurodegeneration: The Molecular Pathology of Dementia and Movement Disorders*, 2nd ed.; Dickson, D.W., Weller, R.O., Eds.; Wiley-Blackwell: Chichester, UK, 2011; pp. 165–170.

20. Ahmed, Z.; Bigio, E.H.; Budka, H.; Dickson, D.W.; Ferrer, I.; Ghetti, B.; Giaccone, G.; Hatanpaa, K.J.; Holton, J.L.; Josephs, K.A.; et al. Globular glial tauopathies (GGT): Consensus recommendations. *Acta Neuropathol.* **2013**, *126*, 537–544. [CrossRef] [PubMed]

21. Lowe, J.; Kalaria, R. Dementia. In *Greenfield's Neuropathology*, 9th ed.; Love, S., Budka, H., Ironside, J., Perry, A., Eds.; CRC Press: Boca Raton, FL, USA, 2015; pp. 858–973.

22. Crary, J.F.; Trojanowski, J.Q.; Schneider, J.A.; Abisambra, J.F.; Abner, E.L.; Alafuzoff, I.; Arnold, S.E.; Attems, J.; Beach, T.G.; Bigio, E.H.; et al. Primary age-related tauopathy (PART): A common pathology associated with human aging. *Acta Neuropathol.* **2014**, *128*, 755–766. [CrossRef] [PubMed]

23. Jellinger, K.A.; Alafuzoff, I.; Attems, J.; Beach, T.G.; Cairns, N.J.; Crary, J.F.; Dickson, D.W.; Hof, P.R.; Hyman, B.T.; Jack, C.R., Jr.; et al. PART, a distinct tauopathy, different from classical sporadic Alzheimer disease. *Acta Neuropathol.* **2015**, *129*, 757–762. [CrossRef] [PubMed]

24. Kovacs, G.G. Invited review: Neuropathology of tauopathies: Principles and practice. *Neuropathol. Appl. Neurobiol.* **2015**, *41*, 3–23. [CrossRef] [PubMed]

25. Kovacs, G.G. Tauopathies. In *Neuropathology of Neurodegenerative Diseases: A Practical Guide*; Kovacs, G.G., Ed.; Cambridge University Press: Cambridge, UK, 2015; pp. 109–148.

26. Kovacs, G.G.; Ferrer, I.; Grinberg, L.T.; Alafuzoff, I.; Attems, J.; Budka, H.; Cairns, N.J.; Crary, J.F.; Duyckaerts, C.; Ghetti, B.; et al. Aging-related tau astrogliopathy (ARTAG): Harmonized evaluation strategy. *Acta Neuropathol.* **2016**, *131*, 87–102. [CrossRef] [PubMed]

27. Graff-Radford, J.; Josephs, K.A.; Parisi, J.E.; Dickson, D.W.; Giannini, C.; Boeve, B.F. Globular glial tauopathy presenting as semantic variant PPA. *JAMA Neurol.* **2016**, *73*, 123–125. [CrossRef] [PubMed]

28. Kovacs, G.G.; Lee, V.M.; Trojanowski, J.Q. Protein astrogliopathies in human neurodegenerative diseases and aging. *Brain Pathol.* **2017**, *27*, 675–690. [CrossRef] [PubMed]

29. Kovacs, G.G.; Robinson, J.L.; Xie, S.X.; Lee, E.B.; Grossman, M.; Wolk, D.A.; Irwin, D.J.; Weintraub, D.; Kim, C.F.; Schuck, T.; et al. Evaluating the patterns of aging-related tau astrogliopathy unravels novel insights into brain aging and neurodegenerative diseases. *J. Neuropathol. Exp. Neurol.* **2017**, *76*, 270–288. [CrossRef] [PubMed]

30. Spillantini, M.G.; Goedert, M.; Crowther, R.A.; Murrell, J.R.; Farlow, M.R.; Ghetti, B. Familial multiple system tauopathy with presenile dementia: A disease with abundant neuronal and glial tau filaments. *Proc. Natl. Acad. Sci. USA* **1997**, *94*, 4113–4118. [CrossRef] [PubMed]

31. Iseki, E.; Matsumura, T.; Marui, W.; Hino, H.; Odawara, T.; Sugiyama, N.; Suzuki, K.; Sawada, H.; Arai, T.; Kosaka, K. Familial frontotemporal dementia and parkinsonism with a novel N296H mutation in exon 10 of the tau gene and a widespread tau accumulation in the glial cells. *Acta Neuropathol.* **2001**, *102*, 285–292. [PubMed]

32. Spina, S.; Farlow, M.R.; Unverzagt, F.W.; Kareken, D.A.; Murrell, J.R.; Fraser, G.; Epperson, F.; Crowther, R.A.; Spillantini, M.G.; Goedert, M.; et al. The tauopathy associated with mutation +3 in intron 10 of tau: Characterization of the MSTD family. *Brain* **2008**, *131*, 72–89. [CrossRef] [PubMed]

33. Ghetti, B.; Wszolek, Z.K.; Boeve, B.F.; Spina, S.; Goedert, M. Frontotemporal dementia and parkinsonism linked to chromosome 17. In *Neurodegeneration: The Molecular Pathology of Dementia and Movement Disorders*, 2nd ed.; Dickson, D.W., Weller, R.O., Eds.; Willey-Blackwell: Chichester, UK, 2011; pp. 110–134.

34. Tacik, P.; Sanchez-Contreras, M.; Rademakers, R.; Dickson, D.W.; Wszolek, Z.K. Genetic disorders with tau pathology: A review of the literature and report of two patients with tauopathy and positive family histories. *Neurodegener. Dis.* **2016**, *16*, 12–21. [CrossRef] [PubMed]

35. Tacik, P.; DeTure, M.; Lin, W.L.; Sanchez-Contreras, M.; Wojtas, A.; Hinkle, K.M.; Fujioka, S.; Baker, M.C.; Walton, R.L.; Carlomagno, Y.; et al. A novel tau mutation, p.K317N, causes globular glial tauopathy. *Acta Neuropathol.* **2015**, *130*, 199–214. [CrossRef] [PubMed]

36. Zarranz, J.J.; Ferrer, I.; Lezcano, E.; Forcadas, M.I.; Eizaguirre, B.; Atares, B.; Puig, B.; Gomez-Esteban, J.C.; Fernandez-Maiztegui, C.; Rouco, I.; et al. A novel mutation (K317M) in the *MAPT* gene causes FTDP and motor neuron disease. *Neurology* **2005**, *64*, 1578–1585. [CrossRef] [PubMed]

37. Ferrer, I.; López-González, I.; Carmona, M.; Arregui, L.; Dalfó, E.; Torrejón-Escribano, B.; Diehl, R.; Kovacs, G.G. Glial and neuronal tau pathology in tauopathies: Characterization of disease-specific phenotypes and tau pathology progression. *J. Neuropathol. Exp. Neurol.* **2014**, *73*, 81–97. [CrossRef] [PubMed]

38. Borrego-Écija, S.; Morgado, J.; Palencia-Madrid, L.; Grau-Rivera, O.; Reñé, R.; Hernández, I.; Almenar, C.; Balasa, M.; Antonell, A.; Molinuevo, J.L.; et al. Frontotemporal dementia caused by the P301L mutation in the *MAPT* gene: Clinicopathological features of 13 cases from the same geographical origin in Barcelona, Spain. *Dement. Geriatr. Cogn. Disord.* **2017**, *44*, 213–221. [CrossRef] [PubMed]

39. Duyckaerts, C.; Dickson, D. Neuropathology of Alzheimer's disease. In *Neurodegeneration: The Molecular Pathology of Dementia and Movement Disorders*, 2nd ed.; Dickson, D.W., Weller, R.O., Eds.; Willey-Blackwell: Chichester, UK, 2011; pp. 62–91.

40. Revesz, T.; Rostagno, A.; Plant, G.; Lashley, T.; Frangione, B.; Ghiso, J.; Holton, J.L. Inherited amyloidoses and neurodegeneration: Familial British dementia and Familial Danish dementia. In *Neurodegeneration: The Molecular Pathology of Dementia and Movement Disorders*, 2nd ed.; Dickson, D.W., Weller, R.O., Eds.; Willey-Blackwell: Chichester, UK, 2011; pp. 439–445.

41. Ghetti, B.; Tagliavini, F.; Kovacs, G.G.; Piccardo, P. Gerstmann-Sträussler-Scheinker. In *Neurodegeneration: The Molecular Pathology of Dementia and Movement Disorders*, 2nd ed.; Dickson, D.W., Weller, R.O., Eds.; Willey-Blackwell: Chichester, UK, 2011; pp. 364–377.

42. Rahimi, J.; Kovacs, G.G. Prevalence of mixed pathologies in the aging brain. *Alzheimer's Res. Ther.* **2014**, *6*, 82. [CrossRef] [PubMed]

43. Thal, D.R.; von Arnim, C.A.; Griffin, W.S.; Mrak, R.E.; Walker, L.; Attems, J.; Arzberger, T. Frontotemporal lobar degeneration FTLD-tau: Preclinical lesions, vascular, and Alzheimer-related co-pathologies. *J. Neural Transm.* **2015**, *122*, 1007–1018. [CrossRef] [PubMed]

44. Oikawa, N.; Kimura, N.; Yanagisawa, K. Alzheimer-type tau pathology in advanced aged nonhuman primate brains harboring substantial amyloid deposition. *Brain Res.* **2010**, *1315*, 137–149. [CrossRef] [PubMed]

45. Perez, S.E.; Raghanti, M.A.; Hof, P.R.; Kramer, L.; Ikonomovic, M.D.; Lacor, P.N.; Erwin, J.M.; Sherwood, C.C.; Mufson, E.J. Alzheimer's disease pathology in the neocortex and hippocampus of the western lowland gorilla (*Gorilla gorilla gorilla*). *J. Comp. Neurol.* **2013**, *521*, 4318–4338. [CrossRef] [PubMed]

46. Perez, S.E.; Sherwood, C.C.; Cranfield, M.R.; Erwin, J.M.; Mudakikwa, A.; Hof, P.R.; Mufson, E.J. Early Alzheimer's disease-type pathology in the frontal cortex of wild mountain gorillas (*Gorilla beringei beringei*). *Neurobiol. Aging* **2016**, *39*, 195–201. [CrossRef] [PubMed]

47. Schultz, C.; Dehghani, F.; Hubbard, G.B.; Thal, D.R.; Struckhoff, G.; Braak, E.; Braak, H. Filamentous tau pathology in nerve cells, astrocytes, and oligodendrocytes of aged baboons. *J. Neuropathol. Exp. Neurol.* **2000**, *59*, 39–52. [CrossRef] [PubMed]

48. Rosen, R.F.; Farberg, A.S.; Gearing, M.; Dooyema, J.; Long, P.M.; Anderson, D.C.; Davis-Turak, J.; Coppola, G.; Geschwind, D.H.; Paré, J.F.; et al. Tauopathy with paired helical filaments in an aged chimpanzee. *J. Comp. Neurol.* **2008**, *509*, 259–270. [CrossRef] [PubMed]

49. Edler, M.K.; Sherwood, C.C.; Meindl, R.S.; Hopkins, W.D.; Ely, J.J.; Erwin, J.M.; Mufson, E.J.; Hof, P.R.; Raghanti, M.A. Aged chimpanzees exhibit pathologic hallmarks of Alzheimer's disease. *Neurobiol. Aging* **2017**, *59*, 107–120. [CrossRef] [PubMed]

50. Lemere, C.A.; Oh, J.; Stanish, H.A.; Peng, Y.; Pepivani, I.; Fagan, A.M.; Yamaguchi, H.; Westmoreland, S.V.; Mansfield, K.G. Cerebral amyloid-β protein accumulation with aging in cotton-top tamarins: A model of early Alzheimer's disease? *Rejuvenation Res.* **2008**, *11*, 321–332. [CrossRef] [PubMed]

51. Holzer, M.; Craxton, M.; Jakes, R.; Arendt, T.; Goedert, M. Tau gene (*MAPT*) sequence variation among primates. *Gene* **2004**, *341*, 313–322. [CrossRef] [PubMed]

52. Nishimura, M.; Namba, Y.; Ikeda, K.; Oda, M. Glial fibrillary tangles with straight tubules in the brains of patients with progressive supranuclear palsy. *Neurosci. Lett.* **1992**, *143*, 35–38. [CrossRef]

53. Yamada, T.; McGeer, P.L.; McGeer, E.G. Appearance of paired nucleated, tau-positive glia in patients with progressive supranuclear palsy brain tissue. *Neurosci. Lett.* **1992**, *135*, 99–102. [CrossRef]

54. Nishimura, T.; Ikeda, K.; Akiyama, H.; Kondo, H.; Kato, M.; Li, F.; Iseki, E.; Kosaka, K. Immunohistochemical investigation of tau-positive structures in the cerebral cortex of patients with progressive supranuclear palsy. *Neurosci. Lett.* **1995**, *201*, 123–126. [CrossRef]

55. Feany, M.B.; Dickson, D.W. Widespread cytoskeletal pathology characterizes corticobasal degeneration. *Am. J. Pathol.* **1995**, *146*, 1388–1396. [PubMed]

56. Ikeda, K.; Akiyama, H.; Arai, T.; Nishimura, T. Glial tau pathology in neurodegenerative diseases: Their nature and comparison with neuronal tangles. *Neurobiol. Aging* **1998**, *19* (Suppl. 1), S85–S91. [CrossRef]
57. Komori, T.; Arai, N.; Oda, M.; Nakayama, H.; Mori, H.; Yagishita, S.; Takahashi, T.; Amano, N.; Murayama, S.; Murakami, S.; et al. Astrocytic plaques and tufts of abnormal fibers do not coexist in corticobasal degeneration and progressive supranuclear palsy. *Acta Neuropathol.* **1998**, *96*, 401–408. [CrossRef] [PubMed]
58. Komori, T. Tau-positive glial inclusions in progressive supranuclear palsy, corticobasal degeneration and Pick's disease. *Brain Pathol.* **1999**, *9*, 663–679. [CrossRef] [PubMed]
59. Arai, T.; Ikeda, K.; Akiyama, H.; Shikamoto, Y.; Tsuchiya, K.; Yagishita, S.; Beach, T.; Rogers, J.; Schwab, C.; McGeer, P.L. Distinct isoforms of tau aggregated in neurons and glial cells in brains of patients with Pick's disease, corticobasal degeneration and progressive supranuclear palsy. *Acta Neuropathol.* **2001**, *101*, 167–173. [PubMed]
60. Arai, T.; Ikeda, K.; Akiyama, H.; Tsuchiya, K.; Yagishita, S.; Takamatsu, J. Intracellular processing of aggregated tau differs between corticobasal degeneration and progressive supranuclear palsy. *Neuroreport* **2001**, *12*, 935–938. [CrossRef] [PubMed]
61. Hattori, M.; Hashizume, Y.; Yoshida, M.; Iwasaki, Y.; Hishikawa, N.; Ueda, R.; Ojika, K. Distribution of astrocytic plaques in the corticobasal degeneration brain and comparison with tuft-shaped astrocytes in the progressive supranuclear palsy brain. *Acta Neuropathol.* **2003**, *106*, 143–149. [CrossRef] [PubMed]
62. Iwasaki, Y.; Yoshida, M.; Hattori, M.; Goto, A.; Aiba, I.; Hashizume, Y.; Sobue, G. Distribution of tuft-shaped astrocytes in the cerebral cortex in progressive supranuclear palsy. *Acta Neuropathol.* **2004**, *108*, 399–405. [CrossRef] [PubMed]
63. Arima, K. Ultrastructural characteristics of tau filaments in tauopathies: Immuno-electron microscopic demonstration of tau filaments in tauopathies. *Neuropathology* **2006**, *26*, 475–483. [CrossRef] [PubMed]
64. Mimuro, M.; Yoshida, M.; Miyao, S.; Harada, T.; Ishiguro, K.; Hashizume, Y. Neuronal and glial tau pathology in early frontotemporal lobar degeneration-tau, Pick's disease subtype. *J. Neurol. Sci.* **2010**, *290*, 177–182. [CrossRef] [PubMed]
65. Yoshida, M. Astrocytic inclusions in progressive supranuclear palsy and corticobasal degeneration. *Neuropathology* **2014**, *34*, 555–570. [CrossRef] [PubMed]
66. Ghetti, B.; Oblak, A.L.; Boeve, B.F.; Johnson, K.A.; Dickerson, B.C.; Goedert, M. Invited review: Frontotemporal dementia caused by microtubule-associated protein tau gene (*MAPT*) mutations: A chameleon for neuropathology and neuroimaging. *Neuropathol. Appl. Neurobiol.* **2015**, *41*, 24–46. [CrossRef] [PubMed]
67. Ikeda, K.; Akiyama, H.; Kondo, H.; Haga, C.; Tanno, E.; Tokuda, T.; Ikeda, S. Thorn-shaped astrocytes: Possibly secondarily induced tau-positive glial fibrillary tangles. *Acta Neuropathol.* **1995**, *90*, 620–625. [CrossRef] [PubMed]
68. Schultz, C.; Ghebremedhin, E.; Del Tredici, K.; Rüb, U.; Braak, H. High prevalence of thorn-shaped astrocytes in the aged human medial temporal lobe. *Neurobiol. Aging* **2004**, *25*, 397–405. [CrossRef]
69. Muñoz, D.G.; Woulfe, J.; Kertesz, A. Argyrophilic thorny astrocyte clusters in association with Alzheimer's disease pathology in possible primary progressive aphasia. *Acta Neuropathol.* **2007**, *114*, 347–357. [CrossRef] [PubMed]
70. Kovacs, G.G.; Molnár, K.; László, L.; Ströbel, T.; Botond, G.; Hönigschnabl, S.; Reiner-Concin, A.; Palkovits, M.; Fischer, P.; Budka, H. A peculiar constellation of tau pathology defines a subset of dementia in the elderly. *Acta Neuropathol.* **2011**, *122*, 205–222. [CrossRef] [PubMed]
71. López-González, I.; Carmona, M.; Blanco, R.; Luna-Muñoz, J.; Martínez-Mandonado, A.; Mena, R.; Ferrer, I. Characterization of thorn-shaped astrocytes in white matter of temporal lobe in Alzheimer's disease brains. *Brain Pathol.* **2013**, *23*, 144–153. [CrossRef] [PubMed]
72. Liu, A.K.; Goldfinger, M.H.; Questari, H.E.; Pearce, R.K.; Gentleman, S.M. ARTAG in the basal forebrain: Widening the constellation of astrocytic tau pathology. *Acta Neuropathol. Commun.* **2016**, *4*, 59. [CrossRef] [PubMed]
73. Lingh, H.; Neal, J.W.; Revesz, T. Evolving concepts of chronic traumatic encephalopathy as a neuropathklogical entity. *Neuropathol. Appl. Neurobiol.* **2017**, *43*, 467–476. [CrossRef] [PubMed]
74. Santpere, G.; Ferrer, I. Delineation of early changes in cases with progressive supranuclear palsy-like pathology. Astrocytes in striatum are primary targets of tau phosphorylation and GFAP oxidation. *Brain Pathol.* **2009**, *19*, 177–187. [CrossRef] [PubMed]

75. Ling, H.; Kovacs, G.G.; Vonsattel, J.P.; Davey, K.; Mok, K.Y.; Hardy, J.; Morris, H.R.; Warner, T.T.; Holton, J.L.; Revesz, T. Astrogliopathy predominates the earliest stage of corticobasal degeneration pathology. *Brain* **2016**, *139*, 3237–3252. [CrossRef] [PubMed]

76. Martinez-Maldonado, A.; Luna-Munoz, J.; Ferrer, I. Incidental corticobasal degeneration. *Neuropathol. Appl. Neurobiol.* **2016**, *42*, 659–663. [CrossRef] [PubMed]

77. Iijima, M.; Tabira, T.; Poorkaj, P.; Schellenberg, G.D.; Trojanowski, J.Q.; Lee, V.M.; Schmidt, M.L.; Takahashi, K.; Nabika, T.; Matsumoto, T.; et al. A distinct familial presenile dementia with a novel missense mutation in the tau gene. *Neuroreport* **1999**, *10*, 497–501. [CrossRef] [PubMed]

78. Stanford, P.M.; Halliday, G.M.; Brooks, W.S.; Kwok, J.B.; Storey, C.E.; Creasey, H.; Morris, J.G.; Fulham, M.J.; Schofield, P.R. Progressive supranuclear palsy pathology caused by a novel silent mutation in exon 10 of the tau gene: Expansion of the disease phenotype caused by tau gene mutations. *Brain* **2000**, *123*, 880–893. [CrossRef] [PubMed]

79. Hayashi, S.; Toyoshima, Y.; Hasegawa, M.; Umeda, Y.; Wakabayashi, K.; Tokiguchi, S.; Iwatsubo, T.; Takahashi, H. Late-onset frontotemporal dementia with a novel exon 1 (Arg5His) tau gene mutation. *Ann. Neurol.* **2002**, *51*, 525–530. [CrossRef] [PubMed]

80. Poorkaj, P.; Muma, N.A.; Zhukareva, V.; Cochran, E.J.; Shannon, K.M.; Hurtig, H.; Koller, W.C.; Bird, T.D.; Trojanowski, J.Q.; Lee, V.M.; et al. An R5L tau mutation in a subject with a progressive supranuclear palsy phenotype. *Ann. Neurol.* **2002**, *52*, 511–516. [CrossRef] [PubMed]

81. Kobayashi, T.; Ota, S.; Tanaka, K.; Ito, Y.; Hasegawa, M.; Umeda, Y.; Motoi, Y.; Takanashi, M.; Yasuhara, M.; Anno, M.; et al. A novel L266V mutation of the tau gene causes frontotemporal dementia with a unique tau pathology. *Ann. Neurol.* **2003**, *53*, 133–137. [CrossRef] [PubMed]

82. Ferrer, I.; Pastor, P.; Rey, M.J.; Muñoz, E.; Puig, B.; Pastor, E.; Oliva, R.; Tolosa, E. Tau phosphorylation and kinase activation in familial tauopathy linked to deln296 mutation. *Neuropathol. Appl. Neurobiol.* **2003**, *29*, 23–34. [CrossRef] [PubMed]

83. Van Herpen, E.; Rosso, S.M.; Serverijnen, L.A.; Yoshida, H.; Breedveld, G.; van de Graaf, R.; Kamphorst, W.; Ravid, R.; Willemsen, R.; Dooijes, D.; et al. Variable phenotypic expression and extensive tau pathology in two families with the novel tau mutation L315R. *Ann. Neurol.* **2003**, *54*, 573–581. [CrossRef] [PubMed]

84. Halliday, G.M.; Song, Y.J.; Creasey, H.; Morris, J.G.; Brooks, W.S.; Kril, J.J. Neuropathology in the S305S tau gene mutation. *Brain* **2006**, *129*, E40. [CrossRef] [PubMed]

85. Ros, R.; Thobois, S.; Streichenberger, N.; Kopp, N.; Sanchez, M.P.; Perez, M.; Hoenicka, J.; Avila, J.; Honnorat, J.; de Yébenes, J.G. A new mutation of the tau gene, G303V, in early-onset familial progressive supranuclear palsy. *Arch. Neurol.* **2005**, *62*, 1444–1450. [CrossRef] [PubMed]

86. Malkani, R.; D'Souza, I.; Gwinn-Hardy, K.; Schellenberg, G.D.; Hardy, J.; Momeni, P. A *MAPT* mutation in a regulatory element upstream of exon 10 causes frontotemporal dementia. *Neurobiol. Dis.* **2006**, *22*, 401–403. [CrossRef] [PubMed]

87. Ferrer, I.; Legati, A.; García-Monco, J.C.; Gomez-Beldarrain, M.; Carmona, M.; Blanco, R.; Seeley, W.W.; Coppola, G. Familial behavioral variant frontotemporal dementia associated with astrocyte-predominant tauopathy. *J. Neuropathol. Exp. Neurol.* **2015**, *74*, 370–379. [CrossRef] [PubMed]

88. Botez, G.; Probst, A.; Ipsen, S.; Tolnay, M. Astrocytes expressing hyperphosphorylated tau protein without glial fibrillary tangles in argyrophilicgrain disease. *Acta Neuropathol.* **1999**, *98*, 251–256. [CrossRef] [PubMed]

89. Armstrong, R.A.; Cairns, N.J. Spatial patterns of the tau pathology in progressive supranuclear palsy. *Neurol. Sci.* **2013**, *34*, 337–344. [CrossRef] [PubMed]

90. Milenkovic, I.; Kovacs, G.G. Incidental corticobasal degeneration in a 76-year-old woman. *Clin. Neuropathol.* **2013**, *32*, 69–72. [CrossRef] [PubMed]

91. Irwin, D.J.; Brettschneider, J.; McMillan, C.T.; Cooper, F.; Olm, C.; Arnold, S.E.; van Deerlin, V.M.; Seeley, W.W.; Miller, B.L.; Lee, E.B.; et al. Deep clinical and neuropathological phenotyping of Pick disease. *Ann. Neurol.* **2016**, *79*, 272–287. [CrossRef] [PubMed]

92. Ferrer, I. Diversity of astroglial responses across human neurodegenerative disorders and brain aging. *Brain Pathol.* **2017**, *27*, 645–674. [CrossRef] [PubMed]

93. Shibuya, K.; Yagishita, S.; Nakamura, A.; Uchihara, T. Perivascular orientation of astrocytic plaques and tuft-shaped astrocytes. *Brain Res.* **2011**, *1404*, 50–54. [CrossRef] [PubMed]

94. Higuchi, M.; Ishihara, T.; Zhang, B.; Hong, M.; Andreadis, A.; Trojanowski, J.; Lee, V.M. Transgenic mouse model of tauopathies with glial pathology and nervous system degeneration. *Neuron* **2002**, *35*, 433–446. [CrossRef]

95. Lin, W.L.; Lewis, J.; Yen, S.H.; Hutton, M.; Dickson, D.W. Filamentous tau oligodendrocytes and astrocytes of transgenic mice expressing the human tau isoform with the P301L mutation. *Am. J. Pathol.* **2003**, *162*, 213–218. [CrossRef]

96. Atzori, C.; Ghetti, B.; Piva, R.; Srinivasan, A.N.; Zolo, P.; Delisle, M.B.; Mirra, S.S.; Migheli, A. Activation of the JNK/p38 pathway occurs in diseases characterized by tau protein pathology and is related to tau phosphorylation but not to apoptosis. *J. Neuropathol. Exp. Neurol.* **2001**, *60*, 1190–1197. [CrossRef] [PubMed]

97. Ferrer, I.; Blanco, R.; Carmona, M.; Puig, B. Phosphorylated mitogen-activated protein kinase (MAPK/ERK-P), protein kinase of 38 kDa (p38-P), stress-activated protein kinase (SAPK/JNK-P), and calcium/calmodulin-dependent kinase II (CaM kinase II) are differentially expressed in tau deposits in neurons and glial cells in tauopathies. *J. Neural Transm.* **2001**, *108*, 1397–1415. [PubMed]

98. Ferrer, I.; Blanco, R.; Carmona, M.; Ribera, R.; Goutan, E.; Puig, B.; Rey, M.J.; Cardozo, A.; Viñals, F.; Ribalta, T. Phosphorylated map kinase (ERK1, ERK2) expression is associated with early tau deposition in neurones and glial cells, but not with increased nuclear DNA vulnerability and cell death, in Alzheimer disease, Pick's disease, progressive supranuclear palsy and corticobasal degeneration. *Brain Pathol.* **2001**, *11*, 144–158. [PubMed]

99. Ferrer, I.; Barrachina, M.; Puig, B. Glycogen synthase kinase-3 is associated with neuronal and glial hyperphosphorylated tau deposits in Alzheimer's disease, Pick's disease, progressive supranuclear palsy and corticobasal degeneration. *Acta Neuropathol.* **2002**, *104*, 583–591. [PubMed]

100. Ferrer, I.; Barrachina, M.; Tolnay, M.; Rey, M.J.; Vidal, N.; Carmona, M.; Blanco, R.; Puig, B. Phosphorylated protein kinases associated with neuronal and glial tau deposits in argyrophilic grain disease. *Brain Pathol.* **2003**, *13*, 62–78. [CrossRef] [PubMed]

101. Nishimura, T.; Ikeda, K.; Akiyama, H.; Arai, T.; Kondo, H.; Okochi, M.; Furiya, Y.; Mori, H.; Oda, T.; Kato, M.; et al. Glial tau-positive structures lack the sequence encoded by exon 3 of the tau protein gene. *Neurosci. Lett.* **1997**, *224*, 169–172. [CrossRef]

102. Irwin, D.J.; Cohen, T.J.; Grossman, M.; Arnold, S.E.; McCarty-Wood, E.; Van Deerlin, V.M.; Lee, V.M.; Trojanowski, J.Q. Acetylated tau neuropathology in sporadic and hereditary tauopathies. *Am. J. Pathol.* **2013**, *183*, 344–351. [CrossRef] [PubMed]

103. Grinberg, L.T.; Wang, X.; Wang, C.; Sohn, P.D.; Theofilas, P.; Sidhu, M.; Arevalo, J.B.; Heinsen, H.; Huang, E.J.; Rosen, H.; et al. Argyrophilic grain disease differs from other tauopathies by lacking tau acetylation. *Acta Neuropathol.* **2013**, *125*, 581–593. [CrossRef] [PubMed]

104. Min, S.W.; Cho, S.H.; Zhou, Y.; Schroeder, S.; Haroutunian, V.; Seeley, W.W.; Huang, E.J.; Shen, Y.; Masliah, E.; Mukherjee, C.; et al. Acetylation of tau inhibits its degradation and contributes to tauopathy. *Neuron* **2010**, *67*, 953–966. [CrossRef] [PubMed]

105. Cohen, T.J.; Guo, J.L.; Hurtado, D.E.; Kwong, L.K.; Mills, I.P.; Trojanowski, J.Q.; Lee, V.M. The acetylation of tau inhibits its function and promotes pathological tau aggregation. *Nat. Commun.* **2011**, *2*, 252. [CrossRef] [PubMed]

106. Ferrer, I.; Aguiló García, M.; López González, I.; Diaz Lucena, D.; Roig Villalonga, A.; Carmona, M.; Llorens, F.; Garcia-Esparcia, P.; Martinez-Maldonado, A.; Frau Mendez, M.; et al. Aging-related tau astrogliopathy (ARTAG): Not only tau phosphorylation in astrocytes. *Brain Pathol.* **2018**. [CrossRef] [PubMed]

107. Kimmelberg, H.K. The problem of astrocyte identity. *Neurochem. Int.* **2004**, *45*, 191–202. [CrossRef] [PubMed]

108. Sofroniew, M.V.; Vinters, H.V. Astrocytes: Biology and pathology. *Acta Neuropathol.* **2010**, *119*, 7–35. [CrossRef] [PubMed]

109. Chandrasekaran, A.; Avci, H.X.; Leist, M.; Kobolák, J.; Dinnyés, A. Astrocyte differentiation of human pluripotent stem cells: New tolos for neurological disorder research. *Front. Cell. Neurosci.* **2016**, *10*, 215. [CrossRef] [PubMed]

110. Oberheim, N.A.; Goldman, S.A.; Nedergaard, M. Heterogeneity of astrocytic form and function. *Methods Mol. Biol.* **2012**, *814*, 23–45. [PubMed]

111. Song, Y.J.; Halliday, G.M.; Holton, J.L.; Lashley, T.; O'Sullivan, S.S.; McCann, H.; Lees, A.J.; Ozawa, T.; Williams, D.R.; Lockhart, P.J.; et al. Degeneration in different parkinsonian syndromes relates to astrocyte type and astrocyte protein expression. *J. Neuropathol. Exp. Neurol.* **2009**, *68*, 1073–1083. [CrossRef] [PubMed]

112. Pekny, M.; Nilsson, M. Astrocyte activation and reactive gliosis. *Glia* **2005**, *50*, 427–434. [CrossRef] [PubMed]
113. Seifert, G.; Schilling, K.; Steinhauser, C. Astrocyte dysfunction in neurological disorders: A molecular perspective. *Nat. Rev. Neurosci.* **2006**, *7*, 194–206. [CrossRef] [PubMed]
114. Verkhratsky, A.; Rodríguez, J.J.; Parpura, V. Astroglia in neurological diseases. *Future Neurol.* **2013**, *8*, 149–158. [CrossRef] [PubMed]
115. Verkhratsky, A.; Rodríguez, J.J.; Parpura, V. Neuroglia in ageing and disease. *Cell Tissue Res.* **2014**, *357*, 493–503. [CrossRef] [PubMed]
116. Verkhratsky, A.; Zorec, R.; Rodrıguez, J.J.; Parpura, V. Astroglia dynamics in ageing and Alzheimer's disease. *Curr. Opin. Pharmacol.* **2016**, *26*, 74–79. [CrossRef] [PubMed]
117. Pekny, M.; Pekna, M. Astrocyte reactivity and reactive astrogliosis: Costs and benefits. *Physiol. Rev.* **2014**, *94*, 1077–1098. [CrossRef] [PubMed]
118. Pekny, M.; Pekna, M. Reactive gliosis in the pathogenesis of CNS diseases. *Biochim. Biophys. Acta* **2016**, *1862*, 483–491. [CrossRef] [PubMed]
119. Verkhratsky, A.; Zorec, R.; Parpura, V. Stratification of astrocytes in healthy and diseased brain. *Brain Pathol.* **2017**, *27*, 629–644. [CrossRef] [PubMed]
120. Verkhratsky, A.; Zorec, R.; Rodriguez, J.J.; Parpura, V. Neuroglia: Functional paralysis and reactivity in Alzheimer's disease and other neurodegenerative pathologies. *Adv. Neurobiol.* **2017**, *15*, 427–449. [PubMed]
121. Osborn, L.M.; Kamphuis, W.; Wadman, W.J.; Hol, E.M. Astrogliosis: An integral player in the pathogenesis of Alzheimer's disease. *Prog. Neurobiol.* **2016**, *144*, 121–141. [CrossRef] [PubMed]
122. Pekny, M.; Pekna, M.; Messing, A.; Steinhäuser, C.; Lee, J.M.; Parpura, V.; Hol, E.M.; Sofroniew, M.V.; Verkhratsky, A. Astrocytes: A central element in neurological diseases. *Acta Neuropathol.* **2016**, *131*, 323–345. [CrossRef] [PubMed]
123. Kersaitis, C.; Halliday, G.M.; Kril, J.J. Regional and cellular pathology in frontotemporal dementia: Relationship to stage of disease in cases with and without Pick bodies. *Acta Neuropathol.* **2004**, *108*, 515–523. [CrossRef] [PubMed]
124. Togo, T.; Dickson, D.W. Tau accumulation in astrocytes in progressive supranuclear palsy is a degenerative rather than a reactive process. *Acta Neuropathol.* **2002**, *104*, 398–402. [PubMed]
125. López-González, I.; Aso, E.; Carmona, M.; Armand-Ugon, M.; Blanco, R.; Naudí, A.; Cabré, R.; Portero-Otin, M.; Pamplona, R.; Ferrer, I. Neuroinflammatory gene regulation, mitochondrial function, oxidative stress, and brain lipid modifications with disease progression in Tau P301S transgenic mice as a model of frontotemporal lobar degeneration-Tau. *J. Neuropathol. Exp. Neurol.* **2015**, *74*, 975–999. [CrossRef] [PubMed]
126. Renkawek, K.; Bosman, G.J.; de Jong, W.W. Expression of small heat-shock protein Hsp27 in reactive gliosis in Alzheimer disease and other types of dementia. *Acta Neuropathol.* **1994**, *87*, 511–519. [CrossRef] [PubMed]
127. Dabir, D.V.; Trojanowski, J.Q.; Richter-Landsberg, C.; Lee, V.M.; Forman, M.S. Expression of the small heat-shock protein αB-crystallin in tauopathies with glial pathology. *Am. J. Pathol.* **2004**, *164*, 155–166. [CrossRef]
128. Schwarz, L.; Vollmer, G.; Richter-Landsberg, C. The small heat shock protein HSP25/27 (HspB1) is abundant in cultured astrocytes and associated with astrocytic pathology in progressive supranuclear palsy and corticobasal degeneration. *Int. J. Cell Biol.* **2010**, *2010*, 717520. [CrossRef] [PubMed]
129. López-González, I.; Carmona, M.; Arregui, L.; Kovacs, G.G.; Ferrer, I. αB-crystallin and HSP27 in glial cells in tauopathies. *Neuropathology* **2014**, *34*, 517–526. [CrossRef] [PubMed]
130. Filipcik, P.; Cente, M.; Zilka, N.; Smolek, T.; Hanes, J.; Kucerak, J.; Opattova, A.; Kovacech, B.; Novak, M. Intraneuronal accumulation of misfolded tau protein induces overexpression of Hsp27 in activated astrocytes. *Biochim. Biophys. Acta* **2015**, *1852*, 1219–1229. [CrossRef] [PubMed]
131. Kahlson, M.A.; Colodner, K.J. Glial tau pathology in tauopathies: Functional consequences. *J. Exp. Neurosci.* **2016**, *9*, 43–50. [CrossRef] [PubMed]
132. Verkhratsky, A.; Nedergaard, M. Physiology of astroglia. *Physiol. Rev.* **2018**, *98*, 239–389. [CrossRef] [PubMed]
133. Cahoy, J.D.; Emery, B.; Kaushal, A.; Foo, L.C.; Zamanian, J.L.; Christopherson, K.S.; Xing, Y.; Lubischer, J.L.; Krieg, P.A.; Krupenko, S.A.; et al. A transcriptome database for astrocytes, neurons, and oligodendrocytes: A new resource for understanding brain development and function. *J. Neurosci.* **2008**, *28*, 264–278. [CrossRef] [PubMed]

134. Orre, M.; Kamphuis, W.; Osborn, L.M.; Melief, J.; Kooijman, L.; Huitinga, I.; Klooster, J.; Bossers, K.; Hol, E.M. Acute isolation and transcriptome characterization of cortical astrocytes and microglia from young and aged mice. *Neurobiol. Aging* **2014**, *35*, 1–14. [CrossRef] [PubMed]

135. Darmanis, S.; Sloan, S.A.; Zhang, Y.; Enge, M.; Caneda, C.; Shuer, L.M.; Gephart, M.G.H.; Barres, B.A.; Quake, S.R. A survey of human brain transcriptome diversity at the single cell level. *PNAS* **2015**, *112*, 7285–7290. [CrossRef] [PubMed]

136. Zeisel, A.; Muñoz-Manchado, A.B.; Codeluppi, S.; Lönnerberg, P.; La Manno, G.; Juréus, A.; Marques, S.; Munguba, H.; He, L.; Betsholtz, C.; et al. Brain structure. Cell types in the mouse cortex and hippocampus revealed by single-cell RNA-seq. *Science* **2015**, *347*, 1138–1142. [CrossRef] [PubMed]

137. Zhang, Y.; Sloan, S.A.; Clarke, L.E.; Caneda, C.; Plaza, C.A.; Blumenthal, P.D.; Vogel, H.; Steinberg, G.K.; Edwards, M.S.; Li, G.; et al. Purification and characterization of progenitor and mature human astrocytes reveals transcriptional and functional differences in mouse. *Neuron* **2016**, *89*, 37–53. [CrossRef] [PubMed]

138. Lin, C.C.J.; Yu, K.; Hatcher, A.; Huang, T.W.; Lee, H.K.; Carlson, J.; Weston, M.C.; Chen, F.; Zhang, Y.; Zhu, W.; et al. Identification of diverse astrocyte populations and their malignant analogs. *Nat. Neurosci.* **2017**, *20*, 396–405.

139. Habib, N.; Avraham-Davidi, I.; Basu, A.; Burks, T.; Shekhar, K.; Hofree, M.; Choudhury, S.R.; Aguet, F.; Gelfand, E.; Ardlie, K.; et al. Massively parallel single-nucleus RNA-seq with Dronc-seq. *Nat. Methods* **2017**, *14*, 955–958. [CrossRef] [PubMed]

140. Spaethling, J.M.; Na, Y.-J.; Lee, J.; Ulyanova, A.V.; Baltuch, G.H.; Bell, T.J.; Brem, S.; Chen, H.I.; Dueck, H.; Fisher, S.A.; et al. Primary cell culture of live neurosurgically-resected aged adult human brain cells and single cell transcriptomics. *Cell Rep.* **2017**, *18*, 791–803. [CrossRef] [PubMed]

141. Simpson, J.E.; Ince, P.G.; Shaw, P.J.; Heath, P.R.; Raman, R.; Garwood, C.J.; Gelsthorpe, C.; Baxter, L.; Forster, G.; Matthews, F.E.; et al. Microarray analysis of the astrocyte transcriptome in the aging brain: Relationship to Alzheimer's pathology and APOE genotype. *Neurobiol. Aging* **2011**, *32*, 1795–1807. [CrossRef] [PubMed]

142. Orre, M.; Kamphuis, W.; Osborn, L.M.; Jansen, A.H.; Kooijman, L.; Bossers, K.; Hol, E.M. Isolation of glia from Alzheimer's mice reveals inflammation and dysfunction. *Neurobiol. Aging* **2014**, *35*, 2746–2760. [CrossRef] [PubMed]

143. Yoshiyama, Y.; Zhang, B.; Bruce, J.; Trojanowski, J.Q.; Lee, V.M. Reduction of detyrosinated microtubules and Golgi fragmentation are linked to tau-induced degeneration in astrocytes. *J. Neurosci.* **2003**, *23*, 10662–10671. [CrossRef] [PubMed]

144. Colodner, K.J.; Feany, M.B. Glial fibrillary tangles and JAK/STAT-mediated glial and neuronal cell death in a Drosophila model of glial tauopathy. *J. Neurosci.* **2010**, *30*, 16102–16113. [CrossRef] [PubMed]

145. Ke, Y.D.; Dramiga, J.; Schütz, U.; Kril, J.J.; Ittner, L.M.; Schröder, H.; Götz, J. Tau-mediated nuclear depletion and cytoplasmic accumulation of SFPQ in Alzheimer's and Pick's disease. *PLoS ONE* **2012**, *7*, E35678. [CrossRef]

146. Frost, B.; Hemberg, M.; Lewis, J.; Feany, M.B. Tau promotes neurodegeneration through global chromatin relaxation. *Nat. Neurosci.* **2014**, *17*, 357–366. [CrossRef] [PubMed]

147. Hernández-Ortega, K.; Garcia-Esparcia, P.; Gil, L.; Lucas, J.J.; Ferrer, I. Altered machinery of protein synthesis in Alzheimer's: From the nucleolus to the ribosome. *Brain Pathol.* **2016**, *26*, 593–605. [CrossRef] [PubMed]

148. Forman, M.S.; Lal, D.; Zhang, B.; Dabir, D.V.; Swanson, E.; Lee, V.M.; Trojanowski, J.Q. Transgenic mouse model of tau pathology in astrocytes leading to nervous system degeneration. *J. Neurosci.* **2005**, *25*, 3539–3550. [CrossRef] [PubMed]

149. Dabir, D.V.; Robinson, M.B.; Swanson, E.; Zhang, B.; Trojanowski, J.Q.; Lee, V.M.; Forman, M.S. Impaired glutamate transport in a mouse model of tau pathology in astrocytes. *J. Neurosci.* **2006**, *26*, 644–654. [CrossRef] [PubMed]

150. Piacentini, R.; Li Puma, D.D.; Mainardi, M.; Lazzarino, G.; Tavazzi, B.; Arancio, O.; Grassi, C. Reduced gliotransmitter release from astrocytes mediates tau-induced synaptic dysfunction in cultured hippocampal neurons. *Glia* **2017**, *65*, 1302–1316. [CrossRef] [PubMed]

151. Hallmann, A.L.; Araúzo-Bravo, M.J.; Mavrommatis, L.; Ehrlich, M.; Röpke, A.; Brockhaus, J.; Missler, M.; Sterneckert, J.; Schöler, H.R.; Kuhlmann, T.; et al. Astrocyte pathology in a human neural stem cell model of frontotemporal dementia caused by mutant tau protein. *Sci. Rep.* **2017**, *7*, 42991. [CrossRef] [PubMed]

152. Sidoryk-Wegrzynowicz, M.; Gerber, Y.N.; Ries, M.; Sastre, M.; Tolkovsky, A.M.; Spillantini, M.G. Astrocytes in mouse models of tauopathies acquire early deficits and lose neurosupportive functions. *Acta Neuropathol. Commun.* **2017**, *5*, 89. [CrossRef] [PubMed]

153. Braak, H.; Braak, E. Neuropathological staging of Alzheimer-related changes. *Acta Neuropathol.* **1991**, *82*, 239–259. [CrossRef] [PubMed]

154. Braak, H.; Braak, E. Temporal sequence of Alzheimer's disease-related pathology. In *Cerebral Cortex Vol. 14, Neurodegenerative and Age-Related Changes in Structure and Function of Cerebral Cortex*; Peters, A., Morrison, J.H., Eds.; Kluwer Academic/Plenum Publishers: New York, NY, USA; Boston, MA, USA; Dordrecht, The Netherlands; London, UK; Moscow, Russia, 1999; pp. 475–512.

155. Duyckaerts, C.; Braak, H.; Brion, J.P.; Buée, L.; Del Tredici, K.; Goedert, M.; Halliday, G.; Neumann, M.; Spillantini, M.G.; Tolnay, M.; et al. PART is part of Alzheimer disease. *Acta Neuropathol.* **2015**, *129*, 749–756. [CrossRef] [PubMed]

156. Giaccone, G. The existence of primary age-related tauopathy suggests that not all the cases with early Braak stages of neurofibrillary pathology are Alzheimer's disease. *J. Alzheimer's Dis.* **2015**, *48*, 919–921. [CrossRef] [PubMed]

157. Ferrer, I. Defining Alzheimer as a common age-related neurodegenerative process not inevitably leading to dementia. *Prog. Neurobiol.* **2012**, *97*, 38–51. [CrossRef] [PubMed]

158. Braak, H.; Del Tredici, K. The preclinical phase of the pathological process underlying sporadic Alzheimer's disease. *Brain* **2015**, *138*, 2814–2833. [CrossRef] [PubMed]

159. Braak, H.; Thal, D.R.; Ghebremedhin, E.; Del Tredici, K. Stages of the pathologic process in Alzheimer disease: Age categories from 1 to 100 years. *J. Neuropathol. Exp. Neurol.* **2011**, *70*, 960–969. [CrossRef] [PubMed]

160. Saito, Y.; Ruberu, N.N.; Sawabe, M.; Arai, T.; Tanaka, N.; Kakuta, Y.; Yamanouchi, H.; Murayama, S. Staging of argyrophilic grains: An age-associated tauopathy. *J. Neuropathol. Exp. Neurol.* **2004**, *63*, 911–918. [CrossRef] [PubMed]

161. Nogami, A.; Yamazaki, M.; Saito, Y.; Hatsuta, H.; Sakiyama, Y.; Takao, M.; Kimura, K.; Murayama, S. Early stage of progressive supranuclear palsy: A neuropathological study of 324 consecutive autopsy cases. *J. Nippon Med. Sch.* **2015**, *82*, 266–273. [CrossRef] [PubMed]

162. Brown, J.A.; Hua, A.Y.; Trujllo, A.; Attygalle, S.; Binney, R.J.; Spina, S.; Lee, S.E.; Kramer, J.H.; Miller, B.L.; Rosen, H.J.; et al. Advancing functional disconnectivity and atrophy in progressive supranuclear palsy. *Neuroimage Clin.* **2017**, *16*, 564–574. [CrossRef] [PubMed]

163. Lewis, J.; Dickson, D.W. Propagation of tau pathology: Hypotheses, discoveries, and yet unresolved questions from experimental and human brain studies. *Acta Neuropathol.* **2016**, *131*, 27–48. [CrossRef] [PubMed]

164. Dujardin, S.; Lecolle, K.; Caillierez, R.; Begard, S.; Zommer, N.; Lachaud, C.; Carrier, S.; Dufour, N.; Aurégan, G.; Winderickx, J.; et al. Neuron-to-neuron wild-type tau protein transfer through a trans-synaptic mechanism: Relevance to sporadic tauopathies. *Acta Neuropathol. Commun.* **2014**, *2*, 14. [CrossRef] [PubMed]

165. Calafate, S.; Buist, A.; Miskiewicz, K.; Vijayan, V.; Daneels, G.; de Strooper, B.; de Wit, J.; Verstreken, P.; Moechars, D. Synaptic contacts enhance cell-to-cell tau pathology propagation. *Cell Rep.* **2015**, *11*, 1176–1183. [CrossRef] [PubMed]

166. Wang, Y.; Balaji, V.; Kaniyappan, S.; Krüger, L.; Irsen, S.; Tepper, K.; Chandupatla, R.; Maetzler, W.; Schneider, A.; Mandelkow, E.; et al. The release and trans-synaptic transmission of Tau via exosomes. *Mol. Neurodegener.* **2017**, *12*, 5. [CrossRef] [PubMed]

167. Polanco, J.C.; Scicluna, B.J.; Hill, A.F.; Gotz, J. Extracellular vesicles isolated from the brains of rTg4510 mice seed tau protein aggregation in a threshold-dependent manner. *J. Biol. Chem.* **2016**, *291*, 12445–12466. [CrossRef] [PubMed]

168. Polanco, J.C.; Li, C.; Durisic, N.; Sullivan, R.; Götz, J. Exosomes taken up by neurons hijack the endosomal pathway to spread to interconnected neurons. *Acta Neuropathol. Commun.* **2018**, *6*, 10. [CrossRef] [PubMed]

169. Tardivel, M.; Begard, S.; Bousset, L.; Dujardin, S.; Coens, A.; Melki, R.; Buée, L.; Colin, M. Tunneling nanotube (TNT)-mediated neuron-to neuron transfer of pathological tau protein assemblies. *Acta Neuropathol. Commun.* **2016**, *4*, 117. [CrossRef] [PubMed]

170. Holmes, B.B.; Diamond, M.I. Prion-like properties of tau protein: The importance of extracellular tau as a therapeutic target. *J. Biol. Chem.* **2014**, *289*, 19855–19861. [CrossRef] [PubMed]

171. Guo, J.L.; Lee, V.M. Cell-to-cell transmission of pathogenic proteins in neurodegenerative diseases. *Nat. Med.* **2014**, *20*, 130–138. [CrossRef] [PubMed]

172. Victoria, G.S.; Arkhipenko, A.; Zhu, S.; Syan, S.; Zurzolo, C. Astrocyte-to-neuron intercellular prion transfer is mediated by cell-cell contact. *Sci. Rep.* **2016**, *6*, 20762. [CrossRef] [PubMed]

173. Clavaguera, F.; Bolmont, T.; Crowther, R.A.; Abramowski, D.; Frank, S.; Probst, A.; Fraser, G.; Stalder, A.K.; Beibel, M.; Staufenbiel, M.; et al. Transmission and spreading of tauopathy in transgenic mouse brain. *Nat. Cell Biol.* **2009**, *11*, 909–913. [CrossRef] [PubMed]

174. Clavaguera, F.; Hench, J.; Goedert, M.; Tolnay, M. Invited review: Prion-like transmission and spreading of tau pathology. *Neuropathol. Appl. Neurobiol.* **2015**, *41*, 47–58. [CrossRef] [PubMed]

175. Boluda, S.; Iba, M.; Zhang, B.; Raible, K.M.; Lee, V.M.; Trojanowski, J.Q. Differential induction and spread of tau pathology in young PS19 tau transgenic mice following intracerebral injections of pathological tau from Alzheimer's disease or corticobasal degeneration brains. *Acta Neuropathol.* **2015**, *129*, 221–237. [CrossRef] [PubMed]

176. Clavaguera, F.; Akatsu, H.; Fraser, G.; Crowther, R.A.; Frank, S.; Hench, J.; Probst, A.; Winkler, D.T.; Reichwald, J.; Staufenbiel, M.; et al. Brain homogenates from human tauopathies induce tau inclusions in mouse brain. *Proc. Natl. Acad. Sci. USA* **2013**, *110*, 9535–9540. [CrossRef] [PubMed]

177. Clavaguera, F.; Lavenir, I.; Falcon, B.; Frank, S.; Goedert, M.; Tolnay, M. "Prion-like" templated misfolding in tauopathies. *Brain Pathol.* **2013**, *23*, 342–349. [CrossRef] [PubMed]

178. Narasimhan, S.; Guo, J.L.; Changolkar, L.; Stieber, A.; McBride, J.D.; Silva, L.V.; He, Z.; Zhang, B.; Gathagan, R.J.; Trojanowski, J.Q.; et al. Pathological tau strains from human brains recapitulate the diversity of tauopathies in non-transgenic mouse brain. *J. Neurosci.* **2017**, *37*, 11406–11423. [CrossRef] [PubMed]

179. Guo, J.L.; Narasimhan, S.; Changolkar, L.; He, Z.; Stieber, A.; Zhang, B.; Gathagan, R.J.; Iba, M.; McBride, J.D.; Trojanowski, J.Q.; et al. Unique pathological tau conformers from Alzheimer's brains transmit tau pathology in nontransgenic mice. *J. Exp. Med.* **2016**, *213*, 2635–2654. [CrossRef] [PubMed]

180. Kaufman, S.K.; Sanders, D.W.; Thomas, T.L.; Ruchinskas, A.J.; Vaquer-Alicea, J.; Sharma, A.M.; Miller, T.M.; Diamond, M.I. Tau prion strains dictate patterns of cell pathology, progression rate, and regional vulnerability in vivo. *Neuron* **2016**, *92*, 796–812. [CrossRef] [PubMed]

181. Wharton, S.B.; Minett, T.; Drew, D.; Forster, G.; Matthews, F.; Brayne, C.; Ince, P.G.; MRC Cognitive Function and Ageing Neuropathology Study Group. Epidemiological pathology of tau in the ageing brain: Application of staging for neuropil threads (BrainNet Europe protocol) to the MRC cognitive function and ageing brain study. *Acta Neuropathol. Commun.* **2016**, *4*, 11. [CrossRef] [PubMed]

182. Lee, G.; Cowan, N.; Kirschner, M. The primary structure and heterogeneity of tau protein from mouse brain. *Science* **1988**, *239*, 285–288. [CrossRef] [PubMed]

183. Di Domenico, F.; Sultana, R.; Barone, E.; Perluigi, M.; Cini, C.; Mancuso, C.; Cai, J.; Pierce, W.M.; Butterfield, D.A. Quantitative proteomics analysis of phosphorylated proteins in the hippocampus of Alzheimer's disease subjects. *J. Proteom.* **2011**, *74*, 1091–1103. [CrossRef] [PubMed]

184. Zahid, S.; Oellerich, M.; Asif, A.R.; Ahmed, N. Phosphoproteome profiling of *substantia nigra* and cortex regions of Alzheimer's disease patients. *J. Neurochem.* **2012**, *121*, 954–963. [CrossRef] [PubMed]

185. Triplett, J.C.; Swomley, A.M.; Cai, J.; Klein, J.B.; Butterfield, D.A. Quantitative phosphoproteomic analyses of the inferior parietal lobule from three different pathological stages of Alzheimer's disease. *J. Alzheimer's Dis.* **2016**, *49*, 45–62. [CrossRef] [PubMed]

186. Muntané, G.; Dalfó, E.; Martínez, A.; Rey, M.J.; Avila, J.; Pérez, M.; Portero, M.; Pamplona, R.; Ayala, V.; Ferrer, I. Glial fibrillary acidic protein is a major target of glycoxidative and lipoxidative damage in Pick's disease. *J. Neurochem.* **2006**, *99*, 177–185.

187. Martínez, A.; Portero-Otin, M.; Pamplona, R.; Ferrer, I. Protein targets of oxidative damage in human neurodegenerative diseases with abnormal protein aggregates. *Brain Pathol.* **2010**, *20*, 281–297. [CrossRef] [PubMed]

188. Tagawa, K.; Homma, H.; Saito, A.; Fujita, K.; Chen, X.; Imoto, S.; Oka, T.; Ito, H.; Motoki, K.; Yoshida, C.; et al. Comprehensive phosphoproteome analysis unravels the core signaling network that initiates the earliest synapse pathology in preclinical Alzheimer's disease brain. *Hum. Mol. Genet.* **2015**, *24*, 540–558. [CrossRef] [PubMed]

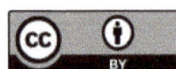

neuroglia

MDPI

Review

NG2 Glia: Novel Roles beyond Re-/Myelination

Roberta Parolisi [1,2] and Enrica Boda [1,2,*]

1   Department of Neuroscience Rita Levi Montalcini, University of Turin, 10126 Turin, Italy;
     roberta.parolisi@unito.it
2   Neuroscience Institute of the Cavalieri Ottolenghi Foundation (NICO), Regione Gonzole 10,
     10043 Orbassano (Turin), Italy
*   Correspondence: enrica.boda@unito.it; Tel.: +39-011-6706615

Received: 10 June 2018; Accepted: 29 June 2018; Published: 4 July 2018

Abstract: Neuron-glia antigen 2-expressing glial cells (NG2 glia) serve as oligodendrocyte progenitors during development and adulthood. However, recent studies have shown that these cells represent not only a transitional stage along the oligodendroglial lineage, but also constitute a specific cell type endowed with typical properties and functions. Namely, NG2 glia (or subsets of NG2 glia) establish physical and functional interactions with neurons and other central nervous system (CNS) cell types, that allow them to constantly monitor the surrounding neuropil. In addition to operating as sensors, NG2 glia have features that are expected for active modulators of neuronal activity, including the expression and release of a battery of neuromodulatory and neuroprotective factors. Consistently, cell ablation strategies targeting NG2 glia demonstrate that, beyond their role in myelination, these cells contribute to CNS homeostasis and development. In this review, we summarize and discuss the advancements achieved over recent years toward the understanding of such functions, and propose novel approaches for further investigations aimed at elucidating the multifaceted roles of NG2 glia.

Keywords: NG2 glia; oligodendrocyte progenitor cells; synapses; neuromodulation; neuroprotection; cell ablation

---

1. Introduction

During central nervous system (CNS) ontogenesis, myelinating oligodendrocytes (OLs) originate from parenchymal precursors expressing the neuron-glia antigen 2 (NG2) chondroitin sulfate proteoglycan, and therefore, commonly referred to as oligodendrocyte precursor cells or NG2-expressing glia (NG2 glia) [1]. These cells persist in the adult CNS parenchyma, where they comprise about 5% of all CNS cells [2], and can serve as a rapidly responding reservoir for new OLs in case of demyelination [1,3,4]. In intact adult nervous tissue, NG2 glia can also be engaged in proliferation and maturation to sustain a certain degree of oligodendrogenesis [5,6] and myelin plasticity [7–11]. Notably, recent in vivo longitudinal two-photon imaging studies showed that, in the murine cortex, OL density continues to increase until two years of age [10], and more than half of the OLs present in middle aged mice are produced during adult life (i.e., after fourmonths of age [9]). The generation of such adult-born OLs is required to maintain proper axonal functions [12], and is involved in the production of new myelin segments [9] and changes of the circuit properties subserving experience-dependent plasticity (i.e., motor skills learning [7,8]). However, in both adult human and rodent CNS, the density, distribution and proliferative rate of NG2 glia seem to be independent of the presence/density of myelinated fibres. NG2 glia distribute homogenously throughout grey and white matter parenchyma. Further, although gray matter cells have a longer cell cycle length than their white matter counterparts [13], NG2 glia proliferative fractions do not differ in highly myelinated vs. non-/poorly myelinated brain regions (i.e., the granular and the molecular layers of the cerebellum, respectively; our unpublished observations). In intact conditions, most NG2 glia appear as "quiescent" cells (i.e., neither progressing along the lineage, nor re-entering the cell cycle), and overall, the fraction of NG2 glia actively engaged in oligodendrogenesis is minimal [14,15]. These observations suggest that in basal conditions such an abundant pool of resident NG2 glia may exert additional roles beyond their functions in oligodendrogenesis and myelin production.

Although the molecular aspects of NG2 glia response to injury are far from being completely understood, data accumulated so far indicate that, phenotypically, NG2 glia provide a stereotypic reaction (i.e., increased NG2 expression, retraction of cell processes, cell body swelling, cell proliferation and migration toward the lesion site) to almost all kind of injury, independently of the extent of myelin loss [14,16–19]. Further, upon experimental demyelination in the subcortical white matter, transient populations of NG2 glia coming from the subventricular zone (SVZ) of the lateral ventricles immediately amplify and invade the lesion site, but ultimately seem not to contribute to myelin repair, and are lost [20–22]. This indicates that the reactivity and amplification of NG2 glia (or at least of some NG2 glia subsets) per se does not simply reflect a regenerative event. The post-injury emergence of transient NG2 glia populations is reminiscent of the developmental scenario, where three waves of NG2 glia are sequentially produced in the forebrain, and the first embryonically-generated cells are entirely replaced during the first week of life [23]. The generation of such cell populations that do not contribute to myelination suggests again that NG2 glia/glial subsets exert additional/alternative functions in specific developmental/post-injury phases.

In line with this view, a subpopulation of NG2 glia has been observed to serve as multipotent progenitors, producing protoplasmic astrocytes as well OLs in the embryonic ventral forebrain or following some kinds of CNS injury [19,24–27]. It has also been proposed that adult NG2 glia may activate spontaneous neurogenic events within restricted brain areas [28]. In view of achieving neuronal replacement in the adult CNS, the idea that NG2 glia can be the source for new neurons is particularly attractive because of their abundance and ubiquitous distribution. However, this has been proven true in vivo only upon specific cell reprogramming approaches, and clear evidence that adult NG2 glia spontaneously contribute to parenchymal neurogenesis or astrogliogenesis is lacking [4,28–30].

Based on these and other findings, four years ago we proposed that, beyond sustaining re-/myelination, NG2 glia may participate in the nervous tissue homeostasis, neuromodulation, developmental and post-injury events [28]. Such a view has recently been substantiated by a growing body of evidence, including descriptive observations and results of functional in vivo/in vitro studies. Here, we summarize and discuss the advancements obtained in the field in the last years and propose novel approaches for further investigations aimed at understanding the multifaceted roles of NG2 glia.

2. NG2 Glia Distribution, Self-Maintenance and Anatomical Relationships with Central Nervous System Cells

Recent studies showed that NG2 glia distribution and density are tightly and homeostatically regulated in adult CNS tissue. In vivo two-photon imaging analyses showed that NG2 glia processes constantly survey their local environment with highly motile filopodia and growth cone-like structures that retract upon contact with other NG2 cells [31,32]. As a result, NG2 glia are arranged in a grid-like manner, where cells are equally spaced and, similar to astrocytes, occupy tridimensional non-overlapping domains. In the mammalian and zebrafish CNS, NG2 glia division and short distance migration are the mechanisms by which these cells maintain their uniform density in space and time: once an individual NG2-expressing cell is "lost" because of maturation (i.e., loss of progenitor features including expression of cell surface signal molecules) or experimental ablation, a neighboring NG2 cell enters the cell cycle and migrate to fill the unoccupied space (Figure 1A) [31–34]. Notably, similar to stem cells, NG2 glia can divide asymmetrically in vivo and give rise to a mixed progeny, either keeping a progenitor phenotype or proceeding to differentiation (Figure 1B) [5,6,35]. This mechanism may allow the generation of OLs, while preventing the progressive exhaustion of NG2 glia during adulthood. NG2 glia maintenance is also regulated by specific synapse-mediated signals received from γ-aminobutyric acid (GABA)-ergic neurons (see also below), as demonstrated by the progressive depletion of the NG2 glia pool lacking the GABA-A receptor subunit γ2 [36]. The discovery of such efficient—and somehow redundant—regulation mechanisms by which a constant population of NG2 glia is homeostatically maintained in time and space, even in non-/poorly-myelinated CNS regions, challenges the assumption that NG2 glia exclusively serve as progenitors for new OLs, and suggests functions related to the surveillance and modulation of the activity of the surrounding neuropil, as formerly assessed for astrocytes and microglia [37–40].

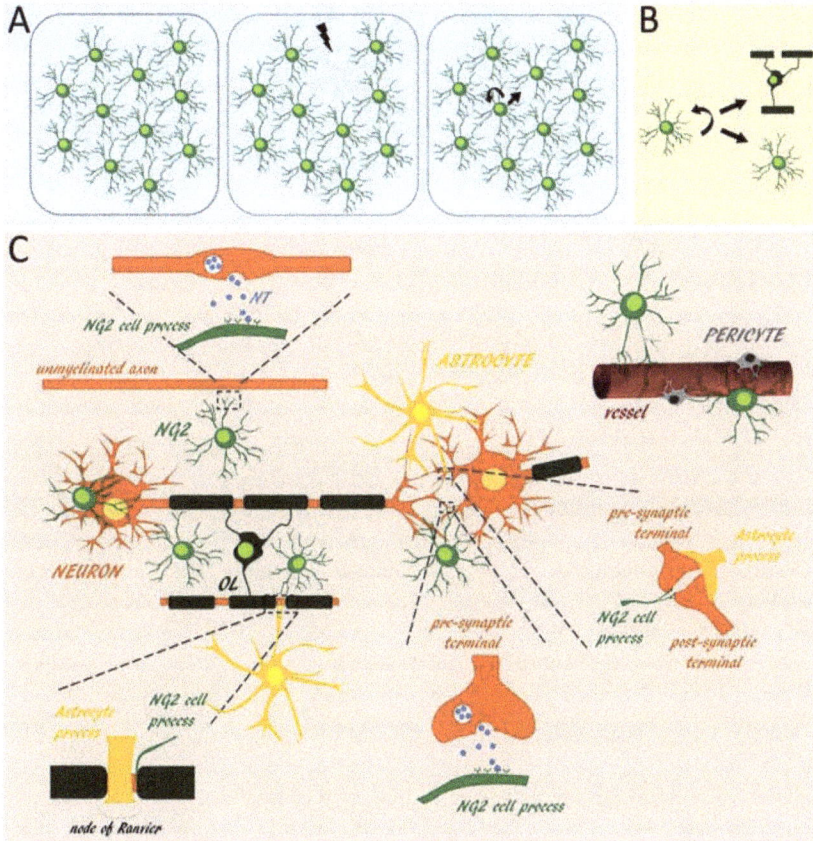

Figure 1. Schematic representation of the mechanisms assuring NG2 glia maintenance and of their physical interactions with neurons and other central nervous system (CNS) cell types (**A**) NG2 glia are distributed in a grid-like manner and occupy non-overlapping domains. When an individual NG2-expressing cell is lost, a neighboring NG2 cell divide and migrate to fill the unoccupied space. (**B**) In the adult and juvenile cortex, NG2 glia can divide asymmetrically and give rise to a mixed progeny either keeping a progenitor phenotype or proceeding to differentiation. (**C**) NG2 glia establish physical contacts with neuronal dendrites, somata, nodes of Ranvier and synapses. NG2 glia and astrocytes often contact the same node of Ranvier or synapse, but the relative processes show distinct localization. NG2 glia also receive functional synaptic contacts from unmyelinated axons and axonal terminals. In the adult CNS, NG2 glia display a perivascular distribution or extend some processes to physically interact with pericytes and blood vessels. NT: Neurotransmitter; OL: Oligodendrocyte.

In line with this view, confocal and electron microscopy studies showed that NG2 glia establish physical contacts with functionally relevant neuronal domains, including dendrites [41,42], somata [14,41,43,44], nodes of Ranvier [45,46] and synapses [47,48] (Figure 1C). About 30–50% of the nodes are contacted by both NG2 glia and astrocyte processes in the optic nerve, corpus callosum, and spinal cord of young adult rodents. Ultrastructural analyses revealed that NG2 glia processes extend fine, finger-like projections that contact the nodal membrane at discrete points, while astrocytes had broader processes that surround the entire nodes [46] (Figure 1C). Similarly, NG2 glia and astrocytes often contact the same axon terminals, with NG2 glia thin processes interdigitating between the pre- and post-synaptic elements and large astrocytic processes ensheating the entire synapses [41,47] (Figure 1C). These observations suggest different roles of the contacts established by the two glial cell types at nodes and synaptic sites.

What makes NG2 glia unique among the glial cells is their connections with neurons through unidirectional neuron-to-NG2 glia synapses. Most, if not all NG2 glia in the grey and white matter receive functional glutamatergic and/or GABAergic synaptic contacts, whose machinery and ultrastructure is remarkably similar to that of conventional neuron-to-neuron synapses. Such organization includes the tight alignment of neuron and NG2 glia cell membranes, the presence of an active zone with accumulation of synaptic vesicles on the neuronal side, and an electron dense postsynaptic density on the NG2 cell side. Notably, neuron-to-NG2 glia synapses are established in parallel with neuronal synaptogenesis [14,49], and are lost during NG2 glia progression in maturation [48,49]; this is in line with a specific role of this form of communication in undifferentiated NG2 glia. Remarkably, while glutamatergic neuron-to-NG2 glia synapses usually derive from long-range axons impinging almost exclusively on NG2 glia processes [50–52], GABAergic synapses derive from local interneurons [49,53] with a specific distribution of the synaptic contacts from fast spiking (located at NG2 glia somata and proximal parts of the processes) and non-fast spiking interneurons (located at the distal parts of NG2 glia processes) [49]. Although both glutamatergic and GABAergic neuron-to-NG2 glia synaptic inputs induce depolarization (since the measured chloride reversal potential in these cells is around $-30/-40$ mV), such well-defined arrangement suggests distinct roles for the different types of synapses impinging onto NG2 glia. In line with this idea, while the glutamatergic inputs onto NG2 glia increase in frequency and amplitude during CNS maturation [54], at least in the cerebral cortex, GABAergic neuron-to-NG2 glia synaptic transmission is a phenomenon restricted to developmental stages [49,55].

Intimate physical interactions also occur between NG2 glia and astrocytes [56,57], microglia [58], and myelinating OLs. Notably, while NG2 glia are never coupled via gap-junctions [59,60], some of them express connexin 32 [61] and partly couple to mature OLs [62]. Further, electron microscopy analysis showed that NG2 glia processes often contact the paranodal loops of myelin [46]. These data suggest a privileged communication between NG2 glia and other elements in the oligodendroglial lineage.

In the embryonic mouse and human brain, NG2 glia are closely associated with the developing blood vessels, by being either positioned at the sprouting tip or tethered along the abluminal surface of the endothelium via the basal lamina [63,64]. Some populations of NG2 glia maintain a perivascular distribution also in the mouse neonatal brain and adult white matter [65–68]. In such perivascular niche, NG2 glia establish direct interactions through their processes or somata with both endothelial cells and pericytes. Beside these perivascular NG2 glia, a large fraction of parenchymal NG2 cells, whose somata are located away from blood vessels, extend some processes to physically interact with pericytes and microvessels [41,46] (Figure 1C). Such a distribution suggests some form of crosstalk among NG2 glia, endothelial cells and pericytes (see below).

3. NG2 Glia as Sensors of Neuronal Activity

NG2 glia contacts/contiguity with functionally relevant neuronal domains put them in a strategic position to monitor the activity of neuronal circuitries, integrate distinct inputs, and possibly respond to changes of the firing patterns of the surrounding neurons [69]. Indeed, a number of studies have shown that NG2 glia dynamically react to alterations in neurotransmission [70]. Pioneer experiments have shown that suppression of neural activity due to intraocular injection of tetrodotoxin (TTX) remarkably reduces NG2 glia proliferation in the optic nerve [71]. Consistently, deprivation of sensory experience (i.e., whisker removal at developmental stages) negatively affects NG2 glia proliferation and survival, and alters their distribution in the somatosensory cortex [6,52]. In contrast, electrical stimulation of the corticospinal tract promotes NG2 cell proliferation and differentiation in the adult rat [72]. Similarly, neuronal activity induced by optogenetic stimulation in Thy1-channelrhodopsin-2 transgenic mice, elicits a mitogenic response in NG2 glia and increases their differentiation [73]. Again in line with an activity-dependent regulation of the number of NG2 glia and OLs, increased rates of NG2 glia proliferation have been observed in response to wheel running and environmental enrichment [74]. However, in later studies, voluntary physical exercise has instead been reported as being accompanied by a reduction of the proliferation rate, premature differentiation, and changes in NG2 glia division modality in the adult mouse brain [5,75,76]. Indeed, a recent study showed that the pattern of neuronal activity, rather than just the presence or absence of activity, determines the activity-dependent behavior of NG2 glia in vivo. By implanting an electrode array into the corpus callosum of adult mice, Nagy and colleagues [77] showed that NG2 glia respond differently when callosal axons are stimulated at 5, 25 or 300 hertz (Hz). Namely, stimulation at 5 Hz promoted NG2 glia maturation, while stimulation at 25 or 300 Hz stimulated NG2 glia proliferation. These findings are particularly noteworthy, because the rate and timing of neuronal firing are the main carriers of information about the features of a task or stimulus, and also because they imply that NG2 glia are somehow capable of discriminating between different patterns of neuronal firing (see below).

How do NG2 glia sense neuronal activity? Indeed, another feature that makes NG2 glia unique among glial cells is the expression of a large repertoire of typically "neuronal" proteins, including ion channels and neurotransmitter receptors. These comprise Ca^{2+}-permeable and impermeable α-amino-3-hydroxy-5-methyl-4-isoxazolepropionicacid (AMPA) and N-methyl-D-aspartate (NMDA) ionotropic glutamate receptors; group I (mGluR1 and mGluR5), group II (mGluR3) and group III (mGluR4) metabotropic glutamate receptors; ionotropic and metabotropic GABA receptors; Ca^{2+}-permeable and impermeable nicotinic acetylcholine receptors (nAChRs); muscarinic acetylcholine receptors (mAChRs); ionotropic glycine receptors (GlyRs); adrenergic, dopamine, serotonin and purinergic receptors [78]. The expression of these receptors is not universal in NG2 cell populations (e.g., only 60% of the callosal NG2 cells are able to respond to NMDA [79]), indicating a certain degree of heterogeneity within NG2 glia as regards their potential to sense and respond to changes in neurotransmission. Despite the fact that some of these neurotransmitter receptors (i.e., AMPA and ionotropic GABA receptors) have been shown to mediate neuron-to-NG2 glia synaptic communication, activation of most of them is thought to occur through extrasynaptic mechanisms [48], and is associated with large, widespread intracellular Ca^{2+} elevations [78].

Beside such activity-dependent "paracrine" interactions with neurons, studies show that NG2 cells are particularly well-suited for exerting a more tight and precise monitoring of the surrounding neuropil. First, NG2 glia are physically integrated in neuronal circuitries, since they receive synapses from collaterals of axons simultaneously impinging on nearby excitatory or inhibitory neurons [50,51,54]. Thus, by receiving paired/synchronous synaptic signals, NG2 glia can operate a real-time control of the incoming inputs onto surrounding neurons. Further, the expression of high levels of "leak" potassium channels and the connection with neurons through conventional synapses make NG2 glia able to sense even small changes in neuronal activity with an extremely high temporal and spatial resolution. Of note, NG2 glia have been reported to detect fine changes of extracellular potassium concentration due to the discharge of a single neuron via the inward-rectifier Kir4.1 potassium channels [78,80]. Similarly, by employing two-photon-based glutamate uncaging to produce very localized and brief release of glutamate onto NG2 glia processes segments, Sun et al. [81] showed that small neurotransmitter release events at neuron-to-NG2 cell synapses can be sensed via the generation of local depolarizations and, consequentially, local Ca^{2+} signals in NG2 glia processes.

The incoming electrical synaptic inputs are temporally and spatially summed and integrated by NG2 glia, by using Ca^{2+} levels to proportionally encode the number of the active synapses [81]. Interestingly, by analysing the properties of ionic currents elicited by repetitive axonal stimulation at glutamatergic neuron-to-NG2 glia synapses, Nagy et al. [77] recently demonstrated that, similar to neurons, NG2 glia are also able to discriminate different patterns of presynaptic axonal activity (i.e., stimulation trains with distinct frequency of pulses). Since in neurons different patterns of incoming inputs induce Ca^{2+} signals with distinct temporal and spatial distribution and the activation of diverse signaling pathways, such discriminative ability is thought to subserve the engagement of NG2 glia in either proliferation or differentiation following stimulation at different frequencies [77].

On the whole, these findings indicate that NG2 glia are specialized "listeners and integrators" of neuronal activity, and adjust their behavior in response to its changes. In this context, intracellular Ca^{2+} transients—generated in different spatial domains of NG2 glia depending on the pattern/type of incoming activity (including synaptic and extrasynaptic inputs)—likely serve distinct roles. Namely, large Ca^{2+} signals involving the entire cell arborization and soma are particularly apt to induce gene expression changes and global cellular actions such as cell division, differentiation, survival or motility [78]. Conversely, beyond allowing the integration of the synaptic activity received by distinct axons, Ca^{2+} transients restricted to specific segments of individual processes may be implicated in more compartmentalized functions, such as the stabilization of contacts between NG2 glia processes and axons [82,83], process motility [31], local protein synthesis [84,85], or secretion. Indeed, NG2 glia produce a wide range of "neuroactive" factors, and the release of some of them is activity-dependent (see below). This suggests that the integration of NG2 glia in neuronal circuitries and their exquisite ability to perceive activity changes/patterns may be instrumental for a neuron-to-NG2 glia-to-neuron communication loop contributing to homeostasis and/or plasticity.

4. Maintenance of NG2 Glia Is Required for Central Nervous System Homeostasis and Development

To unveil the specific contribution of NG2 glia to CNS functions/ontogeny, a wide range of approaches have been developed to study the consequences of their selective ablation from the adult or developing brain. Pioneer studies have exploited the exposure to high-doses of X-rays or the infusion of mitotic blockers (such as Arabinofuranosyl cytidine (AraC)) to ablate cycling cells, including NG2 glia. These approaches lacked cell-type specificity and suffered from side-effects, making it difficult to attribute a phenotype exclusively to NG2 glia loss. Thus, in the most recent studies, NG2 glia ablation has been achieved by the generation of mouse lines expressing a "suicide" gene under a NG2 glia specific promoter. Suicide genes typically encode for an essential protein, for a toxin, or for an enzyme that converts an exogenous drug into a toxic agent [86]. Of note, in all cases the effectiveness of the control mechanisms by which NG2 glia density/distribution are maintained in space and time hampered a long-lasting NG2 glia ablation. Even in the most efficient systems, cells escaping the ablation immediately reacted, entering the cell cycle and replacing the lost cells. Thus, no study has succeeded so far in ablating NG2 glia for long periods, and available data only refer to phenotypes emerging from transient NG2 glia loss. However, despite this limitation, ablation strategies provided important evidence for a NG2 glia specific contribution in CNS physiology and development, beyond their role as OL progenitors.

By using a transgenic mouse model expressing the diphtheria toxin receptor (DTR) under the control of the NG2 promoter (NG2Cre-R26DTR mice), Birey and colleagues [87] showed that the selective ablation of about 50% of NG2 glia in adult mice caused deficits in the glutamatergic neurotransmission (i.e., decreased amplitude and increased decay of the miniature excitatory postsynaptic currents (mEPSC), and an altered postsynaptic glutamate receptor trafficking in pyramidal excitatory neurons), negatively affected the astrocytic extracellular glutamate uptake, and induced depressive-like behaviors in mice. Of note, these effects could be observed only in the prefrontal cortex. No changes were observed in the dorsal striatum, while different electrophysiological phenotypes have been found in the somatosensory cortex (where both mEPSC frequency and decay were increased), indicating a differential contribution of NG2 glia in the regulation of glutamatergic neurotransmission in distinct brain regions. By using this ablation strategy, NG2 glia loss did not result in brain vasculature alterations, inflammation, microglia activation, or neurodegeneration [87].

Conversely, in a transgenic rat model expressing thymidine kinase (TK) (that converts the prodrug ganciclovir into a toxic triphosphate molecule that can be incorporated into the genome during DNA synthesis, leading to the selective ablation of proliferative cells) under the NG2 promoter, Nakano et al. [88] found that NG2 glia loss induced neurodegeneration, microglia activation and neuroinflammation in the adult hippocampus. Reduced levels of the immunomodulatory factor hepatocyte growth factor (HGF) have been proposed to mediate such effects. The different outcomes of NG2 glia ablation in the two studies may be interpreted again as the result of the loss of region-specific functions exerted by NG2 glia, or may be related to the different extent and timing of cell ablation (about 50% of NG2 glia in the cortex after seven days in [87]; about 80% in the hippocampus after one day in [88]). Milder effects reported in Birey et al. [87] may be indicative of the persistence of a sufficient number of NG2 glia contributing to neuronal support in the mouse cortex. However, even in those regions where NG2 ablation reached higher percentages (i.e., 80% in the subcortical white matter and 90% in the striatum after seven days), no sign of neurodegeneration was detected in NG2Cre-R26DTR mice. An alternative explanation could be that the huge mass of NG2 glia simultaneously undergoing cell death in [88] may have triggered a robust microglia response that eventually impacted on hippocampal neuron survival per se (i.e., independently of the possible effects of NG2 glia loss); further studies will clarify this issue. In any case, the inconsistency of the results of these two studies points to the intrinsic limitations of all cell ablation approaches, that must be taken into account in the interpretation of the results obtained by these experimental strategies.

A third recent study [42] used three different methods (i.e., X-irradiation, AraC infusion into the third ventricle and a novel mouse line where Esco2, a protein necessary for cell cycle progression, could be deleted in NG2 glia, inducing cell death in cycling NG2 cells; see also [12]) to ablate NG2 glia in the adult mouse median eminence. Here, NG2 glia ablation caused the degeneration of the dendrites of hypothalamic neurons expressing the leptin receptor. This led to the loss of neuronal responsiveness to leptin, and consequentially, to mouse overeating and obesity. These data showed a specific NG2 glia contribution to the body weight control, likely exerted by providing trophic or structural support to neuronal dendrites.

Cell ablation strategies have also been used to investigate NG2 glia roles during CNS ontogenesis. Recently, Minocha et al. [63] developed two Cre-mouse lines expressing a 'floxed' diphtheria toxin gene under either the Nkx2.1 (Nkx2.1-Cre -R26DTA) or the NG2 (Cspg4-Cre-R26DTA) promoter to ablate the first wave of NG2 glia produced in the forebrain during the embryonic life. In the mouse, these cells originate at E12.5 from Nkx2.1-expressing progenitors of the medial ganglionic eminence and anterior entopeduncular area, and transiently populate the entire telencephalon by E14.5 before disappearing at around postnatal day eight (P8) [84,89,90]. Thus, they do not contribute to myelination and their transient nature raises numerous questions about their possible role/s during CNS development. Interestingly, the ablation of such first wave of NG2 glia severely affected the formation of the blood vessel network by reducing vascular ramifications and connections during the embryonic life. Of note, analyses at postnatal stages did not reveal any such defects, indicating compensatory proangiogenic actions of later appearing NG2 glia or other cell types.

In another study, the ablation of NG2 glia in a transgenic myelin basic protein (MBP)-TK mouse line during the early phases of postnatal development (i.e., at P1) resulted in a rapid increase of axonal sprouting in the cerebellum, changes in the expression of molecules involved in axon plasticity and guidance (i.e., increased levels of the growth-associated protein GAP43, reduced expression of Semaphorin 3a and Netrin 1), and altered localization and function of ionotropic glutamate receptors in Purkinje neurons [91]. These studies showed that during the postnatal and embryonic life, NG2 glia populations are engaged in developmental events well before the onset of myelination, and indicated their active participation in shaping neuronal circuits and blood vessel networks.

5. NG2 Glia-Derived Signals Can Modulate Neuronal and Non-Neuronal Cell Functions in the Central Nervous System

Traditionally, NG2 glia have been considered only as a target for factors produced by neighboring cells: a large repertoire of paracrine signals produced by neurons, astrocytes, microglia, and endothelial cells has been shown to influence NG2 glia during myelination and after injury [68,92]. However, accumulating evidence shows that, depending on the context, NG2 glia can serve as a source for a plethora of secreted molecules which are able to support or interfere with the functions of other CNS cell types. Namely, Sypecka and Sarnowska [93] reported a neuroprotective effect of rat NG2 glia conditioned medium (CM) on organotypic hippocampal slices subjected to oxygen-glucose deprivation. Consistently, rat embryonic cortical neurons showed a marked increase in survival when co-cultured with NG2 glia or exposed to their CM [94,95]. Further, the CM of NG2 glia displayed remarkable pro-angiogenic effects by stimulating proliferation, tip sprouting, tube formation, and expressions of tight-junctions proteins in endothelial cells [65,96,97] and promoting proliferation/survival of pericytes [66]. In contrast, the CM obtained from NG2 glia exposed to inflammatory cytokines weakened endothelial barrier tightness in vitro [67]. These findings indicated that, overall, NG2 glia can provide functionally relevant paracrine signals. However, mechanistic insights about (i) their molecular identity, (ii) the spatio-temporal regulation of their production/release, and (iii) their targeting and relevance in vivo, started to be unveiled only very recently. Indeed, the physical apposition of the tiny NG2 glia processes at specific sites of neuronal and non-neuronal CNS cells suggests a focal release and a precise targeting of NG2 glia-derived signals. Synaptophysin-positive clusters indicative of a 'classical' secretory vesicle accumulation and release machinery have been observed at defined sites along the NG2 glia processes [41]. Other mechanisms of signal transfer have been also reported, including cleavage of fragments of membrane-bound molecules [98] or exosome shedding [99]. Signal transfer through exosomes allows cell-specific targeting by receptor-ligand interactions [100] and assures that a well defined concentration of the signal may be delivered to the target. Thus, this latter form of communication again suggests a specific control of the distribution and intensity of the biological effects elicited by NG2-derived signals.

As regards the molecular identity of NG2 glia secreted factors, in vitro/in vivo analyses of gene expression or of NG2 glia CM showed that they include growth factors, neurotrophins, neuromodulatory and neurosupportive signals, cell adhesion and extracellular matrix (ECM) molecules, matrix metalloproteases and metalloprotease inhibitors, inflammatory cytokines/immunomodulatory factors, morphogens (Table 1).

Table 1. List of the signals produced/released by NG2 glia.

Type of Signal	Name and Abbreviation	Exp. Approach (Source)	Function
Growth factors	Fibroblast growth factor 2, FGF2	Gene expr. study of cultured mouse NG2 glia and expr. in adult mouse NG2 glia in vivo [87]	NG2 glia modulation of glutamatergic neurotransmission and astrocytic extracellular glutamate uptake [87], neuronal protection and CNS repair [101], modulation of synaptic plasticity [102] and astroglial and microglial reactivity [103]
	Platelet-derived growth factor AA, PDGF-AA	CM of cultured mouse NG2 glia [97]	Neuronal protection [104], synaptic plasticity [105] and angiogenesis [106]
	Platelet-derived growth factor BB, PDGF-BB	CM of cultured mouse NG2 glia [97]	Neurotrophic and neuroregulatory functions [107], synaptic plasticity [105]
	Vascular endothelial growth factor, VEGF	CM of cultured mouse NG2 glia [97]	Neurotrophic function [108,109], regulation of adult neurogenesis [108]
	Insulin-like growth factor 1, IGF-1	CM of cultured rat NG2 glia [94]; Gene expr. study of cultured rat NG2 glia [93]	Synaptic maturation [110]
	Hepatocyte growth factor, HGF	In vivo expr. in rat NG2 glia [88]; Protein expr. in cultured rat NG2 glia [111]	Neuronal plasticity [112]
Neurotrophins	Brain derived growth factor, BDNF	CM of cultured rat NG2 glia and protein expr. in adult mouse NG2 glia in vivo [113]; CM of cultured human NG2 glia [114]; Gene expr. study and CM of cultured rat NG2 glia [93]	Neurotrophic function, neurotransmitter modulation and in neuronal plasticity [115]
	Nerve growth factor, NGF	Gene expr. study of cultured mouse NG2 glia [87,116]	Neurotrophic function, brain plasticity [117]
	Neurotrophin-3, NT-3	CM of cultured human NG2 glia [114]; Gene expr. study of cultured rat NG2 glia [93]	Neurotrophic function, neuronal survival and differentiation [118,119]
	Neurotrophin 4/5, NT-4/5	Gene expr. study of cultured mouse NG2 glia [87]	Neurotrophic function, neuronal survival and differentiation [120]
	Glial cell-derived neurotrophic factor, GDNF	Gene expr. study of cultured mouse NG2 glia [87]; Gene expr. study of cultured rat NG2 glia [93]	Neurotrophic function, survival and morphological differentiation of dopaminergic neurons [121]
	Ciliary neurotrophic factor, CNTF	Gene expr. study of cultured rat NG2 glia [93]	Neuronal and oligodendroglial survival [122–124]
Cell adhesion and extracellular matrix molecules	Neuronal cell adhesion molecule, NrCAM	Gene expr. study of freshly sorted adult human NG2 glia [125]	Maintenance of Na+ channels at nodes of Ranvier [126], dendritic spine remodelling [127]
	NCAM	Gene expr. study of freshly sorted adult human NG2 glia [125]	Neuronal plasticity [128], neuritogenesis and synaptogenesis [129], adult neurogenesis [130]
	Down Syndrome Cell Adhesion Molecule, Dscam	Gene expr. study of freshly sorted mouse NG2 glia [131] and freshly sorted adult human NG2 glia [125]	Neurite repulsion [132–135]
	Chondroitin sulphate proteoglycan4, Cspg4/NG2	Gene expr. study of freshly sorted adult human NG2 glia [125,136]	Modulation of synaptic activity and action potential conduction [137], axonal guidance and regenerative processes [138]
	Versican, Vcan	Gene expr. study of freshly sorted adult human NG2 glia [125] and freshly sorted mouse NG2 glia [131]	Assembly, maintenance and function of the nodes of Ranvier [139]
	Brevican	Gene expr. study of freshly sorted mouse NG2 glia [131]	Assembly, maintenance and function of the nodes of Ranvier [140]
	Tenascins	Gene expr. study of freshly sorted adult human NG2 glia [125]; Gene expr. study of freshly sorted mouse NG2 glia [131]	Synaptic plasticity [141]
	Glypican 5, Gpc5	Gene expr. study of freshly sorted mouse NG2 glia [131]	Neuronal plasticity [142,143]

Table 1. *Cont.*

Type of Signal	Name and Abbreviation	Exp. Approach (Source)	Function
Cell adhesion and extracellular matrix molecules	Emilin And Multimerin Domain-Containing Protein 1, Emid1	Gene expr. study of freshly sorted mouse NG2 glia [131]	Blood vessel maintenance [144]
	Syndecan 3, sdc3	Gene expr. study of freshly sorted adult human NG2 glia [125]	Synaptic plasticity [145]
	Spondin 1, Spon1	Gene expr. study of freshly sorted mouse NG2 glia [131]	Neural cell adhesion and neurite outgrowth [146]
	Thrombospondin 2 and 4	Gene expr. study of freshly sorted adult human NG2 glia [125]	Synaptogenesis and synaptic plasticity [147], inflammatory response and repair of the blood brain barrier [148]
	Cerebellin 1, cbln 1	Gene expr. study of cultured mouse NG glia [87]	Synaptic organizer, synapse integrity and synaptic plasticity [149,150]
	SPARC-Related Modular Calcium-Binding Protein 1, SMOC1	Gene expr. study of freshly sorted mouse NG2 glia [131]	Angiogenesis [151]
	Olfactomedin 2, Olfm2	Gene expr. study of freshly sorted mouse NG2 glia [131]	Synaptogenesis and synaptic plasticity [152]
	Neurexophilin 1, Nxph1	Gene expr. study of freshly sorted mouse NG2 glia [131]	Synaptogenesis and synaptic plasticity [150,153]
	Neuronal Pentraxin 2, Nptx2	Gene expr. study of freshly sorted mouse NG2 glia [131] and of cultured and freshly sorted mouse NG2 glia [154]	Synaptogenesis and synaptic plasticity [150,153,155,156], trafficking of glutamate receptors [157]
Matrix metalloproteases and metalloprotease inhibitors	Matrix Metalloprotease 3, MMP3	CM of cultured mouse NG2 glia [26]; Gene expr. study of cultured mouse NG2 glia exposed to Il17 or Tnf [158]	Neuronal and synaptic plasticity [159]
	Matrix Metalloprotease 9, MMP9	CM of cultured mouse NG2 glia [26]; CM of cultured rat NG2 glia and protein expr. in mouse NG2 glia in vivo—adult white matter [67] Gene expr. study of cultured mouse NG2 glia exposed to Il17 or Tnf [158]	Blood vessel remodeling after white matter injury [160]. Remodeling of synaptic networks in adult brain [161]
	Tissue Inhibitor of Metalloprotease 1, TIMP1	CM of cultured mouse NG2 glia [26]	Neuronal death and axonal plasticity [162]
	Tissue Inhibitor of Metalloprotease 4, TIMP4	Gene expr. study of freshly sorted mouse NG2 glia [131]; Gene expr. study of freshly sorted adult human NG2 glia [125]	Tissue remodelling [163,164]
Neuromodulatory/ neurosupportive factors	Neuregulins	Gene expr. study of cultured mouse NG glia [87]; Gene expr. study and CM of cultured rat NG glia [165]	Synaptogenesis and synaptic plasticity [166], oligodendroglial and neuronal survival [167,168]
	Galanin	mRNA and protein expr. in adult mouse NG2 glia [169]	Modulation of neuronal activity [170]
	Chromogranin B, Chgb	Gene expr. study of freshly sorted adult human NG2 glia [125]	Neurotransmission [171,172]
	Chromogranin C, Chgc	Gene expr. study of freshly sorted adult human NG2 glia [125]	Neurite outgrowth [173] and angiogenesis [174].
	Persephin, PSPN	Gene expr. study of cultured mouse NG glia [87]	Neuronal survival [175]

Table 1. *Cont.*

Type of Signal	Name and Abbreviation	Exp. Approach (Source)	Function
Morphogens	Wingless-type MMTV integration site family 4, Wnt4	Gene expr.: study of freshly sorted mouse NG2 glia [176]	Synaptic plasticity [177]
	Wingless-type MMTV integration site family 7a, Wnt7a	Gene expr.: study of freshly sorted mouse NG2 glia [176]; Gene expr.: study and CM of cultured mouse NG2 glia [96]; In vivo expr. in embryonic NG2 glia [64]	Synaptic plasticity [178,179]; NG2 glia regulation of angiogenesis [96]
	Wingless-type MMTV integration site family 7b, Wnt7b	Gene expr.: study of freshly sorted mouse NG2 glia [176]; Gene expr.: study and CM of cultured mouse NG2 glia [96]; In vivo expr. in embryonic NG2 glia [64]	Synaptic plasticity [180]
	Bone morphogenic protein 2, BMP2	Gene expr.: study of freshly sorted adult human NG2 glia [125]	Neuronal survival [181]
	Bone morphogenic protein 7, BMP7	Gene expr.: study of freshly sorted adult human NG2 glia [125]	Maintainance of the identity of catecholaminergic neurons and differentiation of astrocytes [182]
	Retinoic acid, RA	Application of pharmacological inhibitors in cultured mouse NG2 glia and in vivo assays in a model of rat spinal cord injury [99]	NG2 glia regulation of axonal outgrowth [99]
	Slit1	Gene expr.: study of freshly sorted adult human NG2 glia [125]	Regulation of adult SVZ neurogenesis [183], axon outgrowth and glial scar formation [184]
Inflammatory cytokines/ immunomodulatory factors	Interleukin 1 beta, Il-1b	Gene expr.: study of cultured mouse NG2 glia [87]; Gene expr.: study of cultured rat NG2 glia [93]	Synaptic plasticity [185]
	Interleukin 6, Il-6	Gene expr.: study of cultured mouse NG2 glia [87]; Gene expr.: study of cultured rat NG2 glia [93]; Gene expr.: study of cultured mouse NG2 glia exposed to Il17 or Tnf [158]	Regulation of adult neurogenesis [186,187], neuronal protection [187]
	Interleukin 10, Il-10	Gene expr.: study of cultured mouse NG2 glia [87]; Gene expr.: study and CM of cultured rat NG2 glia [93]	Neuronal and glial cell survival [88,88], Anti-inflammatory functions [189]
	Transforming growth factor beta, Tgf-b	Gene expr.: study of cultured mouse NG2 glia [87]; Gene expr.: study of cultured rat NG2 glia and protein expr. in mouse neonatal NG2 glia in vivo [65]	Neuronal survival and modulation of synaptic transmission [190]
	Interleukin 1 Receptor Accessory Protein, Il1rap	Gene expr.: study of freshly sorted mouse NG2 glia [131]	Neuronal survival [191]
	C-X-C Motif Chemokine Ligand 10, CxCl1	Gene expr.: study of cultured mouse NG2 glia exposed to Il17 or Tnf [158,192]	Neuroinflammation [193]
	C-X-C Motif Chemokine Ligand 10, CxCl10	CM of cultured mouse NG2 glia [97]	Neuroinflammation [194]
	C-X3-C Motif Chemokine Ligand 1, Cx3Cl1	CM of cultured mouse NG2 glia [97]	Regulation of synapses activity and plasticity, brain functional connectivity and adult hippocampal neurogenesis [195]
	C-C Motif Chemokine Ligand 7, Ccl7	Gene expr.: study of cultured mouse NG2 glia exposed to Il17 [192]	Neuroinflammation [196–198]
	Granulocyte-Macrophage Colony Stimulating Factor, GM-CSF or Csf2	Gene expr.: study of cultured mouse NG2 glia exposed to Il17 or Tnf [158]	Neurotrophic function [199]

Exp: Experimental; expr: Expression; CM: Conditioned medium; FGF2: Fibroblast growth factor 2; NG2: Neuron–glia antigen 2.

It is noteworthy that NG2 glia express and secrete a large repertoire of 'neuroactive' factors, that can contribute to regulate neuronal survival, maturation and functions. The bioactivity and functional relevance of some these signals have been validated by in vitro or in vivo approaches. Namely, the neutralization of either brain derived growth factor (BDNF) or interleukin (Il)-10 in NG2 glia CM showed that these factors contribute to NG2 glia neuroprotective function in vitro [93]. Birey and colleagues showed that the specific knock-down of fibroblast growth factor 2 (FGF2) in the NG2 glia of the prefrontal cortex suffices to induce depressive-like behaviors in mice, and suggested that the loss of this signal mediates the effects of NG2 cell ablation on glutamatergic transmission [87]. Similarly, by pharmacological and lentiviral inhibition of the retinoic acid (RA) synthesis, Goncalves et al., showed that NG2 glia support axon growth and regeneration by contributing to the conversion of retinal to RA [99].

The enrichment of ECM components and matrix metalloproteases (Table 1) suggests unique interactions of NG2 glia with the ECM compared with other CNS cell types, and specific roles in tissue maintenance and remodeling. Beside this, the regulation of ECM integrity and composition is important for neurotransmitter receptor clustering at synapses [200,201]. Of note, a relatively large repertoire of cell adhesion and ECM-associated molecules expressed by NG2 glia are well known secreted pro-synaptogenic factors and synaptic organizers (e.g., thrombospondins, cerebellin 1, olfactomedin 2, neurexophilin 1, neuronal pentraxin 2). These components may be instrumental to build and maintain neuron-to-NG2 glia synaptic contacts. However, since NG2 glia processes have been observed in close apposition to neuronal dendrites and somata or interdigitating within the synaptic cleft of neuron-to-neuron synapses, this enrichment may be also related to a role of NG2 glia in neuronal synaptogenesis and synaptic plasticity. Similarly, ECM molecules expressed by NG2 glia (i.e., brevican, versican, tenascin R) importantly contribute to the assembly, maintenance and function of the nodes of Ranvier [46], thereby suggesting a specific NG2 glia contribution to neuronal maturation and action potential transmission.

In this context, recent data indicated that the NG2 chondroitin sulfate proteoglycan, whose expression is restricted to NG2 glia among the neural cell types, can serve as a polyvalent regulator of neuronal synaptic activity and action potential conduction. Sakry et al. [98] showed that the ectodomain of the NG2 protein, constitutively released from the NG2 glia surface into the ECM by the ADAM10 secretase, influences AMPA receptor currents and kinetics at glutamatergic synapses of cortical pyramidal neurons. Moreover, the pharmacological inhibition of NG2 cleavage and release from NG2 glia resulted in a large reduction of NMDAR-dependent, long-term potentiation (LTP) at these synapses, indicating a specific role of NG2 in synaptic plasticity [98]. A further neuromodulatory function of NG2 has been attributed to its intracellular domain that regulates the expression of prostaglandin D2 synthase, a secreted enzyme that catalyzes the conversion of prostaglandin H2 to the neuromodulatory form prostaglandin D2 [154]. Finally, in the injured spinal cord, secreted NG2 has been observed to block action potential conduction at the nodes of Ranvier [202].

Transforming growth factor β (TGF-β) and Wingless-type MMTV integration site family 7 (Wnt7) have recently been shown to mediate NG2 glia pro-angiogenetic effects in vivo. The pharmacological inhibition of TGF-b signaling abolished the effect of NG2 glia CM on endothelial cell expression of tight junction proteins in vitro. Consistently, the specific ablation of TGF-b1 in NG2 glia resulted in cerebral hemorrhage and loss of blood brain barrier integrity in neonatal mice [65]. Similar approaches have been used by Yuen et al. [96] to demonstrate that NG2 glia-derived Wnt7 mediates their pro-angiogenic effects in vitro.

Notably, as a part of their plastic nature, NG2 glia dynamically modulate the expression/secretion of specific signals in response to external factors. Importantly, signals inducing NG2 glia depolarization reportedly affected their secretion. Exposure to GABA largely increased the production and secretion of BDNF from adult rat NG2 glia [113]. Consistently, the application of a moderate intensity static magnetic field, with its associated electric field, on human NG2 glia cultures resulted in increased secretion of BDNF and neurotrophin 3 (NT-3) [114]. The release of the NG2 ectodomain from NG2 glia was augmented by treatments with depolarizing agents or glutamate in vitro [98]. Along this line, the expression of the neuromodulatory/neuroprotective peptide galanin significantly increased in NG2 glia upon experimental cortical spreading depression [169]. These observations suggest that activity dependent/synapse-mediated signals converging on NG2 glia may dynamically regulate their secretory activity and homeostatic functions.

In conclusion, although the repertoire of factors expressed/secreted by NG2 glia has not yet been explored in depth, these findings clearly indicate that they can serve as providers of relevant signals for neighboring cells—in particular for neurons—in a context-dependent manner.

6. NG2 Glia Upon Central Nervous System Injury and Stress

The cellular roles of NG2 glia upon pathological conditions remain largely unclear. Notably, in vivo/in vitro exposure to different kinds of stresses or injury-related signals remarkably affects NG2 glia expression profile and secretion. Some of these changes can be interpreted as compensatory attempts aimed at sustaining cell survival/functions and restoring the homeostasis. For example, early after an acute brain injury, such as an ischemic event, BDNF protein expression largely increased in NG2 glia, likely amplifying their neuroprotective potential [113]. However, when the exposure to danger signals or stresses takes place over longer periods, gene expression/secretion alterations in NG2 glia make them sustain or even worsen the pathological condition. In vivo exposure to chronic stress induces profound transcriptional alterations in NG2 glia in specific brain regions (i.e., prefrontal cortex and nucleus accumbens [87,203]), and largely reduces the levels of growth factors (i.e., FGF2) and neurotrophins (i.e., NGF and NT4/5) [87]. After prolonged cerebral hypoperfusion stress, perivascular NG2 glia in the adult white matter increased matrix metalloprotease 9 (MMP9) expression and contributed to blood brain barrier opening [67]. Treatment with sublethal concentrations of the inflammatory cytokine Il-1β also increased MMP9 secretion by cultured NG2 glia [67]. Similarly, exposure to Il-17 or Tnf increased MMP9 and MMP3 expression and elicited a robust inflammatory response in cultured NG2 glia [158]. Consistently, sustained Il-17 signaling in NG2 glia incorporated these cells in the inflammatory pathogenesis of experimental autoimmune encephalomyelitis (EAE) [158]. Complementarily, experimental attenuation of NG2 glia proliferative response after spinal cord lesion was associated with reduced accumulation of activated microglia/macrophages, diminished astrocyte hypertrophy, and eventually with the establishment of a post-injury environment more supportive for tissue repair [204]. This suggests a role for NG2 cells in orchestrating reactive gliosis.

Thus, beyond their role in myelin repair and glial scar formation [205], depending on the circumstances, NG2 glia have been observed either to limit CNS damage or to actively contribute to neuroinflammation/neurotoxicity, as also shown in Amyotrophic Lateral Sclerosis models [206]. To further increase the complexity of this scenario, consistent with previous findings [207,208], in vivo two-photon imaging analyses revealed an assortment of distinct NG2 glia reactions to injury, with some cells starting migration toward the lesion site, others entering cell cycle, and others displaying only hypertrophy and morphological changes [31,86]. Single-cell messenger-RNA (mRNA) profiling of NG2 glia after focal cerebral ischemia also identified at least three subpopulations of cells that could be distinguished according to changes in their expression patterns [19]. Such behavioral and molecular heterogeneity suggests the existence of diverse NG2 glia subsets which respond differently to CNS injury.

7. Concluding Remarks and Open Issues

In this review, we have summarized the advancements obtained over recent years toward the understanding of the roles of NG2 glia in CNS homeostasis and development. Though it is widely accepted that these cells act as precursors for OLs in the developing and mature CNS, accumulating evidence indicates that NG2 glia (or subsets of NG2 glia) can exert additional/alternative functions. Recent studies have shown that NG2 glia establish physical interactions with the other CNS cell types, are integrated in neuronal networks, and possess a repertoire of ion channels and neurotransmitter receptors apt to constantly monitor the activity of the surrounding neurons. In addition to operating as sensors, NG2 glia have features that are expected for active modulators of the neuronal activity, including the expression and release of a complex array of neuromodulatory and neuroprotective factors. Consistently, cell ablation strategies targeting NG2 glia demonstrate that the maintenance of their density contributes to the normal function and development of different CNS regions, beyond their role in myelination.

Although showing some similarities with astrocytes—as regards their physical/functional relationships with neurons and blood vessels, and to a certain extent, gene expression—data available so far point to a distinct contribution of these two glial cell types in CNS homeostasis. NG2 glia specificity relies on the ability to monitor, and perhaps modulate, the activity of the neuronal networks with a resolution in time, space and intensity that cannot be achieved by astroglia. This appears to be related to NG2 glia typical morphology (with fine processes establishing contacts at well defined sites onto neurons) and functional properties (including the ability to sense neuronal activity at the quantal level through neuron-to-NG2 glia synapses). Further, since the roles/features of NG2 glia described above do not emerge as the by-product of the metabolic/gene expression control of typical progenitor functions (i.e., proliferation and differentiation in myelin-producing cells), they cannot simply be interpreted as epiphenomena (i.e., secondary functions) of the role of NG2 glia as OL precursors. Thus, NG2 glia not only represent a transitional stage along the oligodendroglial lineage, but rather, a specific glial cell type endowed with typical properties and functions.

However, this field of research is still in its infancy and the mechanistic nature of NG2 glia functions beyond re-/myelination remains still unclear. Further efforts are needed to overcome the limitations of the experimental strategies employed so far, and to identify the molecular and cellular processes subserving NG2 glia participation in CNS homeostasis, ontogeny, and disease. Namely, the in vivo NG2 glia ablation approaches showed important intrinsic caveats, e.g., the achievement of a partial and transient cell ablation due to the fast repopulation of NG2 glia; region-specific differences in the ablation efficiency due to different cell cycle dynamics and repopulation efficiency of NG2 glia in distinct CNS areas [87]; selective/predominant ablation of specific NG2 glia subsets (i.e., those that are more prone to enter cell cycle; [42,88]); possible interference/superimposition of the reactions of other CNS cell types responding to NG2 glia loss [88]. Such limitations restrict the time window/extent/types of phenotypes that could be attributed to NG2 glia loss, and may also hamper investigation into the underlying molecular mechanisms. Recent studies have started to unveil the cellular processes through which NG2 glia can transfer functionally relevant signals (i.e., conventional vesicle release, exosome shedding, cleavage of extracellular fragments of membrane-bound proteins). Targeting such processes (e.g., by a genetic-based deletion of specific components of the secretory/shedding/cleavage machineries in NG2 glia) may provide an alternative experimental setting to unveil the impact and relevance of NG2 glia to other cell types communication. Further, validation, perhaps using cell type-specific subtractive/deletion approaches (as in [87]), of the effects exerted by NG2 glia-derived factors in vivo is required to define the regulatory signals that are truly unique in mediating NG2 glia functions. The identification of such factors has recently taken advantage of RNA sequencing technologies [131]. The progresses of these strategies will make it possible to study the transcriptomic landscape at the single cell level, thereby possibly unveiling also the heterogeneous nature of NG2 glia [209]. Moreover, since these cells establish contacts with neurons and other cell types at specific sites along processes and somata, and local mRNA localization and translation may be instrumental for their crosstalk (as recently shown for astrocytes, [210]), we envisage that novel approaches of spatial transcriptomics may be also fruitfully exploited to perform high-throughput quantifications while preserving spatial information about the subcellular localization of the analysed transcripts [211].

Indeed, such studies may also open translational perspectives for the implementation of the endogenous neurosupportive/neuroprotective potential of the CNS. In this context, more research is also needed to fully understand NG2 glia participation in pathology. A detailed and comprehensive examination of NG2 glia behaviors/molecular changes upon lesion will likely unveil some elements of cell heterogeneity (see above). Indeed, diverse NG2 glia subpopulations have also been described in the intact CNS based on their origin, proliferative activity, division modality, differentiation potential, expression of diverse transcription factors, Ca^{2+}-binding molecules, neurotransmitter receptors, and ionic currents [5,23,48,69,212]. Thus, it is conceivable that subsets of functionally specialized NG2 glia may be differentially tailored to contribute to distinct aspects of CNS homeostasis, including oligodendrogenesis and additional/alternative functions. This issue deserves to be the focus of future investigations, and adds a further element of complexity on the functioning of this fascinating cell type.

Funding: Our work is supported by the "Cariplo Ricerca Biomedica Giovani Ricercatori" grant from the Cariplo Foundation (ID: 2014-1207) and Individual funding for basic research (Ffabr) granted by the Italian Agency for the Evaluation of University and Research, to EB. This study was also supported by Ministero dell'Istruzione, dell'Università e della Ricerca—MIUR project "Dipartimenti di Eccellenza 2018–2022" to Dept. of Neuroscience "Rita Levi Montalcini".

Acknowledgments: We thank Annalisa Buffo (University of Turin) for insightful comments.

Conflicts of Interest: The authors declare no conflict of interest. The funding sponsors had no role in the interpretation of data or in the writing of the manuscript.

References

1. Boda, E.; Buffo, A. Glial cells in non-germinal territories: Insights into their stem/progenitor properties in the intact and injured nervous tissue. *Arch. Ital. Biol.* **2010**, *148*, 119–136. [PubMed]

2. Dawson, M.R.L.; Polito, A.; Levine, J.M.; Reynolds, R. NG2-expressing glial progenitor cells: An abundant and widespread population of cycling cells in the adult rat CNS. *Mol. Cell. Neurosci.* **2003**, *24*, 476–488. [CrossRef]

3. Assinck, P.; Duncan, G.J.; Plemel, J.R.; Lee, M.J.; Stratton, J.A.; Manesh, S.B.; Liu, J.; Ramer, L.M.; Kang, S.H.; Bergles, D.E.; et al. Myelinogenic plasticity of oligodendrocyte precursor cells following spinal cord contusion injury. *J. Neurosci.* **2017**, *37*, 8635–8654. [CrossRef] [PubMed]

4. Baxi, E.G.; DeBruin, J.; Jin, J.; Strasburger, H.J.; Smith, M.D.; Orthmann-Murphy, J.L.; Schott, J.T.; Fairchild, A.N.; Bergles, D.E.; Calabresi, P.A. Lineage tracing reveals dynamic changes in oligodendrocyte precursor cells following cuprizone-induced demyelination. *Glia* **2017**, *65*, 2087–2098. [CrossRef] [PubMed]

5. Boda, E.; Di Maria, S.; Rosa, P.; Taylor, V.; Abbracchio, M.P.; Buffo, A. Early phenotypic asymmetry of sister oligodendrocyte progenitor cells after mitosis and its modulation by aging and extrinsic factors. *Glia* **2015**, *63*, 271–286. [CrossRef] [PubMed]

6. Hill, R.; Patel, K.D.; Goncalves, C.M.; Grutzendler, J.; Nishiyama, A. Modulation of oligodendrocyte generation during a critical temporal window after NG2 cell division. *Nat. Neurosci.* **2014**, *17*, 1518–1527. [CrossRef] [PubMed]

7. McKenzie, I.A.; Ohayon, D.; Li, H.; Paes de Faria, J.; Emery, B.; Tohyama, K.; Richardson, W.D. Motor skill learning requires active central myelination. *Science* **2014**, *346*, 318–322. [CrossRef] [PubMed]

8. Xiao, L.; Ohayon, D.; McKenzie, I.A.; Sinclair-Wilson, A.; Wright, J.L.; Fudge, A.D.; Emery, B.; Li, H.; Richardson, W.D. Rapid production of new oligodendrocytes is required in the earliest stages of motor-skill learning. *Nat. Neurosci.* **2016**, *19*, 1210–1217. [CrossRef] [PubMed]

9. Hughes, E.G.; Orthmann-Murphy, J.L.; Langseth, A.J.; Bergles, D.E. Myelin remodeling through experience-dependent oligodendrogenesis in the adult somatosensory cortex. *Nat. Neurosci.* **2018**, *21*, 696–706. [CrossRef] [PubMed]

10. Hill, R.A.; Li, A.M.; Grutzendler, J. Lifelong cortical myelin plasticity and age-related degeneration in the live mammalian brain. *Nat. Neurosci.* **2018**, *21*, 683–695. [CrossRef] [PubMed]

11. Wang, S.; Young, K.M. White matter plasticity in adulthood. *Neuroscience* **2014**, *276*, 148–160. [CrossRef] [PubMed]

12. Schneider, S.; Gruart, A.; Grade, S.; Zhang, Y.; Kröger, S.; Kirchhoff, F.; Eichele, G.; Delgado García, J.M.; Dimou, L. Decrease in newly generated oligodendrocytes leads to motor dysfunctions and changed myelin structures that can be rescued by transplanted cells. *Glia* **2016**, *64*, 2201–2218. [CrossRef] [PubMed]

13. Psachoulia, K.; Jamen, F.; Young, K.M.; Richardson, W.D. Cell cycle dynamics of NG2 cells in the postnatal and ageing brain. *Neuron Glia Biol.* **2009**, *5*, 57. [CrossRef] [PubMed]
14. Boda, E.; Buffo, A. Beyond cell replacement: Unresolved roles of NG2-expressing progenitors. *Front. Neurosci.* **2014**, *8*, 122. [CrossRef] [PubMed]
15. Birey, F.; Kokkosis, A.; Aguirre, A. Oligodendroglia-lineage cells in brain plasticity, homeostasis and psychiatric disorders. *Curr. Opin. Neurobiol.* **2017**, *47*, 93–103. [CrossRef] [PubMed]
16. Boda, E.; Viganò, F.; Rosam, P.; Fumagalli, M.; Labat-Gest, V.; Tempia, F.; Abbracchio, M.P.; Dimou, L.; Buffo, A. The GPR17 receptor in NG2 expressing cells: Focus on in vivocell maturation and participation in acute trauma and chronic damage. *Glia* **2011**, *59*, 1958–1973. [CrossRef] [PubMed]
17. Levine, J. The reactions and role of NG2 glia in spinal cord injury. *Brain Res.* **2016**, *1638*, 199–208. [CrossRef] [PubMed]
18. Jin, X.; Riew, T.R.; Kim, H.L.; Choi, J.H.; Lee, M.Y. Morphological characterization of NG2 glia and their association with neuroglial cells in the 3-nitropropionic acid–lesioned striatum of rat. *Sci. Rep.* **2018**, *8*, 5942. [CrossRef] [PubMed]
19. Valny, M.; Honsa, P.; Waloschkova, E.; Matuskova, H.; Kriska, J.; Kirdajova, D.; Androvic, P.; Valihrach, L.; Kubista, M.; Anderova, M. A single-cell analysis reveals multiple roles of oligodendroglial lineage cells during post-ischemic regeneration. *Glia* **2018**, *66*, 1068–1081. [CrossRef] [PubMed]
20. Kazanis, I.; Evans, K.A.; Andreopoulou, E.; Dimitriou, C.; Koutsakis, C.; Karadottir, R.T.; Franklin, R.J.M. Subependymal zone-derived oligodendroblasts respond to focal demyelination but fail to generate myelin in young and aged mice. *Stem Cell Rep.* **2017**, *8*, 685–700. [CrossRef] [PubMed]
21. Guglielmetti, C.; Praet, J.; Rangarajan, J.R.; Vreys, R.; De Vocht, N.; Maes, F.; Verhoye, M.; Ponsaerts, P.; Van der Linden, A. Multimodal imaging of subventricular zone neural stem/progenitor cells in the cuprizone mouse model reveals increased neurogenic potential for the olfactory bulb pathway, but no contribution to remyelination of the corpus callosum. *Neuroimage* **2014**, *86*, 99–110. [CrossRef] [PubMed]
22. Xing, Y.L.; Roth, P.T.; Stratton, J.A.S.; Chuang, B.H.A.; Danne, J.; Ellis, S.L.; Ng, S.W.; Kilpatrick, T.J.; Merson, T.D. Adult neural precursor cells from the subventricular zone contribute significantly to oligodendrocyte regeneration and remyelination. *J. Neurosci.* **2014**, *34*, 14128–14146. [CrossRef] [PubMed]
23. Van Tilborg, E.; de Theije, C.G.M.; van Hal, M.; Wagenaar, N.; de Vries, L.S.; Benders, M.J.; Rowitch, D.H.; Nijboer, C.H. Origin and dynamics of oligodendrocytes in the developing brain: Implications for perinatal white matter injury. *Glia* **2018**, *66*, 221–238. [CrossRef] [PubMed]
24. Zhu, X.; Hill, R.A.; Nishiyama, A. NG2 cells generate oligodendrocytes and gray matter astrocytes in the spinal cord. *Neuron Glia Biol.* **2009**, *4*, 19–26. [CrossRef] [PubMed]
25. Zhu, X.; Bergles, D.E.; Nishiyama, A. NG2 cells generate both oligodendrocytes and gray matter astrocytes. *Development* **2007**, *135*, 145–157. [CrossRef] [PubMed]
26. Huang, W.; Zhao, N.; Bai, X.; Karram, K.; Trotter, J.; Goebbels, S.; Scheller, A.; Kirchhoff, F. Novel NG2-CreERT2 knock-in mice demonstrate heterogeneous differentiation potential of NG2 glia during development. *Glia* **2014**, *62*, 896–913. [CrossRef] [PubMed]
27. Tripathi, R.B.; Rivers, L.E.; Young, K.M.; Jamen, F.; Richardson, W.D. NG2 glia generate new oligodendrocytes but few astrocytes in a murine experimental autoimmune encephalomyelitis model of demyelinating disease. *J. Neurosci.* **2010**, *30*, 16383–16390. [CrossRef] [PubMed]
28. Boda, E.; Nato, G.; Buffo, A. Emerging pharmacological approaches to promote neurogenesis from endogenous glial cells. *Biochem. Pharmacol.* **2017**, *141*, 23–41. [CrossRef] [PubMed]
29. Zuo, H.; Wood, W.M.; Sherafat, A.; Hill, R.A.; Lu, Q.R.; Nishiyama, A. Age-dependent decline in fate switch from NG2 cells to astrocytes after Olig2 deletion. *J. Neurosci.* **2018**, *38*, 2359–2371. [CrossRef] [PubMed]
30. Valny, M.; Honsa, P.; Kriska, J.; Anderova, M. Multipotency and therapeutic potential of NG2 cells. *Biochem. Pharmacol.* **2017**, *141*, 42–55. [CrossRef] [PubMed]
31. Hughes, E.G.; Kang, S.H.; Fukaya, M.; Bergles, D.E. Oligodendrocyte progenitors balance growth with self-repulsion to achieve homeostasis in the adult brain. *Nat. Neurosci.* **2013**, *16*, 668–676. [CrossRef] [PubMed]
32. Kirby, B.B.; Takada, N.; Latimer, A.J.; Shin, J.; Carney, T.J.; Kelsh, R.N.; Appel, B. In vivo time-lapse imaging shows dynamic oligodendrocyte progenitor behavior during zebrafish development. *Nat. Neurosci.* **2006**, *9*, 1506–1511. [CrossRef] [PubMed]

33. Birey, F.; Aguirre, A. Age-dependent netrin-1 signaling regulates NG2+ glial cell spatial homeostasis in normal adult gray matter. *J. Neurosci.* **2015**, *35*, 6946–6951. [CrossRef] [PubMed]
34. Dufour, A.; Gontran, E.; Deroulers, C.; Varlet, P.; Pallud, J.; Grammaticos, B.; Badoual, M. Modeling the dynamics of oligodendrocyte precursor cells and the genesis of gliomas. *PLoS Comput. Biol.* **2018**, *14*, e1005977. [CrossRef] [PubMed]
35. Sugiarto, S.; Persson, A.I.; Munoz, E.G.; Waldhuber, M.; Lamagna, C.; Andor, N.; Hanecker, P.; Ayers-Ringler, J.; Phillips, J.; Siu, J.; et al. Asymmetry-defective oligodendrocyte progenitors are glioma precursors. *Cancer Cell* **2011**, *20*, 328–340. [CrossRef] [PubMed]
36. Balia, M.; Benamer, N.; Angulo, M.C. A specific GABAergic synapse onto oligodendrocyte precursors does not regulate cortical oligodendrogenesis. *Glia* **2017**, *65*, 1821–1832. [CrossRef] [PubMed]
37. Khakh, B.S.; Sofroniew, M.V. Diversity of astrocyte functions and phenotypes in neural circuits. *Nat. Neurosci.* **2015**, *18*, 942–952. [CrossRef] [PubMed]
38. Verkhratsky, A.; Bush, N.; Nedergaard, M.; Butt, A. The special case of human astrocytes. *Neuroglia* **2018**, *1*, 4. [CrossRef]
39. Casano, A.M.; Peri, F. Microglia: Multitasking specialists of the brain. *Dev. Cell* **2015**, *32*, 469–477. [CrossRef] [PubMed]
40. Réu, P.; Khosravi, A.; Bernard, S.; Mold, J.E.; Salehpour, M.; Alkass, K.; Perl, S.; Tisdale, J.; Possnert, G.; Druid, H.; et al. The lifespan and turnover of microglia in the human brain. *Cell Rep.* **2017**, *20*, 779–784. [CrossRef] [PubMed]
41. Wigley, R.; Butt, A.M. Integration of NG2-glia (synantocytes) into the neuroglial network. *Neuron Glia Biol.* **2009**, *5*, 21. [CrossRef] [PubMed]
42. Djogo, T.; Robins, S.C.; Schneider, S.; Kryzskaya, D.; Liu, X.; Mingay, A.; Gillon, C.J.; Kim, J.H.; Storch, K.F.; Boehm, U.; et al. Adult NG2-glia are required for median eminence-mediated leptin sensing and body weight control. *Cell Metab.* **2016**, *23*, 797–810. [CrossRef] [PubMed]
43. März, M.; Schmidt, R.; Rastegar, S.; Strähle, U. Expression of the transcription factor Olig2 in proliferating cells in the adult zebrafish telencephalon. *Dev. Dyn.* **2010**, *239*, 3336–3349. [CrossRef] [PubMed]
44. Boulanger, J.J.; Messier, C. Oligodendrocyte progenitor cells are paired with GABA neurons in the mouse dorsal cortex: Unbiased stereological analysis. *Neuroscience* **2017**, *362*, 127–140. [CrossRef] [PubMed]
45. Butt, A.M.; Duncan, A.; Hornby, M.F.; Kirvell, S.L.; Hunter, A.; Levine, J.M.; Berry, M. Cells expressing the NG2 antigen contact nodes of Ranvier in adult CNS white matter. *Glia* **1999**, *26*, 84–91. [CrossRef]
46. Serwanski, D.R.; Jukkola, P.; Nishiyama, A. Heterogeneity of astrocyte and NG2 cell insertion at the node of Ranvier. *J. Comp. Neurol.* **2017**, *525*, 535–552. [CrossRef] [PubMed]
47. Ong, W.Y.; Levine, J.M. A light and electron microscopic study of NG2 chondroitin sulfate proteoglycan-positive oligodendrocyte precursor cells in the normal and kainate-lesioned rat hippocampus. *Neuroscience* **1999**, *92*, 83–95. [CrossRef]
48. Maldonado, P.P.; Angulo, M.C. Multiple modes of communication between neurons and oligodendrocyte precursor cells. *Neuroscientist* **2015**, *21*, 266–276. [CrossRef] [PubMed]
49. Orduz, D.; Maldonado, P.P.; Balia, M.; Vélez-Fort, M.; de Sars, V.; Yanagawa, Y.; Emiliani, V.; Angulo, M.C. Interneurons and oligodendrocyte progenitors form a structured synaptic network in the developing neocortex. *Elife* **2015**, *4*. [CrossRef] [PubMed]
50. Lin, S.; Huck, J.H.J.; Roberts, J.D.B.; Macklin, W.B.; Somogyi, P.; Bergles, D.E. Climbing fiber innervation of NG2-expressing glia in the mammalian cerebellum. *Neuron* **2005**, *46*, 773–785. [CrossRef] [PubMed]
51. Müller, J.; Reyes-Haro, D.; Pivneva, T.; Nolte, C.; Schaette, R.; Lübke, J.; Kettenmann, H. The principal neurons of the medial nucleus of the trapezoid body and NG2+ glial cells receive coordinated excitatory synaptic input. *J. Gen. Physiol.* **2009**, *134*, 115–127. [CrossRef] [PubMed]
52. Mangin, J.M.; Li, P.; Scafidi, J.; Gallo, V. Experience-dependent regulation of NG2 progenitors in the developing barrel cortex. *Nat. Neurosci.* **2012**, *15*, 1192–1194. [CrossRef] [PubMed]
53. Lin, S.; Bergles, D.E. Synaptic signaling between GABAergic interneurons and oligodendrocyte precursor cells in the hippocampus. *Nat. Neurosci.* **2004**, *7*, 24–32. [CrossRef] [PubMed]
54. Mangin, J.M.; Kunze, A.; Chittajallu, R.; Gallo, V. Satellite NG2 progenitor cells share common glutamatergic inputs with associated interneurons in the mouse Dentate gyrus. *J. Neurosci.* **2008**, *28*, 7610–7623. [CrossRef] [PubMed]

55. Balia, M.; Vélez-Fort, M.; Passlick, S.; Schäfer, C.; Audinat, E.; Steinhäuser, C.; Seifert, G.; Angulo, M.C. Postnatal down-regulation of the GABAA receptor γ2 subunit in neocortical NG2 cells accompanies synaptic-to-extrasynaptic switch in the GABAergic transmission mode. *Cereb. Cortex* **2015**, *25*, 1114–1123. [CrossRef] [PubMed]

56. Hamilton, N.; Vayro, S.; Wigley, R.; Butt, A.M. Axons and astrocytes release ATP and glutamate to evoke calcium signals in NG2-glia. *Glia* **2010**, *58*, 66–79. [CrossRef] [PubMed]

57. Xu, G.; Wang, W.; Zhou, M. Spatial organization of NG2 glial cells and astrocytes in rat hippocampal CA1 region. *Hippocampus* **2014**, *24*, 383–395. [CrossRef] [PubMed]

58. Nishiyama, A.; Yu, M.; Drazba, J.A.; Tuohy, V.K. Normal and reactive NG2$^+$ glial cells are distinct from resting and activated microglia. *J. Neurosci. Res.* **1997**, *48*, 299–312. [CrossRef]

59. Wallraff, A.; Odermatt, B.; Willecke, K.; Steinhäuser, C. Distinct types of astroglial cells in the hippocampus differ in gap junction coupling. *Glia* **2004**, *48*, 36–43. [CrossRef] [PubMed]

60. Butt, A.M.; Hamilton, N.; Hubbard, P.; Pugh, M.; Ibrahim, M. Synantocytes: The fifth element. *J. Anat.* **2005**, *207*, 695–706. [CrossRef] [PubMed]

61. Melanson-Drapeau, L.; Beyko, S.; Davé, S.; Hebb, A.L.O.; Franks, D.J.; Sellitto, C.; Paul, D.L.; Bennett, S.A. Oligodendrocyte progenitor enrichment in the connexin32 null-mutant mouse. *J. Neurosci.* **2003**, *23*, 1759–1768. [CrossRef] [PubMed]

62. Maglione, M.; Tress, O.; Haas, B.; Karram, K.; Trotter, J.; Willecke, K.; Kettenmann, H. Oligodendrocytes in mouse corpus callosum are coupled via gap junction channels formed by connexin47 and connexin32. *Glia* **2010**, *58*, 1104–1117. [CrossRef] [PubMed]

63. Minocha, S.; Valloton, D.; Brunet, I.; Eichmann, A.; Hornung, J.P.; Lebrand, C. NG2 glia are required for vessel network formation during embryonic development. *Elife* **2015**, *4*. [CrossRef] [PubMed]

64. Tsai, H.H.; Niu, J.; Munji, R.; Davalos, D.; Chang, J.; Zhang, H.; Tien, A.C.; Kuo, C.J.; Chan, J.R.; Daneman, R.; et al. Oligodendrocyte precursors migrate along vasculature in the developing nervous system. *Science* **2016**, *351*, 379–384. [CrossRef] [PubMed]

65. Seo, J.H.; Maki, T.; Maeda, M.; Miyamoto, N.; Liang, A.C.; Hayakawa, K.; Pham, L.D.; Suwa, F.; Taguchi, A.; Matsuyama, T.; et al. Oligodendrocyte precursor cells support blood-brain barrier integrity via TGF-β signaling. *PLoS ONE* **2014**, *9*, e103174. [CrossRef] [PubMed]

66. Maki, T.; Maeda, M.; Uemura, M.; Lo, E.K.; Terasaki, Y.; Liang, A.C.; Shindo, A.; Choi, Y.K.; Taguchi, A.; Matsuyama, T.; et al. Potential interactions between pericytes and oligodendrocyte precursor cells in perivascular regions of cerebral white matter. *Neurosci. Lett.* **2015**, *597*, 164–169. [CrossRef] [PubMed]

67. Seo, J.H.; Miyamoto, N.; Hayakawa, K.; Pham, L.D.D.; Maki, T.; Ayata, C.; Kim, K.W.; Lo, E.H.; Arai, K. Oligodendrocyte precursors induce early blood-brain barrier opening after white matter injury. *J. Clin. Investig.* **2013**, *123*, 782–786. [CrossRef] [PubMed]

68. Miyamoto, N.; Pham, L.D.D.; Seo, J.H.; Kim, K.W.; Lo, E.H.; Arai, K. Crosstalk between cerebral endothelium and oligodendrocyte. *Cell. Mol. Life Sci.* **2014**, *71*, 1055–1066. [CrossRef] [PubMed]

69. Hill, R.A.; Nishiyama, A. NG2 cells (polydendrocytes): Listeners to the neural network with diverse properties. *Glia* **2014**, *62*, 1195–1210. [CrossRef] [PubMed]

70. Kato, D.; Eto, K.; Nabekura, J.; Wake, H. Activity-dependent functions of non-electrical glial cells. *J. Biochem.* **2018**, *163*, 457–464. [CrossRef] [PubMed]

71. Barres, B.A.; Raff, M.C. Proliferation of oligodendrocyte precursor cells depends on electrical activity in axons. *Nature* **1993**, *361*, 258–260. [CrossRef] [PubMed]

72. Li, Q.; Brus-Ramer, M.; Martin, J.H.; McDonald, J.W. Electrical stimulation of the medullary pyramid promotes proliferation and differentiation of oligodendrocyte progenitor cells in the corticospinal tract of the adult rat. *Neurosci. Lett.* **2010**, *479*, 128–133. [CrossRef] [PubMed]

73. Gibson, E.M.; Purger, D.; Mount, C.W.; Goldstein, A.K.; Lin, G.L.; Wood, L.S.; Inema, I.; Miller, S.E.; Bieri, G.; Zuchero, J.B.; et al. Neuronal activity promotes oligodendrogenesis and adaptive myelination in the mammalian brain. *Science* **2014**, *344*, 1252304. [CrossRef] [PubMed]

74. Ehninger, D.; Wang, L.P.; Klempin, F.; Römer, B.; Kettenmann, H.; Kempermann, G. Enriched environment and physical activity reduce microglia and influence the fate of NG2 cells in the amygdala of adult mice. *Cell Tissue Res.* **2011**, *345*, 69–86. [CrossRef] [PubMed]

75. Simon, C.; Götz, M.; Dimou, L. Progenitors in the adult cerebral cortex: Cell cycle properties and regulation by physiological stimuli and injury. *Glia* **2011**, *59*, 869–881. [CrossRef] [PubMed]

76. Tomlinson, L.; Huang, P.H.; Colognato, H. Prefrontal cortex NG2 glia undergo a developmental switch in their responsiveness to exercise. *Dev. Neurobiol.* **2018**. [CrossRef] [PubMed]

77. Nagy, B.; Hovhannisyan, A.; Barzan, R.; Chen, T.J.; Kukley, M. Different patterns of neuronal activity trigger distinct responses of oligodendrocyte precursor cells in the corpus callosum. *PLoS Biol.* **2017**, *15*, e2001993. [CrossRef] [PubMed]

78. Larson, V.A.; Zhang, Y.; Bergles, D.E. Electrophysiological properties of NG2$^+$ cells: Matching physiological studies with gene expression profiles. *Brain Res.* **2016**, *1638*, 138–160. [CrossRef] [PubMed]

79. Ziskin, J.L.; Nishiyama, A.; Rubio, M.; Fukaya, M.; Bergles, D.E. Vesicular release of glutamate from unmyelinated axons in white matter. *Nat. Neurosci.* **2007**, *10*, 321–330. [CrossRef] [PubMed]

80. Maldonado, P.P.; Velez-Fort, M.; Levavasseur, F.; Angulo, M.C. Oligodendrocyte precursor cells are accurate sensors of local K$^+$ in mature gray matter. *J. Neurosci.* **2013**, *33*, 2432–2442. [CrossRef] [PubMed]

81. Sun, W.; Matthews, E.A.; Nicolas, V.; Schoch, S.; Dietrich, D. NG2 glial cells integrate synaptic input in global and dendritic calcium signals. *Elife* **2016**, *5*. [CrossRef] [PubMed]

82. Hines, J.H.; Ravanelli, A.M.; Schwindt, R.; Scott, E.K.; Appel, B. Neuronal activity biases axon selection for myelination in vivo. *Nat. Neurosci.* **2015**, *18*, 683–689. [CrossRef] [PubMed]

83. Mensch, S.; Baraban, M.; Almeida, R.; Czopka, T.; Ausborn, J.; El Manira, A.; Lyons, D.A. Synaptic vesicle release regulates myelin sheath number of individual oligodendrocytes in vivo. *Nat. Neurosci.* **2015**, *18*, 628–630. [CrossRef] [PubMed]

84. Wake, H.; Lee, P.R.; Fields, R.D. Control of local protein synthesis and initial events in myelination by action potentials. *Science* **2011**, *333*, 1647–1651. [CrossRef] [PubMed]

85. Haberlandt, C.; Derouiche, A.; Wyczynski, A.; Haseleu, J.; Pohle, J.; Karram, K.; Trotter, J.; Seifert, G.; Frotscher, M.; Steinhäuser, C.; et al. Gray matter NG2 cells display multiple Ca^{2+}-signaling pathways and highly motile processes. *PLoS ONE* **2011**, *6*, e17575. [CrossRef] [PubMed]

86. Jäkel, S.; Dimou, L. Glial cells and their function in the adult brain: A journey through the history of their ablation. *Front. Cell. Neurosci.* **2017**, *11*, 24. [CrossRef] [PubMed]

87. Birey, F.; Kloc, M.; Chavali, M.; Hussein, I.; Wilson, M.; Christoffel, D.J.; Chen, T.; Frohman, M.A.; Robinson, J.K.; Russo, S.J.; et al. Genetic and stress-induced loss of NG2 glia triggers emergence of depressive-like behaviors through reduced secretion of FGF2. *Neuron* **2015**, *88*, 941–956. [CrossRef] [PubMed]

88. Nakano, M.; Tamura, Y.; Yamato, M.; Kume, S.; Eguchi, A.; Takata, K.; Watanabe, Y.; Kataoka, Y. NG2 glial cells regulate neuroimmunological responses to maintain neuronal function and survival. *Sci. Rep.* **2017**, *7*, 42041. [CrossRef] [PubMed]

89. Kessaris, N.; Fogarty, M.; Iannarelli, P.; Grist, M.; Wegner, M.; Richardson, W.D. Competing waves of oligodendrocytes in the forebrain and postnatal elimination of an embryonic lineage. *Nat. Neurosci.* **2006**, *9*, 173–179. [CrossRef] [PubMed]

90. Van Tilborg, E.; Achterberg, E.J.M.; van Kammen, C.M.; van der Toorn, A.; Groenendaal, F.; Dijkhuizen, R.M.; Heijnen, C.J.; Vanderschuren, L.J.M.J.; Benders, M.N.J.L.; Nijboer, C.H.A. Combined fetal inflammation and postnatal hypoxia causes myelin deficits and autism-like behavior in a rat model of diffuse white matter injury. *Glia* **2018**, *66*, 78–93. [CrossRef] [PubMed]

91. Doretto, S.; Malerba, M.; Ramos, M.; Ikrar, T.; Kinoshita, C.; De Mei, C.; Tirotta, E.; Xu, X.; Borrelli, E. Oligodendrocytes as regulators of neuronal networks during early postnatal development. *PLoS ONE* **2011**, *6*, e19849. [CrossRef] [PubMed]

92. Clemente, D.; Ortega, M.C.; Melero-Jerez, C.; de Castro, F. The effect of glia-glia interactions on oligodendrocyte precursor cell biology during development and in demyelinating diseases. *Front. Cell. Neurosci.* **2013**, *7*, 268. [CrossRef] [PubMed]

93. Sypecka, J.; Sarnowska, A. The neuroprotective effect exerted by oligodendroglial progenitors on ischemically impaired hippocampal cells. *Mol. Neurobiol.* **2014**, *49*, 685–701. [CrossRef] [PubMed]

94. Wilkins, A.; Chandran, S.; Compston, A. A role for oligodendrocyte-derived IGF-1 in trophic support of cortical neurons. *Glia* **2001**, *36*, 48–57. [CrossRef] [PubMed]

95. Wilkins, A.; Majed, H.; Layfield, R.; Compston, A.; Chandran, S. Oligodendrocytes promote neuronal survival and axonal length by distinct intracellular mechanisms: A novel role for oligodendrocyte-derived glial cell line-derived neurotrophic factor. *J. Neurosci.* **2003**, *23*, 4967–4974. [CrossRef] [PubMed]

96. Yuen, T.J.; Silbereis, J.C.; Griveau, A.; Chang, S.M.; Daneman, R.; Fancy, S.P.J.; Zahed, H.; Maltepe, E.; Rowitch, D.H. Oligodendrocyte-encoded HIF function couples postnatal myelination and white matter angiogenesis. *Cell* **2014**, *158*, 383–396. [CrossRef] [PubMed]

97. Huang, J.; Xiao, L.; Gong, X.; Shao, W.; Yin, Y.; Liao, Q.; Meng, Y.; Zhang, Y.; Ma, D.; Qiu, X. Cytokine-like molecule CCDC134 Contributes to CD8+ T-cell effector functions in cancer immunotherapy. *Cancer Res.* **2014**, *74*, 5734–5745. [CrossRef] [PubMed]

98. Sakry, D.; Neitz, A.; Singh, J.; Frischknecht, R.; Marongiu, D.; Binamé, F.; Perera, S.S.; Endres, K.; Lutz, B.; Radyushkin, K.; et al. Oligodendrocyte precursor cells modulate the neuronal network by activity-dependent ectodomain cleavage of glial NG2. *PLoS Biol.* **2014**, *12*, e1001993. [CrossRef] [PubMed]

99. Goncalves, M.B.; Wu, Y.; Trigo, D.; Clarke, E.; Malmqvist, T.; Grist, J.; Hobbs, C.; Carlstedt, T.P.; Corcoran, J.P.T. Retinoic acid synthesis by NG2 expressing cells promotes a permissive environment for axonal outgrowth. *Neurobiol. Dis.* **2018**, *111*, 70–79. [CrossRef] [PubMed]

100. Théry, C.; Ostrowski, M.; Segura, E. Membrane vesicles as conveyors of immune responses. *Nat. Rev. Immunol.* **2009**, *9*, 581–593. [CrossRef] [PubMed]

101. Yun, Y.R.; Won, J.E.; Jeon, E.; Lee, S.; Kang, W.; Jo, H.; Jang, J.H.; Shin, U.S.; Kim, H.W. Fibroblast growth factors: Biology, function, and application for tissue regeneration. *J. Tissue Eng.* **2010**, *2010*, 218142. [CrossRef] [PubMed]

102. Zechel, S.; Unsicker, K.; von Bohlen und Halbach, O. Fibroblast growth factor-2 deficiency affects hippocampal spine morphology, but not hippocampal catecholaminergic or cholinergic innervation. *Dev. Dyn.* **2009**, *238*, 343–350. [CrossRef] [PubMed]

103. Goddard, D.R.; Berry, M.; Kirvell, S.L.; Butt, A.M. Fibroblast growth factor-2 induces astroglial and microglial reactivity in vivo. *J. Anat.* **2002**, *200*, 57–67. [CrossRef] [PubMed]

104. Cheng, B.; Mattson, M.P. PDGFs protect hippocampal neurons against energy deprivation and oxidative injury: Evidence for induction of antioxidant pathways. *J. Neurosci.* **1995**, *15*, 7095–7104. [CrossRef] [PubMed]

105. Peng, F.; Yao, H.; Bai, X.; Zhu, X.; Reiner, B.C.; Beazely, M.; Funa, K.; Xiong, H.; Buch, S. Platelet-derived growth factor-mediated induction of the synaptic plasticity gene *Arc/Arg3.1*. *J. Biol. Chem.* **2010**, *285*, 21615–21624. [CrossRef] [PubMed]

106. Risau, W.; Drexler, H.; Mironov, V.; Smits, A.; Siegbahn, A.; Funa, K.; Heldin, C.H. Platelet-derived growth factor is angiogenic in vivo. *Grow. Factors* **1992**, *7*, 261–266. [CrossRef]

107. Sasahara, A.; Kott, J.N.; Sasahara, M.; Raines, E.W.; Ross, R.; Westrum, L.E. Platelet-derived growth factor B-chain-like immunoreactivity in the developing and adult rat brain. *Dev. Brain Res.* **1992**, *68*, 41–53. [CrossRef]

108. Rosenstein, J.M.; Krum, J.M.; Ruhrberg, C. VEGF in the nervous system. *Organogenesis* **2010**, *6*, 107–114. [CrossRef] [PubMed]

109. Tovar-y-Romo, L.B.; Tapia, R. Delayed administration of VEGF rescues spinal motor neurons from death with a short effective time frame in excitotoxic experimental models in vivo. *ASN Neuro* **2012**, *4*. [CrossRef] [PubMed]

110. Nieto-Estévez, V.; Defterali, Ç.; Vicario-Abejón, C. IGF-I: A key growth factor that regulates neurogenesis and synaptogenesis from embryonic to adult stages of the brain. *Front. Neurosci.* **2016**, *10*, 52. [CrossRef] [PubMed]

111. Yan, H.; Rivkees, S.A. Hepatocyte growth factor stimulates the proliferation and migration of oligodendrocyte precursor cells. *J. Neurosci. Res.* **2002**, *69*, 597–606. [CrossRef] [PubMed]

112. Kato, T.; Funakoshi, H.; Kadoyama, K.; Noma, S.; Kanai, M.; Ohya-Shimada, W.; Mizuno, S.; Doe, N.; Taniguchi, T.; Nakamura, T. Hepatocyte growth factor overexpression in the nervous system enhances learning and memory performance in mice. *J. Neurosci. Res.* **2012**, *90*, 1743–1755. [CrossRef] [PubMed]

113. Tanaka, Y.; Tozuka, Y.; Takata, T.; Shimazu, N.; Matsumura, N.; Ohta, A.; Hisatsune, T. Excitatory GABAergic activation of cortical dividing glial cells. *Cereb. Cortex* **2009**, *19*, 2181–2195. [CrossRef] [PubMed]

114. Prasad, A.; The, D.B.L.; Blasiak, A.; Chai, C.; Wu, Y.; Gharibani, P.M.; Yang, I.H.; Phan, T.T.; Lim, K.L.; Yang, H.; et al. Static magnetic field stimulation enhances oligodendrocyte differentiation and secretion of neurotrophic factors. *Sci. Rep.* **2017**, *7*, 6743. [CrossRef] [PubMed]

115. Bathina, S.; Das, U.N. Brain-derived neurotrophic factor and its clinical implications. *Arch. Med. Sci.* **2015**, *11*, 1164–1178. [CrossRef] [PubMed]

116. Byravan, S.; Foster, L.M.; Phan, T.; Verity, A.N.; Campagnoni, A.T. Murine oligodendroglial cells express nerve growth factor. *Proc. Natl. Acad. Sci. USA* **1994**, *91*, 8812–8816. [CrossRef] [PubMed]

117. Varon, S.; Conner, J.M. Nerve growth factor in CNS repair. *J. Neurotrauma* **1994**, *11*, 473–486. [CrossRef] [PubMed]

118. Hodgetts, S.I.; Harvey, A.R. Neurotrophic factors used to treat spinal cord injury. *Vitam. Horm.* **2017**, *104*, 405–457. [CrossRef] [PubMed]

119. Gao, W.Q.; Dybdal, N.; Shinsky, N.; Murnane, A.; Schmelzer, C.; Siegel, M.; Keller, G.; Hefti, F.; Phillips, H.S.; Winslow, J.W. Neurotrophin-3 reverses experimental cisplatin-induced peripheral sensory neuropathy. *Ann. Neurol.* **1995**, *38*, 30–37. [CrossRef] [PubMed]

120. Rabacchi, S.A.; Kruk, B.; Hamilton, J.; Carney, C.; Hoffman, J.R.; Meyer, S.L.; Springer, J.E.; Baird, D.H. BDNF and NT4/5 promote survival and neurite outgrowth of pontocerebellar mossy fiber neurons. *J. Neurobiol.* **1999**, *40*, 254–269. [CrossRef]

121. Lin, L.F.; Doherty, D.H.; Lile, J.D.; Bektesh, S.; Collins, F. GDNF: A glial cell line-derived neurotrophic factor for midbrain dopaminergic neurons. *Science* **1993**, *260*, 1130–1132. [CrossRef] [PubMed]

122. Barres, B.A.; Burne, J.F.; Holtmann, B.; Thoenen, H.; Sendtner, M.; Raff, M.C. Ciliary neurotrophic factor enhances the rate of oligodendrocyte generation. *Mol. Cell. Neurosci.* **1996**, *8*, 146–156. [CrossRef] [PubMed]

123. Giess, R.; Holtmann, B.; Braga, M.; Grimm, T.; Müller-Myhsok, B.; Toyka, K.V.; Sendtner, M. Early onset of Severe Familial Amyotrophic Lateral Sclerosis with a SOD-1 mutation: Potential impact of CNTF as a candidate modifier gene. *Am. J. Hum. Genet.* **2002**, *70*, 1277–1286. [CrossRef] [PubMed]

124. Talbott, J.F.; Cao, Q.; Bertram, J.; Nkansah, M.; Benton, R.L.; Lavik, E.; Whittemore, S.R. CNTF promotes the survival and differentiation of adult spinal cord-derived oligodendrocyte precursor cells in vitro but fails to promote remyelination in vivo. *Exp. Neurol.* **2007**, *204*, 485–489. [CrossRef] [PubMed]

125. Sim, F.J.; Lang, J.K.; Waldau, B.; Roy, N.S.; Schwartz, T.E.; Pilcher, W.H.; Chandross, K.J.; Natesan, S.; Merrill, J.E.; Goldman, S.A. Complementary patterns of gene expression by human oligodendrocyte progenitors and their environment predict determinants of progenitor maintenance and differentiation. *Ann. Neurol.* **2006**, *59*, 763–779. [CrossRef] [PubMed]

126. Amor, V.; Feinberg, K.; Eshed-Eisenbach, Y.; Vainshtein, A.; Frechter, S.; Grumet, M.; Rosenbluth, J.; Peles, E. Long-term maintenance of Na+ channels at nodes of ranvier depends on glial contact mediated by gliomedin and NrCAM. *J. Neurosci.* **2014**, *34*, 5089–5098. [CrossRef] [PubMed]

127. Demyanenko, G.P.; Mohan, V.; Zhang, X.; Brennaman, L.H.; Dharbal, K.E.S.; Tran, T.S.; Manis, P.B.; Maness, P.F. Neural cell adhesion molecule NrCAM regulates Semaphorin 3F-induced dendritic spine remodeling. *J. Neurosci.* **2014**, *34*, 11274–11287. [CrossRef] [PubMed]

128. Rønn, L.C.; Bock, E.; Linnemann, D.; Jahnsen, H. NCAM-antibodies modulate induction of long-term potentiation in rat hippocampal CA1. *Brain Res.* **1995**, *677*, 145–151. [CrossRef]

129. Tessier-Lavigne, M.; Goodman, C.S. The molecular biology of axon guidance. *Science* **1996**, *274*, 1123–1133. [CrossRef] [PubMed]

130. Gascon, E.; Vutskits, L.; Kiss, J.Z. The role of PSA-NCAM in adult neurogenesis. *Adv. Exp. Med. Biol.* **2010**, *663*, 127–136. [CrossRef] [PubMed]

131. Zhang, Y.; Chen, K.; Sloan, S.A.; Bennett, M.L.; Scholze, A.R.; O'Keeffe, S.; Phatnani, H.P.; Guarnieri, P.; Caneda, C.; Ruderisch, N.; et al. An RNA-sequencing transcriptome and splicing database of glia, neurons, and vascular cells of the cerebral cortex. *J. Neurosci.* **2014**, *34*, 11929–11947. [CrossRef] [PubMed]

132. Hattori, D.; Demir, E.; Kim, H.W.; Viragh, E.; Zipursky, S.L.; Dickson, B.J. Dscam diversity is essential for neuronal wiring and self-recognition. *Nature* **2007**, *449*, 223–227. [CrossRef] [PubMed]

133. Hattori, D.; Chen, Y.; Matthews, B.J.; Salwinski, L.; Sabatti, C.; Grueber, W.B.; Zipursky, S.L. Robust discrimination between self and non-self neurites requires thousands of Dscam1 isoforms. *Nature* **2009**, *461*, 644–648. [CrossRef] [PubMed]

134. Soba, P.; Zhu, S.; Emoto, K.; Younger, S.; Yang, S.J.; Yu, H.H.; Lee, T.; Jan, L.Y.; Jan, Y.N. Drosophila sensory neurons require dscam for dendritic self-avoidance and proper dendritic field organization. *Neuron* **2007**, *54*, 403–416. [CrossRef] [PubMed]

135. Hughes, M.E.; Bortnick, R.; Tsubouchi, A.; Bäumer, P.; Kondo, M.; Uemura, T.; Schmucker, D. Homophilic Dscam interactions control complex dendrite morphogenesis. *Neuron* **2007**, *54*, 417–427. [CrossRef] [PubMed]

136. Schneider, S.; Bosse, F.; D'Urso, D.; Muller, H.; Sereda, M.W.; Nave, K.; Niehaus, A.; Kempf, T.; Schnolzer, M.; Trotter, J. The AN2 protein is a novel marker for the Schwann cell lineage expressed by immature and nonmyelinating Schwann cells. *J. Neurosci.* **2001**, *21*, 920–933. [CrossRef] [PubMed]

137. Hunanyan, A.S.; Garcia-Alias, G.; Alessi, V.; Levine, J.M.; Fawcett, J.W.; Mendell, L.M.; Arvanian, V.L. Role of chondroitin sulfate proteoglycans in axonal conduction in mammalian spinal cord. *J. Neurosci.* **2010**, *30*, 7761–7769. [CrossRef] [PubMed]

138. Yi, J.H.; Katagiri, Y.; Susarla, B.; Figge, D.; Symes, A.J.; Geller, H.M. Alterations in sulfated chondroitin glycosaminoglycans following controlled cortical impact injury in mice. *J. Comp. Neurol.* **2012**, *520*, 3295–3313. [CrossRef] [PubMed]

139. Dours-Zimmermann, M.T.; Maurer, K.; Rauch, U.; Stoffel, W.; Fassler, R.; Zimmermann, D.R. Versican V2 assembles the extracellular matrix surrounding the nodes of Ranvier in the CNS. *J. Neurosci.* **2009**, *29*, 7731–7742. [CrossRef] [PubMed]

140. Bekku, Y.; Rauch, U.; Ninomiya, Y.; Oohashi, T. Brevican distinctively assembles extracellular components at the large diameter nodes of Ranvier in the CNS. *J. Neurochem.* **2009**, *108*, 1266–1276. [CrossRef] [PubMed]

141. Dityatev, A.; Schachner, M. Extracellular matrix molecules and synaptic plasticity. *Nat. Rev. Neurosci.* **2003**, *4*, 456–468. [CrossRef] [PubMed]

142. Hagino, S.; Iseki, K.; Mori, T.; Zhang, Y.; Sakai, N.; Yokoya, S.; Hikake, T.; Kikuchi, S.; Wanaka, A. Expression pattern of glypican-1 mRNA after brain injury in mice. *Neurosci. Lett.* **2003**, *349*, 29–32. [CrossRef]

143. Hagino, S.; Iseki, K.; Mori, T.; Zhang, Y.; Hikake, T.; Yokoya, S.; Takeuchi, M.; Hasimoto, H.; Kikuchi, S.; Wanaka, A. Slit and glypican-1 mRNAs are coexpressed in the reactive astrocytes of the injured adult brain. *Glia* **2003**, *42*, 130–138. [CrossRef] [PubMed]

144. Shimodaira, M.; Nakayama, T.; Sato, N.; Naganuma, T.; Yamaguchi, M.; Aoi, N.; Sato, M.; Izumi, Y.; Soma, M.; Matsumoto, K. Association Study of the elastin microfibril interfacer 1 (EMILIN1) gene in essential hypertension. *Am. J. Hypertens.* **2010**, *23*, 547–555. [CrossRef] [PubMed]

145. Kaksonen, M.; Pavlov, I.; Võikar, V.; Lauri, S.E.; Hienola, A.; Riekki, R.; Lakso, M.; Taira, T.; Rauvala, H. Syndecan-3-deficient mice exhibit enhanced LTP and impaired hippocampus-dependent memory. *Mol. Cell. Neurosci.* **2002**, *21*, 158–172. [CrossRef] [PubMed]

146. Feinstein, Y.; Borrell, V.; Garcia, C.; Burstyn-Cohen, T.; Tzarfaty, V.; Frumkin, A.; Nose, A.; Okamoto, H.; Higashijima, S.; Soriano, E.; et al. F-spondin and mindin: Two structurally and functionally related genes expressed in the hippocampus that promote outgrowth of embryonic hippocampal neurons. *Development* **1999**, *126*, 3637–3648. [PubMed]

147. Wang, B.; Guo, W.; Huang, Y. Thrombospondins and synaptogenesis. *Neural Regen. Res.* **2012**, *7*, 1737–1743. [CrossRef] [PubMed]

148. Tian, W.; Sawyer, A.; Kocaoglu, F.B.; Kyriakides, T.R. Astrocyte-derived thrombospondin-2 is critical for the repair of the blood-brain barrier. *Am. J. Pathol.* **2011**, *179*, 860–868. [CrossRef] [PubMed]

149. Matsuda, K.; Yuzaki, M. Cbln family proteins promote synapse formation by regulating distinct neurexin signaling pathways in various brain regions. *Eur. J. Neurosci.* **2011**, *33*, 1447–1461. [CrossRef] [PubMed]

150. Yuzaki, M. Two classes of secreted synaptic organizers in the central nervous system. *Annu. Rev. Physiol.* **2018**, *80*, 243–262. [CrossRef] [PubMed]

151. Awwad, K.; Hu, J.; Shi, L.; Mangels, N.; Abdel Malik, R.; Zippel, N.; Fisslthaler, B.; Eble, J.A.; Pfeilschifter, J.; Popp, R.; et al. Role of secreted modular calcium-binding protein 1 (SMOC1) in transforming growth factor β signalling and angiogenesis. *Cardiovasc. Res.* **2015**, *106*, 284–294. [CrossRef] [PubMed]

152. Pettem, K.L. New Synaptic Organizing Proteins and Their Roles in Excitatory and Inhibitory Synapse Development. Ph.D. Thesis, University of British Columbia, Vancouver, BC, Canada, 2012.

153. Dean, C.; Dresbach, T. Neuroligins and neurexins: Linking cell adhesion, synapse formation and cognitive function. *Trends Neurosci.* **2006**, *29*, 21–29. [CrossRef] [PubMed]

154. Sakry, D.; Yigit, H.; Dimou, L.; Trotter, J. Oligodendrocyte precursor cells synthesize neuromodulatory factors. *PLoS ONE* **2015**, *10*, e0127222. [CrossRef] [PubMed]

155. Tucsek, Z.; Noa Valcarcel-Ares, M.; Tarantini, S.; Yabluchanskiy, A.; Fülöp, G.; Gautam, T.; Orock, A.; Csiszar, A.; Deak, F.; Ungvari, Z. Hypertension-induced synapse loss and impairment in synaptic plasticity in the mouse hippocampus mimics the aging phenotype: Implications for the pathogenesis of vascular cognitive impairment. *GeroScience* **2017**, *39*, 385. [CrossRef] [PubMed]

156. Pelkey, K.A.; Barksdale, E.; Craig, M.T.; Yuan, X.; Sukumaran, M.; Vargish, G.A.; Mitchell, R.M.; Wyeth, M.S.; Petralia, R.S.; Chittajallu, R.; et al. Pentraxins coordinate excitatory synapse maturation and circuit integration of parvalbumin interneurons. *Neuron* **2016**, *90*, 661. [CrossRef] [PubMed]

157. Elbaz, I.; Lerer-Goldshtein, T.; Okamoto, H.; Appelbaum, L. Reduced synaptic density and deficient locomotor response in neuronal activity-regulated pentraxin 2a mutant zebrafish. *FASEB J.* **2015**, *29*, 1220–1234. [CrossRef] [PubMed]

158. Kang, Z.; Wang, C.; Zepp, J.; Wu, L.; Sun, K.; Zhao, J.; Chandrasekharan, U.; DiCorleto, P.E.; Trapp, B.D.; Ransohoff, R.M.; et al. Act1 mediates IL-17–induced EAE pathogenesis selectively in NG2$^+$ glial cells. *Nat. Neurosci.* **2013**, *16*, 1401–1408. [CrossRef] [PubMed]

159. Van Hove, I.; Lemmens, K.; Van de Velde, S.; Verslegers, M.; Moons, L. Matrix metalloproteinase-3 in the central nervous system: A look on the bright side. *J. Neurochem.* **2012**, *123*, 203–216. [CrossRef] [PubMed]

160. Pham, L.D.D.; Hayakawa, K.; Seo, J.H.; Nguyen, M.N.; Som, A.T.; Lee, B.J.; Guo, S.; Kim, K.W.; Lo, E.H.; Arai, K. Crosstalk between oligodendrocytes and cerebral endothelium contributes to vascular remodeling after white matter injury. *Glia* **2012**, *60*, 875–881. [CrossRef] [PubMed]

161. Reinhard, S.M.; Razak, K.; Ethell, I.M. A delicate balance: Role of MMP-9 in brain development and pathophysiology of neurodevelopmental disorders. *Front. Cell. Neurosci.* **2015**, *9*, 280. [CrossRef] [PubMed]

162. Jourquin, J.; Tremblay, E.; Bernard, A.; Charton, G.; Chaillan, F.A.; Marchetti, E.; Roman, F.S.; Soloway, P.D.; Dive, V.; Yiotakis, A.; et al. Tissue inhibitor of metalloproteinases-1 (TIMP-1) modulates neuronal death, axonal plasticity, and learning and memory. *Eur. J. Neurosci.* **2005**, *22*, 2569–2578. [CrossRef] [PubMed]

163. Leco, K.J.; Apte, S.S.; Taniguchi, G.T.; Hawkes, S.P.; Khokha, R.; Schultz, G.A.; Edwards, D.R. Murine tissue inhibitor of metalloproteinases-4 (Timp-4): CDNA isolation and expression in adult mouse tissues. *FEBS Lett.* **1997**, *401*, 213–217. [CrossRef]

164. Melendez-Zajgla, J.; Del Pozo, L.; Ceballos, G.; Maldonado, V. Tissue inhibitor of metalloproteinases-4. The road less traveled. *Mol. Cancer* **2008**, *7*, 85. [CrossRef] [PubMed]

165. Raabe, T.D.; Clive, D.R.; Wen, D.; DeVries, G.H. Neonatal oligodendrocytes contain and secrete neuregulins in vitro. *J. Neurochem.* **2002**, *69*, 1859–1863. [CrossRef]

166. Buonanno, A.; Kwon, O.B.; Yan, L.; Gonzalez, C.; Longart, M.; Hoffman, D.; Vullhorst, D. Neuregulins and neuronal plasticity: Possible relevance in Schizophrenia. *Novartis Found. Symp.* **2008**, *289*, 165–177, discussion 177–179, 193–195. [PubMed]

167. Canoll, P.D.; Musacchio, J.M.; Hardy, R.; Reynolds, R.; Marchionni, M.A.; Salzer, J.L. GGF/neuregulin is a neuronal signal that promotes the proliferation and survival and inhibits the differentiation of oligodendrocyte progenitors. *Neuron* **1996**, *17*, 229–243. [CrossRef]

168. Bermingham-McDonogh, O.; McCabe, K.L.; Reh, T.A. Effects of GGF/neuregulins on neuronal survival and neurite outgrowth correlate with erbB2/neu expression in developing rat retina. *Development* **1996**, *122*, 1427–1438. [PubMed]

169. Shen, K.Z.; Zhu, Z.T.; Munhall, A.; Johnson, S.W. Dopamine receptor supersensitivity in rat subthalamus after 6-hydroxydopamine lesions. *Eur. J. Neurosci.* **2003**, *18*, 2967–2974. [CrossRef] [PubMed]

170. Hökfelt, T.; Broberger, C.; Diez, M.; Xu, Z.Q.; Shi, T.; Kopp, J.; Zhang, X.; Holmberg, K.; Landry, M.; Koistinaho, J. Galanin and NPY, two peptides with multiple putative roles in the nervous system. *Horm. Metab. Res.* **1999**, *31*, 330–334. [CrossRef] [PubMed]

171. Zhang, K.; Biswas, N.; Gayen, J.R.; Miramontes-Gonzalez, J.P.; Hightower, C.M.; Mustapic, M.; Mahata, M.; Huang, C.T.; Hook, V.Y.; Mahata, S.K.; et al. Chromogranin B: Intra- and extra-cellular mechanisms to regulate catecholamine storage and release, in catecholaminergic cells and organisms. *J. Neurochem.* **2014**, *129*, 48–59. [CrossRef] [PubMed]

172. Shin, J.G.; Kim, J.H.; Park, C.S.; Kim, B.J.; Kim, J.W.; Choi, I.G.; Hwang, J.; Shin, H.D.; Woo, S.I. Gender-specific associations between *CHGB* genetic variants and Schizophrenia in a Korean population. *Yonsei Med. J.* **2017**, *58*, 619. [CrossRef] [PubMed]

173. Gasser, M.C.; Berti, I.; Hauser, K.F.; Fischer-Colbrie, R.; Saria, A. Secretoneurin promotes pertussis toxin-sensitive neurite outgrowth in cerebellar granule cells. *J. Neurochem.* **2003**, *85*, 662–669. [CrossRef] [PubMed]

174. Kirchmair, R.; Gander, R.; Egger, M.; Hanley, A.; Silver, M.; Ritsch, A.; Murayama, T.; Kaneider, N.; Sturm, W.; Kearny, M.; et al. The neuropeptide secretoneurin acts as a direct angiogenic cytokine in vitro and in vivo. *Circulation* **2004**, *109*, 777–783. [CrossRef] [PubMed]

175. Milbrandt, J.; de Sauvage, F.J.; Fahrner, T.J.; Baloh, R.H.; Leitner, M.L.; Tansey, M.G.; Lampe, P.A.; Heuckeroth, R.O.; Kotzbauer, P.T.; Simburger, K.S.; et al. Persephin, a novel neurotrophic factor related to GDNF and neurturin. *Neuron* **1998**, *20*, 245–253. [CrossRef]

176. Cahoy, J.D.; Emery, B.; Kaushal, A.; Foo, L.C.; Zamanian, J.L.; Christopherson, K.S.; Xing, Y.; Lubischer, J.L.; Krieg, P.A.; Krupenko, S.A.; et al. A transcriptome database for astrocytes, neurons, and oligodendrocytes: A new resource for understanding brain development and function. *J. Neurosci.* **2008**, *28*, 264–278. [CrossRef] [PubMed]

177. Farías, G.G.; Godoy, J.A.; Cerpa, W.; Varela-Nallar, L.; Inestrosa, N.C. Wnt signaling modulates pre- and postsynaptic maturation: Therapeutic considerations. *Dev. Dyn.* **2009**, *239*, 94–101. [CrossRef] [PubMed]

178. Hall, A.C.; Lucas, F.R.; Salinas, P.C. Axonal remodeling and synaptic differentiation in the cerebellum is regulated by WNT-7a signaling. *Cell* **2000**, *100*, 525–535. [CrossRef]

179. Oliva, C.A.; Vargas, J.Y.; Inestrosa, N.C. Wnts in adult brain: From synaptic plasticity to cognitive deficiencies. *Front. Cell. Neurosci.* **2013**, *7*, 224. [CrossRef] [PubMed]

180. Ahmad-Annuar, A.; Ciani, L.; Simeonidis, I.; Herreros, J.; Fredj, N.B.; Rosso, S.B.; Hall, A.; Brickley, S.; Salinas, P.C. Signaling across the synapse: A role for Wnt and Dishevelled in presynaptic assembly and neurotransmitter release. *J. Cell Biol.* **2006**, *174*, 127–139. [CrossRef] [PubMed]

181. Hattori, A.; Katayama, M.; Iwasaki, S.; Ishii, K.; Tsujimoto, M.; Kohno, M. Bone morphogenetic protein-2 promotes survival and differentiation of striatal GABAergic neurons in the absence of glial cell proliferation. *J. Neurochem.* **2002**, *72*, 2264–2271. [CrossRef]

182. Kusakawa, Y.; Mikawa, S.; Sato, K. BMP7 expression in the adult rat brain. *IBRO Rep.* **2017**, *3*, 72–86. [CrossRef]

183. Nguyen-Ba-Charvet, K.T.; Picard-Riera, N.; Tessier-Lavigne, M.; Baron-Van Evercooren, A.; Sotelo, C.; Chédotal, A. Multiple roles for slits in the control of cell migration in the rostral migratory stream. *J. Neurosci.* **2004**, *24*, 1497–1506. [CrossRef] [PubMed]

184. Wehrle, R.; Camand, E.; Chedotal, A.; Sotelo, C.; Dusart, I. Expression of *netrin-1*, *slit-1* and *slit-3* but not of *slit-2* after cerebellar and spinal cord lesions. *Eur. J. Neurosci.* **2005**, *22*, 2134–2144. [CrossRef] [PubMed]

185. Hewett, S.J.; Jackman, N.A.; Claycomb, R.J. Interleukin-1β in central nervous system injury and repair. *Eur. J. Neurodegener. Dis.* **2012**, *1*, 195–211. [PubMed]

186. Bauer, S.; Kerr, B.J.; Patterson, P.H. The neuropoietic cytokine family in development, plasticity, disease and injury. *Nat. Rev. Neurosci.* **2007**, *8*, 221–232. [CrossRef] [PubMed]

187. Deverman, B.E.; Patterson, P.H. Cytokines and CNS development. *Neuron* **2009**, *64*, 61–78. [CrossRef] [PubMed]

188. Strle, K.; Zhou, J.H.; Shen, W.H.; Broussard, S.R.; Johnson, R.W.; Freund, G.G.; Dantzer, R.; Kelley, K.W. Interleukin-10 in the brain. *Crit. Rev. Immunol.* **2001**, *21*, 427–449. [CrossRef] [PubMed]

189. Garcia, J.M.; Stillings, S.A.; Leclerc, J.L.; Phillips, H.; Edwards, N.J.; Robicsek, S.A.; Hoh, B.L.; Blackburn, S.; Doré, S.L. Role of interleukin-10 in acute brain injuries. *Front. Neurol.* **2017**, *8*, 244. [CrossRef] [PubMed]

190. Dobolyi, A.; Vincze, C.; Pál, G.; Lovas, G. The neuroprotective functions of transforming growth factor βproteins. *Int. J. Mol. Sci.* **2012**, *13*, 8219–8258. [CrossRef] [PubMed]

191. Smith, D.E.; Lipsky, B.P.; Russell, C.; Ketchem, R.R.; Kirchner, J.; Hensley, K.; Huang, Y.; Friedman, W.J.; Boissonneault, V.; Plante, M.M.; et al. A central nervous system-restricted isoform of the interleukin-1 receptor accessory protein modulates neuronal responses to interleukin-1. *Immunity* **2009**, *30*, 817–831. [CrossRef] [PubMed]

192. Wang, C.; Zhang, C.J.; Martin, B.N.; Bulek, K.; Kang, Z.; Zhao, J.; Bian, G.; Carman, J.A.; Gao, J.; Dongre, A.; et al. IL-17 induced NOTCH1 activation in oligodendrocyte progenitor cells enhances proliferation and inflammatory gene expression. *Nat. Commun.* **2017**, *8*, 15508. [CrossRef] [PubMed]

193. Marro, B.S.; Grist, J.J.; Lane, T.E. Inducible expression of CXCL1 within the central nervous system amplifies viral-induced demyelination. *J. Immunol.* **2016**, *196*, 1855–1864. [CrossRef] [PubMed]

194. Klein, R.S. Regulation of neuroinflammation: The role of CXCL10 in lymphocyte infiltration during autoimmune encephalomyelitis. *J. Cell. Biochem.* **2004**, *92*, 213–222. [CrossRef] [PubMed]

195. Paolicelli, R.C.; Bisht, K.; Tremblay, M.È. Fractalkine regulation of microglial physiology and consequences on the brain and behavior. *Front. Cell. Neurosci.* **2014**, *8*, 129. [CrossRef] [PubMed]

196. Hesselgesser, J.; Horuk, R. Chemokine and chemokine receptor expression in the central nervous system. *J. Neurovirol.* **1999**, *5*, 13–26. [CrossRef] [PubMed]

197. Ransohoff, R.M.; Tani, M. Do chemokines mediate leukocyte recruitment in post-traumatic CNS inflammation? *Trends Neurosci.* **1998**, *21*, 154–159. [CrossRef]

198. Mennicken, F.; Maki, R.; de Souza, E.B.; Quirion, R. Chemokines and chemokine receptors in the CNS: A possible role in neuroinflammation and patterning. *Trends Pharmacol. Sci.* **1999**, *20*, 73–78. [CrossRef]

199. Schäbitz, W.R.; Krüger, C.; Pitzer, C.; Weber, D.; Laage, R.; Gassler, N.; Aronowski, J.; Mier, W.; Kirsch, F.; Dittgen, T.; et al. A neuroprotective function for the hematopoietic protein granulocyte-macrophage colony stimulating factor (GM-CSF). *J. Cereb. Blood Flow Metab.* **2008**, *28*, 29–43. [CrossRef] [PubMed]

200. Frischknecht, R.; Heine, M.; Perrais, D.; Seidenbecher, C.I.; Choquet, D.; Gundelfinger, E.D. Brain extracellular matrix affects AMPA receptor lateral mobility and short-term synaptic plasticity. *Nat. Neurosci.* **2009**, *12*, 897–904. [CrossRef] [PubMed]

201. Michaluk, P.; Mikasova, L.; Groc, L.; Frischknecht, R.; Choquet, D.; Kaczmarek, L. Matrix metalloproteinase-9 controls NMDA receptor surface diffusion through integrin β1 signaling. *J. Neurosci.* **2009**, *29*, 6007–6012. [CrossRef] [PubMed]

202. Petrosyan, H.A.; Hunanyan, A.S.; Alessi, V.; Schnell, L.; Levine, J.; Arvanian, V.L. Neutralization of inhibitory molecule NG2 improves synaptic transmission, retrograde transport, and locomotor function after spinal cord injury in adult rats. *J. Neurosci.* **2013**, *33*, 4032–4043. [CrossRef] [PubMed]

203. Liu, J.; Dietz, K.; Hodes, G.E.; Russo, S.J.; Casaccia, P. Widespread transcriptional alternations in oligodendrocytes in the adult mouse brain following chronic stress. *Dev. Neurobiol.* **2018**, *78*, 152–162. [CrossRef] [PubMed]

204. Rodriguez, J.P.; Coulter, M.; Miotke, J.; Meyer, R.L.; Takemaru, K.I.; Levine, J.M. Abrogation of catenin signaling in oligodendrocyte precursor cells reduces glial scarring and promotes axon regeneration after CNS Injury. *J. Neurosci.* **2014**, *34*, 10285–10297. [CrossRef] [PubMed]

205. Adams, K.L.; Gallo, V. The diversity and disparity of the glial scar. *Nat. Neurosci.* **2018**, *21*, 9–15. [CrossRef] [PubMed]

206. Kang, S.H.; Li, Y.; Fukaya, M.; Lorenzini, I.; Cleveland, D.W.; Ostrow, L.W.; Rothstein, J.D.; Bergles, D.E. Degeneration and impaired regeneration of gray matter oligodendrocytes in amyotrophic lateral sclerosis. *Nat. Neurosci.* **2013**, *16*, 571–579. [CrossRef] [PubMed]

207. Hampton, D.; Rhodes, K.; Zhao, C.; Franklin, R.J.; Fawcett, J. The responses of oligodendrocyte precursor cells, astrocytes and microglia to a cortical stab injury, in the brain. *Neuroscience* **2004**, *127*, 813–820. [CrossRef] [PubMed]

208. Lytle, J.M.; Chittajallu, R.; Wrathall, J.R.; Gallo, V. NG2 cell response in the CNP-EGFP mouse after contusive spinal cord injury. *Glia* **2009**, *57*, 270–285. [CrossRef] [PubMed]

209. Marques, S.; Zeisel, A.; Codeluppi, S.; van Bruggen, D.; Mendanha Falcão, A.; Xiao, L.; Häring, M.; Hochgerner, H.; Romanov, R.A.; Gyllborg, D.; et al. Oligodendrocyte heterogeneity in the mouse juvenile and adult central nervous system. *Science* **2016**, *352*, 1326–1329. [CrossRef] [PubMed]

210. Sakers, K.; Lake, A.M.; Khazanchi, R.; Ouwenga, R.; Vasek, M.J.; Dani, A.; Dougherty, J.D. Astrocytes locally translate transcripts in their peripheral processes. *Proc. Natl. Acad. Sci. USA* **2017**, *114*, E3830–E3838. [CrossRef] [PubMed]

211. Crosetto, N.; Bienko, M.; van Oudenaarden, A. Spatially resolved transcriptomics and beyond. *Nat. Rev. Genet.* **2015**, *16*, 57–66. [CrossRef] [PubMed]

212. Dimou, L.; Simons, M. Diversity of oligodendrocytes and their progenitors. *Curr. Opin. Neurobiol.* **2017**, *47*, 73–79. [CrossRef] [PubMed]

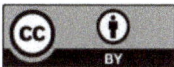

neuroglia

MDPI

Article

Expression of Kir2.1 Inward Rectifying Potassium Channels in Optic Nerve Glia: Evidence for Heteromeric Association with Kir4.1 and Kir5.1

Csilla Brasko [1,2] and Arthur M. Butt [1,*]

[1]   Institute of Biology and Biomedical Sciences, School of Pharmacy and Biomedical Sciences, University of Portsmouth, St Michael's Building, White Swan Road, Portsmouth PO1 2DT, UK; csilla.brasko@yahoo.co.uk
[2]   Department of Physiology, University of Szeged, Szeged Hungary Közép fasor 52, 6726 Szeged, Hungary
*   Correspondence: arthur.butt@port.ac.uk

Received: 25 May 2018; Accepted: 4 July 2018; Published: 10 July 2018

Abstract: Inward rectifying potassium (Kir) channels comprise a large family with diverse biophysical properties. A predominant feature of central nervous system (CNS) glia is their expression of Kir4.1, which as homomers are weakly rectifying channels, but form strongly rectifying channels as heteromers with Kir2.1. However, the extent of Kir2.1 expression and their association with Kir4.1 in glia throughout the CNS is unclear. We have examined this in astrocytes and oligodendrocytes of the mouse optic nerve, a typical CNS white matter tract. Western blot and immunocytochemistry demonstrates that optic nerve astrocytes and oligodendrocytes express Kir2.1 and that it co-localises with Kir4.1. Co-immunoprecipitation analysis provided further evidence that Kir2.1 associate with Kir4.1 and, moreover, Kir2.1 expression was significantly reduced in optic nerves and brains from Kir4.1 knock-out mice. In addition, optic nerve glia express Kir5.1, which may associate with Kir2.1 to form silent channels. Immunocytochemical and co-immunoprecipitation analyses indicate that Kir2.1 associate with Kir5.1 in optic nerve glia, but not in the brain. The results provide evidence that astrocytes and oligodendrocytes may express heteromeric Kir2.1/Kir4.1 and Kir2.1/Kir5.1 channels, together with homomeric Kir2.1 and Kir4.1 channels. In astrocytes, expression of multiple Kir channels is the biophysical substrate for the uptake and redistribution of K^+ released during neuronal electrical activity known as 'potassium spatial buffering'. Our findings suggest a similar potential role for the diverse Kir channels expressed by oligodendrocytes, which by way of their myelin sheaths are intimately associated with the sites of action potential propagation and axonal K^+ release.

Keywords: inward rectifying potassium channel; glia; astrocyte; oligodendrocyte; white matter; potassium regulation

1. Introduction

Inward rectifying potassium (Kir) channels comprise of several well-defined subfamilies, including weakly rectifying Kir4.1 channels and strongly voltage-dependent Kir2.1 channels, which play key roles in setting the membrane potential in central nervous system (CNS) glia and regulating their key functions [1]. In particular, the Kir4.1 subtype plays a central role in the astrocyte function of potassium spatial buffering, which is essential for maintaining extracellular $[K^+]$ in the face of continuous K^+ release from electrically active neurons [2]. Oligodendrocytes are the myelin-forming cells of the CNS and also express Kir4.1 [3–5], although expression appears to be heterogeneous [3,6], and is most highly expressed in certain white matter regions, including the optic nerve [4,5]; genomic analysis by the Barres group confirms that Kir4.1 (*Kcnj10*) is expressed throughout the oligodendroglial lineage, although at a lower level than in astrocytes (https://web.stanford.edu/group/barres_lab/cgi-bin/igv_cgi_2.py?lname=Kcnj10). Astrocytes and oligodendrocytes have also been shown to express strongly rectifying Kir2.1 [7–10], although in situ hybridization analyses failed to detect significant glial expression of Kir2.1 in rat brain [11], consistent with genomic analyses that, overall, Kir2.1 (*Kcnj2*) is expressed by astrocytes and myelinating oligodendrocytes to a much lesser extent than Kir4.1 (https://web.stanford.edu/group/barres_lab/cgi-bin/igv_cgi_2.py?lname=kcnj2). In Müller glia of the retina, Kir2.1 expression is highly localized in processes that contact neurons, and their strong rectifying properties indicate they have a specific role in K$^+$ uptake during neuronal activity [12]. In hippocampal astrocytes, Kir2.1 are dramatically increased by kainic acid-induced seizure, suggesting a key role in protecting against K$^+$ accumulation caused by neuronal hyperexcitability [8].

The functional diversity of Kir is increased by the formation of heteromeric channels [1,13]. Kir2.1 and Kir4.1 are co-localized in Müller glia [12], and changes in Kir2.1 and Kir4.1 during pathophysiology suggest common mechanisms of regulation and co-assembly [8,14]. In addition, multiple lines of evidence indicate widespread astroglial expression of Kir5.1 [12,15–21], which on their own do not form functional channels, but by co-assembly with Kir4.1 form highly pH sensitive channels [22,23] that are important for astrocyte-driven central chemoreception [18]. Recently, we also provided evidence that oligodendrocytes express Kir4.1/Kir5.1 channels [5]; genomic analysis indicates Kir5.1 (*Kcnj16*) is expressed at similar levels as Kir2.1 (*Kcnj2*) and more highly in immature oligodendrocytes than myelinating oligodendrocytes (https://web.stanford.edu/group/barres_lab/cgi-bin/igv_cgi_2.py?lname=kcnj2). Here, we have examined the expression of Kir2.1 and its association with Kir4.1 and Kir5.1 in white matter astrocytes and oligodendrocytes of the mouse optic nerve. The results show that oligodendrocytes, like astrocytes, express Kir2.1, although to a far lesser extent than Kir4.1, and co-immunolabeling and co-immunoprecipitation analyses support the possibility that Kir2.1 may co-assemble with Kir4.1 and Kir5.1. The distinct properties of homomeric Kir2.1 and heteromeric Kir2.1/Kir4.1 and Kir2.1/Kir5.1 channels provide a biophysical basis for efficient K$^+$ spatial buffering in oligodendrocytes, as well as astrocytes, during the large shifts in K$^+$ to which they are exposed during action potential propagation.

2. Materials and Methods

2.1. Animals and Optic Nerve Explant Cultures

The mice used were of the C57 strain, or transgenic mice in which the oligodendroglial myelin gene proteolipid protein (PLP) drives expression of *Discosoma* sp. red fluorescent protein (DsRed) (PLP-DsRed; from Prof. Frank Kirchhoff, University of Saarland, Homburg, Germany), or Kir4.1 knock-out (KO) mice (from Prof. Christian Steinhäuser, University of Bonn, Germany; originally generated by Kofuji et al.) [24]. Mice were killed humanely by cervical dislocation, approved by the Home Office of the United Kingdom under the Animals (Scientific Procedures) Act, 1986, licence number 70/7733.

2.2. Optic Nerve Explant Cultures

Mice aged postnatal day (P)7–11 were used to prepare mixed glial cultures from optic nerve explants [25]. Optic nerves were carefully removed to dissecting media, comprised of Dulbecco's Modified Eagle Medium (DMEM) (Sigma-Aldrich, Irvine, UK), supplemented with 4 mM L-glutamate, 10% fetal bovine serum (FBS; Invitrogen, Paisley, UK) and 0.1% gentamicin (Invitrogen). Nerves were cut into 1–2 mm fragments prior to trituration and transference onto poly-L-lysine (Sigma-Aldrich) coated coverslips and incubated at 37 °C in 5% CO_2. After 24 h, cultures were placed in low serum (0.5%) modified Bottenstein and Sato (B&S) culture medium, supplemented with 10 ng/ml recombinant human platelet-derived growth factor (PDGF)-AA (R&D Systems, Abingdon, UK) and 0.1% gentamicin. After 3–4 days in vitro (DIV), the medium was changed to B&S supplemented with 0.5 mM dibutyryl cAMP for up to 10 DIV, to promote oligodendrocyte differentiation, then B&S media with 0.1% gentamicin for up to 15 DIV, changing media every 3–5 days.

2.3. Immunocytochemistry

After 11–15 DIV, optic nerve explant cultures were fixed in 1% paraformaldehyde in phosphate buffered saline (PBS, pH 7.4) for 10 min at room temperature (RT). Following washes in PBS, coverslips were incubated in blocking solution (5% normal goat serum, NGS, in PBS) for 1 h at RT and then permeabilized in 5% NGS in PBS with 0.2% Triton for 15–30 min, prior to incubation overnight at 4 °C in primary antibodies diluted in PBS (chicken anti-GFAP, 1:500, Chemicon, UK; in-house rabbit anti-Kir4.1, 1:400 [4,5]; rabbit anti-Kir5.1, 1:300, Alomone Labs Ltd., Jerusalem, Israel; goat anti-Kir2.1, 1:100, (Santa Cruz Biotechnology, TX, USA). Following washes, coverslips were incubated for 1 h at RT in secondary antibodies diluted in PBS (goat-anti rabbit Alexafluor 488, 1:400, Molecular Probes; donkey anti-goat 488, Molecular Probes; donkey anti-chicken Alexafluor 568, Molecular Probes UK; donkey anti-chicken Dylight 405, 1:400, Stratech, Ely, UK; donkey anti-rabbit Dylight 647, 1:200, Stratech). Finally, coverslips were washed and mounted on slides with Vectasheild® (VectorLabs, Peterborough, UK). Negative controls were carried out for all antibodies, using pre-incubation with appropriate antigens for Kir2.1 and Kir5.1, according to manufacturer's recommendations, and for Kir4.1 specificity was confirmed using tissue from Kir4.1 knock-out mice.

2.4. Image Capture and Analysis

Immunolabelled coverslips were imaged on a Zeiss LSM 710 confocal microscope (Zeiss, Oberkochen, Germany), using the ×40, ×63, or ×100 oil immersion objectives. Fluorescence was detected using excitation wavelengths of 488 nm (green), 568 nm (red), 633 nm (far red) and 405 nm (blue), with argon, HeNe1 and diode lasers, respectively. Images were captured using optimal settings for pinhole diameter (0.13–0.3 μm), detector gain and offset acquisition to detect the positive signal with minimal background, and multi-track capture of separate channels was used to prevent 'bleed'. Z-stacks comprising 4–15 optical sections (1024 × 1024 pixels) were used to generate three-dimensional images (voxel size 43–76 nm xy/76–283 nm z), using Zen 2009 Light software version x (Zeiss). Identical settings were used to image negative controls. Co-localization analysis was carried out using Volocity 6.1 software (PerkinElmer, USA), by measuring signal overlap from the degree of separation between pixels from the red and green channels in single z-sections, as described by Barlow et al. and used in our previous studies [5,26]. Images were thresholded to separate the positive signal (positive immunolabelling) from background, by measuring the background intensity value for each channel in negative control sections and setting the threshold as the mean background intensity plus three standard deviations (averaged from a minimum of six images). The thresholded Pearson's correlation coefficient (PCC) was used to measure the degree of overlap between the red and green channels, to generate a co-localization channel in three-dimensions and the number of voxels in which the two channels overlap with the same intensity.

2.5. Western Blot and Co-Immunoprecipitation

Whole brains or optic nerves dissected from young adult mice aged 20–30 days old were homogenized in buffer containing 12.5 mM NaCl, pH ~8, 2 mM Tris/HCl, 0.2 mM phenyl-methyl sulphonyl fluoride (PMSF), distilled water and 1× complete mini protease inhibitor cocktail (Roche, Basel, Switzerland), on ice. Samples were centrifuged at 12,000 rpm for 5 min at 4 °C and the aspirated supernatant was placed in a fresh tube on ice. Quantification of protein concentration was carried out with bicinchoninic acid assay (Sigma-Aldrich) with a standard bovine serum albumin (BSA) concentration curve and ultraviolet (UV) spectrophotometer absorbance readings at 550 nm. Samples were used either as whole lysates or subcellular fractions were prepared, as described below.

Western blot was performed on whole tissue lysates, prepared as above, or subcellular fractions prepared, as detailed previously [5]. In brief, whole brains and optic nerves of wild type and Kir4.1 KO animals were homogenized in subcellular fractionation buffer (250 mM sucrose, 20 mM HEPES, 10 mM KCl, 1.5 mM MgCl$_2$, 1 mM ethylenediaminetetraacetic acid (EDTA), 1 mM EGTA, 1 DTT and 1× protease inhibitor cocktail), then centrifuged at 4 °C with 750× g for 10 min to remove the nuclear fraction; the supernatant was then placed in a new centrifuge tube and centrifuged with 10,000× g at 4 °C two times to remove the mitochondrial fraction and the supernatant was placed in an ultracentrifuge tube and centrifuged with 40,000× g at 4 °C for 1 h to leave the pellet containing the crude plasma membrane fraction, which was re-suspended in 400 µL fractionation buffer using a 25× g needle and centrifuged at 40,000× g at 4 °C for 45 min and then the pellet was re-suspended in lysis buffer. Subsequently, total lysates and subcellular fractions were treated the same and prepared for sodium dodecyl sulfate polyacrylamide gel electrophoresis (SDS-PAGE); samples were mixed with Laemmli sample buffer and heated at 95 °C for 5 min with β-mercaptoethanol and loaded for 10% acrylamide SDS-PAGE, submerged in electrophoresis buffer pH ~8 containing of 25 mM Tris base 190 mM glycine 0.1%. Proteins were then electrophoretically transferred to a polyvinyllidene difluoride membrane (Amersham) that had been incubated for 1 h in blocking solution of 5% dried milk in Tris buffered saline (TBS; 150 mM NaCl 10 mM Tris pH 7.4) with 0.05% Tween 20, and incubated in primary overnight at 4 °C in antibodies diluted in 5% dried milk and Tris buffered saline: rabbit anti-Kir4.1, 1:1000 [4], rabbit anti-Kir2.1, 1:300 (Alomone Labs Ltd.), goat anti-Kir2.1, 1:300 (Santa Cruz Biotechnology). Following washes, incubation in horseradish peroxidase-conjugated secondary antibodies diluted in 5% dried milk and Tris buffered saline was carried out for 1 h at RT: rabbit anti-goat, 1:3000 (Dako,), goat anti-mouse, 1:10,000 (Dako), swine anti-rabbit 1:2000 (Dako). Extensive washing of the membranes in TBS with ice cold 0.05% Tween20 was performed after each incubation and immunocomplexes were visualized using an enhanced chemiluminescence method (Amersham).

Co-immunoprecipitation analysis was performed on whole tissue lysates prepared as above, using µMACS™ Protein A/G MicroBead kits (Miltenyi Biotec, Bergisch Gladbach, Germany) according to the manufacturers recommendations [25]. In brief, lysates were centrifuged at 4 °C with 10,000× g 2 times to remove cell debris and 3 µg polyclonal or 2 µg monoclonal antibody was added to the proteins and incubated overnight at 4 °C; for negative controls, proteins were mixed with pre-absorbed antibodies for Kir2.1 and Kir5.1 and Kir4.1 KO tissue was used to confirm the specificity of Kir4.1 antibodies. Then, Protein G MicroBeads were added to the samples to form magnetically labeled immune complexes (50 µL for monoclonal antibody or 100 µL for polyclonal antibody was used for the precipation) for 30 min on ice. Homogenates were then run through a µ Column placed in the magnetic field of the µMACS™ separator and the immune complex was eluted by applying pre-heated (95 °C) 1× Laemelli sample buffer to the column. The drop on the column tip containing the eluted immunoprecipitate was collected and stored on ice or at −80 °C until it was analyzed by SDS-PAGE.

3. Results

Optic nerve explants cultures from P7–11 mice [5,25] were examined after 15 DIV to determine the expression of Kir2.1 in oligodendrocytes, identified by their expression of the PLP-DsRed reporter (Figure 1A), and astrocytes, identified by co-immunostaining for glial fibrillary acidic protein (GFAP) (Figure 1B). Immunostaining for Kir2.1 was punctate (Figure 1Ai,Bi) and in oligodendrocytes was localized to the tips of their processes (Figure 1Aiii), whereas in astrocytes immunostaining was localized to the cell somata and primary processes (Figure 1Biii). No immunostaining was observed in negative controls pre-incubated in the blocking peptides (Figure 1C) and as a further test of the specificity, in the absence of Kir2.1 knock-out tissue, we used two separate antibodies [27], namely a rabbit polyclonal anti-Kir2.1 antibody (Alomone Labs Ltd.) raised against amino acid sequence 393-411 (Accession AAI37842.1), and a goat polyclonal anti-Kir2.1 antibody (C-20, Santa Cruz Biotechnology, Dallas, TX, USA) raised against amino acid sequence 378-427 (Accession P63252); immunostaining was equivalent for the two antibodies in both oligodendrocytes and astrocytes (not illustrated). Furthermore, Western blot analysis of Kir2.1 in brain and optic nerve lysates using either antibody detected a predicted band at ~45 kDa, the molecular weight (MW) of Kir2.1, with an additional band at ~60 kDa, which is considered to be the fully glycosylated plasma membrane bound Kir2.1 protein (Figure 1D). In support of this, 60 kDa Kir2.1 was enriched in the optic nerve plasma membrane fraction (Figure 1D), which also demonstrates that Kir2.1 is localized to glial cell membranes, where it can form functional channels.

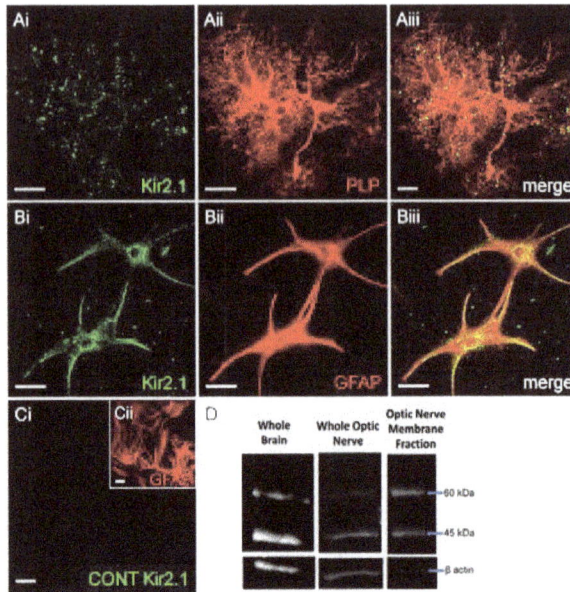

Figure 1. Expression of Kir2.1 (inward rectifying potassium channel 2.1) in optic nerve glia. (**A–C**) Optic nerves from P7-11 mice were maintained in explant culture for 15 days in vitro (DIV) and immunolabelled for Kir2.1 ((**Ai,Bi**), green) in oligodendrocytes, identified by expression of the proteolipid protein, *Discosoma* sp. red fluorescent protein (PLP-DsRed) reporter ((**Aii**), red), and astrocytes, identified by glial fibrillary acidic protein (GFAP) immunolabelling ((**Bii**), red); merged images show co-localisation ((**Aiii,Biii**), co-expression appears yellow) and no signal was detected in negative controls (**C**). Scale bars = 20 μm. (**D**) Western blot analyses for Kir2.1 in lysates of whole brain (left-hand panel) and optic nerve (middle panel), together with optic nerve plasma membrane fraction (right-hand panel), from young adult mice aged P2-30; bands were detected at ~45 kDa as predicted from the molecular weight of the Kir2.1 protein, together with a band at ~60 kDa that was more enriched in the plasma membrane fraction and is considered to be the fully glycosylated Kir2.1 protein.

Next, we used double immunofluorescence in optic nerve explants cultures to demonstrate that Kir2.1 are co-expressed with Kir4.1 in oligodendrocytes (Figure 2Ai–Aiii) and astrocytes (Figure 2Bi–Biii); immunostaining was not observed in negative controls (Figure 2Bix,Bx). To determine the extent of co-localization of Kir2.1 and Kir4.1, we used the technique of Barlow and colleagues [26], as previously described [5,28], to generate a co-localization channel of the voxels in which fluorescence is at equal intensity from the green (Kir2.1) and red (Kir4.1) channels (Figure 2Aiv,Biv). The results demonstrate a high degree of co-localization in oligodendrocytes (Figure 2Aiv–Avi) and astrocytes (Figure 2Biv–Bvi), predominantly on the processes of both cell types (Figure 2Avii–Aix, Bvii–Bviii). Quantification demonstrated greater overall expression of Kir2.1 in astrocytes compared to oligodendrocytes, and markedly less than Kir4.1 in both cell types (Figure 2C,D); ~50% of immunostaining for Kir2.1 was co-localized with Kir4.1 in both cell types (astrocytes: 24,839 ± 11,445 Kir2.1$^+$/Kir4.1$^+$ voxels per cell, compared to 47,152 ± 22,079 Kir2.1$^+$ voxels and 149,541 ± 58,462 Kir4.1$^+$ voxels per cell (n = 13); oligodendrocytes: 32,755 ± 15,080 Kir4.1+/Kir2.1+ voxels per cell, compared to 68,294 ± 34,663 Kir2.1$^+$ voxels and 189,959 ± 100,143 Kir4.1+ voxels per cell (n = 12). Co-immunoprecipitation analyses of total lysates from brain and optic nerve of P20-30 mice provides further evidence that Kir2.1 associate with Kir4.1 (Figure 2F–H). The 45 kDa protein immunoprecipitated with the Kir2.1 antibody (Figure 2F) co-immunoprecipated with Kir4.1 antibody specifically at ~42 kDa, the MW for Kir4.1 (Figure 2G), and the reverse co-immunoprecipitation gave equivalent results (Figure 2H); this was confirmed in four experiments, all unequivocally demonstrating the same result, and no co-immunoprecipitation was detected in negative controls.

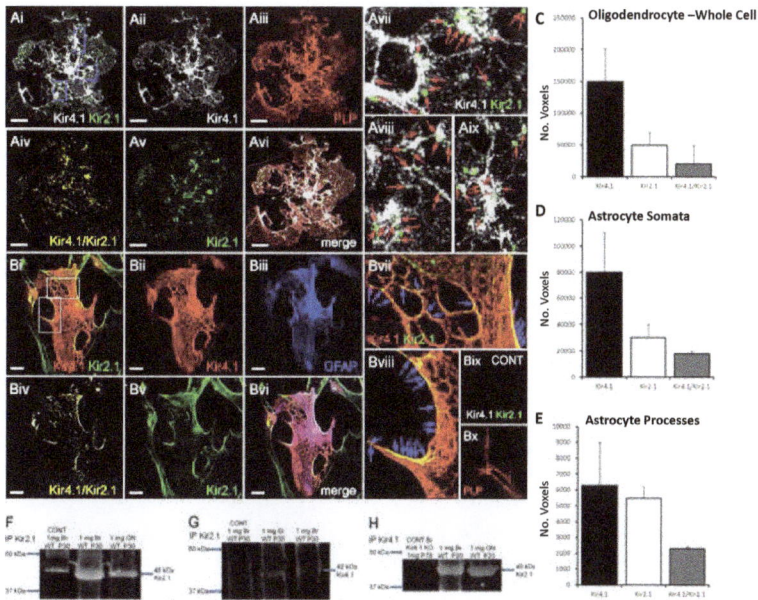

Figure 2. Co-expression of Kir2.1 and Kir4.1 in optic nerve glia. (**A,B**) Double immunofluorescence labeling in optic nerve glia isolated from P11 optic nerve cultured for 11 DIV: (**A**) Kir4.1 (far red, appears white) and Kir2.1 (green) in oligodendrocytes identified by expression of the PLP-DsRed reporter (red); (**B**) Kir4.1 (red) and Kir2.1 (green) in astrocytes identified by immunolabelling for GFAP (blue). Co-localization channels for Kir2.1/Kir4.1 are illustrated (**Aiv,Biv**), together with high magnification merged images indicating co-localization in processes (**Avii–Aix,Bvii–Bvii**); no signal was detected in negative controls (**Bix–Bx**). Scale bars = 20 μm. (**C–E**) Kir4.1/Kir2.1 co-localization analysis in oligodendrocytes (**C**), astrocytes (**D**) and astrocyte processes (**E**); data are means + standard error of the mean (SEM), n = 13. (**F–H**) Co-immunoprecipitation analysis of Kir2.1 and Kir4.1 from lysates of whole brain and optic nerve from mice aged P20–30 detected predicted bands at ~45 kDa for the anti-Kir2.1 antibody (**F**) and at ~42 kDa when co-immunprecipated with anti-Kir4.1 antibody (**G**), with equivalent results when immunoprecipated first with the anti-Kir4.1 antibody and then co-immunoprecipated with the anti-Kir2.1 antibody (**H**); no bands were detected in negative controls.

The results indicate that Kir4.1 and Kir2.1 subunits co-assemble in optic nerve glia and to further investigate this, we determined whether Kir2.1 expression is altered in Kir4.1 knock-out mice, in which we and others have previously demonstrated Kir4.1 to be absent in the brain and optic nerve [5,29,30]. Comparison of whole lysates from brain and optic nerve in controls (Figure 3A) and Kir4.1 KO mice (Figure 3B) demonstrates a significant decrease in expression of the 45 kDa Kir2.1 protein in the absence of Kir4.1 (unpaired t-tests, p values indicated on graph). Conversely, the 60 kDa glycosalted band in the plasma membrane fraction was significantly increased in Kir4.1 KO brain to 1.47 ± 0.52 compared to 0.95 ± 0.098 in wild-type (Figure 3B; $p < 0.01$, unpaired t-test). These data suggest that mechanisms of regulation for Kir2.1 and Kir4.1 are closely inter-related.

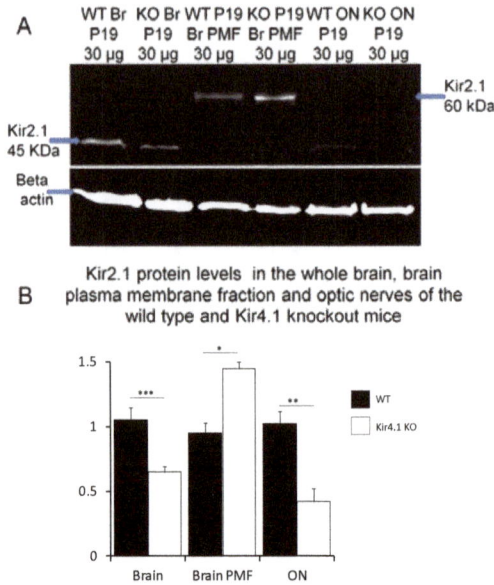

Figure 3. Kir2.1 protein levels are altered in the absence of Kir4.1. (**A**) Western blot analysis of Kir2.1 in total brain lysate (lanes 1, 2), brain plasma membrane fraction (lanes 3, 4) and total optic nerve lysate (lanes 5, 6), from P19 wild-type (WT) and (lanes 1, 3, 5) and Kir4.1 knock-out (KO) mice (lanes 2, 4, 6); predicted bands were detected at ~45 kDa in whole lysates (lanes 1, 2, 5, 6) and a ~60 kDa band for the fully glycosylated plasmalemmal channel enriched in the plasma membrane fraction (PMF) (lanes 3, 4). (**B**) Mean (±SEM, $n = 3$) density of the 45 kDa band for brain and optic nerve, and 60 kDa band for brain plasma membrane fraction, normalized against β-actin; * $p < 0.05$, ** $p < 0.01$, *** $p < 0.001$, unpaired *t*-tests.

Finally, we investigated the possibility of an association between Kir2.1 and Kir5.1, since it has been reported they may form heteromers [31] and we recently showed optic nerve glia express Kir5.1 that did not entirely co-localize with Kir4.1 [5], with which Kir5.1 preferentially form heteromers [23]. Double immunofluorescence labeling of optic nerve explant cultures demonstrates Kir2.1 and Kir5.1 are co-expressed in oligodendrocytes (Figure 4A) and astrocytes (Figure 4B), with a high degree of co-localization in both cell types (Figure 4Aiv–Avi,Biv–Bvi); ~40% of Kir2.1 voxels co-localised with Kir5.1 (Figure 4C,D), whereas conversely only 25% of Kir5.1 were co-localized with Kir2.1 in oligodendrocytes and 16% in astrocytes, consistent with Kir5.1 mainly associating with Kir4.1 [5,23]. Immunoprecipitation of whole brain and optic nerve lysates from P23-27 mice with anti-Kir5.1 antibody identified a specific ~48 kDa protein, the MW of Kir5.1, and co-immunoprecipitation with anti-Kir2.1 antibody identified the predicted 45 kDa protein in the optic nerve, but in the brain (Figure 4F); results were confirmed in four experiments, all unequivocally demonstrating the same result, and no bands were detected in negative controls. The data suggest Kir2.1 may co-assemble with Kir5.1 in optic nerve glia.

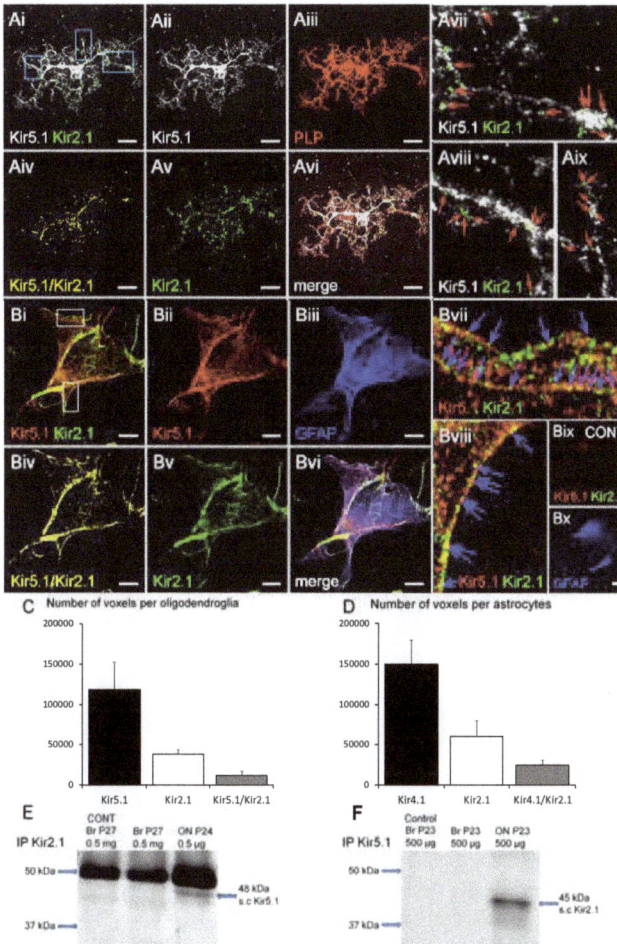

Figure 4. Co-expression of Kir2.1 and Kir5.1 in optic nerve glia. (**A,B**) Double immunofluorescence labeling in optic nerve glia from P11 optic nerve cultured for 11 DIV: (**A**) Kir5.1 (far red, appears white) and Kir2.1 (green) in oligodendrocytes identified by expression of the PLP-DsRed reporter (red); (**B**) Kir5.1 (red) and Kir2.1 (green) in astrocytes identified by immunolabelling for GFAP (blue). Co-localisation channels for Kir5.1/Kir2.1 are illustrated (**Aiv,Biv**), together with high magnification merged images indicating co-localization in processes (**Avii–Aix,Bvii–Bvii**); no signal was detected in negative controls (**Bix–Bx**). Scale bars = 20 μm. (**C–E**) Kir5.1/Kir2.1 co-localization analysis in oligodendrocytes (**C**) and astrocytes (**D**); data are means ± SEM, $n = 13$. (**E,F**) Co-immunoprecipitation analysis of Kir5.1 with Kir2.1 from lysates of whole brain and optic nerve from mice aged P20-30 detected predicted bands at ~48 kDa for the anti-Kir5.1 antibody (**E**) and at ~45 kDa when co-immunoprecipated with anti-Kir2.1 antibody in optic nerve, but not brain (**G**). No bands were detected in negative controls.

4. Discussion

In glia, Kir2.1 are considered to have an important role in the astroglial function of K^+ clearance, due to their strong rectifying properties and cellular expression on processes of Müller glia and Schwann cells that contact neurons and axons [12,32]. Here, we demonstrate that in CNS white matter of the mouse optic nerve, both oligodendrocytes and astrocytes express Kir2.1 and provide evidence they exist alone and in association with Kir4.1 and Kir5.1. The results support the possibility that in CNS white matter homomeric Kir2.1 and heteromeric Kir2.1/Kir4.1 and Kir2.1/Kir5.1 channels interact to play an important role in K$^+$ regulation in astrocytes and oligodendrocytes.

Expression of Kir2.1 in optic nerve glia supports studies in other CNS regions [7–10]. Compared to Kir4.1 expression, Kir2.1 immunostaining was weak, which is consistent with retinal astrocytes, where Kir2.1 expression is 12 times lower than Kir4.1 [14], and with genomic analyses that Kir2.1 (*Kcnj2*) is expressed by astrocytes and myelinating oligodendrocytes to a much lesser extent than Kir4.1 (*Kcnj10*) (https://web.stanford.edu/group/barres_lab/cgi-bin/igv_cgi_2.py?lname=kcnj2). The relatively low expression of Kir2.1 in glia may also help explain why in situ hybridization analyses failed to detect significant glial expression of Kir2.1 in rat brain [11]. Due to technical reasons, immunoblot analyses were performed on tissue from P20-30 mice and immunocytochemical analyses were performed on optic nerve explant cultures from P7-11 mice after 11–15 DIV, hence the ages were compatible. It remains a possibility that the relative expression levels of different Kir subunits may change with age, but the immunocytochemistry and immunoblot data are in accord that in the brain and optic nerve Kir2.1 is strongly associated with Kir4.1, which is almost exclusively glial in the CNS [1,6], providing strong supporting evidence that glia express Kir2.1.

It is known that Kir2.1 channels form functional heteromeric channels with Kir4.1, changing the latter from weak rectifying to strongly rectifying channels [33]. Our results support other studies showing co-localization of Kir2.1 and Kir4.1 in astrocytes and Müller glia [8,12,14], and for the first time demonstrate Kir2.1/Kir4.1 co-localization in oligodendrocytes. Expression of Kir2.1 was significantly decreased in Kir4.1 KO mice, suggesting a high degree of inter-dependence and common mechanisms of regulation and function. Moreover, plasmalemmal Kir2.1 was relatively greater in the absence of Kir4.1, suggesting a role for Kir4.1 in the cellular localization of Kir2.1. Previous studies confirmed the expression of Kir2.1 subunit in the retina from Kir4.1 KO mice, although they did not detect significant changes in the expression of Kir2.1 in Müller glia from Kir4.1 KO mice [12]. In the condition termed proliferative vitreoretinopathy that is associated with proliferative gliosis, Kir4.1 and Kir2.1 were found to be inactivated by mislocalisation in retinal Müller cells [14]. In hippocampal astrocytes, where Kir4.1 is the predominant K$^+$ channel subunit [34], the accumulation of extracellular K$^+$ caused by neuronal hyperexcitability results in the loss of the perivascular weak inward rectifying Kir4.1 channels [35] and an elevation of strong inward rectifying Kir2.1 [8]. Together, these studies demonstrate an inter-dependence of Kir4.1 and Kir2.1 expression in glial cells.

An association between Kir2.1 and Kir5.1 was also demonstrated in optic nerve glia. Co-assembly of Kir2.1 and Kir5.1 subunits has been demonstrated in *Xenopus* oocytes [31], but another study did not find that Kir5.1 can associate with Kir2.1 [23]. We did not find evidence that Kir2.1 associated with Kir5.1 in the brain, but only in the optic nerve. In contrast, here and in a recent study [5], evidence of Kir2.1/Kir4.1 and Kir4.1/Kir5.1 was found in both brain and optic nerve. Overall, the results are consistent with co-assembly of Kir2.1 and Kir5.1 being a special feature of optic nerve glia. In contrast, Kir2.1/Kir4.1 and Kir4.1/Kir5.1 channels appear to be widely expressed throughout the brain [5,8,12,14–21] and respectively form strongly rectifying and highly pH sensitive channels [22,23]. Notably, co-assembly of Kir2.1 with Kir5.1 results in the formation of an electrically silent channel [31]. Thus, Kir5.1 potentially have a major regulatory role in glia, by silencing Kir2.1 and removing them from forming strongly rectifying channels, as homers or heteromers with Kir4.1, which in the absence of Kir2.1 would otherwise form weakly rectifying channels. Interestingly, we previously showed that plasmalemmal Kir5.1 persist in the absence of Kir4.1 [5] and now show the same is true for plasmalemmal Kir2.1. Since Kir5.1 cannot form functional homomeric channels, these results suggest that in the absence of Kir4.1, Kir2.1 may co-assemble with Kir5.1 to form electrically silent channels. This possibility is supported by the almost complete loss of inward rectifying potassium currents in astrocytes and oligodendrocytes upon the genetic deletion of Kir4.1 gene [29,30,36,37], despite our evidence of continued expression of strongly rectifying Kir2.1 in the absence of Kir4.1. The absence of

Neuroglia **2018**, *1*

co-immunoprecipitation for Kir2.1 and Kir5.1 in brain lysates, comprising mainly cortex, suggests that Kir5.1 may not have an equivalent regulatory function in cortical glia, where Kir4.1 have been shown to the dominant potassium channel, although our analyses may not be sufficiently sensitive to detect low levels of co-expression. Together, the results indicate close interactions between Kir2.1, Kir4.1 and Kir5.1 that determine their localization and function in optic nerve glia.

In summary, this study identifies expression of Kir2.1 and Kir2.1/Kir4.1 channels in oligodendrocytes as well as astrocytes, and provides the first evidence of an association between Kir2.1 and Kir5.1, which may be a special feature of optic nerve glia, although further studies are required to determine whether these may be features of white matter glia throughout the CNS. Interestingly, co-assembly of Kir2.1 with Kir4.1 forms a strongly rectifying channel, whereas co-assembly with Kir5.1 results in the formation of an electrically silent channel. Thus, the plasmalemmal expression of Kir2.1 and Kir4.1 as homomeric channels or as heteromeric channels with each other or with Kir5.1 would determine glial membrane properties and their capacity for K^+ uptake and provide a potential mechanism for K^+ spatial buffering. At sites of high neuronal activity, K^+ released into the extracellular space would be taken up via strongly rectifying Kir2.1 and Kir2.1/Kir4.1 channels, whereas K^+ would be released back into the extracellular space at sites of low K^+; for example, during low neuronal activity or at blood vessels, via weakly rectifying Kir4.1 channels combined with silencing of Kir2.1 channels by their co-assembly with Kir5.1.

Author Contributions: A.M.B. and C.B. both contributed to the design and analysis of the data; experiments were performed by C.B.; the paper was written by A.M.B. and C.B.; funding was to A.M.B.

Funding: This research was funded by the BBSRC (BB/J016888) and MRC (MR/P025811/1).

Conflicts of Interest: The authors declare no conflict of interest. The founding sponsors had no role in the design of the study; in the collection, analyses, or interpretation of data; in the writing of the manuscript, and in the decision to publish the results.

References

1. Butt, A.M.; Kalsi, A. Inwardly rectifying potassium channels (Kir) in central nervous system glia: A special role for Kir4.1 in glial functions. *J. Cell. Mol. Med.* **2006**, *10*, 33–44. [CrossRef] [PubMed]

2. Kofuji, P.; Connors, N.C. Molecular substrates of potassium spatial buffering in glial cells. *Mol. Neurobiol.* **2003**, *28*, 195–208. [CrossRef]

3. Poopalasundaram, S.; Knott, C.; Shamotienko, O.G.; Foran, P.G.; Dolly, J.O.; Ghiani, C.A.; Gallo, V.; Wilkin, G.P. Glial heterogeneity in expression of the inwardly rectifying K^+ channel, Kir4.1, in adult rat CNS. *Glia* **2000**, *30*, 362–372. [CrossRef]

4. Kalsi, A.S.; Greenwood, K.; Wilkin, G.; Butt, A.M. Kir4.1 expression by astrocytes and oligodendrocytes in CNS white matter: A developmental study in the rat optic nerve. *J. Anat.* **2004**, *204*, 475–485. [CrossRef] [PubMed]

5. Brasko, C.; Hawkins, V.; De La Rocha, I.C.; Butt, A.M. Expression of Kir4.1 and Kir5.1 inwardly rectifying potassium channels in oligodendrocytes, the myelinating cells of the CNS. *Brain Struct. Funct.* **2017**, *222*, 41–59. [CrossRef] [PubMed]

6. Tang, X.; Taniguchi, K.; Kofuji, P. Heterogeneity of Kir4.1 channel expression in glia revealed by mouse transgenesis. *Glia* **2009**, *57*, 1706–1715. [CrossRef] [PubMed]

7. Howe, M.W.; Feig, S.L.; Osting, S.M.; Haberly, L.B. Cellular and subcellular localization of Kir2.1 subunits in neurons and glia in piriform cortex with implications for K^+ spatial buffering. *J. Comp. Neurol.* **2008**, *506*, 877–893. [CrossRef] [PubMed]

8. Kang, S.J.; Cho, S.H.; Park, K.; Yi, J.; Yoo, S.J.; Shin, K.S. Expression of Kir2.1 channels in astrocytes under pathophysiological conditions. *Mol. Cells* **2008**, *25*, 124–130. [PubMed]

9. Schröder, W.; Seifert, G.; Hüttmann, K.; Hinterkeuser, S.; Steinhäuser, C. AMPA receptor-mediated modulation of inward rectifier K^+ channels in astrocytes of mouse hippocampus. *Mol. Cell. Neurosci.* **2002**, *19*, 447–458. [CrossRef] [PubMed]

10. Stonehouse, A.H.; Pringle, J.H.; Norman, R.I.; Stanfield, P.R.; Conley, E.C.; Brammar, W.J. Characterisation of Kir2.0 proteins in the rat cerebellum and hippocampus by polyclonal antibodies. *Histochem. Cell Biol.* **1999**, *112*, 457–465. [CrossRef] [PubMed]

11. Prüss, H.; Derst, C.; Lommel, R.; Veh, R.W. Differential distribution of individual subunits of strongly inwardly rectifying potassium channels (Kir2 family) in rat brain. *Mol. Brain Res.* **2005**, *139*, 63–79. [CrossRef] [PubMed]

12. Kofuji, P.; Biedermann, B.; Siddharthan, V.; Raap, M.; Iandiev, I.; Milenkovic, I.; Thomzig, A.; Veh, R.W.; Bringmann, A.; Reichenbach, A. Kir potassium channel subunit expression in retinal glial cells: Implications for spatial potassium buffering. *Glia* **2002**, *39*, 292–303. [CrossRef] [PubMed]

13. Hibino, H.; Inanobe, A.; Furutani, K.; Murakami, S.; Findlay, I.A.N.; Kurachi, Y. Inwardly rectifying potassium channels: Their structure, function, and physiological roles. *Physiol. Rev.* **2010**, *90*, 291–366. [CrossRef] [PubMed]

14. Ulbricht, E.; Pannicke, T.; Hollborn, M.; Raap, M.; Goczalik, I.; Iandiev, I.; Härtig, W.; Uhlmann, S.; Wiedemann, P.; Reichenbach, A.; et al. Proliferative gliosis causes mislocation and inactivation of inwardly rectifying K+ (Kir) channels in rabbit retinal glial cells. *Exp. Eye Res.* **2008**, *86*, 305–313. [CrossRef] [PubMed]

15. Hibino, H.; Fujita, A.; Iwai, K.; Yamada, M.; Kurachi, Y. Differential assembly of inwardly rectifying K+ channel subunits, Kir4.1 and Kir5.1, in brain astrocytes. *J. Biol. Chem.* **2004**, *279*, 44065–44073. [CrossRef] [PubMed]

16. Ishii, M.; Fujita, A.; Iwai, K.; Kusaka, S.; Higashi, K.; Inanobe, A.; Hibino, H.; Kurachi, Y. Differential expression and distribution of Kir5.1 and Kir4.1 inwardly rectifying K+ channels in retina. *Am. J. Physiol. Cell Physiol.* **2003**, *285*, C260–C267. [CrossRef] [PubMed]

17. Lichter-Konecki, U.; Mangin, J.M.; Gordish-dressman, H.; Hoffman, E.P.; Gallo, V. Gene expression profiling of astrocytes from hyperammonemic mice reveals altered pathways for water and potassium homeostasis in vivo. *Glia* **2008**, *56*, 365–377. [CrossRef] [PubMed]

18. Mulkey, D.K.; Wenker, I.C. Astrocyte chemoreceptors: Mechanisms of H+ sensing by astrocytes in the retrotrapezoid nucleus and their possible contribution to respiratory drive. *Exp. Physiol.* **2011**, *96*, 400–406. [CrossRef] [PubMed]

19. Puissant, M.M.; Mouradian, G.C., Jr.; Liu, P.; Hodges, M.R. Identifying candidate genes that underlie cellular pH sensitivity in serotonin neurons using transcriptomics: A potential role for Kir5.1 channels. *Front. Cell. Neurosci.* **2017**, *11*, 34. [CrossRef] [PubMed]

20. Raap, M.; Biedermann, B.; Braun, P.; Milenkovic, I.; Skatchkov, S.N.; Bringmann, A.; Reichenbach, A. Diversity of Kir channel subunit mRNA expressed by retinal glial cells of the guinea-pig. *Neuroreport* **2002**, *13*, 1037–1040. [CrossRef] [PubMed]

21. Schirmer, L.; Srivastava, R.; Kalluri, S.R.; Böttinger, S.; Herwerth, M.; Carassiti, D.; Srivastava, B.; Gempt, J.; Schlegel, J.; Kuhlmann, T.; Korn, T. Differential loss of KIR4.1 immunoreactivity in multiple sclerosis lesions. *Ann. Neurol.* **2014**, *75*, 810–828. [CrossRef] [PubMed]

22. Pessia, M.; Imbrici, P.; D'Adamo, M.C.; Salvatore, L.; Tucker, S.J. Differential pH sensitivity of Kir4.1 and Kir4.2 potassium channels and their modulation by heteropolymerisation with Kir5.1. *J. Physiol.* **2001**, *532*, 359–367. [CrossRef] [PubMed]

23. Konstas, A.A.; Korbmacher, C.; Tucker, S.J. Identification of domains that control the heteromeric assembly of Kir5.1/Kir4.0 potassium channels. *Am. J. Physiol. Cell Physiol.* **2003**, *284*, C910–C917. [CrossRef] [PubMed]

24. Kofuji, P.; Ceelen, P.; Zahs, K.R.; Surbeck, L.W.; Lester, H.A.; Newman, E.A. Genetic inactivation of an inwardly rectifying potassium channel (Kir4.1 subunit) in mice: Phenotypic impact in retina. *J. Neurosci.* **2000**, *20*, 5733–5740. [CrossRef] [PubMed]

25. Greenwood, K.; Butt, A.M. Evidence that perinatal and adult NG2-glia are not conventional oligodendrocyte progenitors and do not depend on axons for their survival. *Mol. Cell. Neurosci.* **2003**, *23*, 544–558. [CrossRef]

26. Barlow, A.L.; MacLeod, A.; Noppen, S.; Sanderson, J.; Guérin, C.J. Colocalization analysis in fluorescence micrographs: Verification of a more accurate calculation of Pearson's correlation coefficient. *Microsc. Microanal.* **2010**, *16*, 710–724. [CrossRef] [PubMed]

27. Lorincz, A.; Nusser, Z. Specificity of immunoreactions: The importance of testing specificity in each method. *J. Neurosci.* **2008**, *28*, 9083–9086. [CrossRef] [PubMed]

28. Hawkins, V.; Butt, A. TASK-1 channels in oligodendrocytes: A role in ischemia mediated disruption. *Neurobiol. Dis.* **2013**, *55*, 87–94. [CrossRef] [PubMed]

29. Neusch, C.; Rozengurt, N.; Jacobs, R.E.; Lester, H.A.; Kofuji, P. Kir4.1 potassium channel subunit is crucial for oligodendrocyte development and in vivo myelination. *J. Neurosci.* **2013**, *21*, 5429–5438. [CrossRef]

30. Bay, V.; Butt, A.M. Relationship between glial potassium regulation and axon excitability: A role for glial Kir4.1 channels. *Glia* **2003**, *60*, 651–660. [CrossRef] [PubMed]

31. Derst, C.; Karschin, C.; Wischmeyer, E.; Hirsch, J.R.; Preisig-Müller, R.; Rajan, S.; Engel, H.; Grzeschik, K.; Daut, J.; Karschin, A. Genetic and functional linkage of Kir5.1 and Kir2.1 channel subunits. *FEBS Lett.* **2001**, *491*, 305–311. [CrossRef]

32. Mi, H.; Deerinck, T.J.; Jones, M.; Ellisman, M.H.; Schwarz, T.L. Inwardly rectifying K^+ channels that may participate in K+ buffering are localized in microvilli of Schwann cells. *J. Neurosci.* **1996**, *16*, 2421–2429. [CrossRef] [PubMed]

33. Fakler, B.; Schultz, J.H.; Yang, J.; Schulte, U.; Brandle, U.; Zenner, H.P.; Jan, L.Y.; Ruppersberg, J.P. Identification of a titratable lysine residue that determines sensitivity of kidney potassium channels (ROMK) to intracellular pH. *EMBO J.* **1996**, *15*, 4093–4099. [PubMed]

34. Seifert, G.; Hüttmann, K.; Binder, D.K.; Hartmann, C.; Wyczynski, A.; Neusch, C.; Steinhäuser, C. Analysis of astroglial K+ channel expression in the developing hippocampus reveals a predominant role of the Kir4.1 subunit. *J. Neurosci.* **2009**, *29*, 7474–7488. [CrossRef] [PubMed]

35. Heuser, K.; Eid, T.; Lauritzen, F.; Thoren, A.E.; Vindedal, G.F.; TaubÃll, E.; Gjerstad, L.; Spencer, D.D.; Ottersen, O.P.; Nagelhus, E.A.; et al. Loss of perivascular Kir4.1 potassium channels in the sclerotic hippocampus of patients with mesial temporal lobe epilepsy. *J. Neuropathol. Exp. Neurol.* **2012**, *71*, 814–825. [CrossRef] [PubMed]

36. Djukic, B.; Casper, K.B.; Philpot, B.D.; Chin, L.-S.; McCarthy, K.D. Conditional knock-out of Kir4.1 leads to glial membrane depolarization, inhibition of potassium and glutamate uptake, and enhanced short-term synaptic potentiation. *J. Neurosci.* **2007**, *27*, 11354–11365. [CrossRef] [PubMed]

37. Neusch, C.; Papadopoulos, N.; Muller, M.; Maletzki, I.; Winter, S.M.; Hirrlinger, J.; Handschuh, M.; Bahr, M.; Richter, D.W.; Kirchhoff, F.; et al. Lack of the Kir4.1 channel subunit abolishes K^+ buffering properties of astrocytes in the ventral respiratory group: Impact on extracellular K^+ regulation. *J. Neurophysiol.* **2006**, *95*, 1843–1852. [CrossRef] [PubMed]

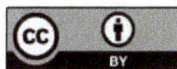

neuroglia

MDPI

Commentary

The History of the Decline and Fall of the Glial Numbers Legend

Alexei Verkhratsky [1,2,*] and Arthur M. Butt [3,*]

1   Faculty of Biology, Medicine and Health, University of Manchester, Manchester M13 9PT, UK
2   Center for Basic and Translational Neuroscience, Faculty of Health and Medical Sciences, University of Copenhagen, 2200 Copenhagen, Denmark
3   Institute of Biomedical and Biomolecular Sciences, School of Pharmacy and Biomedical Science, University of Portsmouth, Portsmouth PO1 2UP, UK
*   Correspondence: Alexej.Verkhratsky@manchester.ac.uk (A.V.); arthur.butt@port.ac.uk (A.M.B.)

Received: 2 July 2018; Accepted: 4 July 2018; Published: 17 July 2018

Abstract: In the field of neuroscience and, more specifically glial cell biology, one of the most fundamentally intriguing and enduring questions has been "how many neuronal cells—neurones and glia—are there in the human brain?". From the outset, the driving force behind this question was undoubtedly the scientific quest for knowledge of why humans are more intelligent than even our nearest relatives; the 'neuronal doctrine' dictated we must have more neurones than other animals. The early histological studies indicated a vast space between neurones that was filled by 'nervenkitt', later identified as neuroglia; arguably, this was the origin of the myth that glia massively outnumber neurones in the human brain. The myth eventually became embedded in ideology when later studies seemed to confirm that glia outnumber neurones in the human cortex—the seat of humanity—and that there was an inevitable rise in the glia-to-neurone ratio (GNR) as we climbed the evolutionary tree. This could be described as the 'glial doctrine'—that the rise of intelligence and the rise of glia go hand-in-hand. In many ways, the GNR became a mantra for working on glial cells at a time when the neuronal doctrine ruled the world. However, the work of Suzana Herculano-Houzel which she reviews in this first volume of *Neuroglia* has led the way in demonstrating that neurones and glia are almost equal in number in the human cortex and there is no inexorable phylogenetic rise in the GNR. In this commentary we chart the fall and decline of the mythology of the GNR.

Keywords: neuroglia; glia to neurone ratio; human brain; astrocytes

"The various models of worship which prevailed … were all considered by the people as equally true; by the philosopher as equally false"

Edward Gibbon (1776), *The Decline and Fall of the Roman Empire* Volume 1, Chapter 2.

One of the most enduring and fundamentally important misconceptions in neuroscience is the number of glial cells in the human brain, purportedly outnumbering neurones by a factor of 10 or even 50 [1–4]. Unfortunately, the notion of a glia-to-neurone ratio (GNR) in the human brain of 10 or more became 'general knowledge' and commonplace in glial literature over several decades. In a way, this myth became a cornerstone of glial research, and, regrettably, the authors of this commentary used the same statement in our textbook in 2007 [5]. Like other glial cell biologists before us, we fell into the trap of blind belief of the accepted doctrine. In our defence, we amended this error in our second, more comprehensive book on glial cell physiology and pathology [6]. What was most surprising to us was that the perception of the high GNR of the human brain was not based on direct counts and experimental observations; rather, it was the result of several conjectures based on limited observation. Interestingly, the very first calculation of GNR made in 1936 defined it as 1.5 [7], which is very far from subsequent speculations and very close to the numbers accepted today. The GNR legend was challenged only about a decade ago by the efforts of the Brazilian neuroanatomist Suzana Herculano-Houzel, who was armed with a powerful cell counting tool known as the 'isotropic fractionator' [8–11]. This technique counts numbers of cell nuclei from homogenised nervous tissue and was initially developed in the middle of 20th century [12–14], and subsequently greatly improved by Suzana Herculano-Houzel; she recalls seeing a paper from the 1970s on attempts to isolate DNA from whole brains and thought "don't count DNA, count nuclei!" This issue of *Neuroglia* contains a personal account of the dramatic history of glial numbers written by Suzana Herculano-Houzel [15].

The early concept of a high glial content of the human brain had wide repercussions. First and foremost, the high GNR of the human brain has been widely believed to reflect the evolutionary progress of the nervous system (this idea was initially suggested by Franz Nissl [16]), whereby the advance in glial numbers was considered to be directly linked to the rise in intelligence [17–19]. These ideas led to even further extremes, when some neuroscientists comprehended glia as the main element of information processing. The most outspoken was Robert Galambos who was convinced that neuroglia represent the primary seat of intelligence, and by extension 'humanity':

> Glia is … conceived as genetically charged to organize and program neuron activity so that the best interests of the organism will be served; the essential product of glia action is visualized to be what we call innate and acquired behavioural responses. In this scheme, neurons in large part merely execute the instructions glia give them. [20]

Galambos also authored the most popular misquote of Fritjof Nancen, "glia is the seat of intelligence as it increases in size from the lower to the higher forms of animal", which never occurred in Nancen's original book [21].

The evolutionary advance of glia is far more complicated, and humans are by no means in possession of the largest GNR (Figure 1). The number of glia varies substantially between different species and the GNR does not simply increase with increasing brain size. The nervous system of invertebrates has, as a rule, relatively smaller numbers of glial cells, with a GNR between 0.001 and 0.1 (56 glia per 302 neurones in *Caenorhabditis elegans* [22,23]; 10 glial cells per 400–700 neurones in every ganglion of the leech [24]; ~9000 glial cells per 90,000 neurones in the central nervous system (CNS) of Drosophila [25,26]). At the same time, the buccal ganglia of the great ramshorn snail *Planorbis corneus* contains 298 neurones and 391 glial cells [27], thus having a GNR of 1.3, very similar to that of humans. Similarly, in vertebrates there is no hard-and-fast increase in the GNR with increasing brain size; for example, in the cortex, the GNR is about 0.3–0.4 in rodents, ~1.1 in cat; ~1.2 in horse, 0.5–1.0 in rhesus monkey, 2.2 in Göttingen minipig, ~1.5 in humans, and as high as 4–8 in elephants and the fin whale [28–34]. The largest absolute number of glial cells has been counted in the neocortex of whales [31,35]; sterological cell counts in the neocortex of the long-finned pilot whale (*Globicephala melas*) brain determined there are approximately 37.2×10^9 neurons and 127×10^9 glial cells [35], and this gives a high GNR of 3.4 which is as expected from neuronal density [36]. In the human brain, the total number of glia is comparable (or even slightly less) with the number of neurones—i.e., the neuronal counts are in a range of ~80 billions—whereas neuroglia are ~60 billions with substantial regional differences. However, it should be noted that the variance in numbers is remarkably high, with numbers of neurones in the neocortex, for example, varying between 20 and 30 billions in cognitively preserved individuals [37]. Remarkably, when compared to the evolutionary new brain, the more primitive parts of the human brain have a higher proportion of neuroglia, with a GNR approaching 7–10 in the brainstem, or even more according to some studies [10,38]; very recent observations, using both stereology and isotropic fractionation, gave a GNR of ~5 in the spinal cord of cynomolgus monkey and almost 7 in humans [39]. These trends argue against the concept that a high GNR reflects evolutionary advance and increased intelligence. Nonetheless, it is important to be aware that evolution brought with it substantial changes in the morphology and complexity of astroglia in the human cortex, which also contains several idiosyncratic types of glial cell [40–42]. However, astrocyte three-dimensional morphology has been systematically studied in too few species so far and none in brains larger than humans. How large and complex astrocytes of whales might be remains unknown. Possibly (though not necessarily), the differences between astrocytes are related to brain size, not clade, but that is a different story.

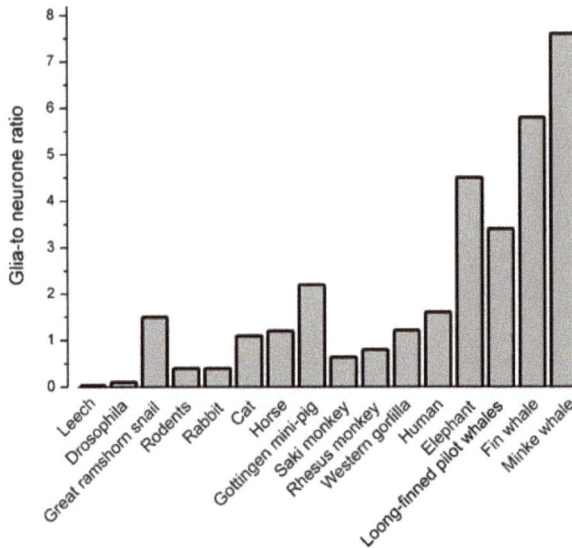

Figure 1. Glia-to-neurone ratio in invertebrates and vertebrates. The glia-to-neurone ratio (GNR) is not clearly related to phylogeny; the great ramshorn snail has a GNR equivalent to the human cortex, and the GNR is over five-times greater in the Minke whale.

Another unexpected consequence of the erroneous perceptions arising from the GNR in the human brain concerns the relative number of the main glial cell types—astrocytes, oligodendrocytes and microglia. Again, the numerical prevalence of astroglia is repeatedly stated in many papers, but this appears to be based on no observations whatsoever (see Table 6 in [10]). Seemingly the most numerous glia are oligodendrocytes (40–60%), with astrocytes accounting for 20–40% and microglia for ~10%, although there is of course considerable variability between brain regions, developmental stage and species. For example, in area 17 of young monkeys, astrocytes account for 40% of total glia, oligodendrocytes for 53% and microglia for ~7%. In cortical layers 1 to 3 of adult monkey astrocytes were calculated at 57%, oligodendrocytes at 36% and microglia at 7%, whereas in the layer 4 (which has higher degree of myelination) 30% of glia are astrocytes, 62% are oligodendroglia and the remaining 8% are microglia [43].

In conclusion, legends, myths and superstitions are arguably the most long-lasting and resilient forms of conserving and passing on false knowledge. Without doubt, this has greatly affected the evolution of humanity and continues to shape the progress of natural science. It is hoped that the work highlighted in this commentary and Suzana Herculano-Houzel's review article [15] will help reverse one of the most enduring misconceptions that glial cells massively outnumber neurones in the human brain. We opened this commentary with a quote from Gibbon's *The Decline and Fall of the Roman Empire*; we think it is fitting to end with a quote from Darwin on the vicissitudes of ignorance and false knowledge.

Neuroglia **2018**, *1*

"Ignorance more frequently begets confidence than does knowledge: it is those who know little, and not those who know much, who so positively assert that this or that problem will never be solved by science.".

Charles Darwin (1871), *The Descent of Man*, Volume 1 (Introduction)

Author Contributions: All authors participated equally in writing this commentary.

Conflicts of Interest: The authors declare no conflict of interest.

References

1. Hyden, H. Dynamic aspects of the neuron-glia relationship—A study with microchemical methods. In *The Neuron*; Hyden, H., Ed.; Elsevier: Amsterdam, The Netherlands, 1967; pp. 179–217.
2. Kandel, E.R.; Schwartz, J.H.; Jessell, T.M. *Principles of Neural Science*; McGrawhill: New York, NY, USA, 2000.
3. Bear, M.F.; Connors, B.W.; Paradiso, M.A. *Exploring the Brain*; Lippincott Williams & Wilkins: Philadelphia, PA, USA, 2007.
4. Darlington, C.L. *The Female Brain*; CRC Press: Boca Raton, FL, USA, 2009.
5. Verkhratsky, A.; Butt, A. *Glial Neurobiology: A Textbook*; John Wiley & Sons: Chichester, UK, 2007.
6. Verkhratsky, A.; Butt, A.M. *Glial Physiology and Pathophysiology*; Wiley-Blackwell: Chichester, UK, 2013; p. 560.
7. Mühlmann, M. About the question of glia formation. Zur neurogliabildungsfrage. *Beitr. Pathol. Anat. Allg. Pathol.* **1936**, *96*, 361–374.
8. Herculano-Houzel, S.; Lent, R. Isotropic fractionator: A simple, rapid method for the quantification of total cell and neuron numbers in the brain. *J. Neurosci.* **2005**, *25*, 2518–2521. [CrossRef] [PubMed]
9. Azevedo, F.A.; Carvalho, L.R.; Grinberg, L.T.; Farfel, J.M.; Ferretti, R.E.; Leite, R.E.; Jacob Filho, W.; Lent, R.; Herculano-Houzel, S. Equal numbers of neuronal and nonneuronal cells make the human brain an isometrically scaled-up primate brain. *J. Comp. Neurol.* **2009**, *513*, 532–541. [CrossRef] [PubMed]
10. Von Bartheld, C.S.; Bahney, J.; Herculano-Houzel, S. The search for true numbers of neurons and glial cells in the human brain: A review of 150 years of cell counting. *J. Comp. Neurol.* **2016**, *524*, 3865–3895. [CrossRef] [PubMed]
11. Andrade-Moraes, C.H.; Oliveira-Pinto, A.V.; Castro-Fonseca, E.; da Silva, C.G.; Guimaraes, D.M.; Szczupak, D.; Parente-Bruno, D.R.; Carvalho, L.R.; Polichiso, L.; Gomes, B.V.; et al. Cell number changes in Alzheimer's disease relate to dementia, not to plaques and tangles. *Brain* **2013**, *136*, 3738–3752. [CrossRef] [PubMed]
12. Nurnberger, J.I.; Gordon, M.W. The cell density of neural tissues: Direct counting method and possible applications as a biologic referent. *Prog. Neurobiol.* **1957**, *2*, 100–128. [PubMed]
13. Brizzee, K.R.; Vogt, J.; Kharetchko, X. Postnatal changes in glia/neuron index with a comparison of methods of cell enumeration in the white rat. *Prog. Brain Res.* **1964**, *4*, 136–149.
14. Zamenhof, S. Final number of purkinje and other large cells in the chick cerebellum influenced by incubation temperatures during their proliferation. *Brain Res.* **1976**, *109*, 392–394. [CrossRef]
15. Herculano-Houzel, S.; Dos Santos, S. You don't mess with the glia. *Neuroglia* **2018**, *1*, 13.
16. Nissl, F. Nervenzellen und graue substanz. *Munch. Med. Wochenschr.* **1898**, *45*, 988–992.
17. Friede, R. Der quantitative anteil der glia and der cortexentwicklung. *Acta Anat. (Basel)* **1954**, *20*, 290–296. [CrossRef] [PubMed]
18. Pfrieger, F.W.; Barres, B.A. What the fly's glia tell the fly's brain. *Cell* **1995**, *83*, 671–674. [CrossRef]
19. Fields, R.D. *The Other Brain*; Simon & Schuster: New York, NY, USA, 2009.
20. Galambos, R. A glia-neural theory of brain function. *Proc. Natl. Acad. Sci. USA* **1961**, *47*, 129–136. [CrossRef] [PubMed]
21. Nansen, F. *The Structure and Combination of the Histological Elements of the Central Nervous System*; John Grieg: Bergen, Norway, 1886.
22. Stout, R.F., Jr.; Verkhratsky, A.; Parpura, V. Caenorhabditis elegans glia modulate neuronal activity and behavior. *Front. Cell. Neurosci.* **2014**, *8*, 67. [CrossRef] [PubMed]
23. Oikonomou, G.; Shaham, S. The glia of caenorhabditis elegans. *Glia* **2011**, *59*, 1253–1263. [CrossRef] [PubMed]

24. Deitmer, J.W.; Rose, C.R.; Munsch, T.; Schmidt, J.; Nett, W.; Schneider, H.P.; Lohr, C. Leech giant glial cell: Functional role in a simple nervous system. *Glia* **1999**, *28*, 175–182. [CrossRef]

25. Edwards, T.N.; Meinertzhagen, I.A. The functional organisation of glia in the adult brain of Drosophila and other insects. *Prog. Neurobiol.* **2010**, *90*, 471–497. [CrossRef] [PubMed]

26. Kremer, M.C.; Jung, C.; Batelli, S.; Rubin, G.M.; Gaul, U. The glia of the adult Drosophila nervous system. *Glia* **2017**, *65*, 606–638. [CrossRef] [PubMed]

27. Pentreath, V.W.; Radojcic, T.; Seal, L.H.; Winstanley, E.K. The glial cells and glia-neuron relations in the buccal ganglia of *Planorbis corneus* (L.): Cytological, qualitative and quantitative changes during growth and ageing. *Philos. Trans. R. Soc. Lond. B Biol. Sci.* **1985**, *307*, 399–455. [CrossRef] [PubMed]

28. Christensen, J.R.; Larsen, K.B.; Lisanby, S.H.; Scalia, J.; Arango, V.; Dwork, A.J.; Pakkenberg, B. Neocortical and hippocampal neuron and glial cell numbers in the rhesus monkey. *Anat. Rec. (Hoboken)* **2007**, *290*, 330–340. [CrossRef] [PubMed]

29. Lidow, M.S.; Song, Z.M. Primates exposed to cocaine in utero display reduced density and number of cerebral cortical neurons. *J. Comp. Neurol.* **2001**, *435*, 263–275. [CrossRef] [PubMed]

30. Pakkenberg, B.; Gundersen, H.J. Neocortical neuron number in humans: Effect of sex and age. *J. Comp. Neurol.* **1997**, *384*, 312–320. [CrossRef]

31. Eriksen, N.; Pakkenberg, B. Total neocortical cell number in the mysticete brain. *Anat. Rec. (Hoboken)* **2007**, *290*, 83–95. [CrossRef] [PubMed]

32. Hawkins, A.; Olszewski, J. Glia/nerve cell index for cortex of the whale. *Science* **1957**, *126*, 76–77. [CrossRef] [PubMed]

33. Jelsing, J.; Nielsen, R.; Olsen, A.K.; Grand, N.; Hemmingsen, R.; Pakkenberg, B. The postnatal development of neocortical neurons and glial cells in the gottingen minipig and the domestic pig brain. *J. Exp. Biol.* **2006**, *209*, 1454–1462. [CrossRef] [PubMed]

34. Tower, D.B. Structural and functional organization of mammalian cerebral cortex; the correlation of neurone density with brain size; cortical neurone density in the fin whale (*Balaenoptera Physalus* L.) with a note on the cortical neurone density in the indian elephant. *J. Comp. Neurol.* **1954**, *101*, 19–51. [CrossRef] [PubMed]

35. Mortensen, H.S.; Pakkenberg, B.; Dam, M.; Dietz, R.; Sonne, C.; Mikkelsen, B.; Eriksen, N. Quantitative relationships in delphinid neocortex. *Front. Neuroanat.* **2014**, *8*, 132. [CrossRef] [PubMed]

36. Kazu, R.S.; Maldonado, J.; Mota, B.; Manger, P.R.; Herculano-Houzel, S. Cellular scaling rules for the brain of Artiodactyla include a highly folded cortex with few neurons. *Front. Neuroanat.* **2014**, *8*, 128. [CrossRef] [PubMed]

37. Pelvig, D.P.; Pakkenberg, H.; Stark, A.K.; Pakkenberg, B. Neocortical glial cell numbers in human brains. *Neurobiol. Aging* **2008**, *29*, 1754–1762. [CrossRef] [PubMed]

38. Pakkenberg, B.; Gundersen, H.J. Total number of neurons and glial cells in human brain nuclei estimated by the disector and the fractionator. *J. Microsc.* **1988**, *150*, 1–20. [CrossRef] [PubMed]

39. Bahney, J.; von Bartheld, C.S. The cellular composition and glia-neuron ratio in the spinal cord of a human and a nonhuman primate: Comparison with other species and brain regions. *Anat. Rec. (Hoboken)* **2018**, *301*, 697–710. [CrossRef] [PubMed]

40. Verkhratsky, A.; Oberheim Bush, N.A.; Nedergaard, M.; Butt, A. The special case of human astrocytes. *Neuroglia* **2018**, *1*, 4. [CrossRef]

41. Oberheim, N.A.; Takano, T.; Han, X.; He, W.; Lin, J.H.; Wang, F.; Xu, Q.; Wyatt, J.D.; Pilcher, W.; Ojemann, J.G.; et al. Uniquely hominid features of adult human astrocytes. *J. Neurosci.* **2009**, *29*, 3276–3287. [CrossRef] [PubMed]

42. Verkhratsky, A.; Nedergaard, M. Physiology of astroglia. *Physiol. Rev.* **2018**, *98*, 239–389. [CrossRef] [PubMed]

43. Peters, A.; Verderosa, A.; Sethares, C. The neuroglial population in the primary visual cortex of the aging rhesus monkey. *Glia* **2008**, *56*, 1151–1161. [CrossRef] [PubMed]

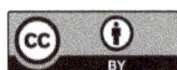

neuroglia

MDPI

Review
You Do Not Mess with the Glia

Suzana Herculano-Houzel [1,2,3,]* and Sandra E. Dos Santos [1]

[1] Department of Psychology, Vanderbilt University, Nashville, TN 37240, USA;
    sandra.e.dos.santos@vanderbilt.edu
[2] Department of Biological Sciences, Vanderbilt University, Nashville, TN 37240, USA
[3] Vanderbilt Brain Institute, Vanderbilt University, Nashville, TN 37240-7817, USA
*   Correspondence: suzana.herculano@vanderbilt.edu

Received: 8 June 2018; Accepted: 3 July 2018; Published: 17 July 2018

Abstract: Vertebrate neurons are enormously variable in morphology and distribution. While different glial cell types do exist, they are much less diverse than neurons. Over the last decade, we have conducted quantitative studies of the absolute numbers, densities, and proportions at which non-neuronal cells occur in relation to neurons. These studies have advanced the notion that glial cells are much more constrained than neurons in how much they can vary in both development and evolution. Recent evidence from studies on gene expression profiles that characterize glial cells—in the context of progressive epigenetic changes in chromatin during morphogenesis—supports the notion of constrained variation of glial cells in development and evolution, and points to the possibility that this constraint is related to the late differentiation of the various glial cell types. Whether restricted variation is a biological given (a simple consequence of late glial cell differentiation) or a physiological constraint (because, well, you do not mess with the glia without consequences that compromise brain function to the point of rendering those changes unviable), we predict that the restricted variation in size and distribution of glial cells has important consequences for neural tissue function that is aligned with their many fundamental roles being uncovered.

Keywords: evolution; glia/neuron ratio; glial density; cell size

---

1. Introduction

The glue that keeps together the tendinous strings that permeate the body: that is a loose but literal translation of the term Neuroglia. Virchow's original reference to connecting material (*Nervenkitt*), which he considered to be a true connective tissue (*Zwischenmasse*), is now known to be an underrepresentation of the role of these cells in nervous tissue [1,2]. To be fair, nerve cells have also kept their designation as "neurons", even though both terms—one from the Latin, *nervus*, the other from the Greek, *neuron*—also grossly misrepresent what these cells actually are or do, for they literally mean tendon, cable, or sinew.

That both neurons and glia are still named after things they are not is a useful reminder of the achievements of scientific research. Persistence and inquisitiveness did bring the field a long way in understanding the actual roles of neurons and glial cells in animals. However, one simple, repeated observation could, or should, have raised much earlier suspicions of a fundamental role of glial cells in the nervous system: that every animal known to have neurons that are well differentiated from the ectoderm also has glial cells of some sort [3]. No matter what criteria are used to define glia, whatever their evolutionary or developmental origins, whether conserved across all animal clades, the fact remains that neurons do not come alone.

The developmental mechanisms that originate glial cells do appear to be shared and conserved across vertebrates, or even invertebrates, going back at least 500 million years [3–7]. Moreover, across a wide range of mammalian species, new evidence indicates that the mechanisms that regulate glial cell diversity and how they are added to brain tissue are indeed highly conserved in evolution.

This conservation is the focus of this review: the remarkable constancy in some key characteristics regarding mammalian glial cells points to either strict biological constraints or the fundamental physical properties of these cells. In the face of abundant neuronal diversity, it becomes clear that, whatever the source of glial constancy, nature has not been able to mess with the glia.

1.1. The More Some Things Change, the More Others Stay the Same

In its simplest definition, biological evolution means change in the characteristics of life over geological time. Whereas it was once proposed that all nervous systems were derived by multiple, independent alterations starting from a single ancestral form [8–10], it now appears more likely that nervous systems organized multiple times independently during animal evolution [11,12]. A consequence of great relevance to comparative studies of brain tissue organization is that the two most widely used animal models for research—the fruit fly and the lab mouse—do not share homologous nervous systems derived from a common urbilaterian ancestor [12]. The lack of homology is the case even if many similar genes are expressed during the development of both vertebrates and invertebrates, which is to be expected given that the basic genetic toolkit of all animals appears to be shared from Cambrian ancestors [12].

If there is not a universal layout of the nervous system from which all versions derived, could they all still share homologous cell types? That is, are glia and neurons ancient cell types that predate animal diversity, and are they formed via the same, conserved developmental pathways in the various vertebrate and invertebrate species? Phylogenetic comparisons indicate that the machinery that allows synaptic transmission and gliotransmission did appear before the differentiation of specialized excitable cells in animals that employ them in particular ways [13]. Glial cells, and also neurons, do express similar markers across multiple vertebrate and invertebrate species, and radial glia-like cells are found in both protostomes and deuterostomes [14]. However, until phylogenomic analyses are performed systematically in a large enough number of species covering all major phyla, it is too early to draw a conclusion on whether all neurons, all radial glial types, and all myelinating cells share a conserved developmental program.

All vertebrates, however, do share a common ancestor exclusive to all of them [15–19], and, therefore, their nervous systems can be safely considered homologous in their organization and in the origin of the cell types that compose them, especially amongst amniotes (mammals and reptiles, including birds). That does not mean that the nervous systems of amniotes are identical; although most glutamatergic neurons are generated from radial progenitors through similar cascades of gene expression in all species examined, comparative studies of the composition of brain tissue across vertebrate species indicate that some neuronal phenotypes are particular to some clades [20]. Sauropsids (avian and non-avian reptiles), for instance, do not have commissural neurons in their cortex or pallium; those neurons are characteristic of placental mammals [21]. Callosal neurons, like other upper-layer neurons, presumably appeared during mammalian evolution with the diversification of transcription factors expressed in newly differentiated neurons in development [20].

Neuronal cell types are, indeed, enormously diverse across brain structures and species in vertebrates, as illustrated in Figure 1. The much wider variation of neuronal compared to glial cell phenotypes is evident in a basic feature of nervous tissue: neurons are not distributed evenly in the tissue, instead agglomerated in clumps (nuclei), layers (cortices), or lattices (reticular formations), in which they form directional circuits. On the other hand, glial cells of different types are distributed much more homogeneously in nervous tissue and generate signals that remain local or spread little and concentrically through gap junctions [22]. Examples of clustering of neuronal, but not glial, cells are shown in Figure 2. Within glial networks, the component cells are considered equivalent in form and function; within neuronal networks, the component cells typically differ in chemical phenotype, electrophysiological properties, and connectivity patterns, endowing each part of the network with a different function.

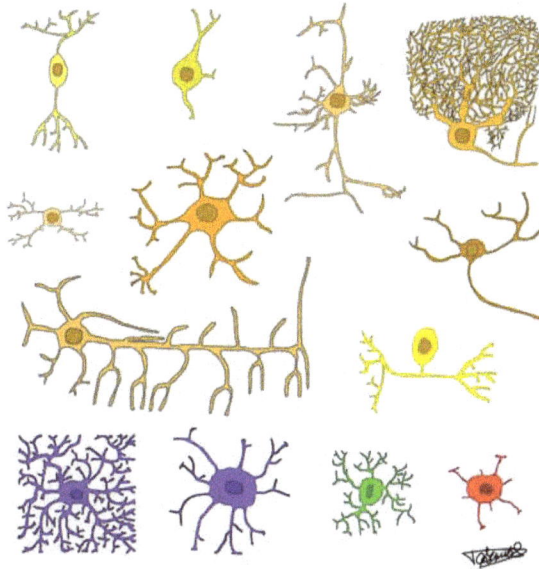

Figure 1. Morphological neuronal types are more numerous than morphological glial cell types. Non-exhaustive representations of some morphological neuronal types in shades of yellow-orange (top three rows) and glial cells (bottom row) in purple, green, and red. First row, left to right: bipolar cell, short axon cell, pyramidal cell, Purkinje cell. Second row, left to right: amacrine cell, multipolar/motor cell, granule cell. Third row, left to right: basket cell, unipolar cell. Bottom row, left to right: protoplasmic astrocyte, like those found in grey matter; fibrous astrocyte, like those found in white matter; microglia; oligodendrocyte. Drawings inspired by those of Ramon y Cajal and del Rio-Hortega [23–26].

Indeed, neurons can express multiple combinations of excitatory, inhibitory, or modulatory transmitters, whereas astrocyte cells appear to use mostly glutamate, purines, and D-serine [27]. It remains possible that interest in gliotransmission has been so recent that not many substances have been identified as mediators (just like there once were only two known neurotransmitters, acetylcholine and noradrenaline), but given the wide range of tools and resources available now to glia-minded researchers, a much greater degree of diversity should have been unveiled by now, if it existed. Similarly, while neurons may be large and highly branched with specifically targeted or widely diffuse projections, small with only local projections, or anything between those extremes, with both dendrites and axons highly intertwined with those of other neurons, glial cells, whether astrocytes, oligodendrocytes, or microglial in type, tend to have many, but only local, branches that form bricks that subdivide the parenchyma into mostly non-overlapping territories or tiles [28] (Figure 1). Such territories are consistent with known contact-mediated inhibition of proliferation of glial cell precursors [29].

Although cell type classification is currently a much-debated issue, recent gene expression-based studies of the cell types found in brain tissue confirm that neuronal cell type diversity, gauged by unsupervised clustering analysis of single-cell transcriptomics, is much greater than that of non-neuronal cell types [30]. Using single-cell RNA sequencing (RNAseq), such studies have found that individual neurons in the mouse cerebral cortex and hippocampus express on average 4-fold more RNA and almost twice as many different genes than non-neuronal cells [31]. These studies have also identified various classes of neuronal cell types based on the clusters of co-expressed genes, which have been uncovered across thousands of cells examined. While the number of brain structures analyzed is still small, and so far, has been restricted to mouse, human, and zebrafish [32–34], a clear pattern already emerges of many more neuronal than non-neuronal cell types. Whereas neurons in mouse primary visual cortex can be subdivided into 42 subtypes, grouped as either excitatory (19 subtypes) or inhibitory neurons (23 subtypes), the number of non-neuronal cell subtypes in the same cortex is only seven, comprising a single type of astrocyte, a single type of oligodendrocyte (which may be subdivided in three stages of differentiation), a single type of microglial cell, and two types of vasculature-associated cells [31] (Figure 3). While that study was biased towards neurons, an unbiased single-cell RNAseq study in mouse somatosensory cortex and hippocampus found similar results: 13 subtypes of pyramidal neurons, 16 subtypes of interneurons, but only 2 subtypes of astrocytes, 1 subtype of microglia, and 6 subtypes of oligodendrocytes that actually correspond to different maturation stages, so are not true cell subtypes [32]. That study confirmed the finding that individual neurons contain more RNA than glia, and a larger number of detectable genes [32]. Even in the juvenile zebrafish brain, as many as 45 neuronal subtypes were identified, but only 3 oligodendrocyte and 1 microglial subtype(s) [34]. Having highly diverse neuronal cell types but very few glial cell types is thus a feature of both fish and mammals.

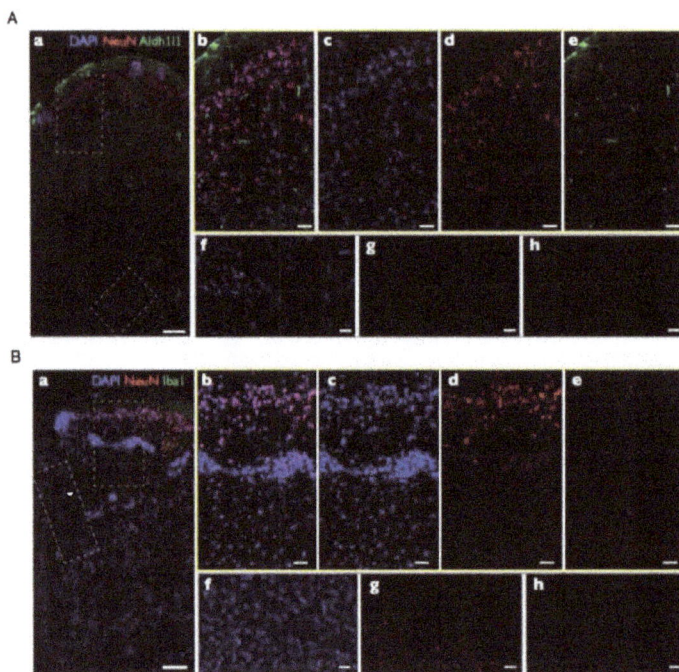

Figure 2. Homogeneous distribution of glial cells, but not neurons, across the cerebral cortex. (**A**) Neuronal nuclei (NeuN) and aldehyde dehydrogenase 1 family member L1 (Aldh1l1) immunoreactivity in the mouse cerebral cortex are shown at 63× magnification with all cells stained with 4′,6-diamidino-2-phenylindole (DAPI) (**c,f**), neurons stained for NeuN in red (**d,g**), astrocytes stained for Aldh1l1 in green (**e,h**), and both labels merged in (**a,b**). Inserts in (**a**) are enlarged in (**b**) and (**f**) and illustrate a portion of the grey matter (**b–e**) and of the white matter (**f–h**); (**B**) NeuN and ionized calcium-binding adapter molecule 1 (Iba1) immunoreactivity in the mouse cerebral cortex are shown at 63× magnification with all cells stained with DAPI (**c,f**), neurons stained for NeuN in red (**d,g**), microglia stained for Iba1 in green (**e,h**), and both labels merged in (**a,b**). Inserts in (**a**) are enlarged in (**b–e**) and (**f–h**) and illustrate a portion of the grey and white matter, respectively. Scale bars: 150 μm (**a** in **A** and **B**), 50 μm (**b–h** in **A** and **B**).

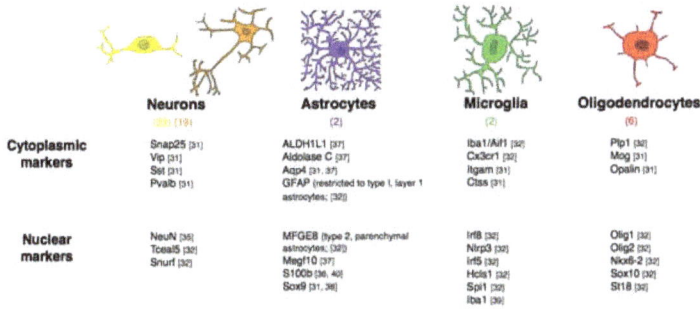

	Neurons	Astrocytes	Microglia	Oligodendrocytes
	(18) [18]	(2)	(2)	(6)
Cytoplasmic markers	Snap25 [31] Vip [31] Sst [31] Pvalb [31]	ALDH1L1 [37] Aldolase C [37] Aqp4 [31, 37] GFAP (restricted to type I, layer 1 astrocytes; [32])	Iba1/Aif1 [32] Cx3cr1 [32] Itgam [31] Ctss [31]	Plp1 [32] Mog [31] Opalin [31]
Nuclear markers	NeuN [35] Tceal5 [32] Snurf [32]	MFGE8 (type 2, parenchymal astrocytes; [32]) Megf10 [37] S100b [36, 40] Sox9 [31, 38]	Irf8 [32] Nlrp3 [32] Irf5 [32] Hcls1 [32] Spi1 [32] Iba1 [39]	Olig1 [32] Olig2 [32] Nkx6-2 [32] Sox10 [32] St18 [32]

Figure 3. Single-cell transcriptomics identify many clusters of interneurons and of excitatory neurons, but only a few glial cell subtypes. Numbers of cell subtypes in each cluster are indicated in parentheses. Oligodendrocyte subtypes appear to be different maturation stages along the same lineage. A non-exhaustive list of specific cytoplasmic and nuclear markers is provided for neurons and each glial cell type. Data from [31,32,35–40]. Snap25: Synaptosomal-associated protein 25; Vip: Vasoactive intestinal peptide; Sst: Neuropeptide somatostatin; Pvalb: Parvalbumin; ALDH1L1: Aldehyde dehydrogenase 1 family member L1; Aqp4: Aquaporin-4; GFAP: Glial fibrillary acidic protein; Cx3cr1: Chemokine (C-X3-C motif) receptor 1; Itgam: Integrin subunit alpha M; Ctss: Cathepsin S; Plp1: Proteolipid protein 1; Mog: Myelin oligodendrocyte glycoprotein; Opalin: Oligodendrocytic myelin paranodal and inner loop protein; NeuN: Neuronal nuclei; Tceal5: Transcription elongation factor A like 5; Snurf: SNRPN upstream reading frame; MFGE8: Milk fat globule-EGF factor 8 protein; Megf10: Multiple EGF like domains 10; S100b: S100 calcium binding protein B; Sox9: SRY (sex determining region Y)- box 9; Irf8: Interferon regulatory factor 8; Nlrp3: NLR family pyrin domain containing 3; Irf5: Interferon regulatory factor 5; Hcls1: Hematopoietic cell-specific Lyn substrate 1; Spi1: Spi-1 proto-oncogene; Iba1: Ionized calcium binding adaptor molecule 1; Olig1: Oligodendrocyte transcription factor 1; Olig2: : Oligodendrocyte transcription factor 2; Nkx6-2: NK6 homeobox 2; Sox10: SRY (sex determining region Y)- box 10; St18: Suppression of tumorigenicity 18.

Gene expression-based estimates of the high diversity of neuronal cell types have been confirmed by more complete analyses of combined morphological, functional, and biochemical types of interneurons [41]. Although some studies have preferentially targeted neuronal cell types [31,33], others have aimed at being at least semiquantitative, capturing the proportions of cells found in the tissue examined, as discussed below [32,34]. While these studies are powerful in the depth and breadth of single-cell transcriptomic analysis, they will probably remain limited to mouse, rat, zebrafish, or human brains, for practical reasons, since the current requirement for fresh, unfixed tissue means that the tissue donor must be alive during tissue collection (but see below). Still, the rising evidence already indicates that, at least across vertebrates, neurons must have been free to change and diverge into multiple phenotypes as brains evolved, whereas glial cells have been more restricted.

1.2. Quantitative Neuroanatomy: Counting Cells by Turning Brains into Soup

Maybe neuronal cell types were most numerous, but non-neuronal cells still outnumbered neurons as a whole—or so it was long stated in the literature [42]. For a couple of decades, scientists and journalists could get away with unreferenced claims, typically in the opening lines of original papers and reviews, that glial cells as a whole, or astrocytes in particular, are the most common cell type in the brain [43–47]. That those claims made it through peer review and editorial processes is a testament to how widely they were believed to represent actual facts—or to extoll the virtues of the underestimated other cells of the nervous system. The view that glial cells far outnumbered neurons was found in one of the most important and influential modern textbooks [48] and maintained, in a toned-down but still incorrect version, in the most recent 5th edition [49].

The underlying problem was that, in a scientific game of telephone, glia/neuron ratios in a few brain structures had been mistaken as representative of the whole human brain [42]. While quantitative data to the contrary were not abundant for a long time, they certainly existed, and not just in the human brain. For instance, a compilation of estimates of neuronal and glial cell density available in the cerebral cortex of mammalian species showed that those densities were clearly in the same range, with no obvious preponderance of glial cells [50], and that glial cell densities were quite stable across species [51]. Even Reinhard Friede's first (incorrect) description that there were more glial cells per neuron in more advanced species still listed only fewer than two glial cells per neuron in the human cerebral cortex [52].

Over the last 12 years, we and our collaborators have generated a wealth of data on the numbers of neuronal and non-neuronal cells that compose brain structures in over 50 species of mammals [53–64]. Our systematic approach to determine the cellular composition of brain structures in a manner that was readily comparable across species, using reproducible dissection criteria, employed a quantitative technique that we developed—the isotropic fractionator [65]. This method consists in first dissolving dissected, fixed regions of interest into a soup of free-floating cell nuclei, whose density can be quickly determined in a cell-counting chamber under a fluorescence microscope. Multiplying the density of nuclei in suspension by the volume of the suspension yields the total number of nuclei in the original structure, and, therefore, the total number of cells (assuming that mammalian brain cells have one and only one nucleus per cell). Finally, morphological criteria or immunocytochemical markers, such as the universal neuronal nuclear marker NeuN [35], can be used to determine the proportion of nuclei that belong to particular cell types. Importantly, this cell quantification technique has been found by three independent groups to yield results that are comparable to those obtained with unbiased stereology, but are much faster to obtain and far less prone to user error and undersampling [66–68]. The consistency of the approach and technique across studies allowed us to collect data that could be compared systematically across structures in individual brains; across individuals of the same species; across species within a clade; across mammalian clades (Figure 4); and even across mammals, birds, and non-avian reptiles [53–64,69–71]. While published results have so far been limited to numbers of neuronal and non-neuronal cells, one advantage of the isotropic fractionator is that, because all tissue heterogeneities in cell distribution are literally dissolved, only very small samples are required for counting, which allows for storage of the remaining suspension at $-20\,^{\circ}\text{C}$ for later studies employing new markers or morphological criteria [65]. Because the cell cytoplasm is lost, counting specific cell types in this way requires markers expressed in the cell nucleus. However, the growing wealth of single-cell transcriptomic data has been rapidly providing cell type-specific markers that can be used for this purpose in our stored collection of processed brain samples, which will be used as we are able to validate them as reliable, cell type-specific, and universal markers across species and clades (see below).

So far, we have defined neurons as nuclei (confirmed by compatible size, shape, and presence of 4',6-diamidino-2-phenylindole (DAPI)-stained DNA) that express NeuN [72], and non-neuronal or other cells as all remaining nuclei, by exclusion of the NeuN-expressing fraction. This procedure leaves no cell unaccounted for, that is, the sum of NeuN-positive and -negative nuclei is the total number of nuclei, and therefore of cells, in the tissue of origin. While a few neuronal cell subtypes are known to not express NeuN, such as photoreceptors, Purkinje cells, mitral cells, and some hypothalamic neurons [35], those are such a small minority amongst all cells that, for the purposes herein of reporting and comparing total numbers in different structures and species, any misrepresentation of NeuN-negative neurons as non-neuronal cells can be considered negligible.

Dividing the total number of neuronal and other cells by the mass of the dissected structure of origin yields densities of neurons and other cells, respectively, expressed as number of cells per milligram of tissue. If brain tissue were made of a single type of cell, then cell density, even though calculated as number of nuclei per volume or mass, would mathematically equal the inverse of average cell size (including soma, all dendrites, all axonal arbors, and the enveloping extracellular space). The advantage of using cell densities over cell sizes is that the former are much more tractable experimentally, because even if cell integrity is, by definition, lost in our method, the number of nuclei per mass of original tissue amounts to the density of cells that composed that tissue. In contrast, measuring full three-dimensional (3D) cell size directly is a much more complicated and still impractical endeavor.

With tissue defined as being composed of neuronal and non-neuronal cells, the relationship between density and average cell size for each of the two classes of cells depends on the proportion of tissue mass that is occupied by each. Using a simple mathematical model of how densities relate to masses in this case, and building on the finding that densities of non-neuronal cells are much less variable than neuronal densities (see below), we were able to estimate that the average volume of non-neuronal cells indeed is proportional to the inverse of non-neuronal cell densities across mammalian brain structures and species [73] (see below).

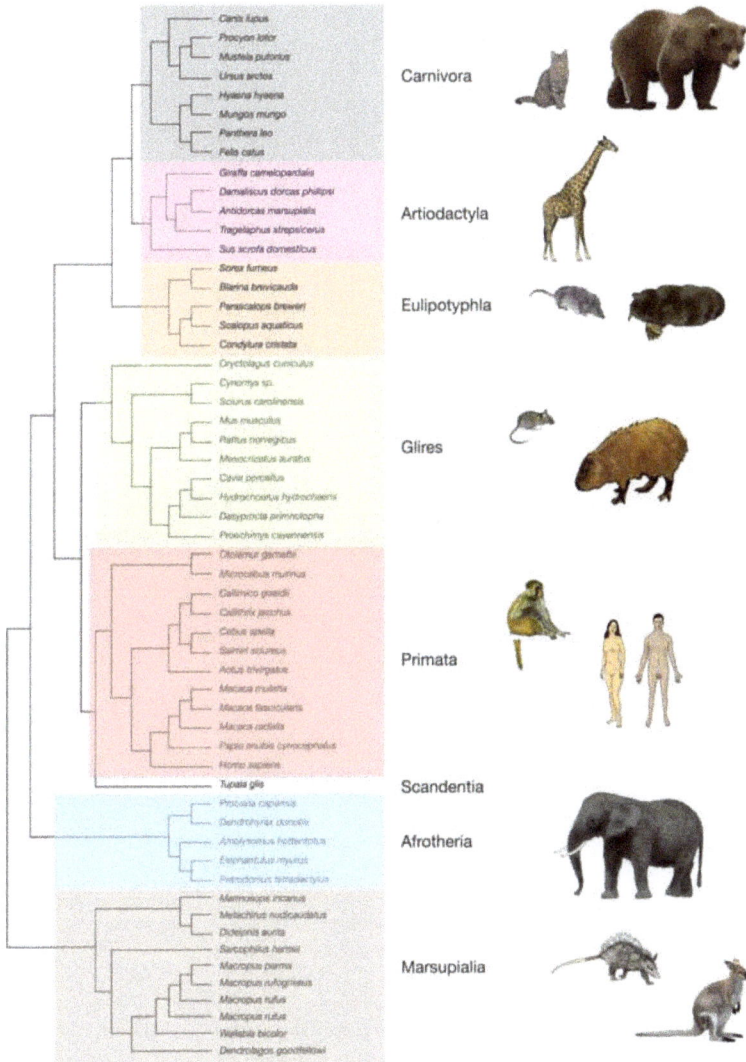

Figure 4. Phylogeny of the mammalian species for which numbers of neuronal and non-neuronal cells presented in this review have been reported. Clades are color-coded similarly in all figures. Drawings by Lorena Kaz.

2. Neurons Are Highly Variable in Density; Other Cells, Not So Much

Although several other groups have published independent, isolated estimates of cell densities using other methods in the same period, all data reported heretofore are limited to those acquired by our group and collaborators using the isotropic fractionator and consistent anatomical criteria, which ensure that all data are directly comparable across brain structures in all species indicated in Figure 4. In all of our studies, cerebral cortex includes the hippocampus, all cortex lateral to the rhinal sulcus, and the underlying subcortical white matter; in a growing number of studies, gray and white matter have been examined separately, and that is mentioned explicitly in this review, where applicable. Cerebellum includes the cerebellar peduncles, subcortical white matter, and deep nuclei; rest of brain is the ensemble of hindbrain-midbrain-striatum-diencephalon (not including the cerebellum) [74]. The olfactory bulbs are counted separately, when available, which they often are not due to the difficulty of collecting them intact.

To put non-neuronal cell densities into context: we find that neuronal density varies by about 1000-fold across brain structures and species, from as few as a couple thousand neurons/mg in cerebral cortex or rest of brain structures to as many as one million neurons/mg in the cerebellum (Figure 5A). Within each structure, neuronal densities may or may not vary systematically across species: for instance, neuronal densities in the cerebellum of eulipotyphlans are consistently high (Figure 5A, orange squares) and are equally constant, albeit at lower values, across primate species (Figure 5A, red squares), whereas neuronal densities decrease systematically with increasing numbers of neurons in the cerebellum of species of other mammalian clades (Figure 5A, other squares). In the cerebral cortex, neuronal densities decrease systematically with increasing numbers of neurons across non-primate species but fail to do so across primates [75] (Figure 5A, red and other circles).

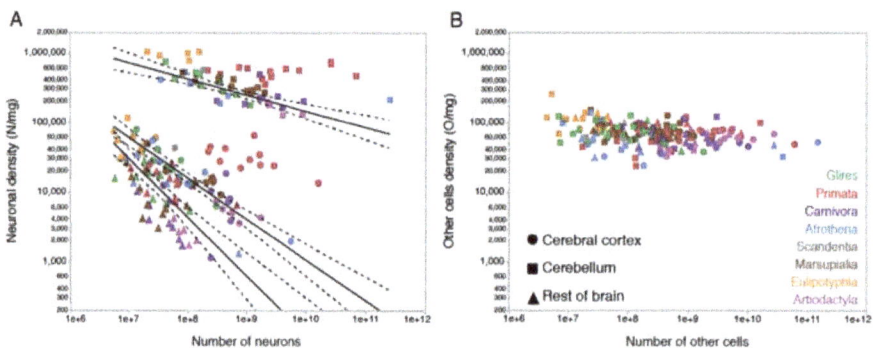

Figure 5. Density of non-neuronal cells is much less variable then neuronal densities in the mammalian brain. (**A**) Neuronal densities per milligram of tissue are enormously variable across brain structures and mammalian species. Each point represents the neuronal density in one structure (cerebral cortex, circles; cerebellum, squares; or rest of brain, triangles) in one of 60 mammalian species belonging to 8 different clades, as indicated, plotted against the total number of neurons found in that brain structure. (**B**) Other cell densities per milligram of tissue vary little across the same brain structures and species. Each point represents the neuronal density in the brain structures and species as shown in the left, plotted as a function of the total number of non-neuronal cells found in that structure. All data obtained with the isotropic fractionator. Data from [53–57,59–64].

In contrast, the density of other cells varies by not even 10-fold across the same structures and species as their numbers of other cells increase, mostly concentrating around 50,000–90,000 cells/mg (Figure 5B, shown in the same scale as A). The much smaller variation in the density of other cells is not due to lack of variation in total numbers of non-neuronal cells in the brain across species; as seen in Figure 5B, absolute numbers of other cells are exactly as variable across mammalian species and brain structures as the absolute numbers of neurons in those structures, by a factor of 100,000. Thus, regardless of how many neurons are found in 1 mg of brain tissue, a similar number of non-neuronal cells are found in that same 1 mg, in any brain tissue (including white matter; see below), in any mammalian species. Intuitively, the most likely scenario that accounts for this finding is that, in 1 mg of any brain tissue in any mammalian species, non-neuronal cells have a similar overall average size (defined as cell body plus any and all ramifications), while neuronal cells can range from very small (as in the cerebellum) to very large (as in the cerebral cortex and rest of brain). The simple mathematical model described above confirmed that the average neuronal and non-neuronal cell size can indeed be estimated as the inverse of neuronal and non-neuronal cell densities, respectively, as detailed below.

Across mammalian species, direct examination of neuronal and non-neuronal densities in different brain structures shows how the former span three orders of magnitude, whereas the latter are concentrated within a single order of magnitude, whether in the cerebellum, cerebral cortex, or rest of brain (Figure 6A). Within a single species (Swiss mouse), neuronal and non-neuronal densities vary together (as assumed in our model that estimates average cell volume from density [69]), such that those individuals with higher neuronal densities in a given brain structure also have higher non-neuronal cell densities in the structure, although always within a much-restricted range, than across species (Figure 6B, shades of orange/magenta; [69]). Neuronal and non-neuronal cell densities are positively correlated across individuals within each of the main brain structures (cerebral cortex, cerebellum, and the rest of brain), despite the much higher neuronal densities in the cerebellum [69]. Consistently, neuronal and non-neuronal densities were also positively correlated across different cortical areas identified by cytoarchitectural features in four C57B/6J mouse individuals (Figure 6B, shades of blue and green; [76]) and in one human cerebral cortex (Figure 7; [77]).

Importantly, despite the much higher neuronal densities found in the cerebellum of the same mouse individuals, densities of other cells there were similar to those found in the cerebral cortex and rest of brain (Figure 6B, compare the squares in shades of red/magenta with other shapes of similar color). Non-neuronal cell densities are similar across brain structures and species as distinct in brain size and distant in evolutionary kinship as the lab mouse and the African elephant, as illustrated in Figure 6B, despite neuronal densities being about 10-fold higher in the Swiss mouse cerebral cortex (orange/magenta circles) than in the gray matter of the elephant cerebral cortex (black circles).

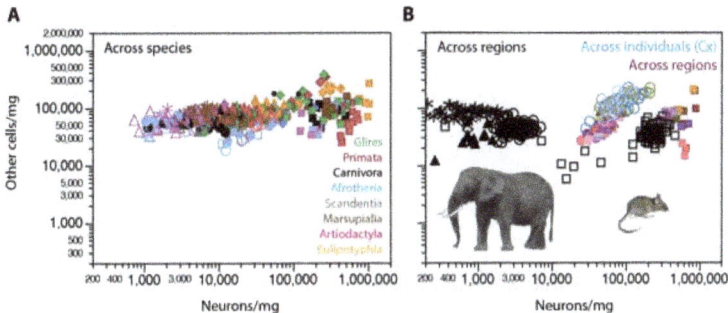

Figure 6. Density of non-neuronal cells per milligram of tissue varies little in the mammalian brain. (**A**) Neuronal densities (horizontal axis), but not other cell densities (vertical axis), are enormously variable across brain structures and mammalian species. Each point represents the neuronal and other cell (non-neuronal) density in one structure (cerebral cortex, cerebellum, and rest of brain, the latter being composed of medulla, pons, mesencephalon, striatum, and diencephalon) in one of 60 mammalian species belonging to eight different clades, as indicated. Filled circles, whole cerebral cortex (including subcortical white matter and hippocampus); empty circles, gray matter of cerebral cortex (including hippocampus); asterisks, white matter of cerebral cortex; filled triangles, rest of brain; empty triangles, substructures of rest of brain, as above; filled squares, cerebellum; empty squares, hippocampus. (**B**) Neuronal and other cell densities across brain structures and regions in the mouse and elephant brains, and in individual mice. Each point in black represents neuronal and other cell density in different structures, cortical regions, or subsections of the cerebellum in one African elephant brain hemisphere [61]; each point in shades of orange to magenta represents neuronal and other cell density in the cerebral cortex (circles), cerebellum (squares), or rest of brain (triangles) of one hemisphere of each of 19 individual male mice of similar age [69]. Each point in one of four shades of blue or green represents neuronal and other cell density in one of 19 cortical areas in the brain in one of four mouse individuals [76].

A similar pattern also applies across sites in a single human cerebral cortex [77], where neuronal densities vary by as much as ten-fold across the anterior–posterior axis, but non-neuronal densities vary by only virca (ca.) three-fold and remain in the same range as non-neuronal densities in the elephant and mouse cortex (Figure 7).

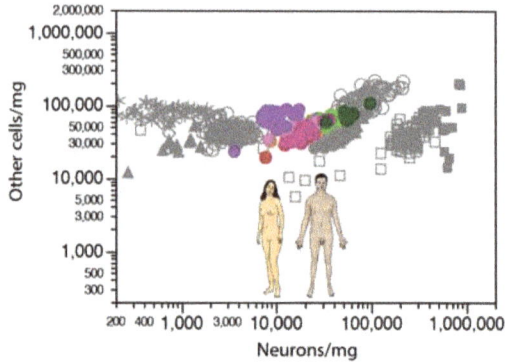

Figure 7. Density of non-neuronal cells varies little across sites in the gray matter of the human cerebral cortex. Same as in Figure 6, right, with the addition of data for the gray matter of the human cerebral cortex [77], for which each point represents the neuronal and other cell (non-neuronal) densities in one 2 mm thick coronal section. In each section, the gray matter of the cerebral cortex was separated into prefrontal (red, anterior to callosum), frontal (orange, anterior to central sulcus), parietal (blue, posterior to central sulcus), occipital (green, posterior 1/3), V1 (dark green, within occipital region), temporal (pink), insular (magenta), and hippocampal (lavender).

Average non-neuronal cell densities within the gray or white matter of the cerebral cortex, separately, are also very stable across species, as shown in Figure 8 across 27 species of marsupials, primates, scandentia, afrotherians, and artiodactyls. The average density of non-neuronal cells is lower in gray matter than in subcortical white matter, at $53,398 \pm 15,793$ cells/mg and $85,867 \pm 18,053$ cells/mg, respectively (Wilcoxon, $p < 0.0001$; Figure 8, compare stars and circles). However, given the high concentration of neuronal cell bodies in the gray matter, a lower average density of non-neuronal cells in the gray matter is still to be expected if the average size of glial cells is identical in both tissues. Only direct, systematic measurements of glial cell size in gray and white matter of different species will be able to settle this issue.

To estimate the experimentally elusive average cell sizes from the densities of neuronal and non-neuronal cells in brain structures that are easily measured with the isotropic fractionator, we used chi-square minimization of a simple model that related variations in those two densities, which allowed us to calculate average masses of individual neuronal and non-neuronal cells in the tissue analyzed [73]. Cell size (mass) in this model includes the soma, all arbors, and pericellular space of each cell, so that all tissue mass is accounted for by either neuronal or non-neuronal cells. The model considers that the relationship between the inverse of neuronal density and average neuronal cell mass depends on the fraction of tissue composed by neurons (that is, the neuronal mass fraction of the tissue). Using chi-square minimization to solve the set of equations relating measured densities and estimated average cell sizes and neuronal mass fraction, and applying the results to our most current dataset, we estimate that while the average mass of individual neuronal cells is highly variable across structures and species, spanning three orders of magnitude (from 0.6 to nearly 600 ng), the average mass of individual non-neuronal cells varies little, centered around 4.5 ng (Figure 9). For instance, we estimate that average neuronal cell mass in the cerebral cortex (including the white matter) is 8.3 ng in the mouse, 48.8 ng in the human species, and 338.8 ng in the African elephant, while the average non-neuronal cell weighs an estimated 4.4, 5.0, and 5.8 ng in the three species, respectively. According to these estimates, the average neuron in the human cerebral cortex has a similar mass to the average neuron in the cerebral cortex of the agouti (49.8 ng). Thus, even in a single structure, such as the cerebral cortex, neurons vary in their three-dimensional size from very small to very large in different mammalian species, while non-neuronal cells remain, on average, fairly small. It will be interesting to see how this enormous variation in predicted average neuronal cell size in the face of very steady average glial cell sizes relates to differences in gene expression across cell types uncovered by single-cell transcriptomics studies as they expand to a wider range of species.

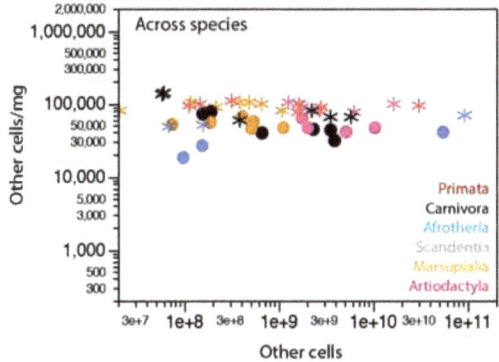

Figure 8. Average density of non-neuronal cells in the gray and white matter of the cerebral cortex varies little across mammalian species. Each point represents the total number and average density of other cells (non-neuronal) in the gray matter (unfilled circles) or in the white matter (asterisks) of the cerebral cortex of 1 of 27 mammalian species belonging to six different clades, as indicated by the colors. Data from [59,60,62,63].

Importantly, our model led to the realization that a consequence of the small variation in non-neuronal cell density, and thus average non-neuronal cell mass, is that the fractional neuronal mass of brain tissue is also remarkably similar across widely different brain structures and species, centered around 0.69 ± 0.09: that is, in 50% of all brain structures and mammalian species studied, the percentage of tissue mass composed by neurons varies narrowly between 63% and 74%. A useful mental picture of fractional neuronal and non-neuronal mass (or volume) of brain structures is the relative size of the piles of neurons and non-neuronal cells that would be obtained by passing the brain structure through a magical sieve that sorted individual cells neatly into two piles. According to our estimates, the neuronal and non-neuronal piles would amount to about 2/3 and 1/3 of any brain structure, in any mammalian species. Our estimates of average neuronal and non-neuronal individual cell mass and neuronal mass fraction for the current set of mammalian species can be found in Supplementary Table S1.

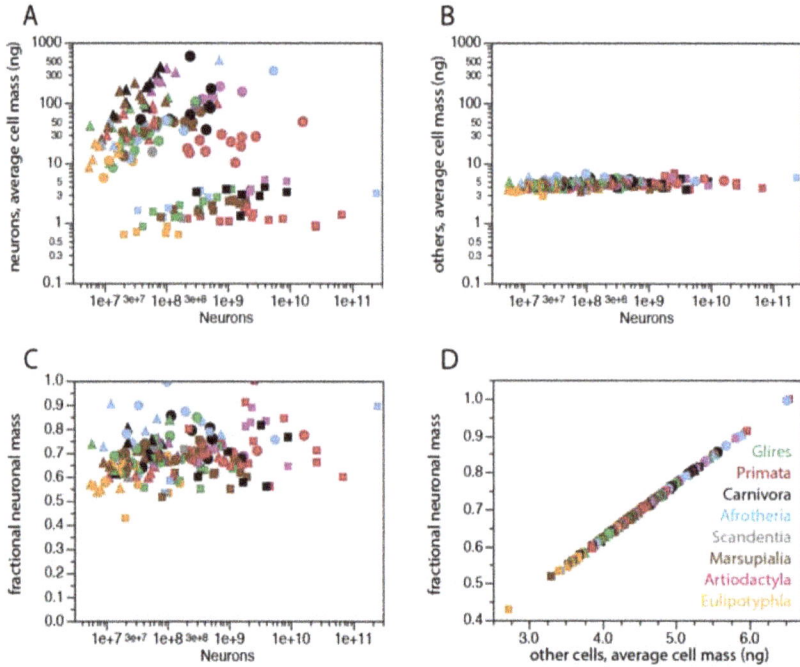

Figure 9. Estimated average mass of neuronal and non-neuronal cells and neuronal fraction in brain structures across mammalian species. (**A**) Average mass of individual neurons in each brain structure, estimated as $0.649 \times (N/ng)^{-1.004}$ according to [73], plotted as a function of number of neurons in the structure for each species; (**B**) average mass of individual non-neuronal (other) cells in each brain structure, estimated as $1.648 \times (O/ng)^{-1.370}$ according to [73], plotted as a function of number of neurons in the structure for each species, and shown in same scale as in (**A**); (**C,D**) fraction of structure mass composed by neuronal cells, estimated as $0.265 \times (O/ng)^{-1.356}$ according to [73], plotted as a function of the number of neurons in the structure (**C**) or of the estimated average mass of individual non-neuronal cells in the same structure (**D**). Each point represents values in one structure (cerebral cortex, cerebellum, rest of brain in one of 60 mammalian species belonging to eight different clades, as indicated. Filled circles, whole cerebral cortex (including subcortical white matter and hippocampus); filled triangles, rest of brain; filled squares, cerebellum.

2.1. Relative Frequencies of Glial Cell Subtypes

Of course, non-neuronal cells are a collection of a few different cell types, not all of them glial. Ependymal cells are expected to be largely absent from our dataset, since we physically remove the choroid plexus of all ventricles in our dissections prior to quantification. Dura-mater and arachnoid are also removed in our dissections, but not the pia-mater, so the superficial glia limitans is presumed to be included. Removing the arachnoid excludes all major blood vessels, but endothelial and endothelium-associated cells of capillaries are part of the parenchyma, and as such are necessarily included in our counts. Still, previous estimates that the microvasculature occupies only a very small fraction of the parenchyma suggested that endothelial cells and vasculature-associated cells were a very small minority of all cells in brain tissue [78]. A minority of vascular cells amongst non-neuronal cells was also found by quantitative single-cell RNAseq in mouse somatosensory cortex and hippocampus (six and 15 times as many oligodendrocytes, astrocytes, and microglial cells as endothelial cells, respectively [32]). Upcoming evidence from our lab confirms that both the vascular fraction and the density of endothelial cells are low and fairly constant across structures in the mouse brain [79]. While these same upcoming data indicate that, in all structures, endothelial cells are a larger proportion of all cells than the ca. 2% expected from microvascular volume (which agrees with the impression that endothelial and vascular-associated cells are very small cells, much smaller than neurons and glia), they still are a minority in brain tissue [79]. In the mouse, we found that about 2/3 of non-neuronal cells are glial indeed, and because the microvascular fraction (or capillary density) is believed to be at best constant across species, if not decreasing in larger brains [80], an even larger majority of non-neuronal cells can be expected to be glial in brains larger than the mouse brain.

Considering that the majority of non-neuronal cells are non-ependymal glial cells, and that the volume fraction of brain tissue occupied by capillaries is so small (2–4% at best) that it is virtually negligible, it follows that the invariant density of non-neuronal cells as a whole (as shown in Figure 5A) is likely to reflect an invariant density of glial cells. Using Iba1 as a marker of microglial cells in frozen samples of our previously processed brain samples in a wide range of mammalian species, we have found the density of Iba1 + microglial cells to be invariant and low across brain structures and species, at about 4500–5000 microglial cells per milligram of tissue, on average, or about 7% of all non-neuronal cells [39]. Our upcoming findings across a range of species are consistent with isolated reports that microglial cells are a small minority of glial cells, totaling only about 5% of glial cells in the gray matter of the human cerebral cortex [81]. In this case, there are three major scenarios that would yield the fairly constant non-neuronal cell densities that we observe in the different structures of mammalian brains.

In the first, simplest scenario, all glial cell types have constant densities across brain structures and species, even if densities differ for each cell type (Figure 10A,B). In this case, the relative cell fractions represented by each glial cell type would also be constant, if different across cell types. While many researchers expect or indeed assume that astrocytes are the most common of all glial cell types [43–45,82], there is quantitative evidence to the contrary: in the human cerebral cortical gray matter, oligodendrocytes represent about 75% of all glial cells, and astrocytes are only about 20% [81]. Similarly, many other studies on the rat cerebral cortex found that oligodendrocytes constitute the majority of the glial cell population [83–85]. In this scenario, the average size of each glial subtype remains constant across structures and species.

The second scenario indicates that while one cell type retains a constant average cell size and therefore a constant cell density, another varies, but that second cell type is infrequent enough that the overall non-neuronal density still appears fairly constant (Figure 10C,D). The scenario depicted in Figure 10C would be consistent both with an initial report that some astrocytes are larger in human than in mouse cerebral cortex [86], and the evidence that oligodendrocytes are the predominant glial cell type in the cerebral cortex, at least in some species [81,83–85].

Finally, the third, more complicated scenario is one in which the two main glial cell types, astrocytes and oligodendrocytes, vary in average cell size, and thus in cell density, but in different directions, compensating for each other and yielding a fairly constant overall cell density (Figure 10E,F). In the scenario where astrocytes become smaller as they become more numerous, oligodendrocytes would necessarily become larger at the same time (Figure 10E); alternatively, in the scenario where astrocytes become larger as they become more numerous (as suggested by [86]), oligodendrocytes would necessarily become smaller at the same time (Figure 10F).

At the moment, all of the scenarios above remain plausible. While our data lead us to presume that the same scenario would apply to all brain structures and mammalian species examined, it remains possible that different scenarios apply to different brain structures. However, the finding that non-neuronal cell densities are remarkably consistent not only across species but also across brain structures within the same individuals makes that unlikely.

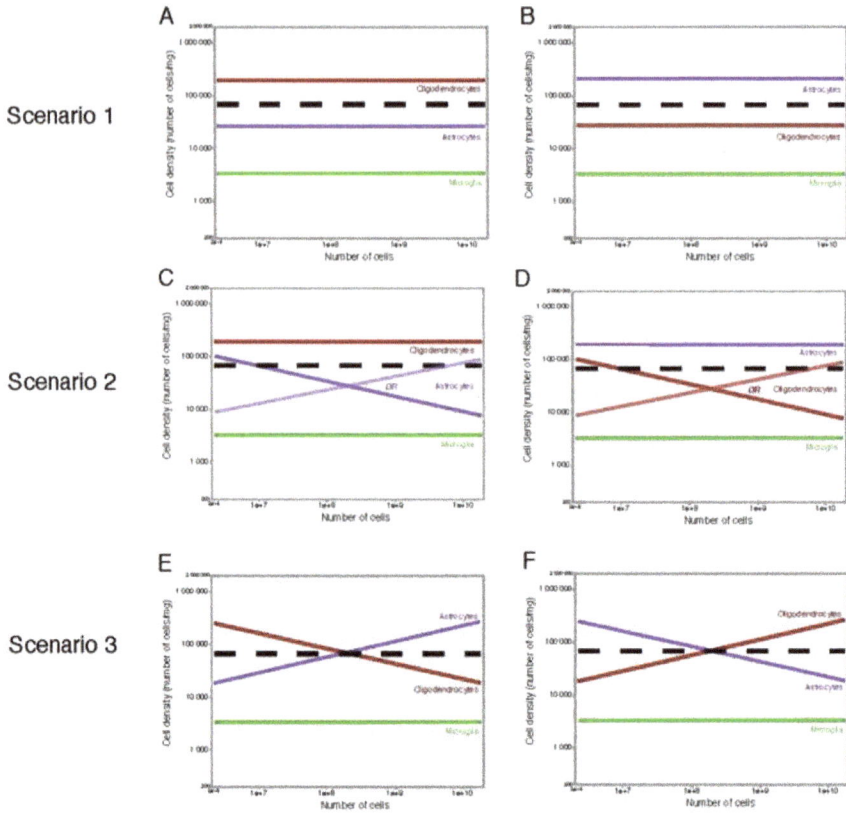

Figure 10. Possible scenarios of variation in densities of glial cell subtypes across mammalian species. Assuming that vasculature-associated cells are a small percentage of non-neuronal cells [78], non-neuronal cell density variation should reflect, almost exclusively, variations in densities of each glial cell subtype and their relative abundance. Each graph shown here represents a possible relationship between cellular density and number of non-neuronal cells in the tissue. Each glial cell type is represented by a color (oligodendrocytes in red, astrocytes in purple, and microglia in green). The invariant density of non-neuronal and glial cells as a whole, as found in previous studies across brain structures and mammalian species, is represented by the black dotted line. Microglial cell density has been found to be constant and low regardless of the number of microglial cells in the structure, across mammalian brain structures and species [39], which implies that the average microglial size tends to stay stable, such that microglial density remains constant, as shown in all three scenarios. **Scenario 1 (A,B)**: Densities of all three glial cell subtypes remain invariant in relation to their number of cells; the predominant glial cell type is either oligodendrocytes (**A**) or astrocytes (**B**). In both scenarios, average cell sizes of each glial cell type remain constant across brain structures and species; the total, constant, density of glial cells as a whole is the simple sum of the densities of each glial cell subtype. **Scenario 2 (C,D)**: One glial cell subtype maintains a constant, and high, density (whether oligodendrocytes, **C**, or astrocytes, **D**), while the other subtype varies in density across brain structures and species, decreasing or increasing systematically with the number of those cells. Decreasing cell densities reflect increasing cell sizes. In these scenarios, the average glial cell density remains constant, as the variation in density of either astrocytes or oligodendrocytes is masked by the high density of the most numerous glial population. **Scenario 3 (E,F)**: Densities of both astrocytes and oligodendrocytes vary as a result of the varying average size of these cells, but they compensate for each other in a way that their added densities remain invariant across structures and species.

Our upcoming data on over 30 mammalian species indicate that astrocytes, identified by ALDH1L1 immunoreactivity that is largely coincident with nuclear expression of S100b, are a somewhat higher percentage of all non-neuronal cells than microglial cells are, but with a more variable percentage across species, although they still occur at fairly invariant densities, with cells spaced apart evenly [40]. These data are so far consistent with oligodendrocytes being the large majority of all non-neuronal cells across brain structures and species, including cortical gray matter [81,87], but possibly also constituting a variable percentage of the non-neuronal cell population. The somewhat variable densities of astrocytes across species are also compatible with the earlier finding that human astrocytes appear larger than mouse astrocytes [86]. However, one must keep in mind that because of the extremely ramified cell morphology, estimates of astrocyte cell size are highly dependent on measuring criteria. In the oft-cited study above, human cortical astrocytes appear more branched than rodent astrocytes when GFAP-positive ramifications are quantified—but those are now known not to represent the entirety of the vast branched ramifications of astrocytes, and, indeed, the images of dye-filled cells in the same study show astrocytes of much more similar sizes in human and mouse cortices [86]. This is an important point to reconciling the findings of higher GFAP-positive branching with ours of nearly invariant cell densities, which relate to the three-dimensional distribution of highly branched cell volume that is known not to be properly captured in GFAP stains. As this point, therefore, our preliminary data suggest that the scenarios depicted in Figure 10A,C are the most likely, where oligodendrocytes predominate among non-neuronal cells in all brain structures, including the gray matter of the cerebral cortex.

2.2. Glia/Neuron Ratio

In several brain structures of several mammalian species, non-neuronal cells are indeed more numerous than neurons. To be clear, however, contrary to many claims in review articles and opening paragraphs of original papers [88–91], the mammalian central nervous system is not composed of 10% neurons and 90% glia, or any variation thereof. Table S1 lists some actual numbers and their sources. For instance, in the human brain, non-neuronal cells do outnumber neurons by 11.2:1 in the ensemble of brainstem, diencephalon and striatum (the rest of brain), and by 3.7:1 in the entire cerebral cortex (including the subcortical white matter), but, conversely, there are only 0.2 non-neuronal cells to every neuron in the cerebellum (Table S1). Because the rest of brain holds not even 1% of all neurons in the human brain, non-neuronal cells are only as numerous as neurons in the human brain as a whole [55]. Importantly, humans fit the pattern that applies to all other species, as discussed below.

The proportion between numbers of glial cells and neurons has been considered a meaningful property of nervous tissue since well before the actual functions of glial cells were understood, if only because this proportion appears to be so variable across species. Observing that human cerebral cortex had a higher proportion of glial cells per neuron than other species, Friede [52] initially proposed that that was a feature of "more advanced" cortices, but the later analysis of other species with even larger cortices indicated that the ratio was rather related to sheer mass [51]. Since then, the idea that has gained traction in the literature is that the glia/neuron ratio (GNR) in the cerebral cortex, sometimes unduly extended to the GNR of the whole brain, increases together with total brain mass: the larger the brain (or the animal), the more glial cells that accompany each neuron [2,51,92,93]. The argument, while intuitive, is convoluted: larger animals tend to have larger brains, which are supposedly made of larger neurons [50,51], which are assumed to have a higher metabolic cost per cell than neurons in smaller brains, which would require more glial cells to supply the energetic requirement of each neuron [92,93]. Importantly, the rationale behind the assumption that larger neurons come with more glial cells per neuron was rooted on another implicit notion: that the vast majority of those glial cells that accompanied each neuron were astrocytes, responsible for providing different types of support to neuronal activity and synaptic transmission.

It will thus be crucial to separate GNRs in different brain structures and species per glial cell type. As mentioned above, a low, stable density of microglial cells in all brain structures that we find across mammalian species [39] suggests that these cells perform functions that are volume-related, which is compatible with the macrophage-like properties of these cells [94,95]. A similar finding for astrocytes would suggest that the function of these cells is also volume-related, with each individual cell capable of servicing only a limited amount of tissue. Concluding our systematic analyses of the densities of astrocytes, oligodendrocytes, and microglial cells separately will allow us to understand what glial cell types occur in numbers that accompany numbers of neurons, density of neurons, volume of tissue, or, eventually, numbers and density of synapses.

Until then, and whatever the biological origin of the much larger variation in neuronal density compared to non-neuronal density across brain structures and species, we could already establish that a mathematical consequence of that difference is that overall GNR varies essentially with the inverse of local neuronal density. Because lower neuronal densities indicate larger neurons, that means that larger neurons are accompanied by more non-neuronal cells than smaller neurons [73,96]. Importantly, the same relationship applies across all brain structures in all mammalian species analyzed so far, as illustrated in Figure 11.

Further, because neuronal densities may differ so much across structures of similar mass, numbers of neurons, and even in brains of similar size (Figure 11A), and considering that the fraction of non-neuronal cells that are not glial cells is minimal, there is no systematic, universal relationship between GNR and brain or structure mass (Figure 11A, top), contrary to common past assertions in both the scientific literature and journalistic reports that larger brains show higher GNRs [89,97,98]. While that initially appeared to be the case for the cerebral cortex alone, at a time when only a handful of species were analyzed [50], systematic examination of species representing all mammalian clades benefitting from the ease of the isotropic fractionator method showed that neuronal densities do not universally decrease with increasing brain size [53–64]—which would have been the requirement for universally increasing GNRs with increasing brain size. Despite the ease with which authors once could claim that the human brain had 10 times more glia than neurons [42,99,100], there are at best similar numbers of neuronal and glial cells in the human brain as a whole [55].

The glia/neuron ratio does vary universally across species, across structures, and even across subregions of the same structure as a function of neuronal density (Figure 11A, bottom). The existence of such a continuum, with no evidence of grade shifts across structures, species, or clades, argues strongly for a highly conserved mechanism governing how glial cells are added to tissue in development and evolution [63,73,96].

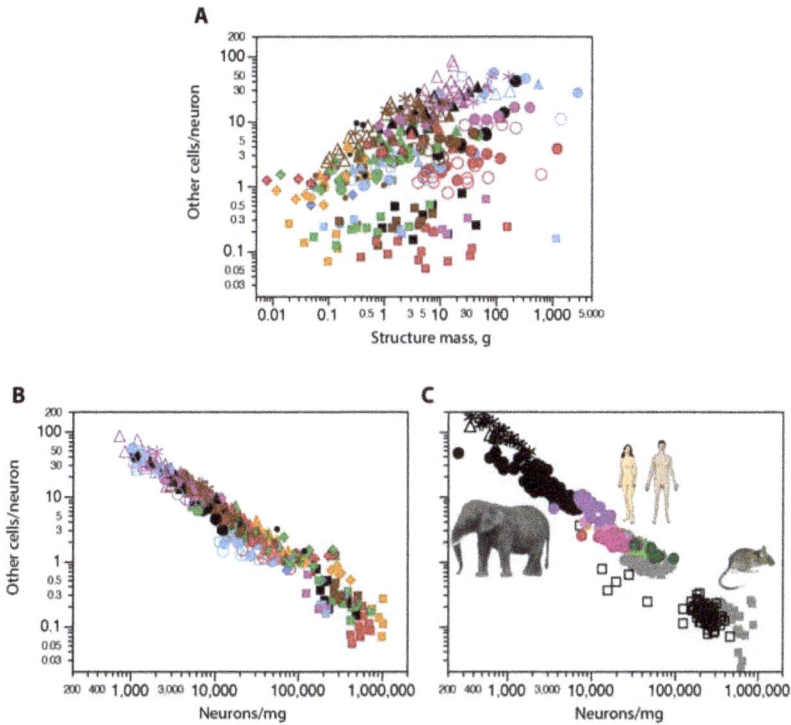

Figure 11. Scaling of the ratio of other (non-neuronal) cells per neuron across species and brain sites. Ratio of non-neuronal cells per neuron varies systematically, not with structure mass (**A**), but with neuronal density across structures and species (**B**), as well as across sites in individual brains (**C**). Each data point represents one brain structure and species, as in Figure 9 (**top**, **left**) or one brain region within the same individual (right: mouse, gray; elephant, black; human cortex, colors), as in Figures 6 and 7. Data from [53–57,59–64,69,77].

We have found recently that different neuronal densities in the cerebral cortex are not accompanied by significantly different energetic costs per neuron [101], which makes it unlikely that the larger glia/neuron ratios that accompany larger neurons are due to a higher metabolism in larger neurons, at least not across species. Instead, as noted above, it is more likely that GNRs vary as a simple consequence of the relative constancy in average glial cell size. In this scenario, glial cells are added to different tissues and species at similar densities, occupying a parenchyma that is initially mostly neuronal, but composed of neurons of highly variable individual cell size. The GNR in any given brain structure within the brain of any mammalian species is thus a simple consequence of the average cell mass of the neurons that formed the initial volume invaded by glial cell precursors, and the precise average cell mass of glial cells [73].

2.3. Why Should Glial Cell Size Be Constrained?

Life spontaneously changes over time—that is, evolves—and it is a rare feature of living beings that is found to remain constant. When one does, it is indicative of a constraint at the physical (mechanical properties of tissue), biochemical (binding site constancy), or biological level (physiology). The degree of folding of any cerebral cortex, for instance, is strictly tied to the combination of cortical surface area and thickness—even though these are free to vary—according to physical minimization of free energy as the tissue forms under uneven pressures [102]. The genetic code is possibly fixed by the matching of the spatial conformation of dinucleotides and amino acid precursors [103]. As suggested above, glial cells of different types might be constrained in size due to a biological limitation imposed by their volume-related function. Astrocytes provide electrolyte homeostasis, neurotransmitter reuptake and turnover, and metabolic support related to synaptic transmission, all strictly local functions, even if coordinated across cells connected electrotonically [2,104]; neurons, by virtue of their long, uneven projections, by definition impact physiology of both near and distant sites. Oligodendrocytes myelinate and provide energy to surrounding axons that contact them once they differentiate from neural/glial antigen 2-positive (NG2+) progenitor cells that actively probe their local environment and respond to loss of contact with oligodendrocytes by proliferating [29,105]. Microglial cells are phagocytic and thus perform volume-related tissue clearance. All of these are highly energy-demanding functions that possibly limit the volume of the individual cells performing them: there is only so much energy that an individual cell can use to perform functions that are determined by the relationship between the volume monitored by the cell and its surface area, which is costly to maintain polarized. While a similar cost applies to neurons, their activity can be self-regulated by decreasing the firing frequency; astrocytes and oligodendrocytes, on the other hand, are forced to accompany that activity. Presumably, astrocytes that became too large might enclose too many synapses to be able to support and maintain them effectively; oligodendrocytes that became too large would come into contact with too many fibers to myelinate; microglial cells that became too large might not have the power required to phagocyte all debris that they encounter.

These constraints might be determined genetically, as any spontaneous variation in genes related to cell size regulation specifically in glial cells leads to negative outcomes that are incompatible with life. Interestingly, though, there is an alternative hypothesis that glial cell size is maintained fairly constant by self-regulation. One likely source of self-regulation is the very energetic cost of maintaining volume-related glial cell function. Another is the fact that the presumed sources of high energy demand, synaptic transmission, are the very synapses which are induced in large numbers by astrocytes themselves [106,107]. Thus, in development, numbers of synapses are initially low; increase in a given tissue volume as that tissue becomes populated by astrocytes, which induce their formation and supports it with cholesterol; then support the increased metabolic demand of those neurons, recycle the transmitters, and maintain ion homeostasis [106–108].

Alternatively, glial cell size might be not self-regulated, but constrained by cell-autonomous means, in which case it would be their restricted size that would impose constraints on neurons. In that scenario, for example, an intrinsic limitation to changes in three-dimensional cell size and surface area of astrocytes might constrain the number of excitatory synapses that can be induced and supported per unit volume in neural tissue, which is consistent with the few reports so far of fairly restricted synaptic densities across species [44,109,110]. That would result in fewer synapses per neuron in a given volume of tissue as neurons became bigger both across brain structures and species, which in turn would contribute to keeping metabolic costs low in those neurons.

Another possibility is that (macro) glial cells are restricted in size and various other characteristics because of the circumstances of their differentiation, late in development, according to the current view that there is progressive restriction to gene expression during development. Indeed, early models of restriction of developmental potential through progressive repression of transcription along cell lineages put forward the counterintuitive notion that progressive diversification of cell types comes with progressive restriction of what each progenitor cell can generate [111]. An alternative proposition held that lineage potentials were expressed individually in a predetermined sequence as progenitor cells matured [112]. Cell lineage studies in brain development soon showed that there is indeed progressive restriction of cell fates, with a narrowing range of cell types and characteristics that culminates in specification of the final, mature identity of different cells [113,114]. Strikingly, in vertebrate brains, macroglial cells are the last cell types to be specified in development [115]: astrocytes in the lineage that earlier gave rise to excitatory neurons, and oligodendrocytes in the lineage that previously formed inhibitory neurons (Figure 12). Our quantitative analyses of developing rats [116,117] and mice [118] show that all brain tissues are indeed 95% neuronal at birth, with significant numbers of non-neuronal cells only appearing during the second postnatal week.

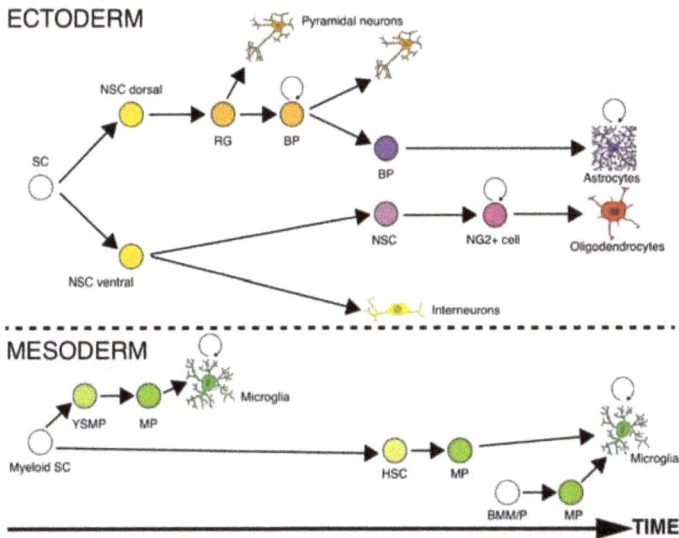

Figure 12. Schematics of the time sequence of generation of different neuronal and non-neuronal cell types in vertebrate brains. Neurons and macroglia (astrocytes and oligodendrocytes) have an ectodermal origin. A single stem-cell gives rise to neural stem-cells that, in turn, depending on their location in the neural tube (dorsal or ventral), give rise to pyramidal neurons and astrocytes or interneurons and oligodendrocytes, respectively. Pyramidal neurons can be generated directly from radial glial cells or from a basal progenitor early during development. Basal progenitors can divide and produce astrocytes later during development. Oligodendrocytes and interneurons are produced from ventral neural stem cells that give rise directly to interneurons early during development and later to oligodendrocytes. Microglia have a mesodermal origin and are produced in several waves throughout development. Embryonic microglia originate from a myeloid stem cell that differentiates into yolk sac macrophage and microglial precursors. This myeloid stem cell also differentiates into hematopoietic stem cells in the fetal liver and later into microglial precursors that originate microglial cells. After birth, the third wave of microglia production has an origin in the bone marrow from monocytes or other progenitors. SC: Stem cell; NSC: Neural stem cells; RG: Radial glia; BP: Basal progenitor; YSMP: Yolk sac macrophage precursor; MP: Microglial precursor; HSC: Hematopoietic stem cell; BMM/P: Bone marrow monocyte/progenitor. Data from [82,119–124].

Progressive restriction of cell fates and cell differentiation occur with global chromatin remodeling that results in progressively compacted, repressed chromatin that corresponds with activation of lineage-specific genes and repression of lineage-inappropriate genes [125–127]. Such progressive restriction of genome transcription is consistent with the recent findings, discussed earlier, that the early-generated neuronal cells express a wider variety of transcripts than the later-generated glial cells [31,32]. However, cells with astrocytic phenotype are known to also function as neural progenitor cells in some regions of the brain [121,128–131], which suggests that, if these are true astrocytes, then their genome is still not irreversibly restricted in its pattern of gene expression.

Finally, while the scenarios above consider that glial cells are the exception in their size-invariance (given the general expectation that biological features tend to diversify over time), the inverse must still be considered: that all cells (or most cell types) are by default constrained in size across species as diverse as mice and elephants, and neurons are the exception in how much they can vary. In line with that possibility, some evidence, compiled from isolated studies using different methods, suggests that many cell types do share similar individual cell volume across species [132,133], but systematic studies of cell size employing the same method across a wide range of species are still lacking. Using the isotropic fractionator, our preliminary findings suggest that, like glial cells, the density of cells that form liver tissue is remarkably similar across species [134].

It has been suggested that constant cell size, accompanied by cellular metabolic rates that decrease with increasing body size, is a property of quickly dividing cells, whereas slowly dividing (or cell-cycle arrested) cells have increasing cell volume but constant cellular metabolic rates [133]. In that case, you do not mess with the glia—or with hardly anything else in the body; only neurons, and maybe a few other cell types, such as adipocytes [133], might escape that limitation. Whatever the scenario that actually applies, the enormous difference in ranges of cell densities in the nervous system indicates that while neurons are free to vary in size, glial cells are not. Two new fundamental questions thus arise regarding the lack of diversity in glial cell types, sizes, and distribution in brain tissue, at least compared to neuronal diversity: how come—and so what?

2.4. What Lies Ahead

The newfound ability to rapidly, reliably, and systematically measure numbers and densities of neuronal and non-neuronal cells in the main brain structures in dozens of mammalian species has provided a wealth of data that finally offer a solid foundation for the field. Those direct measurements have allowed us to estimate how cell sizes vary and compare across brain structures, species, and cell types: neurons are highly diverse in their average cell mass, while non-neuronal cells are hardly variable. These observations match those of budding catalogs of transcripts in single cells that find multiple clusters of neuronal cell types that are rich and diverse in the genes they transcribe, but only a handful of non-neuronal cell types are defined by their much more restricted transcriptomes. With several new hypotheses in hand, informed by the collection of these new developments, future studies that directly investigate the variation in size and three-dimensional complexity of glial cells of different types in different species and clades and how they relate to particular gene transcripts will shed new light on the origins of glial cell diversity or lack thereof. The combination of the two approaches into quantitative studies of the abundance of different cell types according to multiple genes and markers expressed in isolated cells or cell nuclei is an exciting possibility for the near future, particularly taking advantage of novel microscopy techniques such as multiplex ion beam imaging (MIBI) that allow the investigation of the expression of as many as a few dozen markers by the same cells or nuclei in fixed tissue collected from different species. Finally, upcoming methods that allow transcriptomic analysis of fixed cells and isolated nuclei [135] should allow the expansion of those studies to a much wider variety of species and brain structures, also allowing us to take advantage of the ever-growing collection of isolated cell nuclei that we have quantified in our lab. There are exciting times ahead for quantitative neuroanatomists again.

Supplementary Materials: The following are available online at http://www.mdpi.com/2571-6980/1/1/14/s1, Table S1 measured densities and ratios of neuronal and other cells, estimated average mass of individual neuronal (mN) and non-neuronal cells (mO), and estimated neuronal fractional mass of the tissue (fN) according to [73].

Author Contributions: S.H.H. and S.E.D.S. wrote the manuscript, prepared illustrations, and approved the manuscript.

Funding: Supported by Vanderbilt University start-up funds, and James S. McDonnell Foundation grant number 220020232.

Acknowledgments: Thanks to all our collaborators who participated in the original studies that generated the quantitative data mentioned here, in particular to Jon Kaas (Vanderbilt University, USA) and Paul Manger (University of the Witwatersrand, South Africa) for making these studies possible.

Conflicts of Interest: The authors declare no conflict of interest.

References

1. Virchow, R. *Die Cellularpathologie in Ihrer Begründung auf Physiologische und Pathologische Gewebelehre*; Hirschwald: Berlin, Germany, 1858.
2. Allen, N.J.; Barres, B.A. Neuroscience: Glia—more than just brain glue. *Nature* **2009**, *457*, 675–677. [CrossRef] [PubMed]
3. Hartline, D.K. The evolutionary origins of glia. *Glia* **2011**, *59*, 1215–1236. [CrossRef] [PubMed]
4. Umesono, Y.; Agata, K. Evolution and regeneration of the planarian central nervous system. *Dev. Growth Differ.* **2009**, *51*, 185–195. [CrossRef] [PubMed]
5. Younossi-Hartenstein, A.; Ehlers, U.; Hartenstein, V. Embryonic development of the nervous system of the rhabdocoel flatworm Mesostoma lingua (Abilgaard, 1789). *J. Comp. Neurol.* **2000**, *416*, 461–474. [CrossRef]
6. Zhu, B.; Pennack, J.A.; McQuilton, P.; Forero, M.G.; Mizuguchi, K.; Sutcliffe, B.; Gu, C.-J.; Fenton, J.C.; Hidalgo, A. Drosophila neurotrophins reveal a common mechanism for nervous system formation. *PLoS Biol.* **2008**, *6*, e284. [CrossRef] [PubMed]
7. Losada-Perez, M. The evolutionary origins of glia. *Glia* **2018**, *59*, 1215–1236. [CrossRef]
8. De Robertis, E.M.; Sasai, Y. A common plan for dorsoventral patterning in Bilateria. *Nature* **1996**, *380*, 37–40. [CrossRef] [PubMed]
9. Hirth, F.; Kammermeier, L.; Frei, E.; Waldorf, U.; Noll, M.; Reichert, H. An urbilaterian origin of the tripartite brain: Developmental insights from Drosophila. *Development* **2003**, *130*, 2365–2373. [CrossRef] [PubMed]
10. Hirth, F.; Reichert, H. Basic nervous system types: One or many? In *Evolution of Nervous Systems*; Kaas, J.H., Ed.; Academic Press: Amsterdam, The Netherlands, 2007; Volume 1, pp. 55–72.
11. Moroz, L.L. On the independent origins of complex brains and neurons. *Brain Behav. Evol.* **2009**, *74*, 177–190. [CrossRef] [PubMed]
12. Northcutt, R.G. Cladistic analysis reveals brainless Urbilateria. *Brain Behav. Evol.* **2010**, *76*, 1–2. [CrossRef] [PubMed]
13. Ryan, T.J.; Grant, S.G.N. The origin and evolution of synapses. *Nat. Rev. Neurosci.* **2009**, *10*, 701–712. [CrossRef] [PubMed]
14. Helm, C.; Karl, A.; Beckers, P.; Kaul-Strehlow, S.; Ulbricht, E.; Kourtesis, I.; Kuhrt, H.; Hausen, H.; Bartolomaeus, T.; Reichenbach, A.; et al. Early evolution of radial glial cells in Bilateria. *Proc. R. Soc. B* **2017**, *284*, 20170743. [CrossRef] [PubMed]
15. Benton, M.J. *Vertebrate Paleontology*; Chapman and Hall: New York, NY, USA, 1997.
16. Carroll, R.L. *Patterns and Processes of Vertebrate Evolution*; Cambridge Palaeobiology Series; Cambridge University Press: Cambridge, UK, 1997.
17. Cameron, C.B.; Garey, J.R.; Swalla, B.J. Evolution of the chordate body plan: New insights from phylogenetic analyses of deuterostome phyla. *Proc. Natl. Acad. Sci. USA* **2000**, *97*, 4469–4474. [CrossRef] [PubMed]
18. Hedges, S.B. Molecular evidence for the early history of living vertebrates in Major Events. In *Early Vertebrate Evolution: Palaeontology, Phylogeny, Genetics and Development*; Ahlberg, P.E., Ed.; Taylor & Francis: London, UK, 2001; pp. 119–134.
19. Blair, J.E.; Hedges, S.B. Molecular clocks do not support the Cambrian Explosion. *Mol. Biol. Evol.* **2005**, *22*, 387–390. [CrossRef] [PubMed]
20. Greig, L.C.; Woodworth, M.B.; Galazo, M.J.; Padmanabhan, H.; Macklis, J.D. Molecular logic of neocortical projection neuron specification, development and diversity. *Nat. Rev. Neurosci.* **2013**, *14*, 755–769. [CrossRef] [PubMed]
21. Cheung, A.F.; Kondo, S.; Abdel-Mannan, O.; Chodroff, R.A.; Sirey, T.M.; Bluy, L.E.; Webber, N.; DeProto, J.; Karlen, S.J.; Krubitzer, L.; et al. The subventricular zone is the developmental milestone of a 6-layered neocortex: Comparisons in metatherian and eutherian mammals. *Cereb. Cortex* **2010**, *20*, 1071–1081. [CrossRef] [PubMed]
22. Wang, X.; Lou, N.; Xu, Q.; Tian, G.F.; Peng, W.G.; Han, X.; Kang, J.; Takano, T.; Nedergaard, M. Astrocytic Ca^{2+} signaling evoked by sensory stimulation in vivo. *Nat. Neurosci.* **2006**, *9*, 816–823. [CrossRef] [PubMed]
23. Ramon, Y.; Cajal, S. *Histologie du Système Nerveux de 1'Homme et des Vertébrés*; Maloine: Paris, France, 1991; Volume 1, p. 986.
24. Centro Virtual Cervantes Website. Available online: https://cvc.cervantes.es/ciencia/cajal/cajal_recuerdos/recuerdos/laminas.htm (accessed on 7 May 2018).

25. Del Rio, H.P. La microglia y su transformacion en celulas en basoncito y cuerpos granulo-adiposos. *Trab. Lab. Investig. Biol. Madrid.* **1920**, *18*, 37–82.

26. Somjen, G.G. Nervenkitt: Notes on the History of the Concept of Neuroglia. *Glia* **1988**, *1*, 2–9. [CrossRef] [PubMed]

27. Harada, K.; Kamiya, T.; Tsuboi, T. Gliotransmitter release from astrocytes: Functional, developmental, and pathological implications in the brain. *Front. Neurosci.* **2016**, *9*, 499. [CrossRef] [PubMed]

28. Halassa, M.M.; Fellin, T.; Takano, H.; Dong, J.H.; Haydon, P.G. Synaptic islands defined by the territory of a single astrocyte. *J. Neurosci.* **2007**, *27*, 6473–6477. [CrossRef] [PubMed]

29. Hughes, E.G.; Kang, S.H.; Fukaya, M.; Bergles, D.E. Oligodendrocyte progenitors balance growth with self-repulsion to achieve homeostasis in the adult brain. *Nat. Neurosci.* **2013**, *16*, 668–676. [CrossRef] [PubMed]

30. Zeng, H.; Sanes, J.R. Neuronal cell-type classification: Challenges, opportunities and the path forward. *Nat. Rev. Neurosci.* **2017**, *18*, 530–546. [CrossRef] [PubMed]

31. Tasic, B.; Menon, V.; Nguyen, T.N.; Kim, T.K.; Jarsky, T.; Yao, Z.; Levi, B.; Gray, L.T.; Sorensen, S.A.; Dolbeare, T.; et al. Adult mouse cortical cell taxonomy revealed by single cell transcriptomics. *Nat. Neurosci.* **2016**, *19*, 335–346. [CrossRef] [PubMed]

32. Zeisel, A.; Muñoz-Machado, A.B.; Codeluppi, S.; Lönnerberg, P.; La Manno, G.; Juréus, A.; Marques, S.; Munguba, H.; He, L.; Betsholtz, C.; et al. Cell types in the mouse cortex and hippocampus revealed by single-cell RNA-seq. *Science* **2015**, *347*, 1138–1142. [CrossRef] [PubMed]

33. Darmanis, S.; Sloan, S.A.; Zhang, Y.; Enge, M.; Caneda, C.; Shuer, L.M.; Hayden, G.M.G.; Barres, B.A.; Quake, S.R. A survey of human brain transcriptome diversity at the single cell level. *Proc. Natl. Acad. Sci. USA* **2015**, *112*, 7285–7290. [CrossRef] [PubMed]

34. Raj, B.; Wagner, D.E.; McKenna, A.; Pandey, S.; Klein, A.M.; Shendure, J.; Gagnon, J.A.; Schier, A.F. Simultaneous single-cell profiling of lineages and cell types in the vertebrate brain. *Nat. Biotechnol.* **2018**, *5*, 442–450. [CrossRef] [PubMed]

35. Mullen, R.J.; Buck, C.R.; Smith, A.M. NeuN, a neuronal specific nuclear protein in vertebrates. *Development* **1992**, *116*, 201–211. [PubMed]

36. Rothstein, J.D.; Martin, L.; Levey, A.I.; Dykes-Hoberg, M.; Jin, L.; Wu, D.; Nash, N.; Kuncl, R.W. Localization of neuronal and glial glutamate transporters. *Neuron* **1994**, *13*, 713–725. [CrossRef]

37. Cahoy, J.D.; Emery, B.; Kaushal, A.; Foo, L.C.; Zamanian, J.L.; Christopherson, K.S.; Xing, Y.; Lubischer, J.L.; Krieg, P.A.; Krupenko, S.A.; et al. A transcriptome database for astrocytes, neurons, and oligodendrocytes: A new resource for understanding brain development and function. *J. Neurosci.* **2008**, *28*, 264–278. [CrossRef] [PubMed]

38. Sun, W.; Cornwell, A.; Li, J.; Peng, S.; Osorio, M.J.; Aalling, N.; Wang, S.; Benraiss, A.; Lou, N.; Goldman, S.A.; et al. SOX9 is an astrocyte-specific nuclear marker in the adult brain outside the neurogenic regions. *J. Neurosci.* **2017**, *37*, 4493–4507. [CrossRef] [PubMed]

39. Dos Santos, S.E.; Botelho, L.; Medeiros, M.; Porfirio, J.; Herculano-Houzel, S. Invariant microglial cells densities suggest evolutionary conserved developmental mechanisms governing their addition to the brains of mammals. Unpublished work. 2018.

40. Dos Santos, S.E.; Glassburn, L.; Hanflink, A.; Staub, M.; Palan, J.; Wimbiscus, M.; Herculano-Houzel, S. Similar densities of astrocytes found in different brain structures in a wide range of mammalian species. Unpublished work. 2018.

41. Jiang, X.; Shen, S.; Cadwell, C.R.; Berns, P.; Sinz, F.; Ecker, A.S.; Patel, S.; Tolias, A.S. Principles of connectivity among morphologically defined cell types in adult neocortex. *Science* **2015**, *350*, aac9462. [CrossRef] [PubMed]

42. Von Bartheld, C.S.; Bahney, J.; Herculano-Houzel, S. The search for true numbers of neurons and glial cells in the human brain: A review of 150 years of cell counting. *J. Comp. Neurol.* **2016**, *524*, 3865–3895. [CrossRef] [PubMed]

43. Vaughan, D.W.; Peters, A. Neuroglial cells in the cerebral cortex of rats from young adulthood to old age: An electron microscope study. *J. Neurocytol.* **1974**, *3*, 405–429. [CrossRef] [PubMed]

44. O'Kusky, J.; Colonnier, M. A laminar analysis of the number of neurons, glia, and synapses in the visual cortex (area 17) of adult macaque monkeys. *J. Comp. Neurol.* **1982**, *210*, 278–290. [CrossRef] [PubMed]

45. Peters, A.; Josephson, K.; Vincent, S.L. Effects of aging on the neuroglial cells and pericytes within area 17 of the rhesus monkey cerebral cortex. *Anat. Rec.* **1991**, *229*, 384–398. [CrossRef] [PubMed]

46. Kettenmann, H.; Ransom, B.R. *The Concept of Neuroglia: A Historical Perspective*; University Press: Oxford, UK, 2005.

47. Agulhon, C.; Petravicz, J.; McMullen, A.B.; Sweger, E.J.; Minton, S.K.; Taves, S.R.; Casper, K.B.; Fiacco, T.A.; McCarthy, K.D. What is the role of astrocyte calcium in neurophysiology. *Neuron* **2008**, *59*, 932–946. [CrossRef] [PubMed]

48. Kandel, E.R.; Schwartz, J.H.; Jessell, T.M. *Principles of Neural Science*, 3rd ed.; Appleton & Lange: Norwalk, CT, USA, 1991.

49. Kandel, E.R.; Schwartz, J.H.; Jessell, T.M.; Siegelbaum, S.A.; Hudspeth, A.J. *Principles of Neural Science*, 5th ed.; McGraw-Hill: New York, NY, USA, 2013.

50. Haug, H. Brain sizes, surfaces, and neuronal sizes on the cortex cerebri: A stereological investigation of man and his variability and a comparison with some mammals (primates, whales, marsupials, insectivores, and one elephant). *Am. J. Anat.* **1987**, *180*, 126–142. [CrossRef] [PubMed]

51. Tower, D.B.; Young, O.M. The activities of butyrylcholinesterase and carbonic anhydrase, the rate of anaerobic glycolysis, and the question of a constant density of glial cells in cerebral cortices of various mammalian species from mouse to whale. *J. Neurochem.* **1973**, *20*, 260–278. [CrossRef]

52. Friede, R. Der quantitative Anteil der Glia an der Cortex Entwicklung. *Acta Anat.* **1954**, *20*, 290–296. [CrossRef] [PubMed]

53. Herculano-Houzel, S.; Mota, B.; Lent, R. Cellular scaling rules for rodent brains. *Proc. Natl. Acad. Sci. USA* **2006**, *103*, 12138–12143. [CrossRef] [PubMed]

54. Herculano-Houzel, S.; Collins, C.; Wong, P.; Kaas, J.H. Cellular scaling rules for primate brains. *Proc. Natl. Acad. Sci. USA* **2007**, *104*, 3562–3567. [CrossRef] [PubMed]

55. Azevedo, F.A.C.; Carvalho, L.R.B.; Grinberg, L.T.; Farfel, J.M.; Ferretti, R.E.L.; Leite, R.E.P.; Jacob, F.W.; Lent, R.; Herculano-Houzel, S. Equal numbers of neuronal and non-neuronal cells make the human brain an isometrically scaled-up primate brain. *J. Comp. Neurocytol.* **2009**, *513*, 532–541. [CrossRef] [PubMed]

56. Sarko, D.K.; Catania, K.C.; Leitch, D.B.; Kaas, J.H.; Herculano-Houzel, S. Cellular scaling rules of insectivore brains. *Front. Neuroanat.* **2009**, *3*, 8. [CrossRef] [PubMed]

57. Gabi, M.; Collins, C.E.; Wong, P.; Kaas, J.H.; Herculano-Houzel, S. Cellular scaling rules for the brain of an extended number of primate species. *Brain Behav. Evol.* **2010**, *76*, 32–44. [CrossRef] [PubMed]

58. Herculano-Houzel, S.; Kaas, J.H. Gorilla and orangutan brains conform to the primate scaling rules: Implications for hominin evolution. *Brain Behav. Evol.* **2011**, *77*, 33–44. [CrossRef] [PubMed]

59. Herculano-Houzel, S.; Ribeiro, P.F.M.; Campos, L.; da Silva, A.V.; Torres, L.B.; Catania, K.C.; Kaas, J.H. Updated neuronal scaling rules for the brains of Glires (rodents/lagomorphs). *Brain Behav. Evol.* **2011**, *78*, 302–314. [CrossRef] [PubMed]

60. Neves, K., Jr.; Ferreira, F.M.; Tovar-Moll, F.; Gravett, N.; Bennett, N.C.; Kaswera, C.; Gilissen, E.; Manger, P.R.; Herculano-Houzel, S. Cellular scaling rules for the brains of Afrotheria. *Front. Neuroanat.* **2014**, *8*, 5. [CrossRef] [PubMed]

61. Herculano-Houzel, S.; Avelino-de-Souza, K.; Neves, K.; Porfírio, J.; Messeder, D.; Calazans, I.; Mattos, L.; Maldonado, J.; Manger, P.M. The elephant brain in numbers. *Front. Neuroanat.* **2014**, *8*, 46. [CrossRef] [PubMed]

62. Kazu, R.S.; Maldonado, J.; Mota, B.; Manger, P.R.; Herculano-Houzel, S. Cellular scaling rules for the brains of Artiodactyla. *Front. Neuroanat.* **2014**, *8*, 128. [CrossRef] [PubMed]

63. Dos Santos, S.E.; Porfirio, J.; Da Cunha, F.B.; Manger, P.R.; Tavares, W.; Pessoa, L.; Raghanti, M.A.; Sherwood, C.C.; Herculano-Houzel, S. Cellular scaling rules for the brain of marsupials: Not as "primitive" as expected. *Brain Behav. Evol.* **2017**, *89*, 48–63. [CrossRef] [PubMed]

64. Jardim-Messeder, D.; Lambert, K.; Noctor, S.; Marques Pestana, F.; DeCastro Leal, M.E.; Bertelsen, M.F.; Alagaili, A.N.; Mohammad, O.B.; Manger, P.R.; Herculano-Houzel, S. Dogs have the most neurons, though not the largest brain: Trade-off between body mass and number of neurons in the cerebral cortex of large carnivoran species. *Front. Neuroanat.* **2017**, *11*, 118. [CrossRef] [PubMed]

65. Herculano-Houzel, S.; Lent, R. Isotropic fractionator: A simple, rapid method for the quantification of total cell and neuron numbers in the brain. *J. Neurosci.* **2005**, *25*, 2518–2521. [CrossRef] [PubMed]

66. Bahney, J.; von Bartheld, C.S. Validation of the isotropic fractionator: Comparison with unbiased stereology and DNA extraction for quantification of glial cells. *J. Neurosci. Meth.* **2014**, *222*, 165–174. [CrossRef] [PubMed]

67. Miller, D.J.; Balaram, P.; Young, N.A.; Kaas, J.H. Three counting methods agree on cell and neuron number in chimpanzee primary visual cortex. *Front. Neuroanat.* **2014**, *8*, 36. [CrossRef] [PubMed]

68. Ngwenya, A.; Nahirney, J.; Brinkman, B.; Williams, L.; Iwaniuk, A.N. Comparison of estimates of neuronal number obtained using the isotropic fractionator method and unbiased stereology in day old chicks (*Gallus domesticus*). *J. Neurosci. Meth.* **2017**, *287*, 39–46. [CrossRef] [PubMed]

69. Herculano-Houzel, S.; Messeder, D.; Fonseca-Azevedo, K.; Araujo Pantoja, N. When larger brains do not have more neurons: Intraspecific increase in numbers of cells is compensated by decreased average cell size. *Front. Neuroanat.* **2015**, *9*, 64. [CrossRef] [PubMed]

70. Olkowicz, S.; Kocourek, M.; Lucan, R.K.; Portes, M.; Fitch, W.T.; Herculano-Houzel, S.; Nemec, P. Birds have primate-like numbers of neurons in the telencephalon. *Proc. Natl. Acad. Sci. USA* **2016**, *113*, 7255–7260. [CrossRef] [PubMed]

71. Ngwenya, A.; Patzke, N.; Manger, P.R.; Herculano-Houzel, S. Continued growth of the central nervous system without mandatory addition of neurons in the Nile crocodile (*Crocodylus niloticus*). *Brain Behav. Evol.* **2016**, *87*, 19–38. [CrossRef] [PubMed]

72. Herculano-Houzel, S. The Isotropic Fractionator: A fast, reliable method to determine numbers of cells in the brain or other tissues. In *Neuronal Network Analysis Concepts and Experimental Approaches*; Fellin, T., Halassa, M., Eds.; Springer: Berlin, Germany, 2012; pp. 391–403. ISBN 978-1-61779-633-3.

73. Mota, B.; Herculano-Houzel, S. All brains are made of this: A fundamental building block of brain matter with matching neuronal and glial masses. *Front. Neuroanat.* **2014**, *8*, 127. [CrossRef] [PubMed]

74. Herculano-Houzel, S.; Catania, K.; Manger, P.R.; Kaas, J.H. Mammalian brains are made of these: A dataset on the numbers and densities of neuronal and non-neuronal cells in the brain of glires, primates, scandentia, eulipotyphlans, afrotherians and artiodactyls, and their relationship with body mass. *Brain Behav. Evol.* **2015**, *86*, 145–163. [CrossRef] [PubMed]

75. Herculano-Houzel, S.; Manger, P.R.; Kaas, J.H. Brain scaling in mammalian evolution as a consequence of concerted and mosaic changes in numbers of neurons and average neuronal cell size. *Front. Neuroanat.* **2014**, *8*, 77. [CrossRef] [PubMed]

76. Herculano-Houzel, S.; Watson, C.; Paxinos, G. Distribution of neurons in functional areas of the mouse cerebral cortex reveals quantitatively different cortical zones. *Front. Neuroanat.* **2013**, *7*, 35. [CrossRef] [PubMed]

77. Ribeiro, P.F.M.; Ventura-Antunes, L.; Gabi, M.; Mota, B.; Grinberg, L.T.; Farfel, J.M.; Ferretti, R.E.L.; Leite, R.E.P.; Jacob Filho, W.; Herculano-Houzel, S. The human cerebral cortex is neither one nor many: Neuronal distribution reveals two quantitatively different zones in the grey matter, three in the white matter, and explains local variations in cortical folding. *Front. Neuroanat.* **2013**, *7*, 28. [CrossRef] [PubMed]

78. Lauwers, F.; Cassot, F.; Lauwers-Cances, V.; Puwanarajah, P.; Duvernoy, H. Morphometry of the human cerebral cortex microcirculation: General characteristics and space-related profiles. *Neuroimage* **2008**, *39*, 936–948. [CrossRef] [PubMed]

79. Ventura-Antunes, L.; Botelho, L.; Maldonado, J.; Herculano-Houzel, S. Smaller energy availability per neuron in sites with higher neuronal densities in the mouse brain. Unpublished work. 2018.

80. Karbowski, J. Scaling of brain metabolism and blood flow in relation to capillary and neural scaling. *PLoS ONE* **2011**, *6*, e26709. [CrossRef] [PubMed]

81. Pelvig, D.P.; Pakkenberg, H.; Stark, A.K.; Pakkenberg, B. Neocortical glial cell numbers in human brains. *Neurobiol. Aging* **2008**, *29*, 1754–1762. [CrossRef] [PubMed]

82. Ge, W.-P.; Miyawaki, A.; Gage, F.H.; Jan, Y.N.; Han, L.Y. Local generation of glia is a major astrocyte source in postnatal cortex. *Nature* **2012**, *484*, 376–381. [CrossRef] [PubMed]

83. Bass, N.H.; Hess, H.H.; Pope, A.; Thalheimer, C. Quantitative cytoarchitectonic of neurons, glia, and DNA in rat cerebral cortex. *J. Comp. Neurol.* **1971**, *143*, 481–490. [CrossRef] [PubMed]

84. Mori, S. Light and electron microscopic features and frequencies of the glial cells present in the cerebral cortex of the rat brain. *Arch. Histol. Jpn.* **1972**, *34*, 231–244. [CrossRef] [PubMed]

85. Ling, E.-A.; Leblond, C.P. Investigations of glial cells in semithin sections. II Variation with age in the numbers of the various glial cell types in rat cortex and corpus callosum. *J. Comp. Neurol.* **1973**, *149*, 73–81. [CrossRef]

86. Oberheim, N.A.; Takano, T.; Han, X.; He, W.; Lin, J.H.; Wang, F.; Xu, Q.; Wyatt, J.D.; Pilcher, W.; Ojemann, J.G.; et al. Uniquely hominid features of adult human astrocytes. *J. Neurosci.* **2009**, *29*, 3276–3287. [CrossRef] [PubMed]

87. He, Z.; Han, D.; Efimova, O.; Guijarro, P.; Yu, Q.; Oleksiak, A.; Jiang, S.; Anokhin, K.; Velichkovsky, B.; Grünewald, S.; et al. Comprehensive transcriptome analysis of neocortical layers in humans, chimpanzees and macaques. *Nat. Neurosci.* **2017**, *20*, 886–895. [CrossRef] [PubMed]

88. Kandel, E.R.; Schwartz, J.H. *Principles of Neural Science*, 2nd ed.; Elsevier: New York, NY, USA; Amsterdam, The Netherlands; Ofxord, UK, 1985.

89. Nedergaard, M.; Ransom, B.; Goldman, S.A. New roles for astrocytes: Redefining the functional architecture of the brain. *Trends Neurosci.* **2003**, *26*, 523–530. [CrossRef] [PubMed]

90. Ransom, B.; Behar, T.; Nedergaard, M. New roles for astrocytes (stars at last). *Trends Neurosci.* **2003**, *26*, 520–522. [CrossRef] [PubMed]

91. Nishiyama, A.; Yang, Z.; Butt, A. Astrocytes and NG2-glia: What's in a name? *J. Anat.* **2005**, *207*, 687–693. [CrossRef] [PubMed]

92. Sherwood, C.C.; Stimpson, C.D.; Raghanti, M.A.; Wildman, D.E.; Uddin, M.; Grossman, L.I.; Goodman, M.; Redmond, J.C.; Bonar, C.J.; Erwin, J.M.; et al. Evolution of increased glia-neuron ratios in the human frontal cortex. *Proc. Natl. Acad. Sci. USA* **2006**, *103*, 13606–13611. [CrossRef] [PubMed]

93. Hawkins, A.; Olszewski, J. Glia/nerve cell index of the cortex of the whale. *Science* **1957**, *126*, 76–77. [CrossRef] [PubMed]

94. Gehrmann, J.; Matsumoto, Y.; Kreutzberg, G.W. Microglia: Intrinsic immunoeffector cell of the brain. *Brain Res. Rev.* **1995**, *20*, 269–287. [CrossRef]

95. Cunningham, C.L.; Martínez-Cerdeño, V.; Noctor, S.C. Microglia regulate the number of neural precursor cells in the developing cerebral cortex. *J. Neurosci.* **2013**, *33*, 4216–4233. [CrossRef] [PubMed]

96. Herculano-Houzel, S. The glia/neuron ratio: How it varies uniformly across brain structures and species and what that means for brain physiology and evolution. *Glia* **2014**, *62*, 1377–1391. [CrossRef] [PubMed]

97. Kast, B. The best supporting actors. *Nature* **2001**, *412*, 674–676. [CrossRef] [PubMed]

98. Zimmer, C. The dark matter of the human brain. *Discover* **2009**, *30*, 30–31.

99. Banhey, J.; von Bartheld, C.S. The cellular composition and glia-neuron ratio in the spinal cord of a human and a nonhuman primate: Comparison with other species and brain regions. *Anat. Rec.* **2018**, *301*, 697–710. [CrossRef]

100. Von Bartheld, C.S. Myths and truths about the cellular composition of the human brain: A review of influential concepts. *J. Chem. Neuroanat.* **2017**, in press. [CrossRef] [PubMed]

101. Herculano-Houzel, S. Scaling of brain metabolism with a fixed energy budget per neuron: Implications for neuronal activity, plasticity and evolution. *PLoS ONE* **2011**, *6*, e17514. [CrossRef] [PubMed]

102. Mota, B.; Herculano-Houzel, S. Cortical folding scales universally with surface area and thickness, not number of neurons. *Science* **2015**, *349*, 74–77. [CrossRef] [PubMed]

103. Copley, S.D.; Smith, E.; Morowitz, H.J. A mechanism for the association of amino acids with their codons and the origins of the genetic code. *Proc. Natl. Acad. Sci. USA* **2005**, *102*, 4442–4447. [CrossRef] [PubMed]

104. Perea, G.; Navarrete, M.; Araque, A. Tripartite synapses: Astrocytes process and control synaptic information. *Trends Neurosci.* **2009**, *32*, 421–431. [CrossRef] [PubMed]

105. Lee, Y.; Morrison, B.M.; Li, Y.; Lengacher, S.; Farah, M.H.; Hoffman, P.N.; Liu, Y.; Tsingalia, A.; Jin, L.; Zhang, P.-W.; et al. Oligodendroglia metabolically support axons and contribute to neurodegeneration. *Nature* **2012**, *487*, 443–450. [CrossRef] [PubMed]

106. Ullian, E.M.; Sapperstein, S.K.; Chistopherson, K.S.; Barres, B.A. Control of synapse number by glia. *Science* **2001**, *291*, 657–661. [CrossRef] [PubMed]

107. Mauch, D.H.; Nägler, K.; Schumacher, S.; Göritz, C.; Müller, E.-C.; Otto, A.; Pfrieger, F.W. CNS synaptogenesis promoted by glia-derived cholesterol. *Science* **2001**, *294*, 1354–1357. [CrossRef] [PubMed]

108. Magistretti, P.J. Neuron–glia metabolic coupling and plasticity. *J. Exp. Biol.* **2006**, *209*, 2304–2311. [CrossRef] [PubMed]

109. Cragg, B.G. The density of synapses and neurons in the motor and visual areas of the cerebral cortex. *J. Anat.* **1967**, *101*, 639–654. [PubMed]
110. Miki, T.; Fukui, Y.; Itoh, M.; Hisano, S.; Xie, Q.; Takeuchi, Y. Estimation of the numerical densities of neurons and synapses in cerebral cortex. *Brain Res. Protoc.* **1997**, *2*, 9–16. [CrossRef]
111. Caplan, A.I.; Ordahl, C.P. Irreversible gene repression model for control of development. *Science* **1978**, *201*, 120–131. [CrossRef] [PubMed]
112. Brown, G.; Bunce, C.M.; Lord, J.M.; McConnell, F.M. The development of cell lineages: A sequential model. *Differentiation* **1988**, *39*, 83–89. [CrossRef] [PubMed]
113. McConnell, S.K. Constructing the cerebral cortex: Neurogenesis and fate determination. *Neuron* **1995**, *15*, 761–768. [CrossRef]
114. Grimaldi, P.; Carletti, B.; Magrassi, L.; Rossi, F. Fate restriction and developmental potential of cerebellar progenitors. Transplantation studies in the developing CNS. *Prog. Brain Res.* **2005**, *148*, 57–68. [CrossRef] [PubMed]
115. Qian, X.; Shen, Q.; Goderie, S.K.; He, W.; Capela, A.; Davis, A.A.; Temple, S. Timing of CNS cell generation: A programmed sequence of neuron and glial cell production from isolated murine cortical stem cells. *Neuron* **2000**, *28*, 69–80. [CrossRef]
116. Bandeira, F.; Lent, R.; Herculano-Houzel, S. Changing numbers of neuronal and non-neuronal cells underlie postnatal brain growth in the rat. *Proc. Natl. Acad. Sci. USA* **2009**, *106*, 14108–14113. [CrossRef] [PubMed]
117. Dos Santos, S.E.; Noctor, S.C.; Herculano-Houzel, S. Discontinuous addition of cortical cells during embryonic and postnatal rat development. Unpublished work. 2018.
118. Morterá, P.; Dos Santos, S.E.; Noctor, S.; Herculano-Houzel, S. Changing numbers of cells in pre- and postnatal development in the mouse. Unpublished work. 2018.
119. Rowitch, D.H. Glial specification in the vertebrate neural tube. *Nat. Rev. Neurosci.* **2004**, *5*, 409–419. [CrossRef] [PubMed]
120. Chan, W.Y.; Kohsaka, S.; Rezaie, P. The origin and cell lineage of microglia—New concepts. *Brain Res. Rev.* **2007**, *53*, 344–354. [CrossRef] [PubMed]
121. Kriegstein, A.; Alvarez-Buylla, A. The glial nature of embryonic and adult neural stem cells. *Ann. Rev. Neurosci.* **2009**, *32*, 149–184. [CrossRef] [PubMed]
122. Prinz, M.; Mildner, A. Microglia in the CNS: Immigrants from another world. *Glia* **2011**, *59*, 177–187. [CrossRef] [PubMed]
123. Ginhoux, F.; Lim, S.; Hoeffel, G.; Low, D.; Huber, T. Origin and differentiation of microglia. *Front. Cell. Neurosci.* **2013**, *7*, 45. [CrossRef] [PubMed]
124. Ginhoux, F.; Prinz, M. Origin of microglia: Current concepts and past controversies. *Cold Spring Harb. Perspect. Biol.* **2015**, *7*. [CrossRef] [PubMed]
125. Reik, W. Stability and flexibility of epigenetic gene regulation in mammalian development. *Nature* **2007**, *447*, 425–432. [CrossRef] [PubMed]
126. Golkaram, M.; Jang, J.; Hellander, S.; Kosik, K.S.; Petzold, L.R. The role of chromatin density in cell population heterogeneity during stem cell differentiation. *Sci. Rep.* **2017**, *7*, 13307. [CrossRef] [PubMed]
127. Chen, T.; Dent, S.Y.R. Chromatin modifiers and remodelers: Regulators of cellular differentiation. *Nat. Rev. Gen.* **2014**, *15*, 93–106. [CrossRef] [PubMed]
128. Doetsch, F.; Caille, I.; Lim, D.A.; Garcia-Verdugo, J.M.; Alvarez-Buylla, A. Subventricular zone astrocytes are neural stem cells in the adult mammalian brain. *Cell* **1999**, *97*, 703–716. [CrossRef]
129. Seri, B.; Garcia-Verdugo, J.M.; McEwen, B.S.; Alvarez-Buylla, A. Atrocytes give rise to new neurons in the adult mammalian hippocampus. *J. Neurosci.* **2001**, *21*, 7153–7160. [CrossRef] [PubMed]
130. Doetsch, F. The glial identity of neural stem cells. *Nat. Neurosci.* **2003**, *6*, 1127–1134. [CrossRef] [PubMed]
131. Bayraktar, O.A.; Fuentealba, L.C.; Alvarez-Buylla, A.; Rowitch, D.H. Astrocyte development and heterogeneity. *Cold Spring Harb. Perspect. Biol.* **2015**, *5*. [CrossRef] [PubMed]
132. Schmidt-Nielsen, K. Scaling: Why Is Animal Size So Important? Cambridge University Press: Cambridge, UK, 1984.

133. Savage, V.M.; Allen, A.P.; Brown, L.H.; Gillooly, J.F.; Herman, A.B.; Woodruff, W.H.; West, G.B. Scaling of number, size, and metabolic rate of cells with body size in mammals. *Proc. Natl. Acad. Sci. USA* **2007**, *104*, 4718–4723. [CrossRef] [PubMed]

134. Herculano-Houzel, S.; Avelino-de-Souza, K.; Manger, P.R. Constant densities of cells in the liver of reptile and mammalian species irrespective of body size. Unpublished work. 2018.

135. Rosenberg, A.B.; Roco, C.M.; Muscat, R.A.; Kuchina, A.; Sample, P.; Yao, Z.; Graybuck, L.T.; Peeler, D.J.; Mukherjee, S.; Chen, W.; et al. Single-cell profiling of the developing mouse brain and spinal cord with split-pool barcoding. *Science* **2018**, *360*, 176–182. [CrossRef] [PubMed]

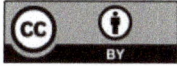

![neuroglia logo] *neuroglia*

MDPI

Article

Ultrastructural Remodeling of the Neurovascular Unit in the Female Diabetic db/db Model—Part I: Astrocyte

Melvin R. Hayden [1,2,*], DeAna G. Grant [3], Annayya R. Aroor [1,2,4] and Vincent G. DeMarco [1,2,4,5]

1   Diabetes and Cardiovascular Center, University of Missouri School of Medicine, Columbia, MO 65212, USA; aroora@health.missouri.edu (A.R.A.); demarcov@missouri.edu (V.G.D.)
2   Division of Endocrinology and Metabolism, Department of Medicine, University of Missouri, Columbia, MO 65211, USA
3   Electron Microscopy Core Facility, University of Missouri, Columbia, MO 65211, USA; GrantDe@missouri.edu
4   Research Service, Harry S. Truman Memorial Veterans Hospital, Columbia, MO 65201, USA
5   Department of Medical Pharmacology and Physiology, University of Missouri, Columbia, MO 65211, USA
*   Correspondence: mrh29pete@gmail.com; Tel.: +1-573-346-3019

Received: 4 July 2018; Accepted: 31 July 2018; Published: 7 August 2018

Abstract: Obesity, insulin resistance, and type 2 diabetes mellitus are associated with cognitive impairment, known as diabetic cognopathy. In this study, we tested the hypothesis that neurovascular unit(s) (NVU) within cerebral cortical gray matter regions display abnormal cellular remodeling. The monogenic ($Lepr^{db}$) female diabetic db/db (BKS.CgDock7^m +/+$Lepr^{db}$/J; DBC) mouse model was utilized for this ultrastructural study. Upon sacrifice (at 20 weeks of age), left-brain hemispheres of the DBC and age-matched non-diabetic wild-type control C57BL/KsJ (CKC) mice were immediately immersion-fixed. We found attenuation/loss of endothelial blood–brain barrier tight/adherens junctions and pericytes, thickening of the basement membrane, aberrant mitochondria, and pathological remodeling of protoplasmic astrocytes. Additionally, there were adherent red blood cells and NVU microbleeds (cortical layer III) in DBC mice, which were not observed in CKC animals. While this study represents only a "snapshot in time", it does allow for cellular remodeling comparisons between DBC and CKC. In this paper, the first of a three-part series, we report the observational ultrastructural remodeling changes of the NVU and its protoplasmic astrocytes in relation to the surrounding neuropil. Having identified multiple abnormal cellular remodeling changes in the DBC as compared to CKC models, we will design future experiments to evaluate various treatment modalities in DBC mice.

Keywords: astrocyte; db/db mouse model; microglia; neuroglia; neurovascular unit; type 2 diabetes

---

1. Introduction

Type 2 diabetes mellitus (T2DM) is a chronic endocrine-metabolic disorder of glucose metabolism characterized by hyperglycemia, insulin resistance or relative lack of insulin and impaired cognition. Type 2 diabetes mellitus is one of the fastest growing public health problems and diseases globally with aging of the global population playing an important role, including the global post-World War II baby boom generation [1]. Concurrently, the prevalence of the age-related neurodegenerative diseases, such as Alzheimer's disease (AD), vascular dementia, and Parkinson's disease (PD), are also increasing [2,3]. Importantly, AD may now be considered a mixed dementia consisting of both neurovascular dysfunction (macrovascular and microvascular disease) and neurodegeneration [4–8].

Type 2 diabetes mellitus and AD are each projected to undergo a marked increase in incidence over the coming decades and may indeed be synergistic [9].

Epidemiologic studies identified T2DM as an independent risk factor for multiple affected target organs, which include neuropathy, retinopathy, nephropathy, cardiomyopathy, and the age-related neurodegenerative diseases, such as diabetic cognopathy and AD [10–13]. Neurovascular unit (NVU) and microvascular small vessel disease remodeling are known to be associated with T2DM and age-related neurodegeneration, which are a growing concern. Thus, we elected to study the ultrastructural remodeling changes of the NVU in the mid-cortical gray matter regions of the obese, insulin-resistant, and diabetic female db/db mice models (DBC), and compared them to the lean, non-diabetic, and aged-matched control models (CKC).

The NVU is a complex functional and anatomical structure comprised of endothelial cells (ECs), pericytes (Pcs), astrocytes (ACs), microglia cells (MGCs), and neurons [14]. The luminal ECs contain the blood–brain barrier (BBB), which is formed by tight junction proteins (TJs; claudin, occludin, and junctional adherens molecule proteins) and adherens junction proteins (AJs; vascular endothelial (VE) cadherins), intertwined to form very electron-dense lines at the overlapping junctional inter-endothelial spaces. The TJ/AJ are anchored by adjacent EC zonula occludens-1 (ZO-1) proteins that bind to EC cytoskeleton proteins, which have a highly selective BBB and a high transendothelial electrical resistance, providing a permeability barrier to hydrophilic molecules and large proteins [5,6,8].

The next component of the NVU (proceeding from the luminal EC), is the EC basal lamina or basement membrane (BM), which splits to encase the Pc, which creates an inner and outer BM of the latter. Pericytes provide the mural structural support of the endothelial capillary and NVU. Importantly, pericytes are known to be contractile cells; however, they allow for the dilatation and relaxation of the capillary, when regional neurons are activated, and of signal pericytes via connecting astrocytes [4–8,13–15].

Astrocytes tightly adhere to the BM of both the EC and Pc via its end-feet basal lamina. Astrocytes are responsible for integrating the vascular mural cells (endothelial cells and pericytes) of the NVU to nearby regional neurons [16]. Astrocytes allow for NVU coupling, which is fundamental for the regulation of regional capillary cerebral blood flow (CBF) by both astrocyte and neuron-derived chemical messengers that provide for functional hyperemia; this link is known as neurovascular coupling [14,16,17]. Astrocytes are surrounded by the neuropil, which, in gray matter, is comprised primarily of dendritic synapses and unmyelinated neurons—interneurons with traversing myelinated neurons and an extracellular matrix (ECM) between these cellular structures (Figure 1; Table 1).

We hypothesized that NVU remodeling in the diabetic DBC models is associated with an attenuation and/or loss of endothelial cell BBB TJ/AJ and pericytes similar to our previous findings in the streptozotocin-induced type 1 diabetes mellitus (T1DM) mouse models [18]. Also, we posited that MGCs might undergo a reactive-activation (M1-type polarization) similar to previous observations in the diet-induced obesity and insulin-resistant Western mouse models with intermittent glucose elevation and impaired glucose tolerance [13]. However, in the DBC we observed additional marked abnormal remodeling in the surrounding neuroglial components including astrocytes, microglia, oligodendrocytes, and myelin in addition to our previous findings in type 1 diabetic models and diet-induced obese Western models. The multiple aberrant cellular phenotypes may be associated with increased vulnerability to other age-related diseases such as AD and (PD) in an aging population, which are known to have an increased risk due to T2DM [13,19]. The multicellular ultrastructure morphologic remodeling observed in this study allowed us to become acutely aware that a single cellular structure does not become abnormally remodeled without affecting the structure, and ultimately, the function of other cells in the mid-cortical gray matter of the DBC models. Furthermore, these observations support the notion that no one cell is an island unto itself, and that single maladaptive cell type and dysfunctional remodeling could have a direct or indirect effect on other cells in the same regions as highlighted by the NVU multicellular remodeling in the DBC [20].

Table 1. Identifying characteristics of cells that form the neurovascular unit by transmission electron microscopy.

	Mural Cells
	Line the entire vascular system (macrovascular and microvascular) in a mononuclear layer.
	The ECs are the first cell one encounters from the vascular lumen as one proceeds from the luminal surface to the outermost abluminal regions of the neurovascular unit (NVU).
	Endothelial cells have an elusive glycocalyx on their luminal cytoplasm; however, this structure is usually eliminated by dehydration in the preparation for microscopy and staining.
Endothelial cell(s) (EC)	The ECs have an intermediate electron-dense cytoplasm and are thin except where one encounters a larger and greater electron-dense nucleus.
	Neurovascular ECs have very few to no pinocytotic vesicles as compared to peripheral capillary ECs with an increase in EC mitochondria. Next one encounters the ECs hyaline basement membrane (BM) with a less electron density.
	The ECs cytoplasm and nuclei are elongated and their terminating cytoplasm ends most commonly with overlapping junctions creating a paracellular–inter-endothelial space that is lined by very election-dense protein staining of tight and adherens junctions that form the brain's specific blood-brain barrier (Figure 1).
	Are the next abluminal encountered cell in the NVU capillary. Pericytes are embedded within the shared BM synthesized by both the ECs and Pcs. The Pcs wrap around (peri-) the ECs of the NVU capillary and those transitioning to very small arterioles with an internal elastic lamina.
Pericyte(s) (Pc)	Similar to the ECs, Pcs have an electron-dense cytoplasm with elongated cytoplasmic processes and nuclei and contain prominent electron-dense lysosomes and mitochondria. Importantly, Pcs are known to be contractile cells that allow for NVU capillary contraction/relaxation to permit relaxation in regions of highly active neurons, which allow for increased regional cerebral blood flow (CBF) and neurovascular coupling (NVC) with intact astrocytes.
	In cross section one sometimes can only identify Pc foot processes (Pcfp) with their encasing inner and outer BMs, whereas in longitudinal sections one can better identify their elongated character (Figure 1)
	Glial Cells
	Are the largest cell of the NVU, which assume a more cuboidal morphology in contrast to ECs and Pcs. The AC are also considered to be the brains connecting cell to regional neurons and form a clear zone, halo or corona around the Pcs and ECs.
Astrocyte cell(s) (AC)	Characteristically, they are the most electron-lucent cell of the NVU and brain cells and one often observes scattered electron-dense line's, which represent their endoplasmic reticulum proteins.
	The ACs electron-dense thinned plasma membranes tightly adhere or abut the outer BMs of the ECs and Pcs.
	The AC completes the third key cell of the neurovascular unit; however, the microglia are also an important part and in both the grey matter and especially the white matter oligodendrocytes become a highly important part of the NVU as well (Figure 1).
	Are the smallest of the glia cells and their cytoplasm is the most electron-dense of the NVU and the brain.
Microglia cells (MGC)	In their non-activated phenotypic state, they have elongated cytoplasmic process in ramified form. They have an extensive endoplasmic reticulum, Golgi body system and contain multiple mitochondria. Their cytoplasmic processes are known to be capable of extending and contracting. They have a unique morphology of their nuclei with an outer stippled chromatin at its neurolemma and a more stippled diffuse chromatin electron dense appearance of the central nuclei (Figure 1).
Oligodendrocyte cell(s) (OL)	As suggested by their name Oligo-, these cells are intermediate in size and their thinned cytoplasm also have an intermediate electron density that is helpful when comparing to AC and MGCs. They also may occur in groups or nests and are more often found in the deeper white matter regions of the brain
	Neurons, Interneurons and the Neuropil
	May be myelinated or unmyelinated.
	Neurons have electron-lucent cytoplasmic axons with a greater electron dense and orderly layered network of neurofilaments and contain the usual cytoplasmic organelles. Neurons are also known to have and axon hillock and very long cytoplasmic axon extensions, which connect to other neurons via their dendritic synapses.
Neurons (N)-interneurons	Sometimes, neurons and especially interneurons can be noted to be closely interacting and in close proximity to the EC, Pc and astrocytes of the NVU.
	Neuronal cytoplasmic axons are also electron-lucent; however, their more electron-dense neurofilaments are layered in an orderly fashion in contrast to the electron densities of the AC, which are randomly scattered throughout the cytoplasm
	Is an all-inclusive term and appears to form the background tissue along with a very thinned extracellular matrix–interstitium within the cortical grey matter, which includes the vast number of dendritic synapses, neurons (myelinated/unmyelinated axons) passing through the neuropil along with other glial cells and processes (Figure 1).
Neuropil–neuropile	The EC, Pc, AC, MGC, oligodendrocytes and neurons–interneurons are the six major cell types that are present within a vast neuropile responsible for forming the NVU within the cortical grey matter

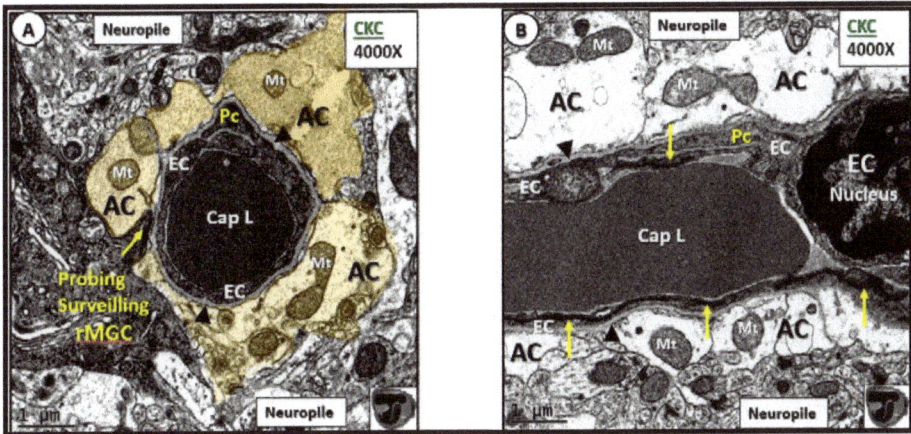

Figure 1. Normal neurovascular unit (NVU) morphology in control wild-type non-diabetic models (C57BL/KsJ; CKC). Panels (**A**) (cross-section) and (**B**) (longitudinal section) illustrate the normal cellular ultrastructure of the NVU. Panel (**A**) depicts an electron-dense ramified microglia cell (rMGC) surveilling the NVU (arrow). The NVU capillary consists of an endothelial cell (EC) encircling a capillary lumen (Cap L) whose basement membrane (BM) splits (arrowheads) to encompass the pericyte (Pc) foot process. Note how the pseudo-colored golden astrocyte (AC) end-feet encompass and tightly abut the capillary EC and Pc BMs. Note that the AC clear zone in panel (**A**) was pseudo-colored golden to emphasize its importance in the NVU, while it exists as a clear-zone with a reduced electron-dense cytoplasm as compared to other cells within the brain, and represents not only a golden halo, but also a clear zone or corona of ACs surrounding the EC and Pc cells of the NVU (panel (**B**)). Panel (**B**) illustrates the electron-lucency of the AC clear zone halo or corona that tightly abuts and encircles the NVU EC and Pc BMs. Note the EC nucleus (far right side) and the highly electron-dense tight junctions/adherens junctions (TJ/AJ) complex that are not readily visible in panel (**A**) (arrows). Also, note that the mitochondria (Mt) have an electron-dense Mt matrix and that cristae may be noted even at this magnification. Note that the NVU is encompassed by the outermost abluminal neuropil (neuropil). In the bottom right-hand corner, note the logo of red blood cells within a capillary NVU that are in the shape of the letter T overlying the letter J, which are used to abbreviate tight junction(s). Magnification ×4000; scale bar = 1 µm.

2. Methods

2.1. Animal Studies

All animal studies were approved by the Institutional Animal Care and Use Committees at the Harry S Truman Memorial Veterans' Hospital and University of Missouri, Columbia, MO, USA (No. 190), and conformed to the Guide for the Care and Use of Laboratory Animals published by the National Institutes of Health (NIH). Eight-week-old female db/db (BKS.Cg-$Dock7^m$+/+$Lepr^{db}$/J; DBC) and wild-type control (C57BLKS/J; CKC) mice were purchased from the Jackson Laboratory (Ann Harbor, MI, USA) and were housed under standard laboratory conditions where room temperature was 21–22 °C, and light and dark cycles were 12 h each. Two cohorts of mice were used: lean non-diabetic controls (CKC, $n = 3$), and obese, insulin-resistant, diabetic db/db (DBC, $n = 3$), which were sacrificed for study at 20 weeks of age. The female model was initially chosen because females have greater impairments in diastolic relaxation and increased aortic stiffness, and may predict future cardiovascular disease events [21]. Furthermore, the female gender is positively associated with dementia/AD risk as compared to men (especially in older age groups) [22].

2.2. Tissue Collection and Preparation for Transmission Electron Microscopy

The left hemisphere was collected immediately upon sacrifice in CKC and DBC models and immediately placed in standard transmission electronic microscopy (TEM) fixative of 2% paraformaldehyde and 2% glutaraldehyde in 100 mM sodium cacodylate buffer (pH = 7.35) for immersion fixation. Approximately 1 mm sections from the mid-cortical gray matter tissue (Figure 2) were then rinsed with 100 mM sodium cacodylate buffer (pH 7.35) containing 130 mM sucrose. Secondary fixation was performed using 1% osmium tetroxide (Ted Pella, Inc., Redding, CA, USA) in cacodylate buffer using a Pelco Biowave (Ted Pella) operated at 100 W for 1 min. Specimens were next incubated at 4 °C for 1 h, then rinsed with cacodylate buffer, and further rinsed with distilled water. En bloc staining was performed using 1% aqueous uranyl acetate and incubated at 4 °C overnight, then rinsed with distilled water. Using the Pelco Biowave, a graded dehydration series (e.g., 100 W for 40 s) was performed using ethanol, transitioned into acetone, and dehydrated tissues were then infiltrated with Epon resin (250 W for 3 min) and polymerized at 60 °C overnight. Ultrathin sections were cut to a thickness of 85 nm using an ultramicrotome (Ultracut UCT, Leica Microsystems, Wetzlar, Germany) and stained using Sato's triple lead solution stain and 5% aqueous uranyl acetate. Multiple images were acquired for study at various magnifications with a JOEL 1400-EX TEM JEOL (JEOL, Peabody, MA, USA) at 80 kV on a Gatan Ultrascan 1000 CCD (Gatan, Inc., Pleasanton, CA, USA).

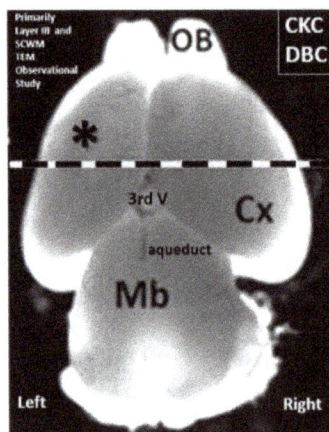

Figure 2. Brain specimens for transmission electron microscopy studies. The left hemisphere was utilized for this study. Cortical gray matter tissue specimens were obtained just cephalad to the mid-cortex dashed line (asterisk). Cx—cerebral cortex; Mb—midbrain; OB—olfactory bulb. TEM—transmission electronic microscopy; V—ventricle; DBC—db/db mice models; SCWM—subcortical with matter.

In regards to utilizing immersion fixation rather than perfusion fixation, the following explanation is in order: in a previous paper, we utilized immersion fixation as a rapid collection and immersion-fixation process of the cortical gray matter study [13]. Since we were interested to provide the same collection and fixation procedures in order to make direct comparisons if necessary, we felt that this collection and fixation method was better suited for our collection team because our previous ultrastructural images appeared to have good penetration of fixative with good fixation for image collection. We are aware and know that perfusion fixation is the preferred method of fixation, and that the immersion fixation is not the most suitable fixation for larger pieces of tissue such as whole brain or the left hemibrain, as in our studies; however, the outermost cortical regions of the brain (layers I–VI and deeper white-matter transitional regions) appear to have fixed nicely via immersion fixation, as can be viewed by our cortical sections in this and our previous paper [13] with distinct ultrastructural morphology. Therefore, because our lab collection team and preparations team previously and successfully supplied previous immersion-fixed specimens with good results, including cellular outline of membranes, cytoplasmic detail of organelles, nuclear detail, and intra-capillary erythrocyte, as well as white-blood-cell morphologic integrity appearance and overall ultrastructure morphology, and overall staining, we decided that this animal model (db/db diabetic female model) allowed us to utilize the rapid immersion fixation as a method of collecting, fixing, and subsequently studying the ultrastructure (fine structure within the cortical gray matter of the present study). Of interest, these same models were being evaluated using light microscopy, immunohistochemistry, and ultrastructure of other organs, which included the myocardium, aorta, and kidney in forthcoming papers to be published in the near future.

3. Results

In regards to the representation of the image data and images shared in this paper, the following factors are important for understanding our image data: three models per group were studied by TEM ($n = 3$ in control CKC models, and $n = 3$ in db/db DBC models). The sections for study (regions of interest) were selected based on the presence of NVU capillaries, which we were able to identify readily in the cortical layer III of the cortical gray matter. Cortical gray matter layer III is identifiable due to the large number of pyramidal neuronal nuclei. A total of 60 NVU capillaries were eventually studied for all models (10 from each model providing 30 NVU capillaries from CKC, and 30 NVU capillaries from DBC models). The marked remodeling changes observed in the diabetic DBC NVUs and their immediate surrounding regions were immediately noted, and therefore, representative comparison images were primarily chosen at varying magnifications for this paper to better illustrate and understand the marked maladaptive ultrastructure remodeling in the obese, diabetic db/db DBC models as compared to the non-obese non-diabetic CKC models. Therefore, the marked ultrastructural remodeling changes that were observed in the DBC were compared to the CKC. The maladaptive NVU capillaries, which included the attenuation and/or loss of endothelial tight and adherens junctions, thickening of basement membranes, attenuation and/or loss of pericytes, and astrocyte detachment or retraction were approximately 80% of the DBC (24 NVU capillaries with maladaptive remodeling versus a total of 30 NVU capillaries) when compared to no abnormalities (0 of 30 NVU capillaries) in CKC models.

3.1. Endothelial Cell Remodeling of the Neurovascular Unit

Because the BBB is formed primarily by the endothelial cells of the NVU, it seems appropriate to begin with EC remodeling and proceed from the luminal to the abluminal regions (inside-out approach). For reference, the normal ultrastructure morphology of the control model (CKC) NVU is shown in Figure 1.

In obese, diabetic DBCs, we observed an abnormal remodeling of the ECs, which consisted of an attenuation and/or loss of BBB EC TJ/AJ when compared to non-diabetic, non-obese control models (CKC; Figure 3). This attenuated, interrupted, and discontinuous TJ/AJ (Figure 3C), as well as the loss of electron-dense TJ/AJ (Figure 3B,D), may contribute to an increase in the permeability of the blood–brain barrier, as well as NVU uncoupling in the cortex and hippocampus [4,5,7]. Incidentally, when the EC NVU is abnormally remodeled and damaged (especially by oxidative stress due to glucotoxicity and loss of BBB TJ/AJ; Figure 3C), the once-probing surveilling ramified microglial cells (that are operative in control CKC models; Figure 1A) undergo a phenotypic remodeling to a more reactive-activated microglia phenotype as a result of danger and damage signals from the NVU. These reactive-activated microglial cells begin to encircle and invade the NVU (Figure 3C) and may be associated not only with the attenuation and/or loss of EC TJ/AJ, but also with the detachment and retraction of astrocytes to the NVU.

We also observed the NVU basement membrane to be thickened and associated with endothelial cell cytoplasmic thinning, vesicles/vacuoles (ranging in size from approximately 50–200 nm), aberrant mitochondria (aMt), and reactive-activated microglial cells (aMGCs; Figures 3C, 4, and 5). Endothelial cells are primarily responsible for the formation of the NVU basement membrane. The basement membrane is composed of collagen IV, fibrinogen, laminin, nidogen, and heparin sulfate proteoglycans (agrin and perlecan) [23,24]. The basement membrane is important for microvascular development, stability, NVU barrier integrity, and encasement of the pericyte (contributing to BM synthesis and maintenance) and provides the surface for the attachment of astrocyte end-feet. The excessive accumulation and thickening of the basement membrane in some images (Figure 5) were somewhat reminiscent of the thickened mesangial matrix expansion found in renal glomerular diabetic models and humans.

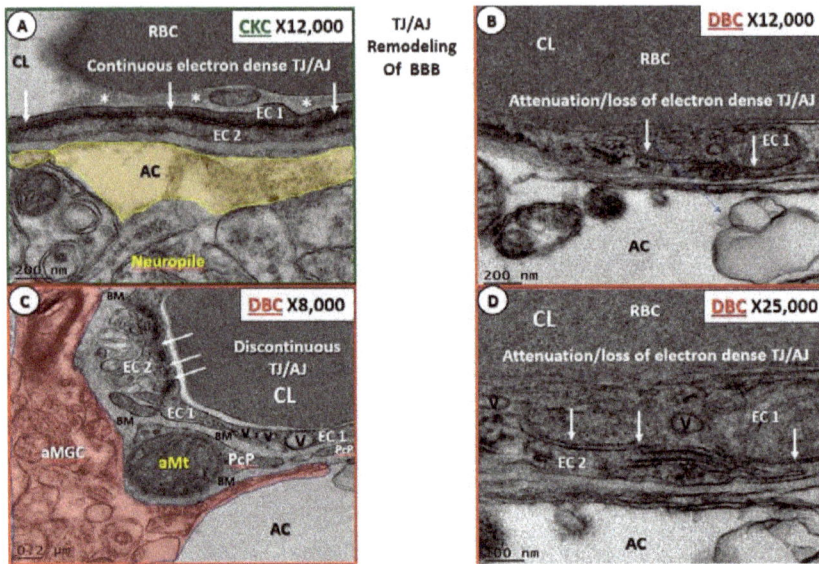

Figure 3. Attenuation and/or loss of tight junctions/adherens junctions (TJ/AJ) in diabetic db/db mice (DBC) models. Panel (**A**) illustrates the normal appearance of the highly electron-dense proteinaceous endothelial cell (EC) tight junction/adherens junction (TJ/AJ) formed between overlapping ECs. EC-1 overlaps EC-2 in the non-diabetic control models (C57BLKS/J; CKC) to form the paracellular blood–brain barrier (BBB; arrows). This image also depicts the elusive endothelial glycocalyx remnants (asterisks) that form the initial EC barrier of the neurovascular unit (not studied in this experiment). Panel (**B**) depicts the loss/attenuation of the highly electron-dense proteinaceous TJ/AJ joining the two overlapping EC layers (arrows) in the diabetic DBC models. Magnification ×12,000; scale bar = 200 nm in panels (**A**,**B**). Panel (**C**) illustrates the attenuated, discontinuous, and interrupted morphology of the EC TJ/AJ (arrows) in the obese, diabetic DBC models. Note the pseudo-colorized red reactive-activated microglial cell (aMGC) and an abbreviated pericyte process (PcP), which contains an aberrant swollen and smudged mitochondria (aMt). Also, note vacuole (V) and vesicles (v) within the EC cytoplasm of EC 1. Magnification ×8000; scale bar = 0.2 μm. Panel (**D**) (higher magnification of panel (**B**)) demonstrates with greater clarity the definite loss of the TJ/AJ electron density depicted in panel (**B**) as compared to the CKC models in Figures 1B and 3A. Magnification ×25,000; scale bar = 100 nm. AC—astrocyte (pseudo-colored golden panel (**A**); CL—capillary lumen; RBC—red blood cell.

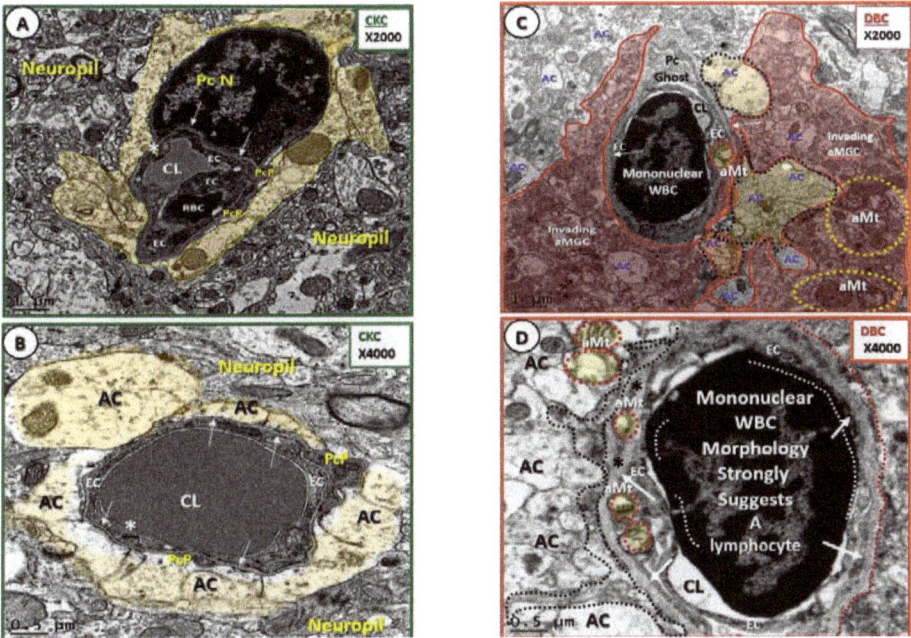

Figure 4. Basement membrane thickening in DBC as compared to control (CKC) models. One can readily observe the thickened ($\geq$200-nm BMs; arrows) in DBC (panels (**C,D**)) as compared to the normal ($\leq$80-nm BMs (in panels (**A,B**) with same magnifications in (**A,C**) and (**B,D**)). Magnification $\times$2000; bar = 1 µm (panel (**A**)), and magnification $\times$4000; bar = 0.5 µm (panel (**B**))). Panel (**C**) depicts a pericyte ghost smudged region superiorly and an invading reactive-activated microglial cell (pseudo-colored red). Note only the two-remaining intact ACs pseudo-colorized golden on the right-hand side of the NVU. Magnification $\times$2000; bar = 1 µm. Panels (**C,D**) also depict an adherent luminal inflammatory mononuclear cell (dashed white lines in panel (**D**) = sites of adherence) to the EC. The size and morphology of this mononuclear suggest a lymphocyte. Also note the EC and AC aMt (pseudo-colored yellow with encompassing red dashed lines) and thinning of the EC cytoplasm, especially noted in panel (**D**) as compared to panel (**B**). Specifically, in panel (**D**), one notes an aMGC cytoplasmic process (black-dashed lines) to the left side of this abnormally inflamed NVU, which also illustrates the detachment of the AC from the NVU BM. These combined maladaptive remodeling changes strongly suggest a morphologically activated-dysfunctional endothelium. Magnification $\times$2000; bar = 1 µm (panel (**C**)), and magnification $\times$4000; bar = 0.5 µm (panel (**D**)). Asterisks—tight junctions/adherens junctions (panels (**A,B**)); PcN—pericyte nucleus.

3.2. Remodeling of Pericytes and Pericyte Foot Processes

Pericytes are essential for proper formation of the NVU and EC BBB TJ/AJ in utero, as well as for NVU maturation and maintenance during adulthood. As previously mentioned, the basement membrane splits to encompass pericytes and their processes to create an inner and outer BM of pericytes in the NVU (Figures 6 and 7). The brain, including the retina, has the highest coverage of vascular endothelial cells by pericytes, which is essential for regulation of BBB permeability [13]. Pericytes not only contribute to EC BBB TJ/AJ function, but also contribute to basement membrane formation and maintenance [13,15]. Pericytes and endothelial cells share a common basement membrane secured by N-cadherins, fibronectin, connexins, and various integrins-(13, 15, 25). Additionally, pericytes induce the synthesis of occludin and claudin in the endothelial cell TJ/AJ complex through the release of angiopoetin-1 [13]. Endothelial cells also signal to pericytes by synthesizing and secreting platelet-derived growth factor β (PDGF-β) to activate the Pc-specific receptor (PDGFR-β), which is important for Pc proliferation, migration, and recruitment of Pc to the endothelium [13,25] (Figures 6 and 7).

Key findings in pericyte remodeling included attenuation and/or loss of pericytes and the retraction or loss of pericyte foot processes, in addition to having aberrant Mt within the cytoplasm and the retraction of pericyte nuclei and of pericyte cytoplasmic processes (Figure 7).

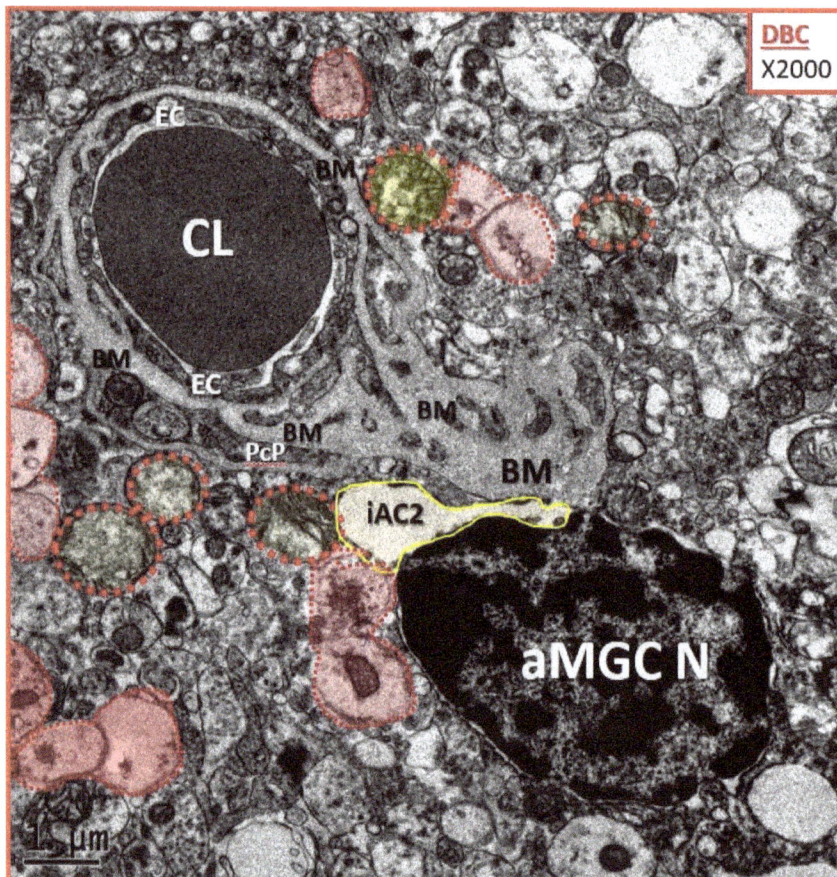

Figure 5. Excessive basement membrane thickening in some DBC models. This image depicts excessive and abundant BM thickening in the NVU of a DBC model. Note that only one intact astrocyte (iAC2) remains in this image (pseudo-colored golden), while the remainder of the ACs are detached and retracted (pseudo-colored red) from the NVU. Note the aMt (pseudo-colored yellow with encapsulating red dashed lines) that are swollen with loss of the electron-dense Mt matrix and loss of cristae. It is important to note the absence of the endothelial cell blood–brain barrier tight and adherent junction complex and pericytes in this image. Importantly, note the detached and retracted astrocytes (pseudo-colored pink with red-dashed outlines). aMGC N—reactive-activated microglial cell nucleus.

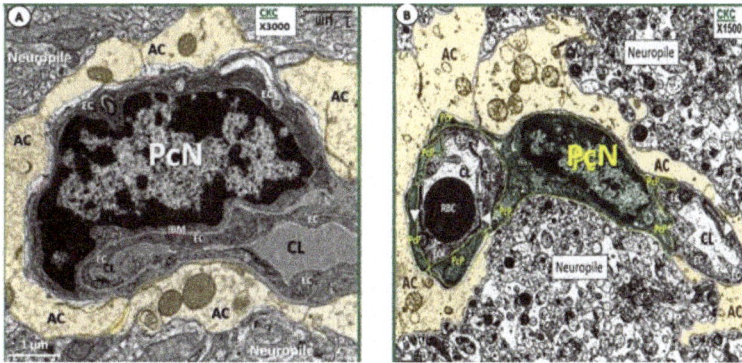

Figure 6. Normal pericyte ultrastructure morphology. Panels (**A,B**) reflect the normal morphology of the Pc in relation to the NVU in control non-diabetic CKC models. While each of these images contains the soma of a Pc with a PcN), Pcs (pseudo-colored green in panel (**B**)) are most often observed as PcP, and they are also defined by an inner (iBM) and outer basement membrane (oBM). The Pc and PcP BMs are abutted by the AC's (pseudo-colored gold) basal lamina. While panel (**A**) demonstrates a single Pc in close relation to the capillary EC of the NVU, one may also observe that Pcs may provide connectivity to two adjacent NVUs as in panel (**B**). Panel (**B**) illustrates prominent tight and adherens junctions (TJ/AJ; arrowheads). Also, one will note that in some NVUs, the neuropil may come into direct contact with the outer BM of Pcs. Magnification ×3000; bar = 1 μm (Panel (**A**)). Magnification ×1500; bar = 1 μm (panel (**B**)).

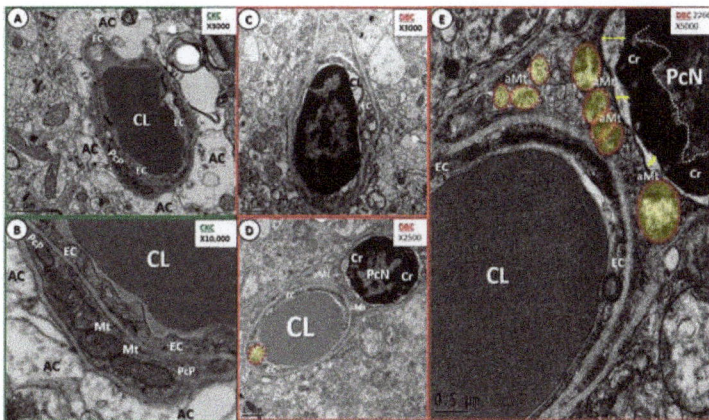

Figure 7. Remodeling of pericytes in diabetic (DBC) models. Panels (**A,B**) illustrate NVU with normal appearing Pc and PcP. Panels (**C–E**) demonstrate some of the abnormal Pc remodeling changes that are observed in the diabetic DBC. Panel (**C**) illustrates the complete loss of PcP in an inflamed abnormally remodeled NVU. Panel (**D**) depicts an abnormal PcN that is retracted from its nuclear membrane at low magnification to illustrate the NVU surroundings in the neuropil. Also, one will note swollen aMt(pseudo-colored yellow with red dashed-line). Panel **€** depicts aMt that are pseudo-colored yellow encapsulated by red dashed lines with abnormal swelling, as well as the loss of Mt matrix electron density and the loss of Mt cristae within the cytoplasm of the Pc. This image also depicts the retraction of the PcN from its nuclear membrane (double arrows), and excessive PcN chromatin (Cr) condensation, strongly suggesting Pc dysfunction and degeneration, and may be in the process of eventual loss in DBC. Panels (**A,C**): magnification ×3000; bar = 1 μm. Panel (**B**): magnification ×10,000; bar = 0.02 μm. Panel (**D**): magnification ×2500; bar = 1 μm. Panel (**E**): magnification ×5000; bar = 0.5 μm.

3.3. Protoplasmic Astrocyte Remodeling in Cortical Gray Matter Diabetic DBC Models

Protoplasmic astrocytes have numerous homeostatic functions in the brain [13,25–27]. Astrocytes are the first glial cells directly abutting the basement membranes of the two mural vascular cells (endothelial cells and pericytes) of the NVU in the healthy brain. This places astrocytes in a unique position for connecting the regional cortical neurons to NVU mural cells. It is this connection between the NVU and the neuron that contributes to a local hyperemia when neurons increase their activity. Additionally, astrocytes act as a major supplier of energy via glycogen storage and glycolysis, as well as of antioxidant reserves (glutathione (GSH) and superoxide dismutase (SOD)), growth factors such as brain-derived growth factor transforming growth factor-β and glial-derived growth factor. Astrocytes also define many aspects of synapse formation, plasticity, protective function, synaptic maintenance, and elimination [26,27]. It is important to note, however, that human studies may not always conform to findings in rodents because human protoplasmic astrocytes in the neocortex are much larger and extend longer than in rodent models [28].

In obese, insulin-resistant, and diabetic DBC, we observed the astrocyte end-feet to detach and retract from the basement membrane, which was especially noted when activated microglia cells were actively encompassing or invading the NVU. The normal morphological relationship of the astrocyte with the two vascular mural cells of the NVU (ECs and Pcs) is shown in Figures 1A,B, 3, 4A,B, 5, 6, and 7A,B. Previous images demonstrating AC detachment include Figures 4C,D, 5, and 7C,D. Herein, we provide additional representative observational findings of the activated AC detachment and retraction from the EC and Pc BMs (Figure 8).

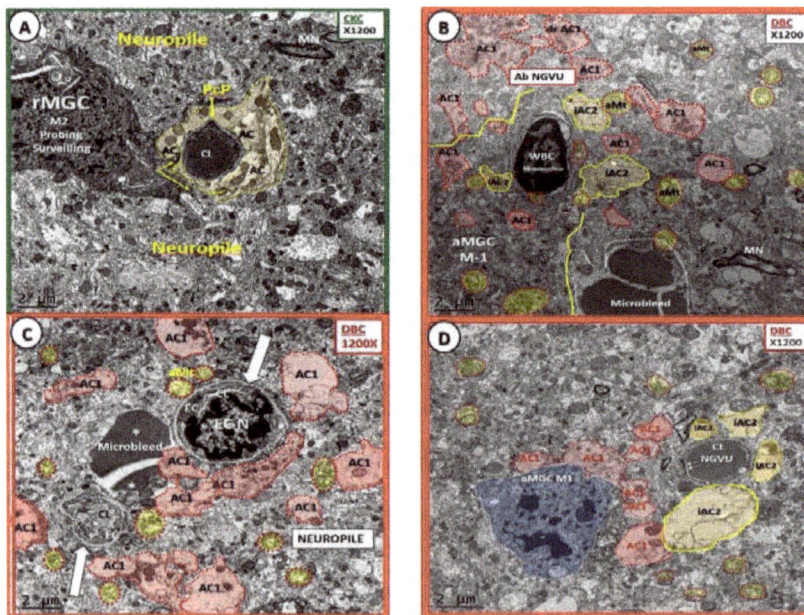

Figure 8. Detachment and retraction of protoplasmic AC in diabetic DBC models. Panel (**A**) depicts the control (CKC) NVU and note that the "golden halos" (corona of the iAC2) tightly about the NVU EC and Pc BMs. Note the nearby ramified microglial cell that is surveilling the NVU (arrows). In panel (**B**), there are still three remaining intact type 2 pseudo-colorized golden in contrast to the detached and retracted AC-1 (pseudo-colored pink with red outlines). Panel (**C**) depicts the total loss of iAC2 and all of the ACs having undergone phenotypic polarization to the detached and retracted AC1-type. Importantly, note the microbleed (asterisks) between the two NVUs (open white arrows), which may

be a contributing factor to the complete absence of the iAC2-type of astrocytes as in the intact AC1 in panel (**A**). Panel (**D**) depicts a aMGCM1 phenotype with abnormal nuclear chromatin condensation, which resembles a blue pseudo-colored "frowning face". The M1 type aMGC may not only contribute to the activation of the polarized-type AC1, but may also result in a structural and possible functional reason for the detachment and retraction of ACs. Indeed, the type 2 iAC2 "golden halos" that used to shine are now gone, detached and retracted from the NVU, and, as a result of their polarized transformation, may contribute to an increased dysfunction and increased permeability of the NVU. Panels (**B–D**) depict the abnormal detachment and retraction of the AC from the NVU in the diabetic DBC. In panel (**B**), there are still three remaining iAC2. Incidentally, panel (**D**) is a lower magnification of Figure 3C. Magnification ×1200; bar = 2 μm. ab NVU—abnormal–aberrant neuroglial vascular unit; MN—myelinated neuron; WBC—monocytic white blood cell.

The large AC cellular presence in the brain and their vast cell–cell communication via gap junctions may be viewed as the brain's functional syncytium [29]. The relationship among the NVU, EC, Pc, and their shared outer basement membrane, as well as the cell–matrix attachments via dystroglycans and integrins to NVU ACs, are essential for proper homeostasis and function [29–31]. Possible mechanisms that may result in AC detachment and retraction are illustrated in Section 4 (Figure 8).

3.4. Sticky, Adhesive Red Blood Cells in the Neurovascular Unit of Diabetic DBC Mice

Occasionally, red blood cells (RBCs) were observed to be adherent to the endothelial cells of the NVU in the cortical gray matter. These NVUs demonstrated highly electron-dense protein staining adhesion plaques between the RBC and the endothelium, which may contribute to sludging of RBCs and hypoxia (Figure 9).

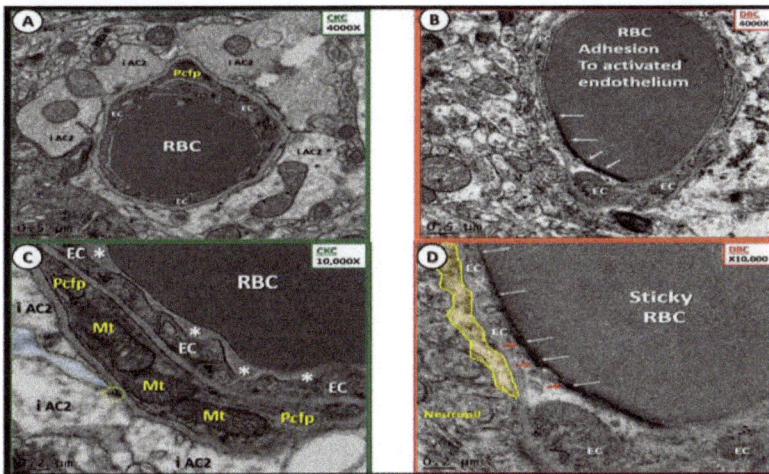

Figure 9. Sticky, adhesive red blood cells (RBCs) in the neurovascular unit of diabetic DBC models. Panels (**B,D**) depict the presence of a marked electron density between the RBC and the luminal EC (arrows). In panel (**D**), there appears to be an electron-dense protein staining in the RBC (white arrows) and also the EC (red arrows) that appear to fuse into one continuous electron-dense RBC/EC adhesion plaque. Also note that the ACs are retracted on the left side of the NVU in panel (**B**). Magnification ×4000 and ×10,000; bar = 0.5 and 0.2 μm, in panels (**B,D**), respectively. Panels (**A,C**) illustrate the relationship between the capillary RBC and the ECs without electron-dense adhesive adherence plaques in CKC models. In panel (**C**), note the compressed endothelial glycocalyces (asterisks), which were not observed in the diabetic NVUs as in panels (**B,D**). Magnification ×4000 and ×10,000; bar = 0.5 and 0.2 μm, in panels (**A,C**), respectively. Pcfp—pericyte foot process

While the elusive endothelial glycocalyx was not specifically studied in these models, it was observed to be compressed between the capillary RBCs and the endothelium only in CKC models (Figure 9C). Notably, the endothelial glycocalyx was not observed in the DBC models.

3.5. Neurovascular Unit Microbleeds in the Diabetic DBC Mice

In the DBC cortical gray matter, we found evidence of microbleeds/microhemorrhages, and these regions were associated with very small capillaries (≤2–3 μm) with notable loss of mural supportive Pcs and detached/retracted ACs (Figures 10 and 11).

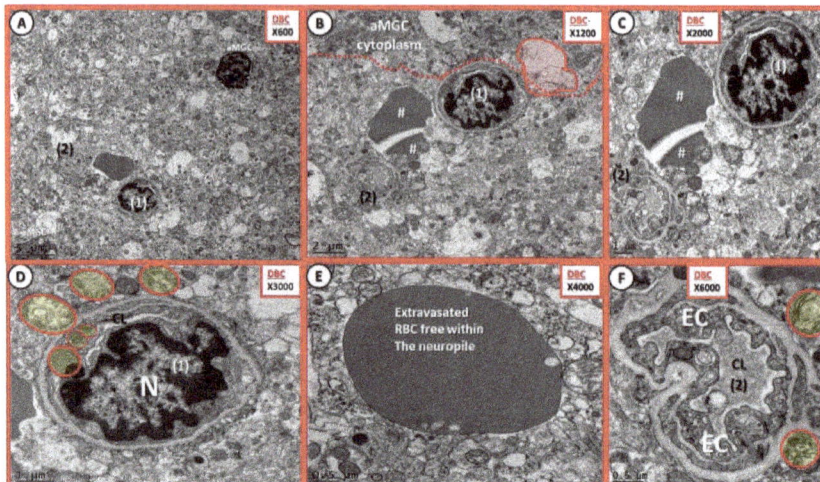

Figure 10. Cortical gray matter microbleeds in diabetic DBC models. Panel (**A**) illustrates a microbleed between two small NVU capillaries (1) and (2) at low magnification ×600; bar = 5 μm. Panel (**B**) depicts this microbleed (#) in a different region of cortical layer III of the gray matter, and note once again that this microbleed resides between two capillary NVUs (1) and (2). Also, note how the electron-lucent ACs are detached and retracted except for the one colored pink with the encircling solid red line (panel (**B**)). Magnification ×1200; bar = 2 μm. Panel (**C**) demonstrates the close proximity of the homogenous microbleed (#) to the paired capillary NVUs. Magnification ×2000; bar = 1 μm. Panel (**D**) at higher magnification depicts aMt, which are pseudo-colored yellow with red lines encircling them. Magnification ×3000; bar = 1 μm. Panel (**E**) allows one to appreciate the rounded homogeneous electron staining that appears similar to a red blood cell or plasma that would be normally located within a capillary lumen; however, this is located outside of any capillary lumen, and is totally surrounded by the neuropil. Magnification ×4000; bar = 0.5 μm. Panel (**F**) also demonstrates aMt in the immediate vicinity of a different NVU similar to panel (**D**), and these aMt may be a result of or contribute to the associated microbleeds. Magnification ×6000; bar = 0.5 μm.

3.6. Nanometer Channels as Possible Origins of the Glymphatic Pathway

While this was not our goal in this study, we were able to observe at least one nanometer-sized channel region that may represent an origin of a glymphatic channel in a transitional region from an NVU capillary with a pericyte lining to an early small arteriole, but with a pericyte lining versus a smooth-muscle-cell lining as in a true arteriole (Figure 12). Additionally, we were able to observe at least six nanometer-sized ultrastructure channels at the NVU that appeared to be bounded by the EC and Pc basal lamina and by the protoplasmic astrocyte basal lamina in the control CKC models (Figure 13). Notably, none of these channels were present in the DBC, which may be due to the previously described AC detachment and separation in diabetic DBC models.

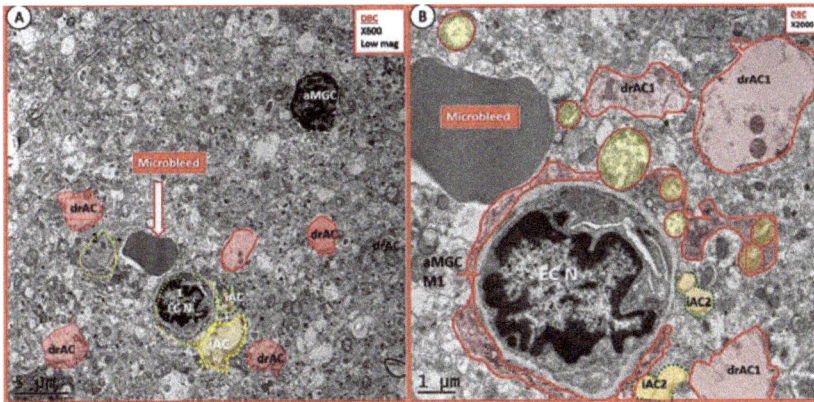

Figure 11. Cortical gray matter microbleeds in diabetic DBC models. Panels (**A,B**) illustrate the detachment and retraction of reactive-activated ACs (drAC1) in the NVU within the immediate proximity of this microbleed (pseudo-colored pink with red outlines). Note in these images that there is only one intact AC2 (golden colored iAC2) remaining. Also, note the aMt (pseudo-colored yellow with red outlines), which could certainly contribute to increased NVU oxidative stress and could support ongoing EC and AC activation, as depicted. Importantly, note the invasion/infiltration by aMGC (pseudo-colored red with encircling red lines) that are almost totally encompassing this NVU. Magnification ×600; bar = 2 μm, and ×2000; bar = 1 μm (panels (**A,B**), respectively). EC N—endothelial cell nucleus.

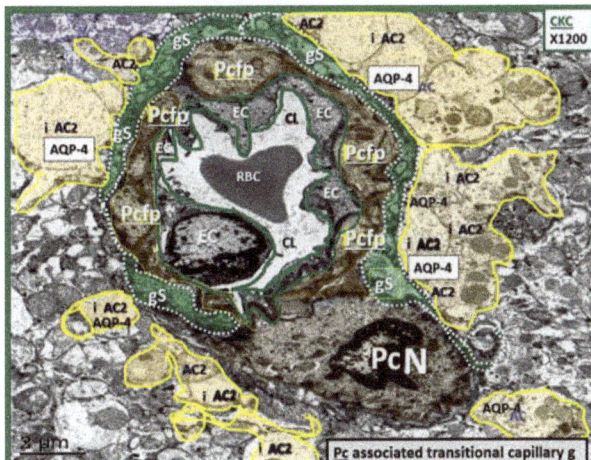

Figure 12. Cortical gray matter NVU capillary may demonstrate a potential paravascular waste clearance channel. This transitional capillary describes one transitioning from a capillary NVU to an arteriole. This NVU capillary EC is still encompassed by a layer of Pcfp with an intact PcN. Between the Pcfp and its basal lamina, and between the surrounding iAC2 and their basal lamina, there is a space that may represent the glymphatic pathway or glymphatic space (gS; pseudo-colored green). This possible glymphatic space may be important for waste clearance from the nanometer channels, and may also represent an ultrastructural origin of the glymphatic pathway in a previous image (Figure 13). The presence of aquaporin 4 (AQP-4) in the basolateral regions of the intact ACs is important for waste clearance. Magnification ×1200; bar = 2 μm.

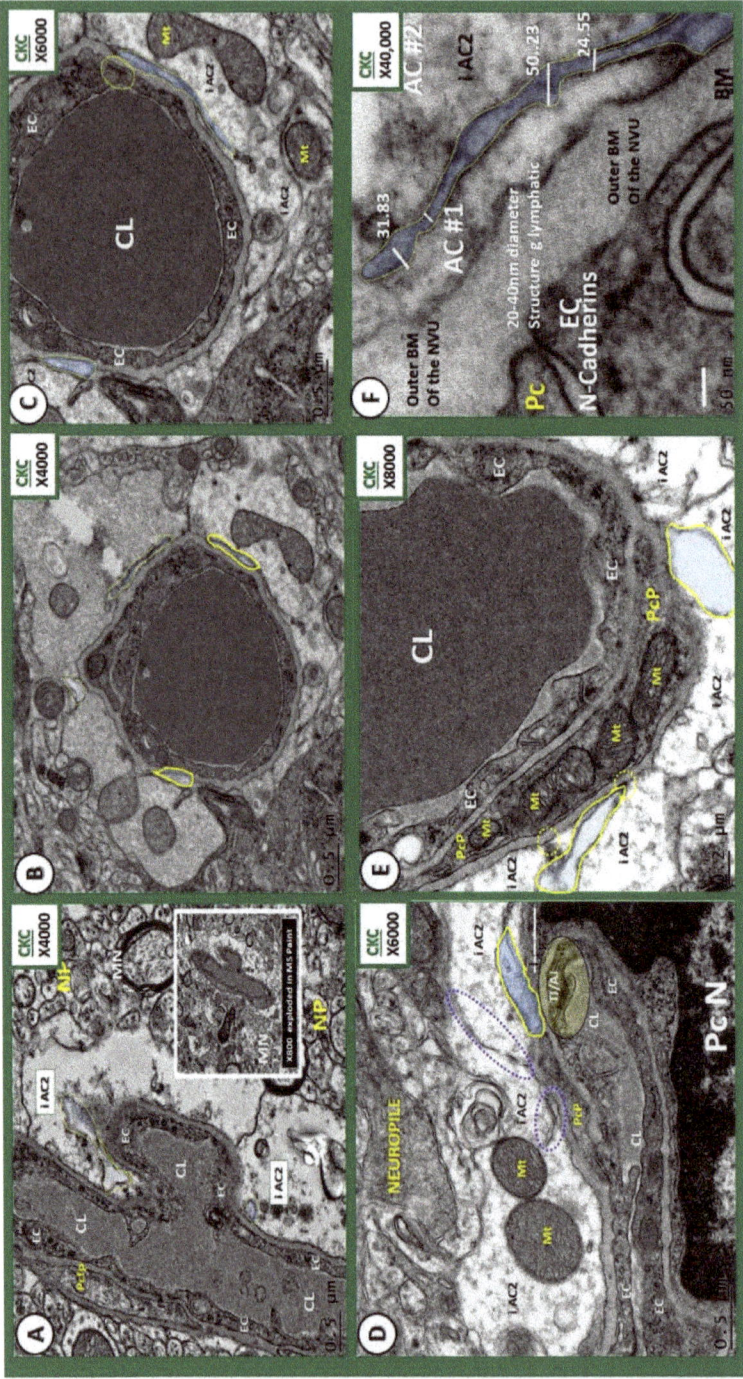

Figure 13. Possible origin of nanometer waste clearance channels adjacent to the NVU in the non-diabetic CKC models. Panels (A–F) illustrate various magnifications of the NVUs with nanometer-sized channels (pseudo-colored blue and outlined by yellow lines) adjacent to EC and Pc BMs. These proposed nanometer waste clearance channels measured 20–50 nm in width, and some were up to 800 nm in length. Magnifications are located in the upper right-hand corner and scale bars in the lower left-hand corner.

4. Discussion

Diabetes-associated cognitive impairment was previously described, and the currently used terminologies include "diabetic encephalopathy", initially described in 1950 [32], "type three diabetes" in 2008 [33], and "diabetic cognopathy" in 2013 [13].

Since capillaries comprise $\geq 60\%$ of the cerebral microvasculature [31], our initial aim was to characterize the capillary NVUs in obese, insulin-resistant, type 2 diabetic female db/db DBC mouse models, and our observational findings demonstrated abnormal, multi-cellular maladaptive ultrastructural remodeling changes in the NVUs of the mid cortical gray matter regions of the brain. These ultrastructure remodeling changes were not previously described in db/db models to the best of our knowledge; however, they may contribute to impaired cognition in the DBC as described in various papers regarding behavioral testing [34–39]. These cognitive impairments include behavioral testing abnormalities of the db/db models (DBC) in the Morris water maze tests, forced swim test, tail suspension test, light/dark box test, olfactory testing, Y-maze, and open-field tests to evaluate learning and memory plus anxiety and/or depression-associated cognitive impairment/deficits.

Understanding the NVU ultrastructural morphology and how this structure maladaptively remodels in the DBC as compared to the CKC models may allow for a better understanding of how the NVU responds to obesity, insulin resistance, and T2DM. Herein, we found concurrent multicellular maladaptive remodeling in the cells comprising the capillary NVU structures: (*i*) endothelial cell BBB TJ/AJ; (*ii*) endothelial cell luminal contents (sticky RBCs) and extraluminal microbleeds; (*iii*) pericytes; (*iv*) BM thickening in the NVU (ECs and encompassed Pcs); (*v*) astrocytes.

i. Endothelial cell BBB TJ/AJ attenuation and/or loss would allow increased permeability (due to dysfunction, attenuation, and/or loss of its permeability barrier), which would allow the accumulation of multiple vasculotoxic and neurotoxic moieties within the NVU parenchyma (Figures 3B–D, 4C,D, 5, 7C,D, 8, and 9) [6]. This compromise of the EC BBB TJ/AJ may aid in the understanding as to why there is concurrent remodeling in the surrounding cellular and extracellular regional constituents of the NVU. Importantly, these ultrastructural maladaptive remodeling changes could also interfere with neurovascular signaling/coupling functions of astrocytes to both pericytes and endothelial cells, which could lead to dysfunction and/or loss of function. As a result, there could also be a reduction in regional cerebral blood flow with regional hypoperfusion and ischemia [4–8].

ii. Luminal RBCs were observed to become adherent (via adherence plaques) in DBC models, which were not observed in the CKC models (Figure 10). Red blood cells become excessively glycated and form advanced glycation end products (AGE) with hemoglobin in human and DBC models of T2DM. Previously, our group showed elevations of hemoglobin A1c (HbA1c) [21], which is known to increase RBC stiffness that is associated with the loss of RBC deformability [40]. The accumulation of AGE in the RBC outer plasma membrane regions will serve as a ligand to the EC AGE receptor (RAGE). Additionally, the inner plasma membrane may translocate phosphatidylserine (PS) to the outer leaflet in the hyperglycemic microenvironment of DBC models. The translocated or "flipped" outer leaflet PS will contribute to the adherence of RBCs to the EC PS receptor, as well as to the EC matrix of thrombospondin, $\alpha v \beta 1$, and CD36, which may add to the increased electron density of the proteinaceous electron-dense adhesion plaques of the RBC and EC [41,42]. Importantly, there were also adherent mononuclear white blood cells within the capillary lumen of NVUs observed in the cortical gray matter in DBC models, as depicted in previous figures (Figures 4C,D, 7C and 8B), which will be discussed in greater detail as they relate to microglia remodeling. While the elusive endothelial glycocalyx was not specifically studied in this experiment, it is known that hyperglycemia results in the loss or shedding of the protective endothelial glycocalyx, and thus, may result in a more vulnerable and activated endothelium with increased inflammation and injury, decreased endothelial bioavailability of nitric oxide, and impaired vasodilation, in addition to becoming a more pro-coagulant surface in the DBC models (Figure 10C,D) [43].

ii.   Microbleeds/microhemorrhages within the gray matter of the cortical layers were observed in DBCs, which certainly could be related to incompetent EC TJ/AJ BBB proteins. These hemoglobin-containing extrusions/microbleeds would contain iron that could promote additional oxidative stress to the NVU and the immediate surrounding tissues (Figures 11 and 12). Importantly, RBC remodeling can result in increasing dysfunction and/or damage to the NVU as a result of adherence, escaping, or loss of deformability within NVU capillary lumen in DBC models. Of note, cerebral microbleeds are being increasingly found on magnetic resonance imaging (MRI) [44]. Currently, the significance of microbleeds in diabetic preclinical models is yet to be evaluated extensively at the transmission electron microscopic ultrastructural level; however, there may be some similarities to retinal microbleeds and hemorrhages [45]. Notwithstanding, these observed microbleeds may be related to remodeled and dysfunctional TJ/AJ. The combination of adherent RBCs and microbleeds in the DBC may have detrimental consequences in local regional blood flow with resultant regional ischemia and loss of neurovascular coupling in the DBC models and may have a predisposition to accelerated neurodegeneration.

iii.   Maladaptive Pc remodeling (Figure 7) in diabetes may contribute to increased BBB TJ/AJ permeability, neuronal dysfunction, injury, and eventual neurodegeneration [13,15,18,25]. Recently, in streptozotozin-induced type 1 diabetes, it was demonstrated that pericytes are also attenuated and/or lost, and that the mitochondrial-specific carbonic anhydrase inhibitor (toprimate) was able to rescue pericyte loss and normalise BBB permeability [46]. Our findings of aberrant mitochondria in DBC pericytes may be playing a detrimental role in our observed pericyte attenuation and/or loss (Figure 7E).

iv.   Capillary NVU BM thickening was observed in the cortical gray matter of DBC (~$\geq$200 nm) as compared to the CKC (~$\leq$80 nm) models (Figures 4 and 5). Capillary BM thickening is a fundamental ultrastructural central finding in most diabetic affected end-organs and nearly a pathognomonic ultrastructural finding in human and rodent models of diabetes. Capillary NVU BM thickening was reported in human diabetics in the cortical regions of the brain [47]. Basement membrane thickening was also reported in the retinas of type 1 diabetic rats (streptozotocin-induced) at six months of age [48], whereas we did not observe BM thickening in our type 1 diabetic mice mid-brain models studied at four months in a previous study [18]. Mechanisms of BM thickening may be related to glucotoxicity, increased protein kinase C, increased vascular endothelial cell growth factor, increased AGE, type IV collagen AGE crosslinking, and oxidative stress [23]. The observed increase in BM thickness may increase NVU permeability and could also play a role in the detachment of ACs from the capillary EC and Pc NVU BM due to an interference in cell–matrix interactions and dysfunctional alterations of BM integrins/dystroglycans. The current finding of BM thickening in DBC models filled in some gaps in our knowledge regarding the lack of BM thickening in diet-induced obesity Western mice models (cortical gray matter) [13] and the type 1 diabetic mice models previously studied (cortical mid-brain) [23]. To the best of our knowledge, we are the first to identify BM thickening in capillary EC/Pc NVU microvessels in the cortical gray matter of the female obese, insulin-resistant, type 2 diabetic db/db mouse model.

v.   Abnormal remodeling changes of the supportive and connecting protoplasmic astrocytes were observed in the DBC models. Astrocytes foot processes were depicted in CKC images as being colored "golden" due to their important function and location as connecting cells between the capillary NVU and their regional neurons when they were observed to have intact connections with the EC and Pc basement membranes. We observed how these connecting intact astrocytes became detached and retracted from the capillary EC and Pc BMs in the DBC, and how they lost their connective essential role of neurovascular coupling. This loss of neurovascular coupling and loss of vasodilation when being actively signaled by regional neurons could result in a loss of function that could result in localized decreased cerebral blood flow, resulting in regional hypoxia with the potential for increased neurodegeneration. In the detached astrocyte, it is possible that the AC soma may remodel its F-actin cytoskeleton such that the AC protoplasmic processes retract toward the soma of the AC in a phenotypic response to injury (brain wounding mechanism), which may result from a combination of excessive reactive oxygen/nitrogen species, toxic cytokines, and ischemia in the DBC models. Some suggested that the activated-reactive detached AC are induced by activated microglia cells [49–51], and furthermore, that these activated microglia may be responsible for the actual physical detachment and subsequent retraction of the capillary NVU astrocytes in the DBC (Figure 4C,D and Figure 5).

Possible mechanisms of astrocyte detachment and retraction may include the invading reactive-aMGC (Figure 14). The aMGCs may physically result in a shearing (bulldozer-like effect) as they invade the NVU, which may result in the physical detachment of ACs. Importantly, these invading aMGCs are known to be capable of secreting excess toxic reactive oxygen/nitrogen species (ROS and oxidative/nitrosative stress) due to the actions of excessive nicotinamide adenine dinucleotide phosphate (NADPH) oxidase and toxic cytokines, which are capable of activating local EC proteolytic matrix metalloproteinases, such as MMP-2. Also, hyperglycemia and resultant excess protein kinase C, ROS production via glucose autoxidation, AGE-RAGE interactions, polyol, and hexosamine flux pathways in the EC will be capable of increasing ROS production. In turn, this excess ROS will further increase not only matrix metalloproteinases (MMP-2) production by ECs, but also inducible (MMP-9) activation by surrounding Pcs and ACs. These above mechanisms may be synergistic with the observed attenuation and/or loss of EC BBB TJ/AJ and pericytes. The detachment and retraction of astrocytes may provide new insights into the loss of neurovascular coupling and eventual neurodegeneration in the DBC (Figure 14).

Early on, the brain was known to lack a classical endothelial-lined lymphatic system as described in the peripheral tissues, and a specific lymphatic-like pathway channel remained somewhat elusive. Recently, the presence of a new paravascular gymphatic pathway/system was described [50–52]. The "g" preceding the word lymphatic, or "glymphatic", is to honor the importance of the glial ACs and their important polarized water channel, aquaporin-4, which is localized to the basal lateral position of ACs that abut and line the EC and Pc basement membranes. Importantly, others suggested that these paravascular channels may potentially extend all the way to the capillary level of the NVU [53]. Concurrent with the above findings, other groups identified lymphatic channels in the meninges, and suggested that the drainage was accomplished via a "perivascular channel" that moves within the basal lamina regions of the outer arteriole smooth muscle cells and adventitia [54]. Of interest, another paper recently discussed the current understanding, significance, and controversy of these waste clearance pathways [55].

A timely publication was released during the preparation of this manuscript (May 2018) regarding the entrance of a cerebral spinal fluid (CSF) tracer (soluble, fluorescent fixable amyloid β (Aβ)) that was introduced via the cisterna magna. These findings demonstrated that the tracer entered the brain along the pial-glial BMs, and reasons for its entry into the extracellular matrix interstitial fluid was not completely clear; however, authors stated there could be multiple reasons [56]. The mixture of the interstitial spinal fluid and CSF was then found to enter the BM regions in capillary walls, before draining further into the BMs of vascular smooth muscle cells within the tunica media in the pial arterioles and arteries within the intramural peri-arterial drainage pathways to the sagittal sinus and cerebral spinal fluid. Also demonstrated in this study was the finding that injected tracers were found to enter and leave the brain along separate peri-arterial basement-membrane pathways [56].

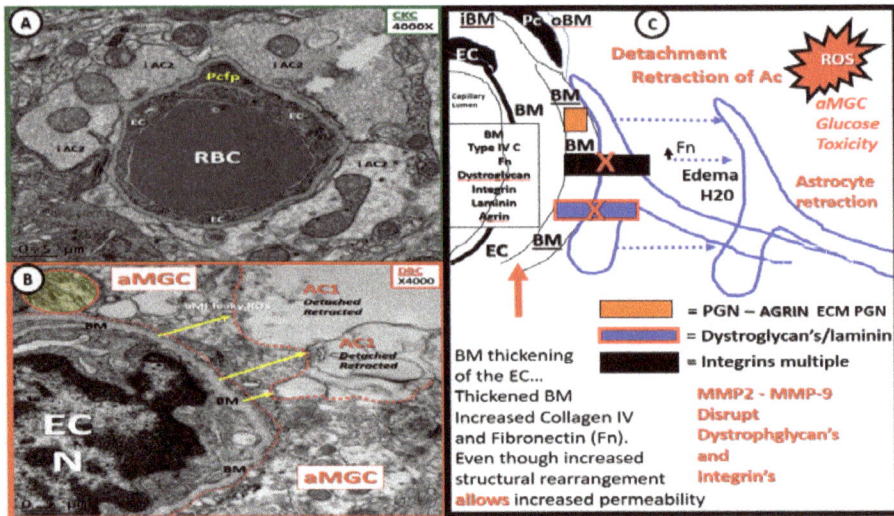

Figure 14. Possible mechanisms for detachment and retraction of astrocytes in diabetic DBC. Panel (**A**) demonstrates the iAC2 in the CKC. Panel (**B**) depicts the near complete loss of iAC2 coverage of the EC and Pcfp. Importantly, note the detachment and retraction (yellow arrows) of phenotypically retracted ACs, labeled AC1, in the DBC. Note the aberrant mitochondria in this image in the detachment zone (pseudo-colored yellow and outlined by red solid line). Also, note the aMGC that is located between the NVU EC BM and the detached AC1 (red dashed lines). Magnification ×4000; scale bar = 0.5 µm. Panel (**C**) contains a cartoon, which may illustrate some of the possible involved mechanisms. C—collagen IVECM—extracellular matrix; Fn—fibronectin; H20—water-edema; MPP2–9—matrix metalloproteinases 2–9; PGN—proteoglycan; ROS—reactive oxygen/nitrogen species.

Interestingly, possible nanometer spaces/channels were observed in both the capillary NVU regions and in pre-arteriole transitional pericyte-lined microvessels of the non-diabetic CKC models (Figures 13 and 14), which were not observed in the diabetic DBC. Whether this is due in part to the outer wall AC detachment and retraction from NVU EC and Pc BMs or the immersion-fixation process utilized in this model remains to be studied in greater detail. It is not certain that these shared images will assist in making any headway or advances; however, they support the discussion that the "glymphatic pathway" may actually have its origin at the capillary NVU to begin the clearance of metabolic toxic waste products from the interstitial fluid of the brain, as seen in Figure 1a that Abbott et al. [53] shared.

The puzzling mechanisms for the clearance of waste products via a specialized glymphatic system of the brain are still far from being completely elucidated, and it may be eventually demonstrated that both the perivascular and paravascular routes for clearance of metabolic byproducts and toxic oligomers of Aβ and other proteins may be cleared via a little bit of both systems currently described in the literature. Regardless, when ACs are detached and retracted from the NVU (in addition to other cellular remodeling changes as found in the cortical gray matter NVUs of DBC models), these changes may result in impaired waste clearance in the DBC models.

Certain limitations apply to this study, which include the following: (i) this study was limited to immersion fixation, which studied only a snap shot in time; however, these images allowed comparisons at the same point in time between healthy normal controls (CKC) and diabetic (DBC), such that maladaptive remodeling changes could be observed; (ii) this study was limited to the cortical gray matter (primarily layer III) and may not apply to other regions of the brain such as the hippocampus, mid-brain, or cerebellum. However, cortical remodeling usually occurs at later time points than hippocampal remodeling, and therefore, may be representative of earlier time points in the expectation of similar remodeling findings in the hippocampal structure); (iii) this study was primarily designed and directed to interrogate the NVU and its immediate surroundings; (iv) this study was limited to only ultrastructural observational findings, and was not supported by functional studies, immunohistochemistry, or protein Western blots. As with any transmission electron microscopic study, the regions studied were very small and limited. Furthermore, this study was not supported by larger regions of study, such as light microscopy, to more closely examine larger areas of tissue remodeling. In general, the above limitations reflect the very nature of TEM studies in general when not accompanied by other functional and light microscopic methods. Given these limitations, however, this study does allow for the ultrastructural comparisons of age-matched CKC to the diseased obese, insulin-resistant, and diabetic DBC at the same time points. Additionally, the authors attempted referencing what other investigators previously established in diabetic models.

While each individual cellular component of the NVU is considered to be a vital element to ensure proper functioning, homeostasis, and integrity, the multicellular remodeling in the brains of the DBC are thought to be of extreme interest. The detachment and retraction of the ACs from the capillary NVUs are thought to be very important novel findings, in that, ACs are the connecting/communicating cell between the regional neurons and capillary microvessels of the NVU, providing neurovascular coupling. This loss of neurovascular coupling could possibly provide novel mechanisms for impaired regional capillary blood flow, cerebral blood flow dynamics, and regional ischemia, which may markedly contribute to the ongoing neurodegenerative progression in this model and the increased vulnerability to age-related neurodegenerative diseases.

The authors observed that, in most of the diabetic end-organs affected by T2DM, there appears to be accelerated/premature aging. These observations suggest that T2DM may induce premature macrovascular and microvascular brain aging and/or negatively interact with the normal aging process [57], which supports the brain reserve hypothesis [58]. Accelerated aging could render these cells highly vulnerable to the effects of other specific neurologic age-related diseases, such as Alzheimer's disease, vascular dementia, and Parkinson's disease. Indeed, other investigators also suggested that T2DM is associated with learning and memory dysfunction, specifically in older adults [59].

In summary, to the best of our knowledge, we are the first group to perform an in-depth ultrastructural study of the brain NVU in obese, insulin-resistant, and diabetic female db/db DBC models with the transmission electron microscope. Ultrastructural observations included an attenuation and/or loss of EC BBB TJ/AJ and Pc, as hypothesized, as well as capillary NVU BM thickening and abnormal remodeling in supportive neuroglia ACs, consisting of detachment and retraction from the NVUs. Also, there were observational findings of sticky red blood cells and microbleeds in the DBC that were not noted in CKC. Additionally, we were not only able to image a possible example of the recently defined glial lymphatic (glymphatic) pathway system at the CKC pre-arteriolar and capillary NVU level, but we were also able to demonstrate a possible nanoscale origin of the glymphatic system for waste clearance.

These observational findings, in whole or in part, appear important to the known impaired cognition in db/db models of T2DM, and certainly suggest that the multicellular remodeling may place a certain credence regarding the saying that the whole may be greater than the sum of its parts. Indeed, this study was certainly a voyage of discovery, and while we may all dance around in a ring and suppose, the secret sits in the middle and knows ("The Secret Sits"—a poem by Robert Frost (1874–1963)). These sage thoughts by Frost suggest that the abnormal cellular remodeling changes may represent the secret sitting in the middle in order for us to better understand the complicated structures of the brain in the diabetic DBC as compared to the control CKC models.

5. Type 2 Diabetes Mellitus Increases the Risk of the Neurodegenerative Diseases, Alzheimer's and Parkinson's Disease

Type 2 diabetes mellitus is known to increase the risk of developing AD. However, the increased clinical risk that T2DM brings to the development of PD was only recently more strongly established during the preparation of this manuscript [60]. Our observational ultrastructural findings of the NVU in T2DM DBC models are quite disturbing, in that, these maladaptive remodeling changes of the NVU in DBC models could lead to predisposition to additional maladaptive remodeling with aging, and the increased vulnerability of the T2DM brain tissue to age-related neurodegenerative diseases.

6. Future Directions

Now that there is an established model of marked ultrastructural remodeling changes in the NVU in the female diabetic DBC, studies utilizing various treatment modalities are certainly of great interest. Multiple treatment modalities may be studied to observe if they can prevent/abrogate the ultrastructural brain remodeling. Additionally, functional studies utilizing light microscopy, immunohistochemistry, and protein and mechanistic studies may be employed. Also, there are newer technologies being utilized even currently, and of course, newer technologies that are yet to be created in the future.

One exciting new modality in current use is the focused ion beam/scanning electronic microscopic (FIB/SEM) instrument [61] that is being increasingly incorporated in core facilities to capture images (Figure 15).

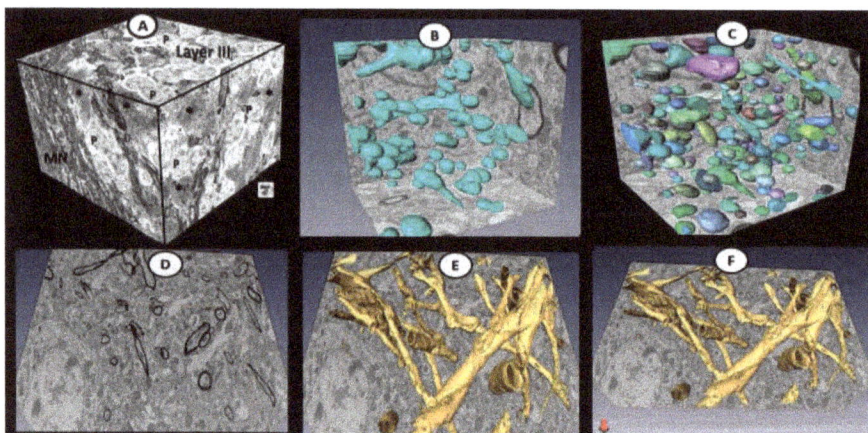

Figure 15. Examples utilizing focused ion beam/scanning electronic microscopic (FIB/SEM) technology to study various models of disease. Panel (**A**) illustrates the use of 3-view system (Gatan, Inc., Pleasanton, CA, USA) with tagged image file format (TIFF) cutouts in diet-induced obesity models of cortical gray matter layer III (P—pyramidal cells; MN). Panels (**B–D**) were obtained by utilizing FIB/SEM technology. Panels (**B,C**) depict randomized pseudo-colorized Mt in control CKC models. Panels (**D–F**) demonstrate myelin. In panel (**D**), note that the myelin is not pseudo-colorized, in contrast to panels (**E,F**), where the myelin is pseudo-colorized golden in control CKC models. No specific magnification or actual scale bars are included in these FIB/SEM images.

Some of the potential capabilities of FIB/SEM technology are actually reminiscent of how computerized axial tomography and MRI technologies expanded some of our most recent new findings and concepts regarding both rodent models and human diseases. Regarding brain barriers and fluid movement, a recent paper commented that there are several ongoing clinical trials underway testing the intrathecal route of drug delivery, which may evolve to become a treatment modality for brain diseases [62]. Indeed, these are exciting times.

Author Contributions: M.R.H. and V.G.D. conceptualized the study; M.R.H. performed the image collection and interpretation; D.G.G. prepared the tissue specimens for transmission electron microscopic studies and assisted M.R.H.; M.R.H. prepared the manuscript; A.R.A. collected tissue specimens; V.G.D., A.R.A., and D.G.G. assisted in editing.

Funding: This study was supported by an integral grant in Excellence in Electron Microscopy grant issued by the University of Missouri Electron Microscopy Core and Office of Research. No external funding was available.

Acknowledgments: Authors wish to thank Tommi White of the University of Missouri Electron Microscopy Core Facility. Authors also wish to thank our mentor James R. Sowers, who inspired us to interrogate, characterize, and understand the secrets that the tissues behold.

Conflicts of Interest: The authors declare no conflict of interest.

References

1. Wild, S.; Roglic, G.; Green, A.; Sicree, R.; King, H. Global prevalence of diabetes: Estimates for the year 2000 and projections for 2030. *Diabetes Care* **2004**, *27*, 1047–1053. [CrossRef] [PubMed]
2. Ott, A.; Breteler, M.M.; van Harskamp, F.; Claus, J.J.; van der Cammen, T.J.; Grobbee, D.E.; Hofman, A. Prevalence of Alzheimer's disease and vascular dementia: Association with education. The Rotterdam study. *BMJ* **1995**, *310*, 970–973. [CrossRef] [PubMed]
3. Reeve, A.; Simcox, E.; Turnbull, D. Ageing and Parkinson's disease: Why is advancing age the biggest risk factor? *Ageing Res. Rev.* **2014**, *14*, 19–30. [CrossRef] [PubMed]
4. Nelson, A.R.; Sweeney, M.D.; Sagare, A.P.; Zlokovic, B.J. Neurovascular dysfunction and neurodegeneration in dementia and Alzheimer's disease. *Biochim. Biophys. Acta* **2016**, *1862*, 887–900. [CrossRef] [PubMed]
5. Snyder, H.M.; Corriveau, R.A.; Craft, S.; Faber, J.E.; Greenberg, S.M.; Knopman, D.; Lamb, B.T.; Montine, T.J.; Nedergaard, M.; Schaffer, C.B.; et al. Vascular contributions to cognitive impairment and dementia including Alzheimer's disease. *Alzheimer's Dement.* **2015**, *11*, 710–717. [CrossRef] [PubMed]
6. Zlokovic, B.V. Neurovascular pathways to neurodegeneration in Alzheimer's disease and other disorders. *Nat. Rev. Neurosci.* **2011**, *12*, 723–738. [CrossRef] [PubMed]
7. Iadecola, C. The pathobiology of vascular dementia. *Neuron* **2013**, *80*, 844–866. [CrossRef] [PubMed]
8. Kisler, K.; Nelson, A.R.; Montagne, A.; Zlokovic, B.V. Cerebral blood flow regulation and neurovascular dysfunction in Alzheimer disease. *Nat. Rev. Neurosci.* **2017**, *18*, 419–434. [CrossRef] [PubMed]
9. Rocca, W.A.; Petersen, R.C.; Knopman, D.S.; Herbert, L.E.; Evans, D.A.; Hall, K.S.; Gao, S.; Unverzawt, F.W.; Langa, K.M.; Larson, E.B.; et al. Trends in the incidence and prevalence of Alzheimer's disease, dementia, and cognitive impairment in the United States. *Alzheimer's Dement.* **2011**, *7*, 80–93. [CrossRef] [PubMed]
10. Leibson, C.L.; Rocca, W.A.; Hanson, V.A.; Cha, R.; Kokmen, E.; O'Brien, P.C.; Palumbo, P.J. Risk of dementia among persons with diabetes mellitus: A population-based cohort study. *Am. J. Epidemiol.* **1996**, *145*, 301–308. [CrossRef]
11. Ott, A.; Stolk, R.P.; van Harskamp, F.; Pols, H.A.; Hofman, A.; Breteler, M.M. Diabetes mellitus and the risk of dementia: The Rotterdam Study. *Neurology* **1999**, *53*, 1937–1942. [CrossRef] [PubMed]
12. Peila, R.; Rodriguez, B.L.; Launer, L.J. Type 2 diabetes, *APOE* gene, and the risk for dementia and related pathologies: The Honolulu-Asia Aging Study. *Diabetes* **2002**, *51*, 1256–1262. [CrossRef] [PubMed]
13. Hayden, M.R.; Banks, W.A.; Shah, G.N.; Gu, Z.; Sowers, J.R. Cardiorenal metabolic syndrome and diabetic cognopathy. *Cardiorenal Med.* **2013**, *3*, 265–282. [CrossRef] [PubMed]
14. McConnell, H.L.; Kersch, C.N.; Woltjer, R.L.; Neuwelt, E.A. The Translational Significance of the Neurovascular Unit. *J. Biol. Chem.* **2017**, *292*, 762–770. [CrossRef] [PubMed]
15. Hall, C.N.; Reynell, C.; Gesslein, B.; Hamilton, N.B.; Mishra, A.; Sutherland, B.A.; O'Farrell, F.M.; Buchan, A.M.; Lauritzen, M.; Attwell, D. Capillary pericytes regulate cerebral blood flow in health and disease. *Nature* **2014**, *508*, 55–60. [CrossRef] [PubMed]
16. Mishra, A.; Reynolds, J.P.; Chen, Y.; Gourine, A.V.; Rusakov, D.A.; Attwell, D. Astrocytes mediate neurovascular signaling to capillary pericytes but not to arterioles. *Nat. Neurosci.* **2016**, *19*, 1619–1627. [CrossRef] [PubMed]

17. Petzold, G.C.; Murthy, V.N. Role of astrocytes in neurovascular coupling. *Neuron* **2011**, *71*, 782–797. [CrossRef] [PubMed]

18. Salameh, T.S.; Shah, G.N.; Price, T.O.; Hayden, M.R.; Banks, W.A. Blood-brain barrier disruption and neurovascular unit dysfunction in diabetic mice: Protection with the mitochondrial carbonic anhydrase inhibitor topiramate. *J. Pharmacol. Exp. Ther.* **2016**, *359*, 452–459. [CrossRef] [PubMed]

19. Hu, G.; Jousilahti, P.; Bidel, S.; Antikainen, R.; Tuomilehto, J. Type 2 diabetes and the risk of Parkinsons's disease. *Diabetes Care* **2007**, *30*, 842–847. [CrossRef] [PubMed]

20. Butt, A.; Mihaila, D.; Verkhratsky, A. Neuroglia: A New Open-Access Journal Publishing All Aspects of Glial Research. *Neuroglia* **2018**, *1*, 1. [CrossRef]

21. Habibi, J.; Aroor, A.R.; Sowers, J.R.; Jia, G.; Hayden, M.R.; Garro, M.; Barron, B.; Mayoux, E.; Rector, R.S.; Whaley-Connell, A.; et al. Sodium glucose transporter-2 (SGLT-2) inhibition with empagliflozin improves cardiac diastolic function in a female rodent model of diabetes. *Cardiovasc. Diabetol.* **2017**, *16*, 9. [CrossRef] [PubMed]

22. Laws, K.R.; Irvine, K.; Gale, T.M. Sex differences in cognitive impairment in Alzheimer's disease. *World J. Psychiatry* **2016**, *6*, 54–65. [CrossRef] [PubMed]

23. Hayden, M.R.; Sowers, J.R.; Tyagi, S.C. The central role of vascular extracellular matrix and basement membrane remodeling in metabolic syndrome and type 2 diabetes: The matrix preloaded. *Cardiovasc. Diabetol.* **2005**, *4*, 9. [CrossRef] [PubMed]

24. Thomsen, M.S.; Routhe, L.J.; Moos, T. The vascular basement membrane in the healthy and pathological brain. *J. Cereb. Blood Flow Metab.* **2017**, *37*, 3300–3317. [CrossRef] [PubMed]

25. Bell, R.D.; Winkler, E.A.; Sagare, A.P.; Singh, I.; LaRue, B.; Deane, R.; Zlokovic, B.V. Pericytes control key neurovascular functions and neuronal phenotype in the adult brain and during brain aging. *Neuron* **2010**, *68*, 409–427. [CrossRef] [PubMed]

26. Verkhratsky, A.; Nedergaard, M. Astroglial cradle in the life of the synapse. *Phil. Trans. R. Soc. Lond. B Biol. Sci.* **2014**, *369*, 20130595. [CrossRef] [PubMed]

27. Verkhratsky, A.; Nedergaard, M. Physiology of Astroglia. *Physiol. Rev.* **2018**, *98*, 239–389. [CrossRef] [PubMed]

28. Verkhratsky, A.; Bush, N.A.; Nedergaard, M.; Butt, A. The Special Case of Human Astrocytes. *Neuroglia* **2018**, *1*, 4. [CrossRef]

29. Scemes, E.; Spray, D.C. Chapter: The astrocytic syncytium. In *Non-Neural Cells in the Nervous System: Function and Dysfunction*; Hertz, L., Ed.; Elsevier: New York, NY, USA, 2004; Volume 31, pp. 165–179.

30. Abbott, N.J.; Rönnbäck, L.; Hansson, E. Astrocyte-endothelial interactions at the blood-brain barrier. *Nat. Rev. Neurosci.* **2006**, *7*, 41–53. [CrossRef] [PubMed]

31. Del Zoppo, G.J.; Milner, R. Integrin–Matrix Interactions in the Cerebral Microvasculature. *Arterioscler. Thromb. Vasc. Biol.* **2006**, *26*, 1966–1975. [CrossRef] [PubMed]

32. Reske-Nielsen, E.; Lundbaek, K. Diabetic Encephalopathy. In *Pathophysiologie und Klinik/Pathophysiology and Clinical Considerations*; Pfeiffer, E.F., Ed.; Springer: Berlin/Heidelberg, Germany, 1971.

33. De la Monte, S.M.; Wands, J.R. Alzheimer's Disease Is Type 3 Diabetes—Evidence Reviewed. *J. Diabetes Sci. Technol.* **2008**, *2*, 1101–1113. [CrossRef] [PubMed]

34. Li, X.L.; Aou, S.; Oomura, Y.; Hori, N.; Fukunaga, K.; Hori, T. Impairment of long-term potentiation and spatial memory in leptin receptor-deficient rodents. *Neuroscience* **2002**, *113*, 607–615. [CrossRef]

35. Zheng, H.; Zheng, Y.; Zhao, L.; Chen, M.; Bai, G.; Hu, Y.; Hu, W.; Yan, Z.; Gao, H. Cognitive decline in type 2 diabetic db/db mice may be associated with brain region-specific metabolic disorders. *Biochim. Biophys. Acta* **2017**, *1863*, 266–273. [CrossRef] [PubMed]

36. Ramos-Rodriguez, J.J.; Ortiz, O.; Jimenez-Palomares, M.; Kay, K.R.; Berrocoso, E.; Murillo-Carretero, M.I.; Perdomo, G.; Spires-Jones, T.; Cozar-Castellano, I.; Lechuga-Sancho, A.M.; et al. Differential central pathology and cognitive impairment in pre-diabetic and diabetic mice. *Psychoneuroendocrinology* **2013**, *38*, 2462–2475. [CrossRef] [PubMed]

37. Andersen, J.V.; Nissen, J.D.; Christensen, S.K.; Markussen, K.H.; Waagepetersen, H.S. Impaired Hippocampal Glutamate and Glutamine Metabolism in the db/db Mouse Model of Type 2 Diabetes Mellitus. *Neural Plast.* **2017**, *2017*, 2107084. [CrossRef] [PubMed]

38. Ernst, A.; Sharma, A.N.; Elased, K.M.; Guest, P.C.; Rahmoune, H.; Bahn, S. Diabetic db/db mice exhibit central nervous system and peripheral molecular alterations as seen in neurological disorders. *Transl. Psychiatry* **2013**, *3*, e263. [CrossRef] [PubMed]

39. Kalani, A.; Chaturvedi, P.; Maldonado, C.; Bauer, P.; Joshua, I.G.; Tyagi, S.C.; Tyagi, N. Dementia-like pathology in type-2 diabetes: A novel microRNA mechanism. *Mol. Cell. Neurosci.* **2017**, *80*, 58–65. [CrossRef] [PubMed]

40. Tomaiuolo, G. Biomechanical properties of red blood cells in health and disease towards microfluidics. *Biomicrofluidics* **2014**, *8*, 051501. [CrossRef] [PubMed]

41. Carelli-Alinovi, C.; Misiti, F. Erythrocytes as Potential Link between Diabetes and Alzheimer's Disease. *Front. Aging Neurosci.* **2017**, *9*, 276. [CrossRef] [PubMed]

42. Yang, Y.; Koo, S.; Lin, C.S.; Neu, B. Macromolecular depletion modulates the binding of red blood cells to activated endothelial cells. *Biointerphases* **2010**, *5*, FA19–FA23. [CrossRef] [PubMed]

43. Nieuwdorp, M.; van Haeften, T.W.; Gouverneur, M.C.; Mooij, H.L.; van Lieshout, M.H.; Levi, M.; Meijers, J.C.; Holleman, F.; Hoekstra, J.B.; Vink, H.; et al. Loss of endothelial glycocalyx during acute hyperglycemia coincides with endothelial dysfunction and coagulation activation in vivo. *Diabetes* **2006**, *55*, 480–486. [CrossRef] [PubMed]

44. Martinez-Ramirez, S.; Greenberg, S.M.; Viswanathan, A. Cerebral microbleeds: Overview and implications in cognitive impairment. *Alzheimers Res. Ther.* **2014**, *6*, 33. [CrossRef] [PubMed]

45. Qiu, C.; Cotch, M.F.; Sigurdsson, S.; Jonsson, P.V.; Jonsdottir, M.K.; Sveinbjrnsdottir, S.; Eiriksdottir, G.; Klein, R.; Harris, T.B.; van Buchem, M.A.; et al. Cerebral microbleeds, retinopathy and dementia: The AGES-Reykjavik study. *Neurology* **2010**, *75*, 2221–2228. [CrossRef] [PubMed]

46. Price, T.O.; Eranki, V.; Banks, W.A.; Ercal, N.; Shah, G.N. Topiramate treatment protects blood-brain barrier pericytes from hyperglycemia-induced oxidative damage in diabetic mice. *Endocrinology* **2012**, *153*, 362–372. [CrossRef] [PubMed]

47. Johnson, P.C.; Brendel, K.; Meezan, E. Thickened cerebral cortical capillary basement membranes in diabetics. *Arch. Pathol. Lab. Med.* **1982**, *106*, 214–217. [PubMed]

48. Cherian, S.; Roy, S.; Pinheiro, A.; Roy, S. Tight Glycemic Control Regulates Fibronectin Expression and Basement Membrane Thickening in Retinal and Glomerular Capillaries of Diabetic Rats. *Investig. Ophthalmol. Vis. Sci.* **2009**, *50*, 943–949. [CrossRef] [PubMed]

49. Liddelow, S.A.; Guttenplan, K.A.; Clarke, L.E.; Bennett, F.C.; Bohlen, C.J.; Schirmer, L.; Bennett, M.L.; Münch, A.E.; Chung, W.S.; Peterson, T.C.; et al. Neurotoxic reactive astrocytes are induced by activated microglia. *Nature* **2017**, *541*, 481–487. [CrossRef] [PubMed]

50. Iliff, J.J.; Wang, M.; Liao, Y.; Plogg, B.A.; Peng, W.; Gundersen, G.A.; Benveniste, H.; Vates, G.E.; Deane, R.; Goldman, S.A.; et al. A Paravascular Pathway Facilitates CSF Flow Through the Brain Parenchyma and the Clearance of Interstitial Solutes, Including Amyloid β. *Sci. Transl. Med.* **2012**, *4*, 147ra111. [CrossRef] [PubMed]

51. Iliff, J.J.; Nedergaard, M. Is there a cerebral lymphatic system? *Stroke* **2013**, *44*, S93–S95. [CrossRef] [PubMed]

52. Jessen, N.A.; Munk, A.S.; Lundgarrd, I.; Nedergaard, M. The glymphatic system—A beginner's guide. *Neurochem. Res.* **2015**, *40*, 2583–2599. [CrossRef] [PubMed]

53. Abbott, N.J.; Pizzo, M.E.; Preston, J.E.; Janigro, D.; Thorne, R.G. The role of brain barriers in fluid movement in the CNS: Is there a 'glymphatic' system? *Acta Neuropathol.* **2018**, *135*, 387–407. [CrossRef] [PubMed]

54. Weller, R.O.; Sharp, M.M.; Christodoulides, M.; Carare, R.O.; Mollgard, K. The meninges as barriers and facilitators for the movement of fluid, cells and pathogens related to the rodent and human CNS. *Acta Neuropathol.* **2018**, *135*, 363–385. [CrossRef] [PubMed]

55. Bacyinski, A.; Maosheng, X.U.; Wang, W.; Hu, J. The paravascular pathway for brain current understanding, significance and controversy. *Front. Neroanat.* **2017**, *11*, 101. [CrossRef] [PubMed]

56. Albargothy, N.J.; Johnston, D.A.; MacGregor-Sharp, M.; Weller, R.O.; Verma, A.; Hawkes, C.A.; Carare, R.O. Convective influx/glymphatic system: Tracers injected into the CSF enter and leave the brain along separate periarterial basement membrane pathways. *Acta Neuropathol.* **2018**. [CrossRef] [PubMed]

57. Nilsson, P.M. Early vascular aging (EVA): Consequences and Prevention. *Vasc. Health Risk Manag.* **2008**, *4*, 547–552. [CrossRef] [PubMed]

58. Wrighten, S.A.; Piroli, G.G.; Grillo, C.A.; Reagan, L.P. A look inside the diabetic brain: Contributors to diabetes-induced brain aging. *Biochim. Biophys. Acta* **2009**, *1792*, 444–453. [CrossRef] [PubMed]

59. Ryan, C.M.; Geckle, M. Why is learning and memory dysfunction in Type 2 diabetes limited to older adults? *Diabetes Metab. Res. Rev.* **2000**, *16*, 308–315. [CrossRef]

60.   De Pablo-Fernandez, E.; Goldacre, R.; Pakpoor, J.; Noyce, A.J.; Warner, T.T. Association between diabetes and subsequent Parkinson disease: A record-linkage cohort study. *Neurology* **2018**. [CrossRef] [PubMed]
61.   Knott, G.; Marchman, H.; Wall, D.; Lich, B. Serial section scanning electron microscopy of adult brain tissue using focused ion beam milling. *J. Neurosci.* **2008**, *28*, 2959–2964. [CrossRef] [PubMed]
62.   Pizzo, M.E.; Wolak, D.J.; Kumar, N.N.; Brunette, E.; Brunnquell, C.L.; Hannocks, M.J.; Abbott, N.J.; Meyerand, M.E.; Sorokin, L.; Stanimirovic, D.B.; et al. Intrathecal antibody distribution in the rat brain: Surface diffusion, perivascular transport and osmotic enhancement of delivery. *J. Physiol.* **2018**, *596*, 445–475. [CrossRef] [PubMed]

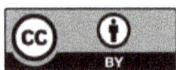

neuroglia

MDPI

Review

An Early History of Neuroglial Research: Personalities

Alexandr Chvátal [1,2],* and Alexei Verkhratsky [3,4,5],*

1   Scimed Biotechnologies, s.r.o., 25241 Zlatníky-Hodkovice, Czech Republic
2   Institute of Pharmacology and Toxicology, Faculty of Medicine in Plzeň, Charles University, 30605 Plzeň, Czech Republic
3   Faculty of Biology, Medicine and Health, The University of Manchester, M13 9PT Manchester, UK
4   Achucarro Center for Neuroscience, IKERBASQUE, Basque Foundation for Science, 48011 Bilbao, Spain
5   Center for Basic and Translational Neuroscience, Faculty of Health and Medical Sciences, University of Copenhagen, 2200 Copenhagen, Denmark
*   Correspondence: chvatal@fastmail.fm (A.C.); Alexej.Verkhratsky@manchester.ac.uk (A.V.)

Received: 16 July 2018; Accepted: 6 August 2018; Published: 16 August 2018

Abstract: Neuroscience, like most other divisions of natural philosophy, emerged in the Hellenistic world following the first experimental discoveries of the nerves connecting the brain with the body. The first fundamental doctrine on brain function highlighted the role for a specific substance, pneuma, which appeared as a substrate for brain function and, being transported through the hollow nerves, operated the peripheral organs. A paradigm shift occurred in 17th century when brain function was relocated to the grey matter. Beginning from the end of the 18th century, the existence of active and passive portions of the nervous tissue were postulated. The passive part of the nervous tissue has been further conceptualised by Rudolf Virchow, who introduced the notion of neuroglia as a connective tissue of the brain and the spinal cord. During the second half of the 19th century, the cellular architecture of the brain was been extensively studied, which led to an in-depth morphological characterisation of multiple cell types, including a detailed description of the neuroglia. Here, we present the views and discoveries of the main personalities of early neuroglial research.

Keywords: neuroglia; neuroscience; history; glial research

1. Brief History of Neuroscience: From Ventricular-Pneumatic Doctrine to Cellular Structure

In the most ancient times, natural philosophy associated human intelligence with the heart and the cardiovascular system. This cardiocentric doctrine was predominant in ancient Egypt, in Judea, and in Persia; it was popular in the Hellenic world, and it remained a mainstream concept in Oriental medicine (most notably in China and in Japan) until the middle of 19th century [1]. In ancient Greece, Aristotle (384–322 B.C.) was the prominent proponent of the cardiovascular doctrine; Aristotle introduced the concept of pneuma, an air-like substance that was produced in the heart and that was distributed through the body. This pneuma, according to Aristotle, was a substrate of intelligence and cognition, and when released from the blood it triggered peripheral voluntary reactions. Within this paradigm, the brain was a bloodless organ that served for cooling pneuma and for moderate passions [2,3].

The first natural philosopher, anatomist, and physiologist who linked the brain with higher cognitive functions was Alcmaeon of Croton (6th–5th centuries B.C.). Alcmaeon defined intelligence as the main factor distinguishing between humans and other animals: "Man differs from other animals, because he alone comprehends, while the other animals perceive but do not understand, because understanding and perception are different things", and realised that "all the senses are connected somehow with the brain" [4]. The brain as an organ of intelligence was recognised by Plato, by Socrates, and in the writings of the Hippocratic school. The Hippocratic corpus (~60 medical texts written by the members of Hippocrates' school in the 5th–4th centuries B.C.) contains a chapter entitled "On the sacred disease", which identifies the brain as an organ of cognition.

"It ought to be generally known that the source of our pleasure, merriment, laughter, and amusement, as of our grief, pain, anxiety, and tears, is none other than the brain. It is specially the organ which enables us to think, see, and hear, and to distinguish the ugly and the beautiful, the bad and the good, pleasant and unpleasant..." [5].

Systematic neuroanatomy was introduced by Herophilus of Chalcedon (335–280 B.C.) and Erasistratus of Cos (304–250 B.C.) who both worked in the Museum of Alexandria (Figure 1A,B). Herophilus identified nerves (including cranial nerves) and found that nerves connect the body with the brain. He further discovered the existence of motor and sensory nerves, and realised that motor nerves originate either in the brain or in the spinal cord. Herophilus was also the first to describe brain ventricles. Erasistratus continued the neuroanatomical studies of his predecessor, and was the first to found the direct relations between complexity of the brain and human intelligence [1,6–8]. Erasistratus was also the first to outline the principles of the ventricular-pneumatic theory of brain function. According to this theory, there are several classes of pneuma; the first type, the vital pneuma, is produced in the lungs from the inhaled air; this vital pneuma is subsequently distributed throughout the body by blood vessels, the vital pneuma diffuses to the tissues and sustains their life. The brain parenchyma converts the vital pneuma into the psychic pneuma, which is concentrated in the ventricles. The psychic pneuma represents the substrate of nervous function, including cognition. From the ventricles, the psychic pneuma is sent to the periphery through the hollow nerves; when released from nerve terminal, the psychic pneuma instigates peripheral responses [1,6–8]. Of note, Democritus (460–370 B.C.) suggested that the "psyche", that is, the substrate of nerve function, is formed by the lightest atoms [3].

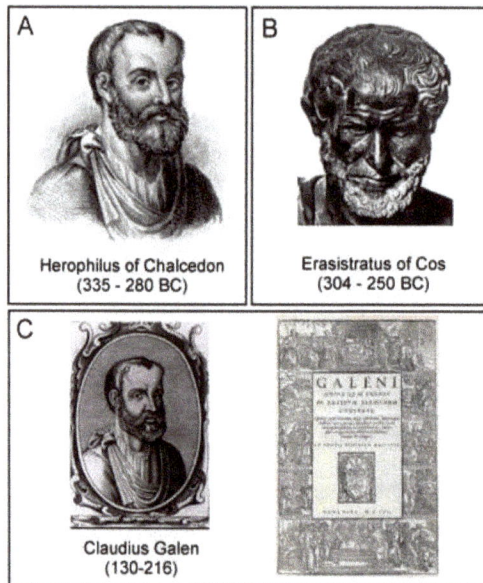

Figure 1. Founders of neuroanatomy and neurophysiology: (**A**) Herophilius, (**B**) Earsistratus, and (**C**) Galen, and the frontispiece of the Renaissance edition of Galen's works (*Galeno. Omnia quae extant opera.* Venezia, eredi di Luca Antonio Giunta, 1556).

The ventricular-pneumatic theory of the brain function was further developed by Claudius Galen of Pergamon (129–200 A.D., Figure 1C). Galen regarded the pneuma as a special fluid that was produced by the brain parenchyma from the "vital spirit" produced by the lungs from the air; the final conversion of vital spirit to pneuma occurred in the choroid plexus, through which pneuma entered the ventricular system. The ventricles worked as a pump, which maintained the movement of pneuma through the motor nerves, and the aspiration of pneuma from the sensory nerves. The pneuma, which completely filled the nerves, made them rigid, which allowed the rapid conduction of signals similar to the pulse wave propagation through blood vessels. Signalling at the sensory nerve endings and motor nerve terminals occurred through microscopic pores that allowed free exchange of pneuma between the nerves and peripheral tissues. At the brain level, pneuma carrying sensory signals is delivered to the anterior ventricles, whereas the afferent signals to the muscles originate from the posterior ventricle [9]. Based on experiments on live animals which involved selective compression or lesioning of different parts of the brain and nerve ligation, Galen contemplated distinct localisation of functions within different anatomical structures. First, he demonstrated that damage to the brain parenchyma *per se* did not cause major deficits unless the ventricle was opened (apparently causing the escape of the pneuma). He also found that compression of anterior ventricle led to blindness, whereas compression of the posterior ventricle resulted in general paralysis. The damage to the ventricles resulted either in serious sensory deficits (anterior ventricle), or in collapse and death (middle and posterior ventricles).

The ventricular-pneumatic doctrine remained the main theory of neuroscience throughout the Middle Ages and the Renaissance. Anatomists and medics from both western world (Albertus Magnus, Tomas Aquinas, Roger Bacon, Petrus de Montagnana, Lodovico Dolce, Ghiradelli of Bologna, and Theodor Gull of Antwerp) and from Arabic countries (Ibn Sīnā and Ibn Rushd, known in Europe as Avicenna and Averroes), added further developments by assigning different functions to different parts of ventricular system (Figure 2). The anterior ventricle was usually associated with sensory input and sensory processing, the middle ventricle was linked to creativity and imagination, cognition and intellect, whereas the posterior ventricle was a seat for memory [9]. Leonardo da Vinci, who was an adept of the ventricular-pneumatic doctrine, made the first three-dimensional cast of the ventricles by filling them with melted wax (Figure 2C); when the wax was set, the brain tissues were removed, thus revealing the ventricular system [10]. According to Leonardo's reckoning the anterior ventricles were responsible for bridging the sensory inputs with *senso commune*, while memory resided in the posterior ventricle.

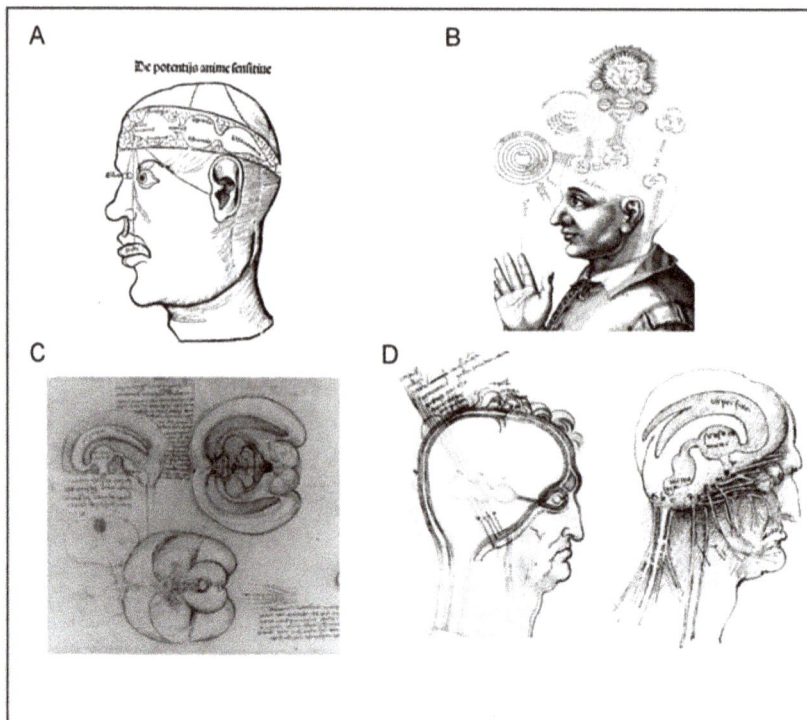

Figure 2. Pneumo-ventricular doctrine of the brain function. (**A**) The conceptual scheme of ventricular localisation of brain functions proposed by Albertus Magnus, as depicted in the later version from the 16th century, made by Gregorius Reisch, who was the Prior of the House of Carthusians at Freiburg and confessor to the Emperor Maximilian, and who published a concise encyclopaedia of knowledge in 1503 [11]. (**B**) Ventricular divisions of brain functions as presented in 'The Art of Memory' by English Paracelcian physician Robert Fludd [12]. (**C**) The three-dimensional depiction of the ventricular system as drawn by Leonardo da Vinci. Leonardo made a mould of the brain ventricles by injecting them with melted wax, which after the removal of soft tissues produced their precise cast [13]. "Make two vent-holes in the horns of the greater ventricles, and insert melted wax with a syringe, making a hole in the ventricle of memory; and through such a hole, fill the three ventricles of the brain. Then when the wax has set, take apart the brain, and you will see the shape of the ventricles exactly." (cited from [10]). (**D**) The concept of brain functions and cross-section of the human head and cranial nerves according to Leonardo da Vinci. Since Leonardo used his left hand for writing and wrote from right to left, his drawings with descriptions are presented mirrored in this figure. On the left is a cross-section of the head with a symbolic image of three ventricles; it is possible to recognize the names of the individual layers, such as the *cerebro* (brain), *dura mater*, and *pia mater* (meninges), the *cranio* (skull), and the *pericranio* (periosteum). On the right is the "cell" theory of brain functions and the cranial nerves. In the first ventricle, Leonardo placed *imprensiva*, a term proposed by himself (and never used by anybody else) for a structure connecting the senses and *senso commune*; in the second ventricle, he placed *senso comune*; and in the third, he placed *memo* (memory) [10].

Rene Descartes (1596–1650), who introduced the concept of reflexes, had his own view on the functioning of the nervous system. He assigned the nervous function to small corpuscles or "a very fine flame" which was released from nerve endings [14]. According to Descartes, peripheral stimulation triggered mechanical displacement of nerves that almost immediately caused the central end of the nerve to twitch. This in turn triggered the release of "animal spirit" or "a very fine flame" that in the form of minute particles, flew to the ventricles. The same particles carried signals through the nerves to the periphery. In the nerve endings, these signalling particles were released through miniature valves and diffused to the muscles, where they were taken up by congruent valves; after entering the muscles, these said particles initiated and regulated contraction. Descartes also suggested that volatile movements originate from the pineal gland surrounded by the cerebrospinal fluid. Small movements of the pineal gland are accordingly able to regulate the flow of the *spiritus animales* through a complex system of pipes and valves (Figure 3A).

The first departures form the ventricular-pneumatic views emerged in the 17th century when Marchello Malpighi and, to a larger extend Thomas Willis, noted the roles for the grey matter and brain parenchyma in nervous function [15,16]. Localisation of functions in the brain was initially performed by numerous phrenologists, including Georg Prochaska, Franz Joseph Gall, Johann Gaspard Spurzheim, and George Combe [17–20]. The first true functional brain centre was discovered by Paul Broca, who identified the area in the posterior-inferior part of the frontal cortex of the dominant hemisphere as a centre of speech [21]. Further advances in the localisation of brain functions were made by Gustav Theodor Fritsch and Edward Hitzig [22], and by systematic studies of Sir David Ferrier, who produced the first map of functional speciality of various brain regions in monkeys, including the motor and sensory (vision, heating and taste) areas [23–25]. The electrophysiological mapping of the motor cortex was finalised by Wilder G. Penfield who invented the concept of the motor and sensory "homunculus" [26].

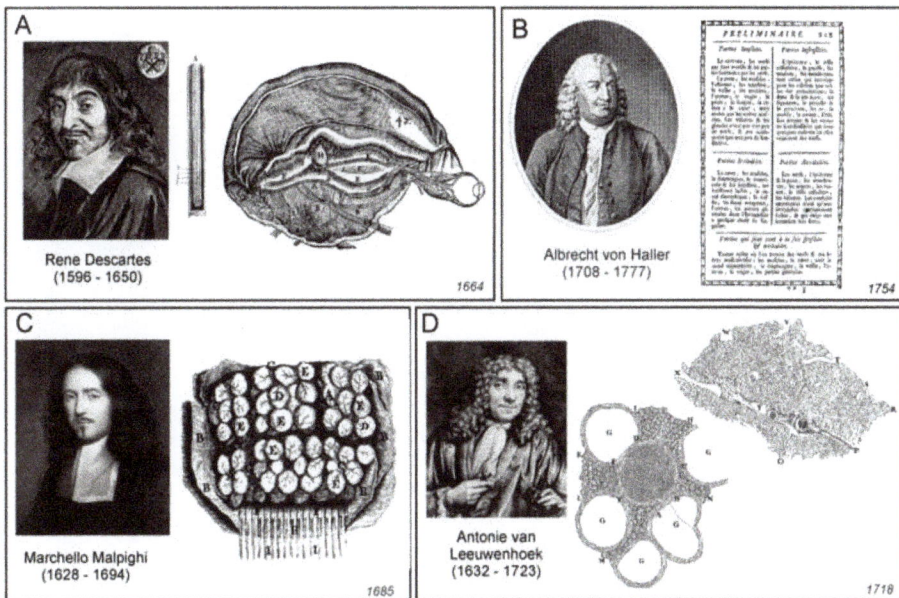

Figure 3. Early morphological studies of the nervous system. (**A**) Nervous structure and the formation of voluntary movements as proposed by René Descartes. On the left is a diagram of the optic nerve comprising hollow tube-like structures [14]. On the right is the formation of voluntary movements regulated by the activity of the pineal gland [27]. (**B**) Albrecht von Haller, and the excerpt of his book *De partibus corporis humani sensilibus et irritabilibus. Commentarii societatis regiae scientiarum gottingensis* [26] in which he introduces the existence of irritable (*irritabilis*) and sensible (*sensibilis*) tissues. (**C**) Globular (gland-like) structures of the brain cortex according to Marcello Malpighi (reproduced from [28]). (**D**) Cross-section of a nerve (left, [29]) and the structure of the brain tissue after Antoni van Leeuwenhoek. On the right is a structure of dried pig brain tissue containing two vesicles [30].

These advances in neuroanatomy coincided with the emergence of neurophysiology. Probably the first true neurophysiologist was Albrecht von Haller, who performed physiological experiments and developed the theory of irritability and sensitivity [31,32]. By systematic injury to all organs and parts of organs by spraying with cold, hot or corrosive substances, by stinging, squeezing, and also by means of electricity, Haller, in observing the stimulus response of the organ part concerned, classified the two categories of irritable (*irritabilis*) and sensible (*sensibilis*) tissues [33]. Haller's stimulation experiments, based on the assignment of the criteria irritable and sensitive, led for the first time to a precise, functional differentiation of the smallest components (fibres) of animal organisms (Figure 3B). Haller also noticed that in addition to the tissues that were directly responsible for irritation and sensitivity, there was another type of tissue which belonged to neither group. Haller called the third type of tissue the "cell tissue fibre" (*Zellgewebsfaser*), constituting "cellular tissue" (*Zellgewebe*). According to him, this was an inert tissue forming a filling or a basic substance, that encompassed all those components of the organism that Haller was unable to identify as either sensitive or irritable [34].

The ideas of cellular nature of the nervous tissue were developed in parallel. Starting from the mid-17th century, the notion of elementary units of life were contemplated by several natural philosophers, most notable by Pierre Gassendi and Robert Boyle. This coincided with the emergence of first microscopes that allowed visualisation of life units. The term "cell" was introduced in 1665 by Robert Hooke [35], who noted the semblance between regular microstructures that he observed in cork, with the monk's cells in the monastery dormitories. The first animal cells were visualised and described by Antonie van Leeuwenhoek (1632–1723), who, by using self-made microscopes, found bacteria (he called them *animalcules* or little animals); he also observed erythrocytes, single muscle fibres, and followed the movements of live spermatozoids [36]. The cellular theory of life was formalised by Theodor Schwann and Matthias Jakob Schleiden [37,38].

In particular, Theodor Schwann (1810–1882), in his famous book devoted to the cell theory [38], summarized the properties of tissues as follows:

> Upon these more or less important modifications of the cell-life the following classification of the tissues is based: 1st. Isolated, independent cells, which either exist in fluids, or merely lie unconnected and moveable, beside each other. 2d. Independent cells applied firmly together, so as to form a coherent tissue. 3d. Tissues, in which the cell-walls (but not the cell-cavities) have coalesced together, or with the intercellular substance. Lastly, tissues in which both the walls and cavities of many cells blend together. In addition to these, however, there is yet another very natural section of the tissues, namely, the fibre-cells, in which independent cells are extended out on one or more sides into bundles of fibres. The naturalness of this group will form my excuse for sacrificing logical classification to it, and inserting it as the fourth class (4th), consequently, that last mentioned, consisting of tissues, in which the cell-walls and cell-cavities coalesce, becomes the fifth (5th). (Cited from English translation; [39] p. 65)

Thus, according to Schwann, all tissues, including nervous and connective tissues, were composed from cells or their constituents; accordingly, all fibres were parts of the cells and they were cellular processes.

Probably the first microscopic observations of the cortex were made by Marcello Malpighi, who noted that nervous tissue is composed from numerous little formations, which he called "globules" or "little glands" ([40] and Figure 3C); similar structures were mentioned by other contemporary microscopists including Antonie van Leeuwenhoek (Figure 3D and [41]). Whether these structures indeed represented neural cells remains unknown. The very first true description of neural cells belongs to Emanuel Swedenborg (1688–1772) who described (in the 1740s) that the "globules" or "cerebellulas" (small brains) were independent functional entities that were interconnected with fibres; these globules and their projected fibres were the substrates for brain function: "From each cortical gland proceeds a single nerve fibre; this is carried down into the body, in order that it may take hold of some part of a sensation or produce some action" (quoted from [41]). Swedenborg's writings unfortunately were not published until 1882 [42] and hence they did not influence the developments of cellular neuroscience. The globular structures of different sizes (which sizes vary between regions of the nervous system) have been also described by Giovanni Maria Della Torre (Figure 4A and [43]).

Peripheral nerves were first observed under microscope by van Leeuwenhoek, who described (in 1717, see [44]) small regular circular structures (that represented single axons) in the sagittal slice of the nerves isolated from cows or sheep (Figure 3D). Felice Gaspar Ferdinand Fontana produced, in 1780, the very first anatomical description of nerve and neural fibres or axons, noting that the nerve is composed "of a large number of transparent, uniform, and simple cylinders. These cylinders seem to be fashioned like a very thin, uniform wall or tunic which is filled, as far as one can see, with transparent, gelatinous fluid insoluble in water" [44].

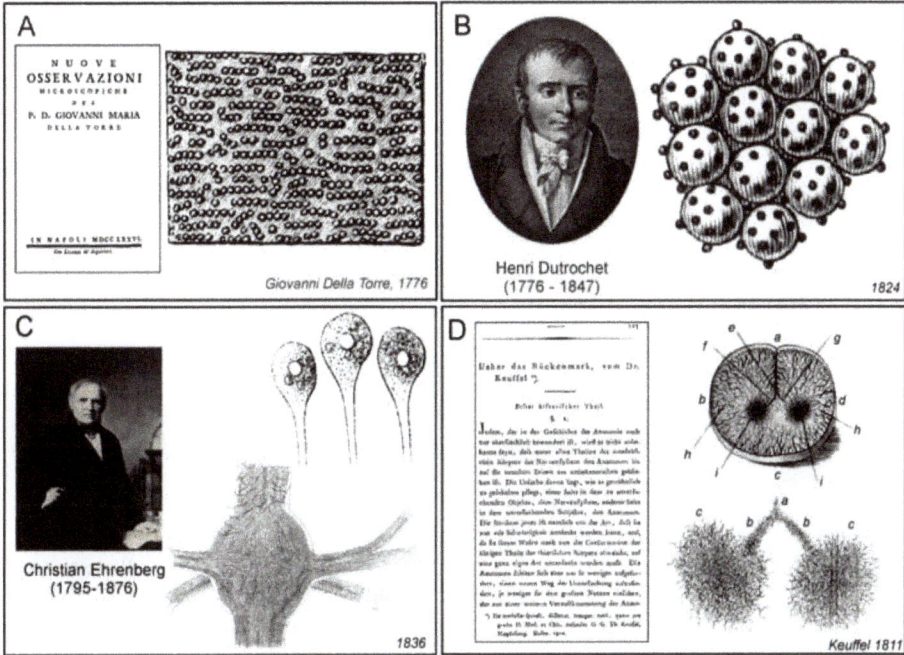

Figure 4. The early studies of the elements of the nervous system. (**A**) Globular structure of the spinal cord tissue according to Giovanni Maria Della Torre, and the frontispiece of his book [36]. (**B**) Henri Dutrochet and his drawings of the globular corpuscules from mollusc cervical ganglia [38]. (**C**) Christian Gottfried Ehrenberg and his image of the nerve cell of the leech [41]. (**D**) Theodor Keuffel and the excerpt of his book on the structure of the spinal cord [45]. Right: the fibrous substance in the thin slice of ox spinal cord (top) and in the grey matter only (bottom) Top: a, b, c, d—the *pia mater*; f, g—two fibres extending from the *pia mater* and splitting into two centres (i); h—neurilem. Bottom: two centres of the grey matter; a—the end of the extension of the *pia mater*; b—the last fibrils into which this extension splits; c—the two centres of grey matter.

One of the earliest description of cellular elements of the central nervous system have been made by Henri Dutrochet (1776–1847), who observed clusters of globular particles (*corpuscules globuleux agglomeres*) in the frog brain, which he suggested were the structural elements of the nervous tissue [46,47]. Dutrochet further concluded that these globular structures (nerve bodies) were "manufacturers of nervous energy", while nerve fibres provided "nervous motion". He further studied cerebral ganglia of molluscs *Helix pomatia* and *Arion rufus*, and reported clusters of spherical cells that were associated with smaller spherical or ovoid particles (Figure 4B). A century later,

František Karel Studnička speculated that Dutrochet described large ganglion neurones surrounded by glial cells, which can be further identified as microglia, and thus Dutrochet was the first discoverer of neuroglia [48]. This inspiring idea however, remains a mere surmise Dutrochet by himself was oblivious to the existence of supportive cells of the nervous system.

The first documented microscopic images of leech neurones (Figure 4C) were obtained by Christian Gottfried Ehrenberg [49], while Jan Evangelista Purkyně identified and imaged nerve cells of the cerebellum [50], and his pupil Gustav Gabriel Valentin observed neurones with nuclei (Figure 5A,B). In those days, the nerve cells were generally called *globules or kugeln* (spheres in German). Robert Bently Todd was the first to name these structures cells; he wrote: "The essential elements of the grey nervous matter are "vesicles" or cells, containing nuclei and nucleoli". They have also been called nerve or ganglion "globules" [51]. In 1873, Camillo Golgi introduced the silver-chromate staining technique [52], which allowed much more detailed microscopic visualisation of neural cells.

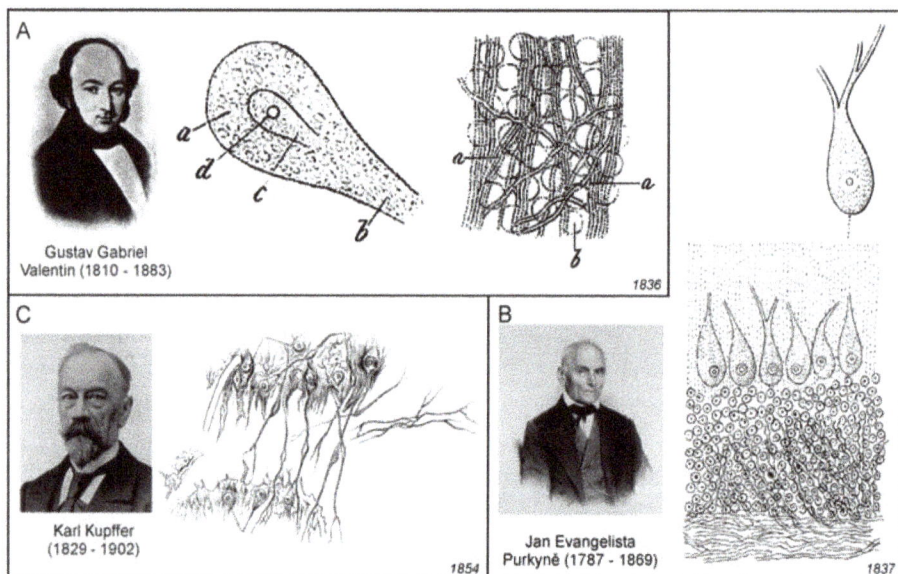

Figure 5. First microscopic images of neural cells. (**A**) The first drawing of neurones with processes and nervous structures, made by Gustav Gabriel Valentin [48]. Middle: single globule of the human yellow matter, terminated by a tail-like process: (a) parenchyma, (b) tail-like process, (c) vesicle-like core similar to the germinal vesicle, and (d) bodies present on the surface. Right: fibres and globules in the sheep spinal cord. A thin section of the spinal cord in the cervical region, *medulla oblongata*: (a) the undulated longitudinal primitive fibres forming plexuses and (b) globules present in the interstitial space. (**B**) Jan Evangelista Purkyně and the first drawings of the Purkinje neurone made by him for the Congress of Physicians and Scientists Conference in Prague, in 1837. (**C**) Karl Kupffer [53] and the first drawing of the cellular elements in the frog spinal cord grey matter, which had "definite connections with undoubted connective tissue fibres".

2. The Concept of Neuroglia. The Birth of the Concept

Albrecht von Haller, in his treatise on irritability and sensitivity (see above) also noted that besides tissues involved in irritation and sensitivity, another type of tissue exists which belong to neither group and which Haller called as "cell tissue fibre" (*Zellgewebsfaser*), constituting "cellular tissue" (*Zellgewebe*). According to him, this was an inert tissue forming a filling or basic substance that encompassed all those components of the organism that Haller was unable to identify as either sensitive or irritable [33].

Haller, most likely for the first time, defined fibre tissue as an inert tissue forming a filling or basic substance in the brain tissue.

Almost 60 years after Haller's work, German anatomist Theodor Keuffel (no personal data are available), who was a student of famous German physician, physiologist, anatomist, and psychiatrist Johann Christian Reil (1759–1813), published a book, based on his PhD thesis, which was dedicated to the histological examination of the central nervous system [45,54]. In the spinal cord slices, he described fine-needled fabric of the finest fibres; the whole fibrous substance was of reticular shape, as it would correspond to a fibrous network consisting of an innumerable amount of finest fibrils, which formed anastomoses between themselves in the most varied ways, and to connect with each other by countless branches (Figure 4D). The fibrous matter in the white, as well as in the grey matter, expressed a completely uniformly net-like structure without any predominant direction. The fibrils of the white and grey matter, merged directly with each other, so that it seemed to Keuffel that the fibrillary mesh ran through the entire cross-section of the spinal cord. The nature of the fibrous substance, according to him, was a compressed animal substance. What he observed, was probably the vascular network of the spinal cord, since by using his methods, all neuroglial cells disappeared and only vessels and the actual connective tissue remained (see also [55]). Thus, the main contribution of Keuffel was the concept of a histological microstructure that existed in the nervous tissue in addition to the nervous elements, which led to the conviction that the brain and spinal cord tissue also contained some sort of fibrillary tissue which was observed in the other organs of the body.

Gabriel Valentin (1810–1883) was a German physiologist; after finishing in the University of Breslau (now Wroclaw in Poland), he worked as an assistant to Jan Evangelista Purkyně. Valentin published results of his investigation of the structure if the nervous tissue, which was done most likely under the influence of Purkyně, in an extensive treatise [56,57]. According to Valentin:

> The whole nervous system consists of two primary masses, namely the isolated spheres of the occupying masses and the isolated, continuous primitive fibres. The former are probably representatives of the creative, active, higher principle, the latter of the receiving and guiding, passive, lower principle. Each of these is enveloped by a cell-tissue sheath, the strength of which determines the intensity of the action of both heterogeneous parts on each other. These are the pure and peculiar formations of the nervous system. ([56]; p. 157)

In Valentin's model, the nervous tissue comprised spheres (*Kugeln der Belegungsmassen*), which represent cell bodies, primitive fibres (*Primitivfasern*), which represent nerve fibres, and intermediate substance (*Zellgewebescheide*) containing fibres or threads, which was most likely identical to what some authors later called as glial sheaths (*Gliascheiden*). In contrast to Keuffel, who considered this substance to be fibrous only, Valentin clearly identified it as cellular tissue (Figure 5A). He also described that the sheaths were always of a cellular nature where the cellular elements were interconnected by threadlike cellular tissue extensions. Valentin proposed that this whole formation evidently had the purpose of inhibiting the mutual direct action of the primitive fibres and the spheres, since he was convinced, on the basis of physiological experiments, that the sheaths had the properties of an insulator. The main contribution of Valentin was therefore the establishment of the concept of the nerve tissue structure, which moved towards the later neuroglial concept in two ways: first, the intermediate filling substance, other than nerve bodies and fibres, had a cellular structure with thread-like extensions, and second, this intermediate filling substance had insulating properties.

Purkyně' was the first to provide topographic description of the ganglionic bodies, which from today's perspective, corresponds to the agglomerations of various classes of nerve cells in different areas of the brain, spinal cord, and ganglia, and in which he described nuclei and nucleoli. Among them were also Purkinje cells, large neurons with many branching dendrites found in the cerebellum (Figure 5B). However, lesser known in fact, was that Purkyně has also a priority in the description of the processes of cells in the brain and spinal cord that were in close relationship with nearby blood vessels. As he pointed out in the extended and less known version of his abstract from the Prague meeting in 1837:

The processes of the ganglionic cells in the brain and in the spinal cord sometimes appear to be related to the large number of surrounding blood vessels, but it has never been proven with certainty, even less could be determined here about the reduction of very fine brain fibres [58].

What Purkyně most likely observed were the processes of perivascular astrocytes, which are closely associated with the brain capillaries.

The general view on the structure of the nervous system was significantly, and for a long period of time, affected by the concept suggested by the German professor emeritus of anatomy and physiology at Heidelberg, Friedrich Arnold (1803–1890). In his handbook of human anatomy [59] he stated, that the base substance (*Grundmasse*), the germinal matter, or the primary substance of the cellular tissue (*Zellgewebe*), is recognized, with the aid of good instruments and with moderate moderation of light, as a dull, finely granulated, molecular substance (*moleculare Substanz*) between the threads and bundles of the connective tissue. Concerning the nerve substance, he was convinced that it was composed of a (i) granular base substance (*körnige Grundmasse*), (ii) spherical, sphere-like and disk-shaped bodies, and (iii) primitive fibres and strips. The granular base substance he characterized as following:

> The granular base substance occurs both in the white and grey matter; but in the latter, it seems, in greater quantity. The fact that it is also found in the marrow mass and here in no small quantity is proved by the examination of the intact upper marrow of small animals. The grains or granules are extremely small, measuring 0.0007‴–0.0005‴ [1.1–1.5 μm] and above, have either a bright and light or a greyish and dark appearance. They lie randomly between and around the closer and the next form components. In this fine-grained mass (*feinkörnigen Masse*), especially in the brain cortex and in the eye retina, one perceives light-yellowish, larger and smaller bodies of very dull appearance, rounded shape, and somewhat dark contours; they appear in different numbers, sometimes more scattered, now in denser masses, and appear in the former case as gaps in the granular base substance. According to their behaviour, they consist of protein and fat. I could not prove a compound of a nucleus and a bark or a skin on them; they are not vesicles, but simple molecular bodies (*molekulare Körper*). ([59] p. 260)

Terms, such as *moleculare Substanz*, *körnige Grundmasse* and *feinkörnigen Masse*, were found throughout numerous works of various authors who described the structure of the nervous tissue in the middle of the 19th century. Most probably, such structures were an artefact resulted from the improper tissue processing methods used by researchers of that time.

Karel Rokytanský (in German Carl Freiherr von Rokitansky, 1804–1878) was a famous Czech physician; he studied medicine and worked until the end of his life in Vienna. Nowadays almost forgotten, Rokytanský extensively studied the pathological changes of the brain connective tissue [60, 61]. In the publication, where he compared the development of tumour stroma with the development of other tissues, he described the similarity of the structure of brain tumours with brain connective tissue (*Bindegewebs-Substanzen*), and also argued for networked cellular formations in brain melanoma metastases [62]. In a publication dealing with general properties of connective tissue [63] Rokytanský also suggested that inflammation may significantly affect nerve connective tissue, which according to him was a storeroom (*Lager*) and scaffold (*Gerüste*) or binding substance (*Bindemasse*) for neural elements. Describing the scar formation in the brain, he stated:

> If, in particular, these conditions are also formed in the brains with the inclusion of the higher sensory nerves and in the spinal cord, this requires the demonstration of a connective tissue substance as the basis and starting point of the new formation. A connective-tissue substance is here present, indeed, as a delicate, soft substance, which in the tissue appears as shagreened, and accumulates more abundantly in the ganglionic substance also containing abundant

nuclei (*Kernen*), in which the elements of the brain-tissue are all embedded. It occurs in the ventricles as the lining of the same, ependyma. But not only here, rather also on the surface of the brain, it appears as a delicate clothing of the cerebral cortex, an outer ependyma formation (*äussere Ependyma-Formation*) that, similarly as in ventricles, is characterized by the appearance of simple and layered amyloid bodies (*amyloider Körperchen*). Accordingly, there is a storage and binding mass in the nervous centre, which forms a sheaths and a lining on the outer surface and in the inner spaces. ([63]; p. 136)

Subsequent work of Rokytanský was dedicated exclusively to pathophysiology of nerve connective tissue [64]. He described different pathological states, when the primary change was an increase in the number of nuclei and the volume of the connective tissue, which separated the nerve cells, their fibres and vessels. In physiological conditions, to the contrary, connective tissue formed an almost homogeneous matrix. In degenerative disorders, he described an increase of the connective tissue volume and its fibrillation (most likely fibromatosis), which compressed nerve cells and their processes, thus instigating their subsequent atrophy and disintegration into fat particles (*Fettkörnchen-Agglomerat*) and colloid or amyloid bodies (*corpora amylacea*). Rokytanský found these degenerative changes in the pons, cerebellar peduncles, cerebral cortex, and even in the cranial nerves. Besides the extensive investigation of the brain connective substance pathology, Rokytanský clearly formulated the concept of the connective tissue as a binding substance, where neural elements are embedded, and a place of the starting point of their new formation. In this sense he might also influenced another famous pathologist of the time, Rudolph Virchow.

Rudolf Virchow (1821–1902) was a person of Renaissance proportion, being a medic, a cell biologist, an anatomist and histologist, an anthropologist, a hygienist, and a statesman. He was born on 13 September 1821 in Schivelbein, which is a small town in Pomerania. Virchow introduced the concept of cellular pathology epitomised in his widely known aphorism "*Omnis cellula e cellula*" ("every cell stems from another cell"; the erroneous belief that this aphorism belongs to Francois-Vincent Raspail [53,65] could not be verified and we could not find this phrase in Raspail's writings). Pathological changes in cells or in cellular groups were, according to this concept, the seat of disease. In addition, Virchow was well known hygienist and advocate of social health. He was a member of the German Reichstag, a member of the municipal council of Berlin, and he organised the construction of modern water and sewage systems in the city of Berlin. Politically, he was at odds with Otto Bismarck, and their arguments led to a legendary duel in which Virchow, being challenged by Bismarck (and the argument was about hygienic values of the cities), chose as their weapons two pork sausages: a cooked sausage for himself, and a cooked sausage tainted with *Trichinellala* larva for Bismarck, who refused to fight under those conditions, considering them too dangerous.

When only 25-year-old, Virchow published a short paper dedicated to the structure of the connective tissue beneath the ependyma of brain ventricles [66]. He confirmed the presence of five basic elements of this tissue, previously described by Rokytanský [67]. In addition, Virchow also described small, round bodies, similar to glass beads or to dew drops, which were relatively densely packed without being interconnected, on the inner surface of the ventricles. If the tissue was well cleaned of blood, it was possible to observe how these units, being star-shaped, were interconnected by fine fibres, so that the entire area was covered by a fine net. Ten years later, Virchow published the same paper again, this time with commentaries [68]; in one of these comments he stated that:

> Thus, according to my investigations, the ependyma consists not merely of an epithelium but essentially of a layer of connective tissue covered with epithelium, and although this can be easily removed from the surface, it forms no isolated membrane in the narrower sense of the word, but only the surface of the interstitial connective of the brain substance protruding above the surface... This connective substance forms in the brain, the spinal cord and the higher sensory nerves a type of putty (neuroglia), in which the nervous elements are immersed and which is the main deposition site for Corpora amylacea... ([68]; p. 890)

However, the term "neuroglia" was not accepted instantly; for a while, many researchers used the term "nerve connective tissue". It is still matter of debate as to whether Virchow also observed cells in what he named neuroglia. In the fresh connective tissue, Virchow have seen fine-grained material with elongated nuclei, which according to him, was mistaken for a special type of nerve substance. These elements, however, are far from the meaning of what we today call neuroglial or glial cells. The same concept of neuroglia, including images (Figure 6), was further elaborated by Virchow in his Opera Magna, *Die Cellularpathologie in ihrer Begründung auf physiologische und pathologische Gewebelehre*, which outlined the foundations of cellular pathophysiology. This book (which was in fact a stenograph of Virchow's 20 lectures for students of Berlin Medical University Charite) was published first in German [69] and shortly afterwards in English [70]. Virchow's concept of connective tissue was very similar to that which was published two years earlier by Rokytanský, who first suggested that the nerve connective tissue is a storeroom, scaffold, and binding material for elements of neural tissue [63]. However, it is evident from giving a special term for it (neuroglia), that Virchow was convinced that it significantly differed from other connective tissues in the body. Virchow's concept of glia become universally acknowledged, and, albeit in a modified form, it has survived up to the present day.

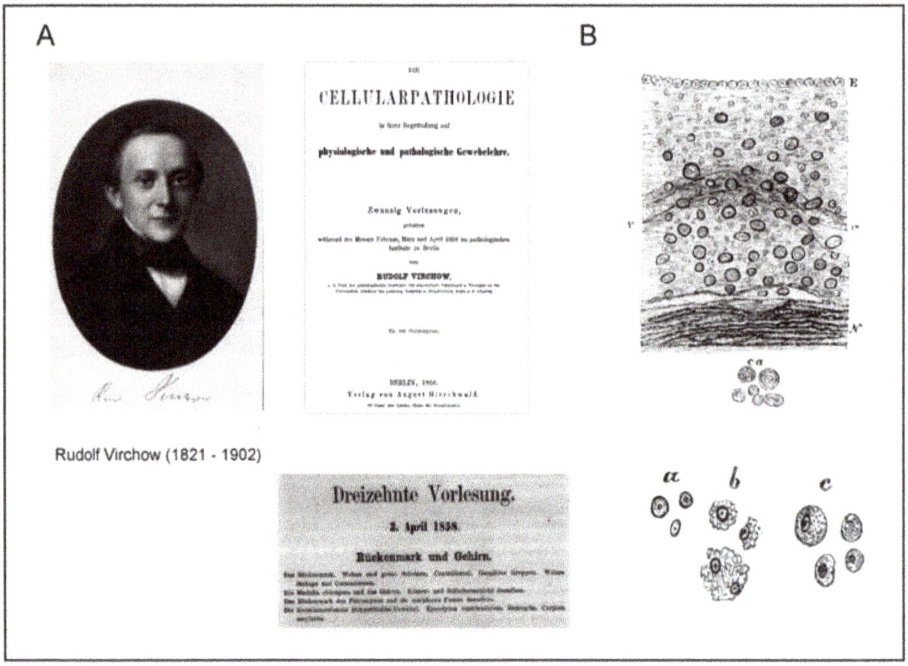

Figure 6. Rudolf Virchow and the concept of neuroglia. (**A**) Rudolf Virchow, the frontispiece of his book *Die cellularpathologie in ihrer begründung auf physiologische und pathologische* [69,70] and the title of lecture 13, in which the concept of neuroglia was presented to the students of the Medical University of Berlin (Charite) on 3 April 1858. (**B**) Top: ependyma and neuroglia in the floor of the fourth ventricle. Between the ependyma and the nerve fibres is "the free portion of the neuroglia with numerous connective tissue corpuscles and nuclei". Numerous *corpora amylacea* are also visible, shown enlarged below the main illustration (*ca*). E—ependymal epithelium; N—nerve fibres; v–w—blood vessels. Bottom: elements of neuroglia from the white matter of the human cerebral hemispheres. A—free nuclei with nucleoli; b—nuclei with partially destroyed cell bodies; c—complete cells. Reproduced from [69].

Another important turning point to the cellular concept of the nervous connective tissue was represented by the research of Baltic-German physiologist and anatomist Georg Bidder (1810–1894) from the University of Dorpat (now Tartu, Estonia) and his students. Bidder, together with his former student Karl Kupffer (1829–1902), published an extensive work devoted to the investigation on the texture of the spinal cord and the development of its form elements [71]. Besides the general historical overviews, they also described their own results, which were obtained mainly in cold-blooded animals, that is, fishes and frogs. Bidder and Kupffer were aware of the importance of the connective tissue in the spinal cord; however, they did not consider elements of the connective tissue to be of nervous origin. Their work also included two large chapters devoted to connective tissue. As with other numerous researchers in the field, they were convinced that what they described as a connective tissue in the brain and in spinal cord shared similar properties with the other connective tissues in the body; therefore, one extensive chapter contained the detailed information on connective tissue in general, and in brain and spinal cord in particular. The second extensive chapter contained information on the methods, and how to distinguish the elements of the connective tissue from neural elements, neural bodies and nerve fibres. The publication is also important due to the fact that it gives most likely the first description of the connective tissue (neuroglial) cell in the grey matter of the spinal cord:

> ...there is also a third type of fibre associated with cells, which are distributed in large numbers throughout the grey matter. It has always been thought that these cells are nerve cells, and they undoubtedly refer to the statement that "the smallest" nerve cells are found in this part of the spinal cord. These are partly round, partly oblong, some without processes, some with two or more processes, and thus angular or star-shaped bodies of 0.003–0.004'" [6.4–8.5 μm] in diameter, with deep dark contours, and a generally sharply delimited nucleus in the middle. They are fairly uniformly distributed throughout the grey matter, and no particular law can be demonstrated in their arrangement. The processes are often so delicate that they do not present two lateral boundary lines, but appear as a simple wavy line. The processes of neighbouring cells often overlap, giving rise to an appearance, as shown by the anastomosing processes of the bony bodies in a thin bone section. Of particular note, however, is the fact that the processes of these cells are sometimes associated with those fibres which emanate from the pointed and grey mass end of the spinal cord epithelial cells. If this connection alone would be sufficient to refute the nerve-cell nature of these elements, then the deficiency of the yellow colour, which in the chromic-acid preparation belongs to the unquestionable nerve-cells, and the missing connection with definite nerve-fibres, speak against it. Thus, these cells are connective tissue corpuscles, and the fibres associated with them are the admixtures to the connective tissue known as spiral or elastic fibres. ([71], p. 45)

Unfortunately, this description had no accompanying figure. However, Kupffer's earlier dissertation [72] contained results indicating that the connective tissue is an integral part of the spinal cord grey matter. Investigating the cellular elements in the frog spinal cord grey matter, Kupffler observed cells which he at first determined to be supposed nerve cells, but afterwards, he also observed that they had definite connections with undoubted connective tissue fibres. He afterwards had to classify the considerable part of these cells not as essential nerve elements, but as connective tissue corpuscles (Figure 5C).

3. Discovery of Glial Cells as Cellular Entities

3.1. Retinal Radial Glia: Samuel Pappenheim, Heinrich Müller, and Max Schultze

Probably the very first description of the histological structure of the retina was published by Samuel Moritz Pappenheim (1811–1882), who was Purkyně's assistant in Wroclaw. They published several papers together on histology and physiology. Pappenheim also published several extensive monographs, one of which was dedicated to the structure of the eye [73]. All findings, especially the description of cellular elements, were based on a long period of research, and on the extensive amount of processed tissues, including bones, eye ball, and eye accessory organs of different species of animals and of humans. This book also contained the very first detailed description of the histological structure of the retina, which included the description of radially oriented cells (most likely radial glial cells, Figure 7A), of dark red granules (probably rhodopsin) and layers of ganglion cells.

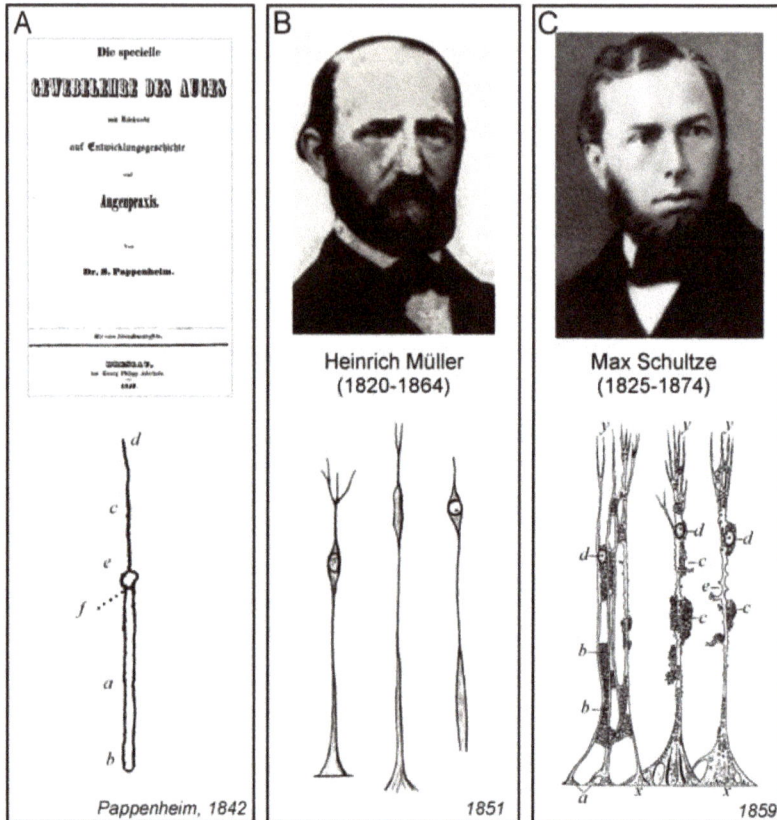

Figure 7. (**A**). Probably the first image of radial astrocytes of the retina or Muller glial cells made by Samuel Pappenheim (a—the inner part, b—part of the retina, e—an outer part with a large spherical base changing into the fibre (c) and into the ending (d), [73], the panel also shows the frontispiece of his book *Die specielle gewebelehre des auges mit rücksicht auf entwicklungsgeschichte und augenpraxis*). (**B**): Radial astrocytes of the retina by Heinrich Müller [74]. (**C**): Radial astrocytes of the retina by Max Schultze [75]. The processes of Müller fibres passing into the outer nuclear layer (s), inner membrane (x) and the holes in membrana limitans interna (a), the holes in the network of fine membranes for optic nerves (b), so-called molecular network (c), the nuclei in Müller fibres (d), the space with the cell nuclei of the inner nuclear layer (e).

Almost 10 years after Pappenheim, Heinrich Müller (1820–1864), who held a chair at the University of Würzburg, published a preliminary communication on the structure of the retina. In this paper, he described in detail the layers of the retina by using chromic acid [74]. He provided a description of the cell layers, of the radial cells extending from the inner to the outer layer, and also of cellular extensions in the granular layer, with these extensions containing the nuclei. Five years later, Müller published further descriptions of the retina [76], which contained figures of individual cellular elements in different species of animals, including radial glial cells, which were subsequently were named after him (Müller glia, Figure 7B).

Three years after Müller's descriptions of the retina, German microscopic anatomist Max Johann Sigismund Schultze (1825–1874), published an advanced treatise on the structure of the retina [75] on the occasion of his appointment as a professor of anatomy and director of the Institute of Anatomy in Bonn. Besides the description of other structures, Schultze devoted the whole chapter to radial glial cells (he named them *fibras Muellerianas* to emphasize that they were described for the first time in detail by Heinrich Müller). The treatise, written in Latin, also contained images of retinal structures, and particularly of radial glial cells, which were of exceptional quality with the minutest details (Figure 7C).

3.2. Carl Bergmann

German anatomist, physiologist, and biologist Carl Georg Lucas Christian Bergmann (1814–1865), who was professor of anatomy and physiology at the University of Rostock, published a short paper about some structural relationships in the cerebellum and spinal cord [77]. In the first part of this paper, Bergmann confirmed previous descriptions of conical cells surrounding the central canal of the spinal cord of frog; processes of these cells entered into the grey matter of the spinal cord and were interconnected with each other (Figure 8A). However, he disagreed with the idea that cell processes were linked to elements of connective tissue. In the second part of the paper, Bergmann described the cellular structure of cerebellum of a newborn kitten, the preparation was stained with chromic acid. Between the grey matter and *pia mater*, he observed a great number of very fine, branched, parallel, and radially arranged fibres:

> The isolated fibres showed short (probably broken) branches starting at acute angles. These have partially the direction toward the periphery, but also partly into the interior of the organ. The latter circumstance may contradict the assumption that the fibrils discussed belong to the branching of the ganglia bodies, whereas there are other reasons as well. (Especially in the case of the kitten, where these fibres are so clear, the processes are hardly to be found directly on the ganglion bodies.) On the other hand, it has become probable for these branches, which are so different in direction, that the fibres in question form a net in grey matter. On an isolated fibre, which protrudes by 0.004‴ [85 μm], is nicely visible ending embedded in the clear substance, the fibre here transients into some finer fibrils. The picture recalls (only noticeably gentler) the behaviour of the radial fibres of the retina, where they approach the *membrana limitans* [77].

Bergmann was the first to describe these fibres of specialized cerebellar astrocytes whose bodies are located in the layer of Purkyně neurons, with their processes running throughout the molecular layer, all the way up to the *pia mater*. These cells are known today as Bergmann glia.

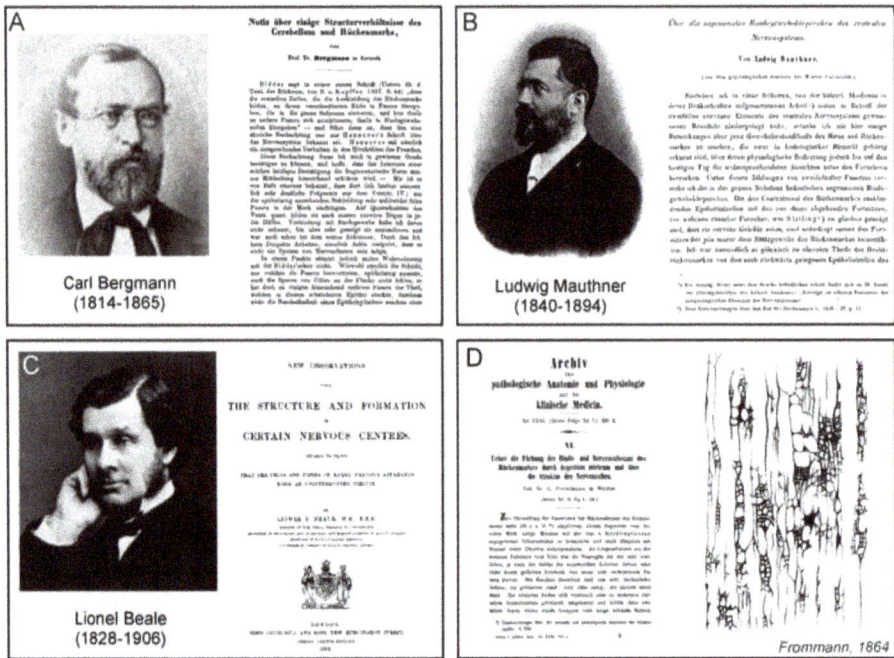

Figure 8. First glioanatomists and their contributions. (**A**) Carl Bergmann and the excerpt of his paper [77] describing the anatomy of the cerebellum, including radial glia (Bergmann glial cells). (**B**) Ludwig Mauthner and his paper on the connective tissue of the brain [78]. (**C**) Lionel Beale and his book: *New observations upon the structure and formation of certain nervous centres* [79]. (**D**) The paper of Carl Frommann [80] and his images of stained neuroglia from the surface of the spinal cord longitudinal cut.

3.3. Ludwig Mauthner

Ludwig Mauthner (1840–1894) who was born in Prague and was professor at Innsbruck University, and subsequently held a chair in ophthalmology in Vienna, described, in 1861, the cellular elements of the connective tissue of the brain and the spinal cord [78] in fishes (Figure 8B). Around the central canal of the spinal cord, he found epithelial cells with large processes (ependymoglial cells) which, without contact with other cell formations, extended to the periphery of the spinal cord and disappeared into the fibres of the spinal meninges. Mauthner observed that connective tissue cells were about 10 times smaller than the ganglion cells (as neurones ware called in those time). Connective tissue cells appeared in clusters in the ventral horns of the spinal cord, and formed a network consisting of their fibre-like processes. Similar cells were also observed in the cerebellar nuclei. Mauthner concluded that connective cells in the grey matter represented the basic elements of connective tissue; furthermore, he considered them as neural cells and not as the particles of connective tissue. He also assumed that the formations, which were previously considered to be connective tissue cells, were in fact larger nuclei of cells whose cytoplasm was so transparent it seemed that that an empty space surrounded the cell nucleus.

3.4. Lionel Beale

Physician and microscopist Lionel Smith Beale (1828–1906) was a professor at King's College in London; he was also a President of the Royal Microscopical Society (Figure 8C). He studied in detail the structure of the nerve tissue, and wrote numerous publications in which he dealt with the development, internal structures, and interconnections of neurons. Beale had an opinion that connective tissue and connective tissue corpuscles are produced from the very same masses of germinal matter as those from which nerve cells and nerve fibres were developed, and that they are the remains of nerve cells, nerve fibres, and vessels which were in a state of functional activity at an earlier period of life. He was also convinced that true nerve fibres, which convey the nerve current do not lose themselves in the connective tissue or blend with it, nor are they connected with its corpuscles, but they form networks. In addition, a normal nerve fibre can always be distinguished from a fibre of connective tissue. However, Beale also considered the connective tissue of the brain in the following, rather philosophical (and prophetic!) manner:

> It is possible that, for many years to come, some observers will persist in terming everything in which they fail to demonstrate distinct structure, connective tissue, and all nuclei which are not seen in their specimens to be in connexion with positive vessels, positive nerve-fibres, or other well-defined tissues besides fibrous tissues, connective-tissue corpuscles; but there is little doubt that when the changes occurring during the development of special tissues shall have been patiently worked out by the use of high powers and better means of preparation, opinions on the connective-tissue question will be completely changed. The idea of the necessity for a supporting tissue or framework will be given up, and many structures now included in "connective tissue" will be isolated, just as new chemical substances year after year are being discovered in the indefinite "extractive matters". ([79]; p. 25)

3.5. Carl Frommann

Carl Friedrich Wilhelm Frommann (1831–1892) was a German physician; in 1870 he habilitated at the University of Heidelberg and became a private lecturer for histology; in 1872 he moved to the University of Jena, where he was, in 1875, appointed as professor. In 1864 (being in Weimar as an ordinary doctor) he published a paper summarizing the results of staining of the spinal cord with silver nitrate [80]. In the longitudinal sections of the white matter of cow spinal cord, the connective tissue, which, as previously was proposed by Virchow, Frommann called "neuroglia", appeared to be a very fine dark-brown network or mesh of interconnected fibres (Figure 8D). The elements of this web were quite variable, the larger were round, oval or square, the smaller one were usually round, and were either isolated or grouped; sometimes they formed long narrow rows. The fibre network was arranged in parallel with the nerve fibres. Cells appeared to be uniformly brown, or with a lighter core, even without sharp contours; sometimes it seemed that the nucleus was a bit darker than the protoplasm. The cells were, by means of their processes, connected to the fibre network, and were also interconnected. On the cross-section of the frozen spinal cord, which was thawed in the silver solution, the neuroglial web was not usually visible, and the shape of its elements resembled a very fine granular mass. Similar findings Frommann were also obtained in the human spinal cord.

Concerning the connective tissue fibres, Frommann believed "that all fibres originate from the cell processes and that they are hollow, and therefore, all white matter connective tissue consists of a continuous network of channels of varying size, which form cellular collectors and centres by numerous connections" ([80]; p. 46). In general, however, his papers and books clearly demonstrate that at his time, there was no clear definition of terms such as "glia", "glia mass" (for which he used *Leim-masse*) and "connective tissue", as evidenced by some of his statements. For instance, Frommann claimed that glial fibres (*Glifasern*) are found inside of the glial mass, or that "it is characteristic of connective tissue cells, unlike neurones, that they are interconnected with their processes to the fibre glial networks..." ([81]; p. 9).

3.6. Otto Friedrich Karl Deiters

German neuroanatomist Otto Friedrich Karl Deiters (1834–1863) spent most of his short professional career in Bonn. Deiters's most famous work was his treatise on the structure of the nervous system, which substantially advanced studies of the cellular structure of the nerve tissue [82].

This book was published two years after Deiter's untimely death (he perished at 29-year-old from typhoid), by his colleague Max Schultze, who, on the basis of several Deiter's illustrations and notes, attempted to organize the results of his histological research as logically as possible. This book contains 13 chapters, and chapter 3 is dedicated to the brain connective tissue (*Bindesubstanz*). Similarly to his contemporaries, who were convinced of the existence of connective tissue in the brain and the spinal cord, Deiters sought to find its characteristic features in order to distinguish them from neurones. He postulated that the connective tissue in the central nervous system (CNS) differed from that in other organs:

> One is accustomed to discuss only the distinction between connective tissue and nervous tissues in the central organs, or to call anything that is not nervous, briefly connective tissue. For the time being it would be more correct, as some wish, to separate nervous elementary parts from those which are not connected with the nervous system. The further distinction is certainly for the moment indifferent. That the non-nervous tissue of the central organs does not readily have the character of ordinary connective tissue is plausible, and here, too, certain conditions are certainly not justified in any way. If, therefore, many people oppose the designation of such parts as connective tissue, this is probably nothing more than that the concept of connective tissue is far from exhausted, and may perhaps reveal unexpected new sides. ([82]; p. 35)

Deiters did not use the term "neuroglia", although he was well acquainted with Virchow's concepts. Deiters provided detailed descriptions of all elements of the nervous connective tissue. The basic structure of this tissue was spongy mass (*schwammige Masse*) or porous mass (*poröse Grundmasse*), containing several types of fibres. These were either connective tissue fibres (*Bindegewebsfibrillen, elastischen Fasern*) or intercellular support fibres (*interzelluläre Stützfasern*) which Deteirs suggest to put:

> ...aside the Mullerian fibres of the retina, and thus to establish another analogy between this tissue and those of the central nervous system... Thus, it may well be assumed that such intercellular support fibres may form an essential link in the whole tissue arrangement... It can generally be established as a law that such a streaky arrangement of the connective tissue mass goes hand in hand with a regular linear arrangement also of the nervous parts; such represents the retina, such in the cerebellum, in the Ammon's horn (hippocampus), etc. ([82]; p. 43)

Deiters also described and discussed the presence of the formations called "free nuclei" which could be in fact some transition forms of cells without detectable cytoplasm and processes. He also described in the connective tissue cellular elements which he named cells of the connective tissue (*Bindesubstanzzelle*):

> Close to the glossy nucleus, which contains no nucleoli, we can see a mass of outgoing fibre tracts, which from the beginning have a firm though delicate appearance, a very sharp, smooth contour, a considerable shine, and which radiate to all sides. These are easily movable, twisting on isolated cells many times, and are not fragile. They divide very soon and then ramify in the most varied way under always forked splitting. I do not think that anyone who sees such an isolated element, will want to think of artifacts, accidental coagulation. ([82]; p. 46)

Deiters observed these cells in both white and grey matter, in the *substantia gelatinosa* of the spinal cord, and in the *medulla oblongata* (Figure 9). Unfortunately, as stated almost 10 years later by Franz Boll (see further in text) "in general it is to be noted that the excellent disputes of Deiters, as well as his positive discovery of the true form of these connective-tissue cells, have been neglected by almost all his successors in an almost irresponsible manner."

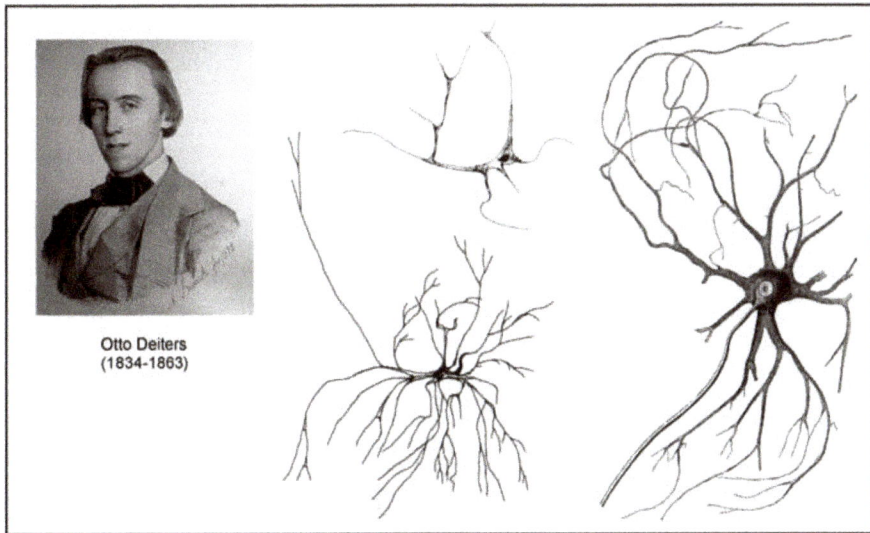

Figure 9. Otto Deiters and his drawings of connective tissue cells (seemingly astrocyte, middle top—from the white matter, middle bottom—from the hypoglossal nucleus grey matter) and (at the right) neurone [82].

3.7. Leopold Besser

German physician Leopold Besser (1820–1906) worked as a provisional intern in the mental illness clinic in Siegburg, Germany. In 1866 he published a paper, which had a great impact on the research of neuroglia; this paper described the development of nerve tissue in the neonate brain with particular emphasis on the role of neuroglia [83]. He demonstrated the emergence of neuroglial cells not only in grey matter but also in the vicinity of capillaries (Figure 10A) and was convinced of its importance during nerve tissue development. Besser particularly noted:

> This mass of connective tissue of central organs, which Rokytanský called "connective tissue of ependymal formation" (*Bindegewebe der Ependym formation*) and Virchow in 1846 suggested to name as "neuroglia", Kölliker referred to as "connective substance forming networks", or "the reticulum" (*netzförmige Bindesubstanz, Reticulum*), whose "spongy part" (*Schwammigen Theil*) were considered by Deiters to be "intercellular substance" (*Intercellularsubstanz*), and Hensen named its multi-nuclear elements "parenchymal cells" (*Parenchymzellen*), has in the brain of newborns so essential meaning and its formative character has a determined dimension and form that I have to name it as "neuroglia of newborns" (*Neuroglia des Neugebornen*) because it has properties that the adult reticulum does not have in its normal condition. ([83]; p.309)

Although Rokytanský and Virchow suggested differences between the neuroglia found in nervous tissue vs connective tissue in the rest of the body (see [84]), the question of connective tissue containing fibres and loose nuclei on the one hand, and neuroglia on the other hand, still remained under debate. Besser adopted Virchow's concept and used term "neuroglia" to emphasize its different properties from the connective tissue of other organs and systems. In particular, he wrote:

> The name neuroglia—*Nervenkitt*—chosen by Virchow could be discussed with a bit of a criticism because this matter is far from being putty, clinging or sticking to cover the nerve elements. It is also not the most important supportive structure because much more closely

arranged vessels are more important for the shape and support of nervous parts. But this matter has such specific features and is so different from all other types of connective tissue formations that it is quite justified to stick to a special name. ([83]; p. 310)

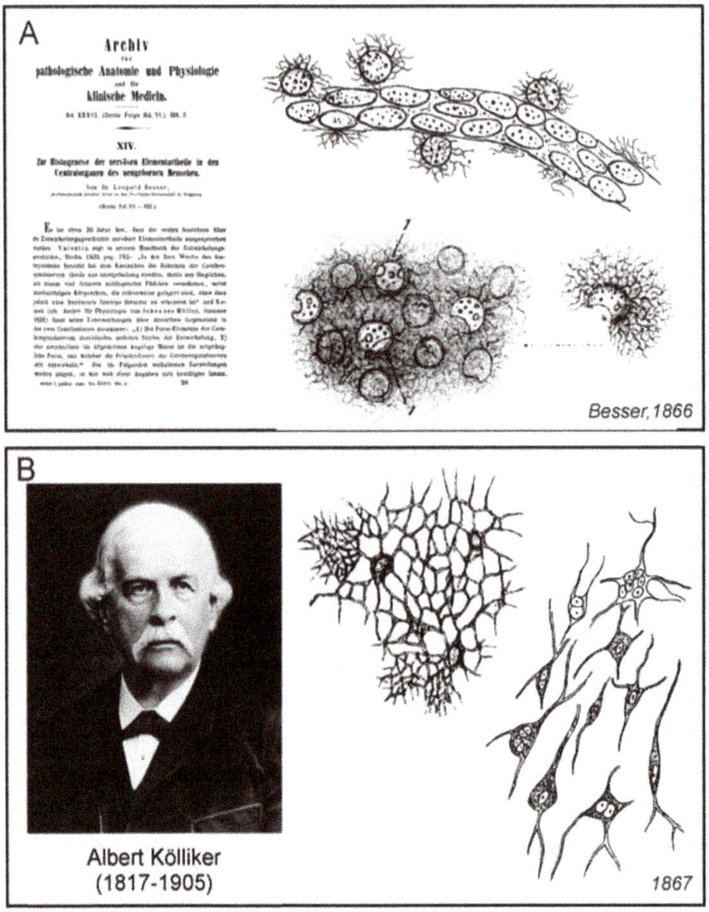

Figure 10. (**A**): Images of connective tissue cells made by Leopold Besser, and the title page of his paper [83]. Top: vascular neoplasms in the brain of the newborn showing the glial formations located on the blood vessels. Bottom: formations on the cut of the neonatal cortex (**left**), including normal and damaged "glial nuclei" (1) during the cutting process; enlarged "glial nucleus" (**right**). (**B**): Images of connective tissue made by Albert Kölliker [85]. Middle: part of the connective tissue reticulum from the dorsal columns of the spinal cord, in two places the finest mesh forming reticulum is shown. Right: connective tissue cells in the grey matter of the human brain.

According to Besser, glial mass contained corpuscles that could be easily observed around evolving blood capillaries. According to him, the glial matter itself consisted of two separate structures, which were, however in a mutual "genetic" relationship. Besser named them as "*Glia-Kern*" (glial nuclei) and "*Glia-Reisernetz*" (glial finely branched nets). Beser's term "net" did not describe networks formed by the glial cell processes, as we know today, but the glial nets attached to "glial cores" and from them, growing fibrous felt. According to him, neuroglial origin, development, transformation, and interrelationship formed the embryology of the nervous basic parts. "Glial nuclei" (which today's we recognise as glial cell bodies) were formed by dividing, and before reaching the size of red blood cells, they remained homogeneous. Shortly thereafter, however, with their growth, a fine granulation emerged on their surface from which developed protuberances and branched processes forming networks. The shape of the delicately branched processes seemed to Besser be round, like the branching of the small twigs of our trees. He was convinced that after death, these branches changed so much that we could not observe them anymore. These networks, however, in the course of further development, according to Besser, separated and gave rise to other structures.

Besser was of the opinion that all nerve elements of the human CNS developed from the part of neuroglia that had morphogenetic properties. According to him, the nuclei of the neurones were transformed glial nuclei, the neuronal bodies were formed from glial branched networks, and the neuronal processes were formed from glial processes. Nerve fibres developed from long branches of proliferating glial nets, and axons were formed by the conversion of fine fibres of branched nets. Besser also described the involvement of glial cells in the capillary development in the cerebellar cortex of newborns. As he noted, thousands of these glial structures touched each other in parallel layers that were stacked together on the capillaries and on the smallest blood vessels. The significance of Besser is that, besides the conviction that the neuroglia in the nervous tissue and the connective tissue were different, he also suggested their importance in the development of the CNS, and for the first time, displayed star-shaped neuroglial cells, probably astrocytes, attached on blood vessels.

3.8. Albert Kölliker

Albert Kölliker (1817–1905), a professor at University of Würzburg, in 1867 published the fifth edition of his extensive manual on the human microscopic anatomy [85]. This handbook, as well as its previous editions, contained a detailed summary of contemporary knowledge about the structure of nerve tissue. Besides the detailed description of the nervous elements of the brain and spinal cord tissue, that is, nerve fibres and nerve cells, Kölliker also dedicated a relatively large section of this handbook to the connective tissue (sometimes he referred to it as the supporting tissue—*Stützsubstanz*). In the spinal cord he described the connective substance as following:

> ...here, apart from the *pia mater* and its processes in the anterior cleft and the adventitia of larger vessels, there is no ordinary fibrillar connective tissue, but only a simple binding substance, consisting entirely of nets of star-shaped connective tissue cells (connective tissue bodies sap cells—*Bindegewebskörperchen Saftzellen*) or of scaffolds of coreless fibres and trabeculae resulting from the cell networks, as described in the general parts (§ 23) as part of the cytogenetic binding substance. These nets and scaffolds, which I denote by the name of the net-like binding substance (*netzförmigen Bindesubstanz*), where they occur singularly as the supporting substance of other tissue elements, are found in the spinal cord in both substances in such a development that they form a very significant part of the whole mass of the organ. In other words, they form a delicate skeleton running through the whole white and grey substance, which I shall call the reticulum of the central nervous system (*Reticulum des zentralen Nervensystemes*), which contains in its numerous gaps the cells and nerve tubes and carries the blood vessels as well. ([85]; p. 266)

Kölliker believed that fine-grained matter containing numerous nuclei and observed by a number of authors in nerve connective tissue, was an artefact. Under much larger (up to 300 times) magnification, he observed that it consisted of connective tissue cells forming a network of structures. Perhaps under the influence of Deitres, who described and visualized connective tissue cells in some areas of the brain and spinal cord, Kölliker called one type of cells, which in earlier issues he named as "cells in the central grey cores of the human spinal cord", connective tissue cells (Figure 10B). He also emphasized the role of the mentioned "reticulum" during pathological states, which, according to him, increased the proportion of interstitial matter that became fibrous.

3.9. Theodor Meynert

Austrian neuroanatomist and psychiatrist Theodor Hermann Meynert (1833–1892) worked together with Karel Rokytanský in Vienna. He studies the cortical structures of the brain cortex, as well as the interconnections of certain regions of the brain, through the neural pathways. Meynert also developed new cell markers and used thin serial slices stained with carmine or gold for quantitative measurements of neurones and investigation of the brain tissue structure. A comprehensive summary of his research was published in Stricker's *Manual of histology* [86]. Concerning connective tissue, Meynert referred to it as to a basement-substance (*Grundgewebe*). Similarly to Besser, he pointed to the inconsistent terminology of his contemporaries, noting:

> This basement-substance is called by Rokytanský ependymal formation (*Ependymformation*), by Virchow, neuroglia, by Kölliker, connective tissue (*Bindesubstanz*), by Deiters, spongy tissue (*schwammige Substanz*), by Henle and R. Wagner, fused ganglion-cell substance (*zusammengeflossene Ganglienzellenmasse*). Occurring in the olfactory lobe and ammon's horn, it receives from Clarke the designation of gelatinous (*gelatinöse*), from Kupfer that of molecular substance (*moleculare Substanz*). (Cited from the English translation [87]; p. 660)

Unlike Deiters, who recognized only loose nuclei in the connective tissue of the cerebral cortex, Meynert insisted "upon the indisputable fact of the occurrence here of the star-shaped cells, with very little protoplasm, and a great number of the finest possible processes" (Figure 11A). Moreover, he also noticed, that "these cells swell up under certain pathological conditions and assume grotesque forms". In addition, Meynert was the first to declare that the basic substance of the grey matter of the cerebral cortex contains spongioform structures made up from the processes of cells other than neurones.

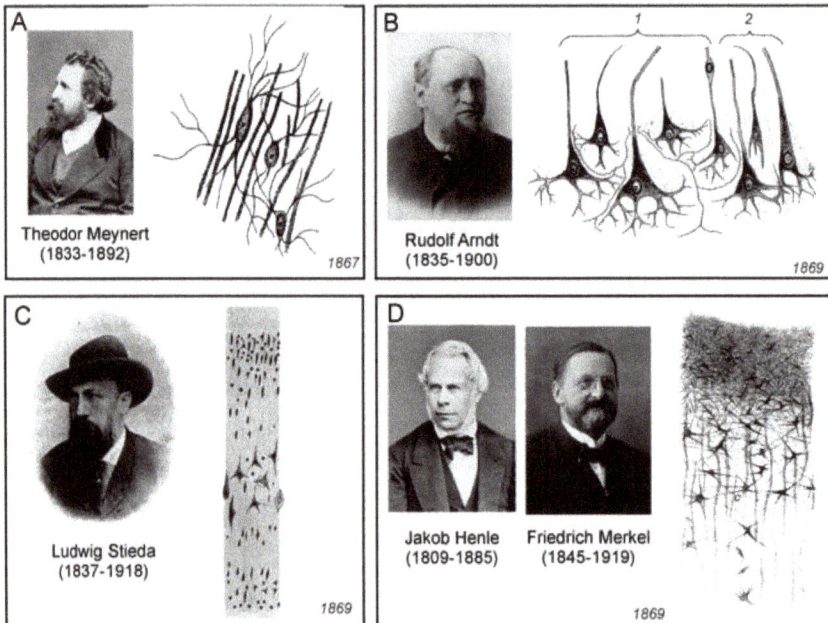

Figure 11. (**A**) Images of connective tissue cells located between the nerve fibres, drawn by Theodor Meynert [88], (**B**) Brain cortex neurones embedded in the fine-grained connective tissue, by Rudolf Arndt [89]. (**C**) Brain cortex neurones embedded in the fine-grained connective tissue, by Ludwig Stieda [90]. (**D**) A surface layer containing fibres of white matter with visible axons and multipolar connective tissue cells, by Jakob Henle and Friedrich Merkel [91].

3.10. Rudolf Arndt

German psychiatrist Rudolf Gottfried Arndt (1835–1900) studied the morphology of the brain tissue of large vertebrates and humans. He summarised his findings in a series of three papers [89,92,93]. In the first paper he described five to six layers in the cortex. In the first layer, there were intertwined parallel fibres, some of which were nervous, another belonging to the fibres of the connective tissue. The second layer, according to Arndt, consisted mainly of neuroglia, which was grainy-fibrous (*körnig-faserigen*) or spongy (*schwammigen*), and which was, according to him, differentiated protoplasm, neither nervous nor connective. In the neuroglia were nuclei and loose thin and thick fibres; some ended with the loops described by Gabriel Valentin. The third layer contained isolated nuclei and nerve cells with a nucleus, all immersed in neuroglia; their shape was either round, elliptical or triangular (Figure 11B). From the latter emerged horizontally and inwardly oriented processes, one thick process pointing to the surface of the cortex, which he considered to be an axon. Whether these processes served to interconnect cells, passed into nerve fibres, or dissolved in neuroglial tissue, Arndt was not certain.

The second paper mostly contained polemic about the works of Besser, Meynert, and others that had been published in the meantime. It also included consideration of the purpose of the corpuscles of the connective matter, which he believed to be a remnant of the development of nervous mass in the foetus. Arndt also accepted Besser's terminology (*Gliakern*, *Gliareiser*) and an idea on the development of nerve tissue elements; he assumed that from these two glial components developed three brain elements: blood vessels, neurons, and nerve fibres. In the third, shorter paper, Arndt confirmed his findings from the previous publications and discussed the functional unity of ganglion bodies and their processes, together with the surrounding granular-fibrous substance:

> Concerning the nerve cell of the central organ of an adult, I believe that according to the foregoing description the ganglion body together with its central processes and the part of granular-fibrous substance, which is genetically related to it, must be understood. Whether we will ever get to know them intact is questionable, indeed highly unlikely. It may not even exist on its own, although this is still quite conceivable, but it is probably so completely merged with adjacent parts, so intimately interwoven with them by their finest threads, that together they are only one, their creation form absolutely indivisible mass. But if this is the case, then we must logically consider the interganglionary granular-fibrous substance, the terminal fibre-network, as it turns out in the adult, to be a coalesced protoplasm modified for definite purposes, as an irritable tissue, the actual carrier of all is central operations. ([89]; p. 329)

Arndt was thus one of the first researchers who hypothesized that the nerve cells and the surrounding granular-fibrous substance are developmentally related and form a single functional unit.

3.11. Ludwig Stieda

The Baltic German Ludwig Stieda (1837–1918) was professor of anatomy in Dorpat and Königsberg. He studied the structure of the neural tissue, predominantly in animals. Stieda published many works and he summarised his findings in two extensive publications [90,94]. According to him, the CNS consisted of nerve cell bodies, nerve fibres, connective tissue, blood vessels, and epithelium. There was no general agreement on the composition and terminology of brain connective tissue or neuroglia, and Stieda absolutely correctly pointed out that there was no agreement on the terminology on the nerve cells as well. As he noted, these formations were named by various names, such as ganglion bodies (*Ganglienkörper*), nerve bodies (*Nervenkörper*), ganglion balls (*Ganglienkugeln*), occupancy balls (*Belegungskugeln*), spinal bodies (*Spinalkörpen*), ganglion cells (*Ganglienzellen*), or nerve cells (*Nervenzellen*). Concerning the connective tissue, Stieda did not distinguished the true fibrous connective tissue in meninges from what was called connective tissue in the grey matter, where it, according to him, had a fine-grained appearance and contained nuclei of the basement substance

(Figure 11C). He also did not consider the basement substance to be nervous, but to be a special category of supportive or connective tissue of the nervous system. Moreover, Stieda could not confirm the presence of the grained basement substance as a network of cells interconnected with anastomoses, as was described by other researchers.

3.12. Jakob Henle and Friedrich Merkel

Four years after the publication of Deiters' monograph on the structure of nerve tissue, Jakob Henle (1809–1885), who was professor of anatomy in Gottingen, and his son-in-law Friedrich Merkel (1845–1919), published a paper dealing with the connective tissue of the CNS [91]. Although this work contained a detailed historical overview of connective tissue research, the authors did not even mention Deiters' findings. The goal of the Henle and Merkel study was to determine whether fine-grained or reticular tissue had the properties of nervous substance, or was only a supportive, connective, essentially cementing substance. For the study of tissues from various regions of the brain and spinal cord of several mammals and humans, they used a variety of histological methods, from carmine staining followed by fixation with chromic acid, to boiling, using differently diluted acids and bases, or alcohol hardening. Henle and Merkel were convinced that the connective tissue consisted of a so-called molecular mass and the elements of the connective tissue (Figure 11D), that is, fibres, cells, and grains or nuclei:

> These connective tissue cells could, according to the analogy of the nerve cells, be called bipolar, as opposed to the multipolar connective tissue cells, from which three or more fibres emanate. From multipolar cells merging with their processes, the above-mentioned reticular connective tissue develops; similar cells, growing in several threads, but usually preferentially in two opposite directions, owe their origin to the confused fibres of the innermost layer of the *pia mater*. The fibres can be traced over long distances and, although they branch out, do not appear to anastomose regularly; they are more of a felt than a net. The cells are observed in this layer only with difficulty, isolated, hardly without the help of Carmin absorption. More clearly, because more scattered and less obscured by fibres, they are found on the border of the *pia mater* and the cortical layer, and in the latter itself. ([91]; p. 57)

Although Henle and Merkel referred to the term "neuroglia" only in relation to Virchow's results and did not use it at all in the description of their own results, they suggested that the fibrous networks described by them could be considered as so-called neuroglia or Kölliker's reticulum.

3.13. Camillo Golgi: Early Studies on Neuroglia

In the early 1870s, Camillo Golgi (1843–1926), while a 27-year-old employee of the University Clinic in Pavia, published his first brief communication on the connective tissue of the brain [95], which a year later, was translated to German [96]. Golgi studied the connective cells of the cortical regions of the human brain, using staining primarily with osmic acid. He observed circular, oval, or star-shaped cells with a large nucleus, from which several very long processes emerged in different directions. He even described anastomoses between the processes of neighbouring cells.

During the same year, Golgi began to publish an expanded three-part version of the previous communication with a detailed description of his findings [97–99]. In the three chapters, it contained a detailed description of the results obtained in the brain, cerebellum, and spinal cord. Golgi did not use the terms "neuroglia" or "glial cells" in these publications. The introductory historical overviews of the findings at the beginning of each chapter are very instructive. Golgi observed the cells described in the previous publication, in various regions of the brain and spinal cord (Figure 12A), and he summarized the results as following:

In summary, with the preparations in osmic acid I have demonstrated:

1. That a very thin superficial layer of the brain cortex is exclusively constituted, except of some bundles of nerve fibres coming from the marrow, from the connective cells provided with a large number of thin, long and for the most part rigid unbranched extensions.
2. That identical cells are scattered in considerable numbers in all the layers of the cortex, forming a continuous support tissue.
3. That many extensions of the connective cells are inserted in the contour of the vessels, and that there is neither the space nor the perivascular lymphatic network... ([97]; p. 344).

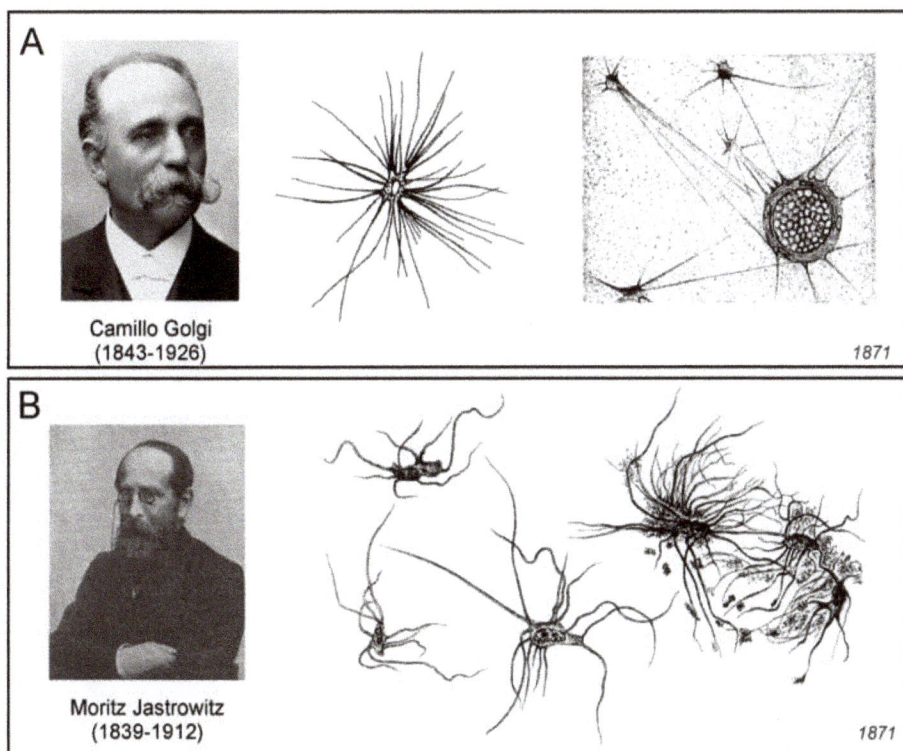

Figure 12. (**A**) Images of connective tissue cell made by Camillo Golgi [96]. Middle: spinal cord cell with long longitudinal processes in deeper layers of white matter. Right: cross section of the capillary showing the connective cell processes closely adjacent to its contour. (**B**) Images of glial cells by Moritz Jastrowitz [100]. Isolated spider-like glial cells from the vicinity of the human brain ventricle ependym.

In addition, Golgi employed several modifications of osmic acid staining, and also described the pericellular lymphatic space. By using different staining methods on very thin slices of the cortex, he was able to observe a large number of "elegant" connective cells with 10–30 very thin and long processes, very rarely branched. These branches separated at a short distance from the cell boundary, and he never observed more than two or three secondary branches, which were also very long and unbranched. Golgi also commented on the contents of the neuropil, which, according to today's findings, is part of the grey matter that fills the space between the perikarya and the vessels, where the nerve fibres, the synapses, and the glial cell processes are located, and which appear to be amorphous under the light microscope. According to Golgi, the so-called fine-grained, possibly mesh-like, spongy or dotted molecular, amorphous or gelatinous matter originated either as a result of changes in the dead body, due to reagents or tissue processing. These effects led to the breakdown of the fibrillary substance, which, in his opinion, was likely to occur not only in the processes of connective tissue cells but also in the finest protoplasmic processes of neurons. It should be noted, however, that the above mentioned findings by Golgi were made before his discovery of the biochemical method of colouring the nerve tissue preparation with potassium dichromate and silver nitrate in 1873 [101], now known as the Golgi method or *reazione nera*.

3.14. Moritz Jastrowitz

German neurologist and psychiatrist Moritz Jastrowitz (1839–1912), working as an assistant at the clinic for mentally and neurotic patients in Berlin, published in 1870–1871 a two-part paper on the structure of nerve tissue during encephalitis and myelitis in children in the early postnatal period. In the first part, he described in detail the anamnesis of patients from whom he took brain tissue, and described the macroscopic tissue changes [102]. In the second part, he examined in detail the individual elements of nerve tissue and neuroglia, which, according to him, also played an important role during encephalitis [100].

Jastrowitz in his paper, clearly distinguished neuroglia and connective tissue, which consisted of spongious structures, fibres, granular (molecular) substances, and also lymphoid cells. The molecular substance, according to Jastrowitz, was associated with the myelination of nerve fibres, since during the development of nerve tissue, it was gradually lost. Therefore, he considered it not only as a supportive matter, but also as an embryonic tissue that was responsible for axonal isolation. Jastrowitz also believed that molecular substance played a more important role than connective matter, and therefore recommended not to include it among the other elements of connective tissue under the common name of "neuroglia".

The most prominent non-nerve cells, which, according to Jastrowitz, no one had mentioned before, he found in the ependyma (Figure 12B). As he noticed, "If Virchow's view, initially expressed by the ependymal layer of the fourth ventricle, that in it the neuroglia comes to light in its purity, also applies to this location, then these would be true prototypes of glial cells". Jastrowitz described these cells as following:

> They generally surpass those of the third layer in volume, not inconsiderably, especially with respect to the diameter of the base, and differ in shape and size from one another. Most are spindle-shaped, but also rounded and angular as well as cylindrical shapes are encountered; they are often narrowed at one end and may be quite pointed at this, sometimes at both ends. Their length is usually double and even three times their width, on average for the smaller ones 0.007–0.01: 0.004–5 [length 15–21 μm, width 8.7–10.6 μm] and for the large ones 0.012–0.017: 0.005–7 [length 25–36 μm, width 10.6–14.8 μm]. The protoplasm is a little more granulated and less transparent, usually it contains very large oval nucleus with several granules larger than nucleoli is often located at one end of the cell, and particularly is intensively coloured, therefore one easily overlooks its contents in the tissue. An immense amount of delicate, bright processes extend from them widely in all directions, often across each other, and finally disappear in the molecular mass, whose particles usually adhere to them in isolation. Despite the long distances they travel, divisions are exceptional, but often kinks and bends. They are chiefly those who give the whole structure a very characteristic appearance, which resembles that of a little spider. ([100]; p. 169)

Jastrowitz, therefore, named these cells as "spider glial cells" (*spinnenähnliche Gliazellen*) or "spider cells" (*Spinnezellen*). Their number increased toward the surface of the brain ventricle so that they finally formed the epithelium of the ependyma. Jastrowitz disagreed with Besser, who believed that the glial elements were made up of separated glial nuclei and glial networks. The glial nuclei observed by Besser, according to Jastrowitz, corresponded in part to embryonic cells, in part to the nuclei of connective tissue cells and neurons, and partially to free nuclei.

3.15. Victor Butzke

Russian psychiatrist Victor Butzke (1845–1904), while collaborating with the German pathologist and histologist Eduard Rindfleisch (see below) at the Pathological-Anatomical Institute in Bonn, published in 1872 a paper dedicated to the fine microscopic structure of nerve cells and glia and their interrelationships [103].

Butzke has extensively described other types of cells than nerve cells. As he stated, "not everything must be considered as a connective substance, or even as a connective tissue, that is not recognized as a ganglion cell or nerve fibre in the central organs of the nervous system" ([103]; p. 590). He questioned the existence of the so-called "free" nuclei, believing that even these were surrounded by protoplasm that often passed into the processes, and he also distinguished glial elements with thin and thicker processes, partially oriented radially, which were found on the surface of the large brain (Figure 13A). Other glial elements were cells with a relatively large nucleus and radially emerging thick processes, which, according to Butzke, were scattered among the well-known real nerve elements of the grey matter of the cerebral cortex, and furthermore, he detached them into a special category, "real connective tissue corpuscles with their thicker and thinner processes" ([103]; p. 591; Figure 13A). In addition, he also expressed a hypothesis on the physiological role of the glial network in the nervous tissue, namely, its role in the formation of new connections between nerve cells:

> The fine-grained fibrous mass is therefore not a simple putty substance (*Kittsubstanz*) for us, which is only intended to adhere the parts together; it is no longer the simple intermediate mass (*Zwischenmasse*) through which the coarser structures pass, but it also contains one enclosed within it highly subtle tissue in the form of a network, which is formed by the end fibrils of the ganglion processes and supported by the processes of the glial corpuscles (*Gliakörperchen*). I now put forward the hypothesis, which has never been formulated sufficiently clearly and sufficiently supported by reasons that the connection between the end branches of the ganglion bodies takes place through this fine irregular network. I have not seen clearly that connection, so I call my view a hypothesis. But if you look right where the finest branches are, and you see a network that starts directly from the final ramifications, what other conclusion could you make?... Nor are we aware of any facts that suggest that not every physiological connection between the elementary centres could be fixed, strengthened, and newly formed: in practice and in learning. But what about the notions of learning, forgetting, practicing, getting used to, etc., if all the connections of the functioning elements were given once and for all in rigid anastomoses, or in the entry and exit of nerve fibres into a ganglion body?... But that is probably no longer so necessary and, in order to come back specifically to the one organ which I subjected to the more detailed examination, I will ask, if not every impression which arrives at the brain through the senses and adheres to it is proof enough that there are suddenly created a hundred new connections that may exist for life? And is not every new thought that comes to us proof enough that out of the old connections that already existed, new ones were formed automatically (that is, without influence from outside), others were strengthened, others disappeared or become weaker? It is, after all, to quote Master Goethe in the end: "the thought factory is a weaver masterpiece, where—one stroke strikes a thousand connections." ([103]; p. 595)

Like Golgi, Butzke also drew attention to the particular funnel-like shape of some of the glial processes that were adjacent to the vessels or the meninges.

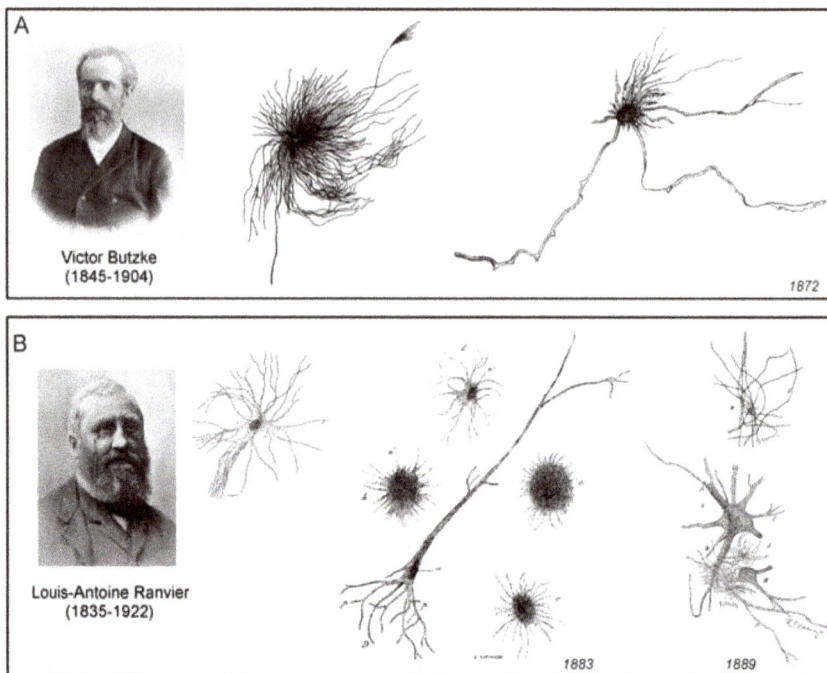

Figure 13. (**A**) Images of glial cell with richly branched processes (middle) and connective tissue cell (right) drawn by Victor Butzke [103]. (**B**) Images of glial cells and neurons drawn by Louis-Antoine Ranvier [104]. Left: neuroglial cell of the lateral cords of the ox spinal cord. Middle: elements of the cortical layer of the cat's brain; a, b, c, and d, four neuroglial cells; n, nerve cell; p its protoplasmic processes, v its axon. Right top: cells and fibres in the spinal cord. Right bottom: two spinal cord neurons (**A,B**) with axons (D) and protoplasmic processes (p), and glial cell (C) between them.

3.16. Louis-Antoine Ranvier

French physician and histologist Louis-Antoine Ranvier (1835–1922), who worked at the Collège de France in Paris, is universally known as a discoverer of the nodes of Ranvier, which are regularly spaced discontinuities of the myelin sheath, occurring at varying intervals along the length of a nerve fibre. It is less known, however, that Ranvier was also interested in the structure of connective tissue. In 1873, he published a brief note on the spinal cord connective elements [105]. Through a golden cannula, he perfused white and grey matter of the spinal cord with osmic acid, and thus in stained longitudinal slices, he visualised homogenous black structures in white matter and marbled black structures in the grey matter. In white matter, he described neural tubes (axons) with myelin sheaths, among which he observed fibrils or bundles of connective tissue fibrils. The small bundles of connective tissue in spinal cord white matter, according to Ranvier, did not produce anastomoses, but at some points four to eight or even more intersected one another. At this crossing, a round or oval flattened nucleus with small nucleoles surrounded by granular mass was often observed. This whole unit Ranvier named as a flattened cell of connective tissue (*cellule plate de tissu conjonctif*). The same structures he also described in detail in grey matter. Consequently, Ranvier noted that the connective tissue of the spinal cord was constituted by bundles of connective fibrils or fibres and flat cells.

Ten years later, Ranvier published an extended paper containing figures, describing his new achievements in neuroglial research [104]. Concerning the term "neuroglia" and the meaning of it, he wrote:

The word neuroglia is detestable and if I use it, it is only because it has passed into the language of histologists. All know that it designates the connective tissue of the nervous centres; but if they agree to adopt it, they do not agree on the organisation of the neuroglia itself, because some believe with Henle and Merkel, that it is formed of elements of the connective tissue ordinary; others, with Gerlach, that it is composed of elastic fibres or analogous to certain elastic fibres, that it consists entirely of branched cells of a special nature of Deiters cells (Boll, Golgi, etc.). Some, finally, think, with Schwalbe, that the cells which are between the nervous elements of the brain, the marrow, and the optic nerve are nothing but the lymphatic cells in migration. I myself have maintained that the marrow neuroglia is composed of fibres of any length, intersecting at certain points, at the levels of which are generally flattened cells. ([104]; p. 177)

Using the method of hardening the nervous tissue of his own, Ranvier was convinced that the neuroglial cells do not have the rudimentary forms attributed to them by Deiters. According to him, their nucleus was well formed, their well-developed cell bodies were membranous, irregularly star-shaped, and showed shape-related accidents that depended to a large extent on the pressures exerted by neighbouring elements (Figure 13B). They had numerous processes which, as Ranvier believed, were nothing but fibres of any length, so distinct in the preparations made by means of the interstitial injections of osmic acid, and which, in these preparations, appeared to be independent of the cells. These fibres which passed through the neuroglial cells did not always follow a rectilinear path; a large number of them described curves or were folded in the shape of a loop.

Ranvier also believed that nerve cells and cells of the neuroglia had a common origin; they both proceeded from the primitive neuroepithelium, and although they may have had absolutely different physiological significances, they retained in their structures certain points that betrayed their common origin. He was also convinced that the granular substance, which various researchers had attached to the neuroglia, did not exist. Ranvier summarized the composition of the nervous tissue as follows:

The grey matter of the brain and that of the spinal cord are thus reduced to the same type. Both are composed of ganglion cells, myelinated nerve fibres, myelin-free nerve fibres, and neuroglia cells, leaving, of course, the blood vessels and their perivascular sheath, which belong to the ordinary connective tissue. ([104]; p. 185)

Concerning the general view on the nerve tissue structure, Ranvier's observations were correct. However, his description of the neuroglial cells as cells through which passed neuroglial fibres, was stepped aside and it significantly influenced neuroglial research in the next decade.

3.17. Eduard Rindfleisch

German pathologist and histologist Eduard Rindfleisch (1836–1908), who attained professorship in Bonn and in Würzburg, recognised the role of nerve connective tissue, which he called *"neuroglia Virchovi"*, especially during pathological processes. In his textbook of pathological histology, the third German edition of which was published in 1873, he dedicated the entire section to neuroglial cells (Figure 14A) [106]. Rindfleisch joined those researchers who discussed the question what known elements of the nervous tissue should be considered as the part of the neuroglia. He was convinced, that

As for the neuroglia of the medullary [white] substance, we may safely affirm that it comprises whatever elements are met with in the white matter, apart from nerve-fibres and blood-vessels; hence all the granules and nuclei in the white substance are neuroglia-cells and nuclei, so the soft fibrous-spongy material into which the nerve fibres are embedded is also neuroglia. Concerning the relation of these parts of neuroglia to each other, a maceration of fresh cerebral substance in 1/10 per cent of super-osmic acid for several days teaches that some of the cells are star-shaped and have numerous, finely branched processes. These cells are arranged at regular intervals and represent a network of connective tissue corpuscles in Virchow's sense. Their finest processes form by numerous anastomoses the mentioned fibrous-spongy material, the actual nervous putty (*Nervenkitt*), so that it can be reasonably not mentioned as a special basic substance of this connective tissue. ([106]; p. 570)

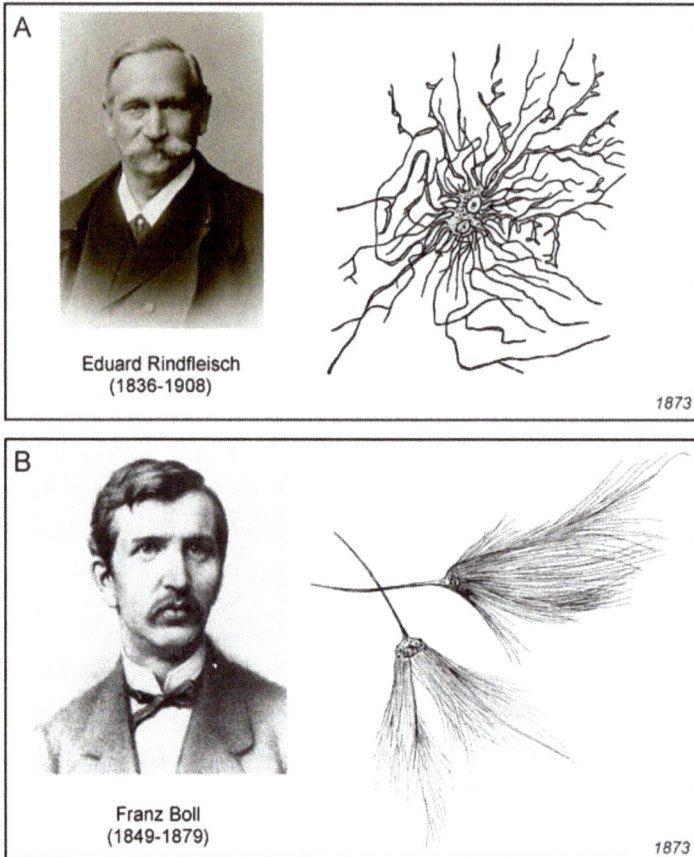

Figure 14. Images of neuroglia drawn by Eduard Rindfleish (**A**, [106]) and Franz Boll (**B** [107]).

Rindfleisch, according to his preface to the first edition, "offered his new textbook to the student-youth of Germany"; therefore, his view on the neuroglia as a connective tissue containing star-shaped cells forming a network, had a big impact on a new generation of researchers dealing with the structure of the nervous tissue.

3.18. Franz Boll

German physiologist and histologist Franz Christian Boll (1849–1879) who held professorships in Genoa and Rome, is universally known as the discoverer of rhodopsin. In 1873, however, he published an extensive work describing in detail the structure and development of the brain and spinal cord [107]. The publication also contained results of his extensive examination of the nervous connective tissue.

Boll was convinced that the connective tissue, besides connective tissue fibres, also contained cells (Figure 14B) which were, as he pointed out, for the first time isolated, described, and illustrated in "their true form" by Deiters. However, he added, the Deiters name and the description of these cells did not appear in the writings of Henle and Merkel, Stieda, Gerlach, Kolliker, and Frommann, but the cells were described and illustrated by Jastrowitz, Golgi, and, to a certain extent, by Rindfleisch. For this reason, Boll was likely to continue to name these cells as the "Deiters' cells" (*Deiters'schen Zellen*); this term was used for some time by other researchers simultaneously with the name "glial cells". Today, however, by the term "Deiters' cells", or phalangeal cells, are named supporting cells of the Corti organ in the inner ear, which are not related to glial cells at all. Describing the glial cells in the ox spinal cord Boll noted that:

> These cells are so peculiar that I cannot give them any analogue from the series of other known histological elements. Characteristic of these is the lack of a body or cell body. At first sight, some seem to imagine only a confused convolution of fine fibres, in the centre of which there is a nucleus-like structure. If, however, in most of these cells the actual cell-body is an absolutely vanishing minimum, the processes of the latter are all the more pronounced. Each of these cells emits a very large number of very long hair-thin processes, comparable to the fineness of connective tissue fibrils, of straight or only slightly tortuous course. The length of these fibrous processes is often very considerable; not infrequently, individuals are drawn through the entire field of view of the microscope and even further. Whether these fine processes ramify, I certainly do not want to decide; I have never received unambiguous pictures of such a place. On the other hand, on the basis of my experience, I do not necessarily dare deny ramification: in any case, such is one of the rarer occurrences. The direction of the processes is subject to countless differences: there are cells from which these fibres emanate multipolarly in all directions; besides, there are other cells where two dense fibrous bundles are detached on two opposing poles, and finally a third main form is not uncommon, where the whole mass of the fibrous processes is directed to one side, while from the opposite pole of the cell depart only very insignificant fibres, so that these cells offer a surprising similarity with a fine hair brush (brush cells—*Pinselzellen*). ([107]; p. 7)

Thus Boll, in addition to the detailed description of glial cell as cells with the long hair-thin processes, also drew attention to the variety of shapes of the glial cells, and attempted to classify them. Boll further analysed the structure of the perivascular space. The presence of terminals of glial processes on the capillary walls before Boll, had already been indicated by Besser, Golgi, and Butzke (see above). Boll, however, described that capillaries in the brain and spinal cord of humans, cows, and sheep were surrounded by rows of "brush cells" of various sizes and shapes spreading numerous processes to the capillary walls. In addition, on the basis of the detailed study of the nerve tissue development, Boll was convinced that both glial and nerve cells were histologically distinct elementary parts of the CNS.

3.19. Hans Gierke

German anatomist Hans Paul Bernhard Gierke (1847–1886) attained professorship at the Imperial University of Tokyo and in Breslau (Wrocław). Already in 1882, he published his paper on the elements of the CNS, where he described nerve cells and neuroglia studied predominantly by the carmine method, which he, based on numerous experiments, considered to be the most suitable for tissue staining [108]. According to Gierke, "The skeleton for the nervous elements of the central organ, the network in which they are embedded, is composed of two different substances, the fibrillar connective tissue and Virchow's so-called neuroglia, which is considered to be a subspecies of the reticular connective tissue." [108]. He also included in his paper a detailed description and pictures of several forms of neuroglial cells (Figure 15), and discussed their relationship to nerve cells and fibres. In addition, Gierke was convinced that: "The neuroglia develops from elements of the ectoderm like the nerve cells and like the cells of the epidermis. Even this histogenetic fact speaks for a peculiar position of the neuroglia, even more so its appearance, its behaviour against reagents and the arrangement of the elements." [108].

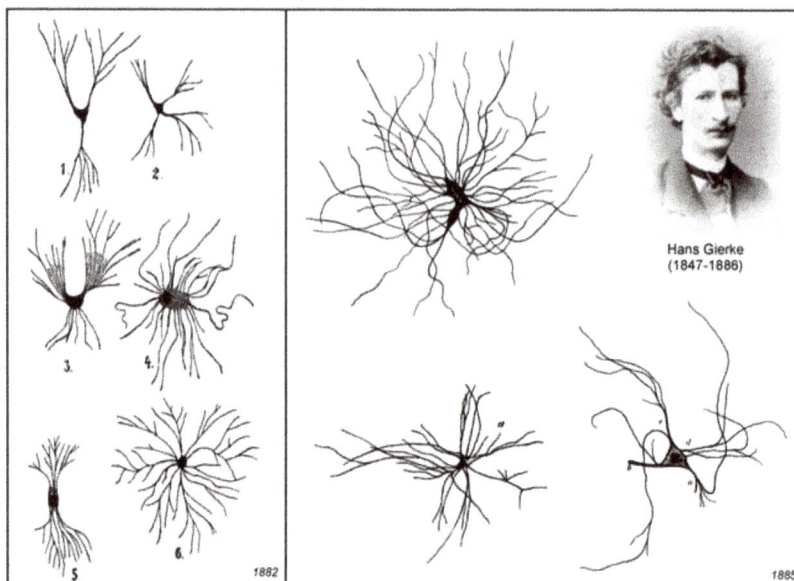

Figure 15. Images of glia drawn by Hans Gierke [108,109]. Left: neuroglial cells from the white matter (1–3) and from the grey matter (4); proliferating neuroglial cell (5,6). Right top: large glial cell from the bottom of the fourth ventricle; bottom left: glial cell from the grey matter of the spinal cord; bottom right: glial cell from the white matter of the spinal cord.

A year later, Gierke published an updated paper devoted to the supportive substance of the nervous system [110]. He described different types of neuroglial cells in the various regions of the brain and spinal cord, and at the same time, he moved forward in questioning what should be considered to be neuroglia:

> The supporting substance consists of unformed and shaped elements, both of which must be grouped under the term Neuroglia. The unformed part, the basic substance (*Grundsubstanz*), has not yet received the due attention it deserves. It is the basis of the grey matter in which everything else is stored and quantitatively occupies about the third part of it... The shaped elements of the supportive substance are cells and their processes. ([110]; p.362)

In two years Gierke published results of the investigation of supportive substance of the CNS in two extensive publications [109,111]. He described in detail many modifications of his carmine staining method, which he still considered to be the best. Gierke made an attempt to clearly define the connective tissue and neuroglia. First of all, he was convinced that free grains observed in the connective tissue by Jastrowitz and Boll did not exist. Concerning the connective tissue, Gierke wrote:

> The nervous elements of the central organs are not directly next to each other, but are separated from each other by a different mass, which can be named with a very indifferent name as a supporting substance (*Stutzsubstanz*) of the central nervous system. It is often called connective tissue (*Bindegewebe*) by the authors, and indeed regarded as "reticular connective tissue" (*retikulären Bindesubstanz*) in terms of its histological significance, and is presented as a subspecies of it in addition to the cytogenous connective substance of the mucous membranes and of many glands and the jelly-tissue ... In any case, it is desirable not to name it that way any longer, but I shall name it in the following to have the shortest possible expression, with the name "neuroglia" (or nerve putty), or glia, introduced by Virchow.

The supporting substance of the central organs consists of two components, the unformed and the shaped substance; both must be grouped together under the name of neuroglia, although of course the term "nerve putty" is less suitable for the cellular elements than for the matrix substance. When we shorten, as is customary, that word, we have in the terms "glial substance" and "glial cells" very convenient names, which I do not find at all like Ranvier in the above-quoted little work "detestable". ([109]; p. 452)

Gierke also tried to find out the general characteristics of the glial cells:

First, what is common to all glial cells? In most cases characteristic of them are the processes. Just as in the central nervous system, no nerve cells without processes occur, so are cells of the support substance without such unthinkable. In order to be able to take part in the formation of the framework for the embedded nervous elements, the glial cells must connect by means of processes with other similar elements. I can also say with the utmost certainty that there are absolutely no glial cells in the central nervous system, which are without processes, and which therefore lie isolated, without connection to the general scaffold. With regard to the number of processes, certain details are not to be specified. Most of the cells have very many, but even with very few occur. Cells with a single process, if they exist at all, are very rare; they might perhaps appear on the surface of the cerebral cortex as an exception. Bipolar cells occur in certain places, especially where long sutures are needed. The cell-body can then grow so much in the formation of the growing processes, that it only makes a small swelling in the middle of them, indeed one finds horn-threads in those places, which have no trace of a cell-body, but detectable in of the imaginary way. . . . Glial cells with three or very few processes proceeding to different sides occur in all parts of the central organ; yet they are much rarer than those with many processes. ([109]; p. 466)

In general, due to the staining methods, which reached its borders, Gierke's investigations did not bring extraordinary new information about the glial cells, if compared to the works of his predecessors. It became evident that the carmine staining has reached its limits, and in the following years, it withdrew its place in favour of the "black reaction" staining invented by Golgi.

4. Recapitulation

The notions of the passive elements of the CNS have emerged in the second half of 18th century, and at the beginning of 19th century. The idea of the brain connective tissue (*Bindegewebs-Substanzen*) was first introduced by Karel Rokytanský, and then it was developed by Rudolf Wirchow into the concept of neuroglia. In the course of the second half of the 19th century, many neuroanatomists dedicated their efforts to study neuroglia; as a result, numerous morphologically distinct cell types have been described. The turn of research toward neuroglia has been precipitated by the development of staining techniques which allowed much more precise morphological analysis of neural cells. This allowed several major types of neuroglia to be distinguished; in addition, the theories of glial roles in the physiology and pathophysiology of the nervous system began to evolve. Detailed descriptions of these studies will be covered in our papers that are to follow.

Author Contributions: All authors participated equally in writing this commentary.

Funding: This research received no external funding.

Conflicts of Interest: The authors declare no conflict of interest.

References

1. Crivellato, E.; Ribatti, D. Soul, mind, brain: Greek philosophy and the birth of neuroscience. *Brain Res. Bull.* **2007**, *71*, 327–336. [CrossRef] [PubMed]
2. Clarke, E. Aristotelian concepts of the form and function of the brain. *Bull. Hist. Med.* **1963**, *37*, 1–14. [PubMed]

3. Gross, C.G. Aristotle on the brain. *Neuroscientist* **1995**, *1*, 245–250. [CrossRef]
4. Codellas, P.S. Alcmaeon of Croton: His life, work, and fragments. *Proc. R. Soc. Med.* **1932**, *25*, 1041–1046. [PubMed]
5. Hippocrates. On the sacred disease. In *The Medical Works of Hippocrates*; Chadwick, J., Mann, W.N.T., Eds.; Blackwells: Oxford, UK, 1950; pp. 179–189.
6. Longrigg, J. *Greek Rational Medicine: Philosophy and Medicine from Alcmaeon to the Alexandrians*; Routledge: New York, NY, USA, 1993.
7. Von Staden, H. *Herophilus: The Art of Medicine in Early Alexandria*; Cambridge University Press: Cambridge, UK, 1989.
8. Wills, A. Herophilus, Erasistratus, and the birth of neuroscience. *Lancet* **1999**, *354*, 1719–1720. [CrossRef]
9. Manzoni, T. The cerebral ventricles, the animal spirits and the dawn of brain localization of function. *Arch. Ital. Biol.* **1998**, *136*, 103–152. [PubMed]
10. Pevsner, J. Leonardo da Vinci's contributions to neuroscience. *Trends Neurosci.* **2002**, *25*, 217–220. [CrossRef]
11. Reisch, G. *Margarita Philosophica*; Johann Schott: Freiburg, Germany, 1503.
12. Fludd, R. *Utriusque Cosmi Majoris Scilicet et Minoris Metaphysica, Physica Atque Technica Historia in duo Volumina Secundum Cosmi Differentiam Divisa. Tomus Primus de Macrososmi Historia in duo Tractatus Divisa*; Oppenhemii, Aere Johan-Theodori de Bry, Typis Hieronymi Galleri: Frankfurt, Germany, 1617–1621.
13. Da Vinci, L. *Corpus of the Anatomical Studies in the Collection of Her Majesty, the Queen, at Windsor Castle*; Harcourt Brace Jovanovich: Windsor, UK, 1978–1980.
14. Descartes, R.; Schuyl, F. *De Homine*; Petrum Leffen, Franciscum Moyardum: Ludguni Batavorum (Leiden), The Netherlands, 1662.
15. Malpighi, M. *Opera Omnia*; Royal SocietyTomis Duobus: London, UK, 1687.
16. Willis, T. *De Anima Brutorum Quae Hominis Vitalis ac Sentitiva est: Exercitationes Duae*; Typis E.F. Impensis Ric. Davis: Oxon, UK, 1672.
17. Combe, G. *The Constitution of Man Considered in Relation to External Objects*, 8th ed.; MacLahlan Steward & Co.: Edinburgh, UK, 1847.
18. Gall, F.J. *On the Functions of the Brain and Each of Its Parts: With Observations on the Possibility of Determining the Instincts, Propensities and Talents, or the Moral and Intellectual Dispositions of Men and Animals, by the Configuration of the Head*, Trans, Winslow Lewis, Jr.; Marsh, Capen & Lyon: Boston, UK, 1835.
19. Gall, F.J.; Spurzheim, J.G. *Anatomie et Physiologie du Système Nerveux en Général et du Cerveau en Particulier Avec des Observations sur la Possibilité de Reconnaître Plusieurs Dispositions Intellectuelles et Morales de L'homme et des Animaux par la Configuration de Leurs Têtes*, 4 Vols., with an Atlas of 100 Engraved Plates; Schoell: Paris, France, 1810–1819.
20. Prochaska, G. *Functions of the Nervous System (English Translation by T. LAYCOCK, 1851)*; Sydenham's Society Series: London, UK, 1784.
21. Broca, P. Perte de la parole, ramollissement chronique et destruction partielle du lobe anterieur gauche du cerveau (sur la siege de la faculte du langage). *Bulletins et Mémoires de la Société D'anthropologie de Paris* **1861**, *2*, 235–238.
22. Fritsch, G.T.; Hitzig, E. Über die electrische erregbarkeit des grosshirns. *Arch. Anat. Physiol. Wiss. Med.* **1870**, *37*, 300–322.
23. Ferrier, D. Experiments in the brain of monkeys. *Proc. R. Soc. Lond. Ser. B.* **1875**, *23*, 409–430. [CrossRef]
24. Ferrier, D. *The Functions of the Brain*; Smith, Elder: London, UK, 1876.
25. Ferrier, D. *The Croonian Lectures on Cerebral Localisation*; Smith, Elder & Co.: London, UK, 1890.
26. Penfield, W.; Bouldrey, E. Somatic motor and sensory representation in the cerebral cortex of man as studied by electrical stimulation. *Brain* **1937**, *60*, 389–443. [CrossRef]
27. Descartes, R. *L'homme, et un Traité de la Formation du Foetus du Mesme Autheur. Avec les Remarques de Louys de la Forge*, 1st ed.; Nicolas Le Gras: Paris, France, 1664.
28. Bidloo, G.; de Lairesse, G. *Anatomia Humani Corporis*; Joannis à Someren, Joannis à Dyk, Henrici & Theodori Boom: Amstelodami, The Netherlands, 1685.
29. Leeuwenhoek, A.V. *Alle de Briefen van Antoni van Leeuwenhoek/The Collected Letters of Antoni van Leeuwenhoek 1673–1696 (Eleven Volumes), Edited, Illustrated, and Annotated by Committees of Dutch Scientists*; Swets & Zeitlinger: Amsterdam, The Netherlands, 1939–1983.

30. Van Leeuwenhoek, A. *Send-Brieven, Zoo aan de Hoog Edele Heeren van de Koninklyke Societeit te Londen*; Adriaan Beman: Te Delft, The Netherlands, 1718.

31. Von Haller, A. *Elementa Physiologiae Corporis Humani, in 8 Volumes*; Marci-Michael Bosquet & Sociorum: Lausanne, Switzerland, 1757–1778.

32. Chvatal, A. Jiri Prochaska (1749–1820): Part 2: "De structura nervorum"—Studies on a structure of the nervous system. *J. Hist. Neurosci.* **2015**, *24*, 1–25. [CrossRef] [PubMed]

33. Von Haller, A. *De Partibus Corporis Humani Sensilibus et Irritabilibus. Commentarii Societatis Regiae Scientiarum Gottingensis*; Vadenhoek: Gottingen, Germany, 1753.

34. Dierig, S. Neuronen-Doktrin und Neuroglia. PhD Thesis, Inaugural-Dissertation, University of Konstanz, Konstanz Germany, 1994.

35. Hooke, R. *Micrographia*; Folio Society: London, UK, 2017.

36. Shapiro, S. Antony van Leeuwenhoek; a review of his life and work. *J. Biol. Photogr. Assoc.* **1955**, *23*, 49–57. [PubMed]

37. Schleiden, M.J. Beiträge zur phytogenesis. *Arc. Anat. Physiol. Wiss. Med.* **1838**, 137–176.

38. Schwann, T. *Mikroskopische Untersuchungen über die Übereinstimmung in der Struktur und dem Wachstum der Tiere und Pflanzen*; Sanderschen Buchhandlung: Berlin, Germany, 1839.

39. Schwann, T. *Microscopical Researches into the Accordance in the Structure and Growth of Animals and Plants*; Sydenham Society: London, UK, 1847.

40. Malpighi, M. De Cerebri Cortice. In *De Viscerum Structura Exercitatio Anatomica*; Giacomo Monti: Bologna, Italy, 1666.

41. Gross, C.G. Emanuel Swedenborg: A neuroscientist before his time. *Neuroscientist* **1997**, *3*, 142–147. [CrossRef]

42. Swedenborg, E. *The Brain, Considered Anatomically, Physiologically and Phylosopically. (Translated and Edited by R.L. Tafel), in 4 Volumes*; James Speirs: London, UK, 1882.

43. Torre, G.M.D. *Nuove Osservazioni Microscopiche*; C. R. Somasco: Napoli, Italy, 1776.

44. Bentivoglio, M. 1896–1996: The centennial of the axon. *Brain Res. Bull.* **1996**, *41*, 319–325. [CrossRef]

45. Keuffel, G.G.T. Ueber das ruckenmark. *Arch. Physiol.* **1811**, *10*, 123–202.

46. Dutrochet, M.H. *Recherches Anatomiques et Physiologiques sur la Structure Intime des Animaux et des Végétaux, et sur leur Motilité*; J.B.Bailliere: Paris, France, 1824.

47. Dutrochet, M.H. *Mémoires Pour Servir a L'historie Anatomique et Physiologique des Végétaux et des Animaux. II*; J.-B. Bailliere: Paris, France, 1837; p. 688.

48. Studnička, F.K. Aus der Vorgeschichte der Zellenteorie. H. Milne edwards, H. Dutrochet, F. Raspail, j.E. Purkinje. *Anatomischer Anzeiger* **1932**, *73*, 390–416.

49. Ehrenberg, C.G. *Beobachtungeiner Auffallenden Bisher Unerkannten Strukfurdes Seelenorgans bei Menschen und Thieren*; Königlichen Akademie der Wissenschchaft: Berlin, Germany, 1836.

50. Purkinje, J.E. Neueste Beobachtungen uber die Struktur des Gehirns. In *Opera omnia*; Purkynova Spolecnost: Prague, Chec Republic, 1837; Volume 2, p. 3.

51. Todd, R.B. *The Descriptive and Physiological Anatomy of the Brain, Spinal Cord, Ganglions and Their Coverings*; Sherwood, Gilbert and Piper: London, UK, 1845.

52. Golgi, C. *Opera Omnia*; Hoepli: Milano, Italy, 1903.

53. Tan, S.Y.; Brown, J. Rudolph virchow (1821–1902): "Pope of pathology". *Singap. Med. J.* **2006**, *47*, 567–568.

54. Keuffel, G.G.T. De Medulla Spinali. Doctoral Dissertation, Halae, Magdeburg, Germay, 1810.

55. Weigert, C. *Kenntnis der Normalen Menschlichen Neuroglia*; Moritz Diesterweg: Frankfurt, Germany, 1895.

56. Valentin, G. Über den verlauf und die letzten enden der nerven. *Nova Acta Academiae Caesareae Leopoldino-Carolinae Germanicae Naturae Curiosorum. Verhandlungen der Kaiserlich Leopoldinisch-Carolinischen Deutschen Akademie der Naturforscher* **1836**, *18*, 51–240.

57. Chvatal, A. Discovering the structure of nerve tissue: Part 2: Gabriel Valentin, Robert Remak, and Jan Evangelista Purkyně. *J. Hist. Neurosci.* **2015**, *24*, 326–351. [CrossRef] [PubMed]

58. Purkyně, J.E. Untersuchungen aus der Nerven-und Hirnanatomie. *Isis* **1838**, 581–584.

59. Arnold, F. *Handbuch der Anatomie des Menschen*; Verlag Herder: Freiburg, Germany, 1844.

60. Rokitansky, C. Ueber die dendritischen Vegetationen auf Synovialhäuten. *Zeitschrift der Kaiserlichen Königlichen Gesellschaft der Aerzte zu Wien* **1851**, *7*, 1–8.

61. Rokitansky, K. Über die Entwickelung der Krebsgerüste mit Hinblick auf das Wesen und die Entwickelung anderer Maschenwerke. *Sitzungsberichte der Kaiserlichen Akademie der Wissenschaften. Mathematisch-Naturwissenschaftliche Classe. Wien* **1852**, *8*, 391–405.

62. Rokitansky, K. Über den Zottenkrebs. *Sitzungsberichte der Kaiserlichen Akademie der Wissenschaften. Mathematisch-Naturwissenschaftliche Classe. Wien* **1852**, *8*, 513–535.

63. Rokitansky, K. Über das auswachsen der Bindegewebs-Substanzen und die Beziehung desselben zur Entzündung. *Sitzungsberichte der Kaiserlichen Akademie der Wissenschaften. Mathematisch-Naturwissenschaftliche Classe. Wien* **1854**, *13*, 122–140.

64. Rokitansky, K. Über Bindegewebs-Wucherung im Nervensysteme. *Sitzungsberichte der Kaiserlichen Akademie der Wissenschaften. Mathematisch-Naturwissenschaftliche Classe. Wien* **1857**, *24*, 517–536.

65. Wright, N.A.; Poulsom, R. *Omnis cellula e cellula* revisited: Cell biology as the foundation of pathology. *J. Pathol.* **2012**, *226*, 145–147. [CrossRef] [PubMed]

66. Virchow, R. Ueber das granulirte Ansehen der Wandungen der Gehirnventrikel. *Allgemeine Zeitschrift für Psychiatrie und Psychisch-Gerichtliche Medicin* **1846**, *3*, 242–250.

67. Rokitansky, C. *Handbuch der Pathologischen Anatomie. II. Band*; Braumüller & Seidel: Wien, Austria, 1844.

68. Virchow, R. Ueber das granulirte Ansehen der Wandungen der Gehirnventrikel. In *Gesammelte Abhandlungen zur Wissenschaftlichen Medicin.*; Virchow, R., Ed.; Meidinger Sohn & Comp.: Frankfurt, Germany, 1856; pp. 885–891.

69. Virchow, R. *Die Cellularpathologie in Ihrer Begründung auf Physiologische und Pathologische Gewebelehre 20 Vorlesungen, Gehalten Während d. Monate Febr., März u. April 1858 im Patholog. Inst. Zu Berlin*; August Hirschwald: Berlin, Germany, 1858.

70. Virchow, R.L.K. *Cellular pathology*; John Churchill: London, UK, 1860; p. 511.

71. Bidder, F.H.; Kupffer, C. *Untersuchungen über die Textur des Rückenmarks und die Entwicklung Seiner Formelemente*; Breikopf und Härtel: Leipzig, Germany, 1857; p. 151.

72. Kupffer, C. *De Medullae Spinalis Textura in Ranis Ratione Imprimis Habita Indolis Substantiae Cinereae*; Typis Viduae, J.C. Schünmanni et C. Mattiesseni: Dorpati Livonorum, 1854.

73. Pappenheim, S. *Die Specielle Gewebelehre des Auges mit Rücksicht auf Entwicklungsgeschichte und Augenpraxis*; Georg Philipp Aderholz: Breslau, Poland, 1842.

74. Müller, H. Zur Histologie der Netzhaut. *Zeitschrift für Wissenschaftliche Zoologie* **1851**, *3*, 234–237.

75. Schulze, M. *Observationes de Retinae Structura Penitiori*; Published Lecture at the Univeesity of Bonn: Bonn, Germany, 1859.

76. Müller, H. *Anatomisch-Physiologische Untersuchungen über die Retina des Menschen und der Wirbelthiere*; Wilhelm Engelmann: Leipzig, Germany, 1856.

77. Bergmann, C. Notiz über einige Structurverhältnisse des Cerebellum und Rückenmarks. *Zeitschrift für Rationelle Medicin* **1857**, *8*, 360–363.

78. Mauthner, L. Über die sogenannten Bindegewehskörperchen des centralen Nervensystems. *Sitzungsberichte der Kaiserlichen Akademie der Wissenschaften. Mathematisch-Naturwissenschaftliche Classe. Wien* **1861**, *43*, 45–54.

79. Beale, L. *New Observations upon the Structure and Formation of Certain Nervous Centres, Tending to Prove That the Cells and Fibres of Every Nervous Apparatus form an Uninterrupted Circuit*; John Churchill and Sons: London, UK, 1864.

80. Frommann, C. Ueber die Färbung der binde- und Nervensubstanz des Rückenmarkes durch Argentum nitricum und über die Struktur der Nervenzellen. *Archiv für Pathologische Anatomie und Physiologie und für Klinische Medicin* **1864**, *31*, 129–153. [CrossRef]

81. Frommann, C. *Untersuchungen über die Normale und Pathologische Anatomie des Rückenmarks. Zweiter Theil*; Friedrich Frommann: Jena, Germany, 1867.

82. Deiters, O. *Untersuchungen über Gehirn und Rückenmark des Menschen und der Säugethiere*; Vieweg: Braunschweig, Germany, 1865.

83. Besser, L. Zur Histogenese der nervösen Elementartheile in den Centralorganen des neugebornen Menschen. *Archiv für Pathologische Anatomie und Physiologie und für Klinische Medicin* **1866**, *36*, 305–334. [CrossRef]

84. Chvatal, A. Discovering the structure of nerve tissue: Part 3: From Jan Evangelista Purkyne to Ludwig Mauthner. *J. Hist. Neurosci.* **2017**, *26*, 15–49. [CrossRef] [PubMed]

85. Kölliker, A. *Handbuch der Gewebelehre des Menschen für ärtze und Studirende*, 5th ed.; Engelmann: Leipzig, Germany, 1867.

86. Meynert, T. Vom Gehirne der Säugethiere. In *Handbuch der Lehre von den Geweben des Menschen und der Thiere. Zweiter Band*; Stricker, S., Ed.; Wilhelm Engelmann: Leipzig, Germany, 1872; pp. 694–809.

87. Meynert, T. The brain of mammals. In *A Manual of Histology*; Stricker, S., Ed.; William Wood & Company: New York, NY, USA, 1872; pp. 650–766.

88. Meynert, T. Der Bau der Gross-Hirnrinde und seine örtlichen Verschiedenheiten, nebst einem pathologisch-anatomischen Corollarium. I. Vierteljahrsschrift für Psychiatrie in ihren Beziehungen zur Morphologie und Pathologie des Central-Nervensystems der physiologischen Psychologie. *Statistik und Gerichtlichen Medicin* **1867**, *1*, 77–124.

89. Arndt, R. Studien über die Architektonik der Grosshirnrinde des Menschen. III. *Archiv für Mikroskopische Anatomie* **1869**, *5*, 317–331. [CrossRef]

90. Stieda, L. Studien uer das centrale Nervensystem der Wirbelthiere. *Zeitschrift für Wissenschaftliche Zoologie* **1869**, *20*, 273–456.

91. Henle, J.; Merkel, F. Uber die sogenannte Bindesubstanz der Centralorgane des Nervensystems. *Z. Med.* **1869**, *34*, 49–82.

92. Arndt, R. Studien über die Architektonik der Grosshirnrinde des Menschen. *Archiv für Mikroskopische Anatomie* **1867**, *3*, 441–476. [CrossRef]

93. Arndt, R. Studien über die Architektonik der Grosshirnrinde des Menschen. II. *Archiv für Mikroskopische Anatomie* **1868**, *4*, 407–526. [CrossRef]

94. Stieda, L. *Studien über das Centrale Nervensystem der Wirbelthiere*; Wilhelm Engelmann: Leipzig, Germany, 1870.

95. Golgi, C. Sulla sostanza connettiva del cervello. *Gazzetta Medica Italiana, Lombardia* **1870**, *19*, 145–146.

96. Golgi, C. Ueber die Bindesubstanz im Gehirne. *Schmidt's Jahrbücher der in-und Ausländischen Gesammten Medicin* **1871**, *150*, 3–4.

97. Golgi, C. Contribuzione alla fina anatomia degli organi centrali del sistema nervoso. I. *Rivista Clinica di Bologna* **1871**, *1*, 338–350.

98. Golgi, C. Contribuzione alla fina anatomia degli organi centrali del sistema nervoso. II. *Rivista Clinica di Bologna* **1871**, *1*, 371–380.

99. Golgi, C. Contribuzione alla fina anatomia degli organi centrali del sistema nervoso. III. *Rivista Clinica di Bologna* **1872**, *2*, 38–46.

100. Jastrowitz, M. Studien über die Encephalitis und Myelitis des ersten Kindesalters. *Archiv für Psychiatrie und Nervenkrankheiten* **1871**, *3*, 162–213. [CrossRef]

101. Golgi, C. Sulla struttura della sostanza grigia del cervello. *Gazzetta Medica Italiana, Lombardia* **1873**, *6*, 244–246.

102. Jastrowitz, M. Encephalitis und Myelitis des ersten Kindersalters. *Archiv für Psychiatrie und Nervenkrankheiten* **1870**, *2*, 389–414. [CrossRef]

103. Butzke, V. Studien uber den feineren Bau der Grosshirnrinde. *Archiv für Psychiatrie und Nervenkrankheiten* **1872**, *3*, 575–600. [CrossRef]

104. Ranvier, L.A. De la névroglie. *Archives de Physiologie Normale et Pathologique* **1883**, *3* S1, 177–185.

105. Ranvier, L.A. Sur les éléments conjonctifs de la moelle épinière. *Comptes Rendus Hebdomadaires des Séances de l'Académie des Sciences* **1873**, *77*, 1299–1302.

106. Rindfleisch, E. *Lehrbuch der Pathologischen Gewebelehre zur Eeinführung in das Studium der Pathologischen Anatomie*; Wilhelm Engelmann: Leipzig, Germany, 1873.

107. Boll, F. Die Histiologie und Histiogenese der nervösen Centralorgane. *Archiv für Psychiatrie und Nervenkrankheiten* **1873**, *4*, 1–138. [CrossRef]

108. Gierke, H. Beiträge zur Kenntniss der Elemente des centralen Nervensystems. *Breslauer Aerztliche Zeitschrift* **1882**, *4*, 157–160, 172–177.

109. Gierke, H. Die Stützsubstanz des Centralnervensystems. I. Theil. *Archiv für Mikroskopische Anatomie* **1885**, *25*, 441–554. [CrossRef]

110. Gierke, H. Die Stützsubstanz des Centralennervensystems. *Neurologisches Centralblatt* **1883**, *2*, 361–369, 385–392.

111. Gierke, H. Die Stützsubstanz des Centralnervensystems. II. Theil. *Archiv für Mikroskopische Anatomie* **1886**, *26*, 129–228. [CrossRef]

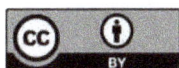

Article

Inflammatory Cytokines Facilitate the Sensitivity of P2X7 Receptors Toward Extracellular ATP at Neural Progenitor Cells of the Rodent Hippocampal Subgranular Zone

Juan Liu [1,2], Muhammad Tahir Khan [1], Yong Tang [2], Heike Franke [1] and Peter Illes [1,2,*]

1   Rudolf-Boehm-Institut für Pharmakologie und Toxikologie, Universität Leipzig, 04107 Leipzig, Germany; liujuan@cdutcm.edu.cn (J.L.); MuhammadTahir.Khan@medizin.uni-leipzig.de (M.T.K.); heike.franke@medizin.uni-leipzig.de (H.F.)
2   Acupuncture and Tuina School, Chengdu University of Traditional Chinese Medicine, Chengdu 610075, China; tangyong@cdutcm.edu.cn
*   Correspondence: peter.illes@medizin.uni-leipzig.de; Tel.: +49-341-9724614; Fax: +49-341-9724609

Received: 26 July 2018; Accepted: 16 August 2018; Published: 22 August 2018

Abstract: Organotypic hippocampal slice cultures were used to model the effects of neuroinflammatory conditions following an epileptic state on functional P2X7 receptors (Rs) of subgranular zone (SGZ) neural progenitor cells (NPCs). The compound, 4-aminopyridine (4-AP), is known to cause pathological firing of neurons, consequently facilitating the release of various transmitter substances including ATP. Lipopolysaccharide (LPS) and interleukin-1β (IL-1β) both potentiated the dibenzoyl-ATP (Bz-ATP)-induced current amplitudes in NPCs, although via different mechanisms. Whereas LPS acted via promoting ATP release, IL-1β acted via its own receptor to directly influence P2X7Rs. Thus, the effect of LPS was inhibited by the ecto-ATPase inhibitor, apyrase, but not by the IL-1β antagonist, interleukin-1RA (IL-1RA); by contrast, the effect of IL-1β was inhibited by IL-1RA, but not by apyrase. Eventually, incubation with 4-AP upregulated the number of nestin/glial fibrillary acidic protein/P2X7R immunoreactive cells and their appropriate staining intensity, suggesting increased synthesis of P2X7Rs at NPCs. In conclusion, inflammatory cytokines accumulating after epilepsy-like neuronal firing may facilitate the effect of endogenous ATP at P2X7Rs of NPCs, thereby probably promoting necrosis/apoptosis and subsequent cell death.

Keywords: neural progenitor cells; extracellular ATP; P2X7 receptors; neuroinflammation; cytokines

1. Introduction

In the adult mammalian brain, the subgranular zone (SGZ) of the hippocampal *dentate gyrus* is one of the regenerative niches where neural progenitor cells (NPCs) are produced to give rise to the three main neural cell linages, i.e., neurons, astrocytes, and oligodendrocytes [1–3]. During their integration into the hippocampal circuits, NPCs pass through various consecutive developmental stages before differentiating to newborn and subsequently mature granule cells (glutamatergic projection neurons to CA3 pyramidal neurons).

The physiological functions of adult neurogenesis comprise emotions, learning, and memory, i.e., temporal separation, pattern separation, fear conditioning, high-resolution memory, and synaptic plasticity [4,5]. Some disease conditions, like Parkinson's disease, Huntington's disease, Alzheimer's disease, multiple sclerosis, stroke, depression, and temporal lobe epilepsy are also connected to abnormal adult neurogenesis [6]. The misbalance between NPC proliferation and disintegration may contribute to the establishment of a pathological pacemaker in the hippocampus after a one-time *status epilepticus* [7,8].

The P2X7 receptor (R) is a ligand-gated non-selective cationic channel, which has a uniquely low affinity for extracellular ATP, and is transformed to a large membrane pore on long-lasting exposure to high ATP concentrations [9,10]. In the central nervous system (CNS), P2X7Rs are present at microglia and astrocytes/oligodendrocytes, as well as NPCs; their existence at neurons is a much-debated issue [10,11]. Neuroinflammation is a common denominator of both epilepsy [12,13] and P2X7R activation [14,15]. Hence, there are good reasons to speculate that the massive outflow of ATP from the epileptic focus may stimulate P2X7Rs, which are linked to the NLRP3/ASC inflammasome assembly, fostering the maturation and release of inflammatory cytokines such as interleukin-1β (IL-1β), especially from microglia [16]. It was proposed that, preceding the activation of P2X7Rs, the stimulation of lipopolysaccharide (LPS)-targeted Toll-like receptors (TLRs) leads to the accumulation of cytoplasmic pro-IL-1β, which is then processed to mature IL-1β under the influence of P2X7Rs [17].

We recently showed that pilocarpine-induced *status epilepticus* in rodents increases the sensitivity of P2X7Rs at SGZ NPCs toward ATP, consequently leading to a decrease in ectopic NPC/granule cell number in the *hilus hippocampi* [2,18]. Electrophysiological measurements in hippocampal slices prepared from such epileptic rats documented an increased sensitivity of their NPCs to ATP/dibenzoyl-ATP (Bz-ATP). This may lead to apoptosis/necrosis initiated via the caspase cascade and the loss of intracellular constituents of vital significance through the dilated P2X7R. When hippocampal slices were incubated with 4-aminopyridine (4-AP), a blocker of the transient outwardly directed potassium current ($I_{K(A)}$), to cause seizure-like activity in neurons, P2X7Rs at NPCs also became functionally upregulated [19].

We hypothesized that the pro-convulsive agent, 4-AP, causing P2X7R activation via endogenously released ATP may stimulate the synthesis and release of inflammatory cytokines which signal back to P2X7Rs and facilitate seizure susceptibility. In fact, incubation of organotypic hippocampal slices with LPS and IL-1β facilitated the P2X7R sensitivity of SGZ NPCs versus agonistic activation. This suggests that long-term P2X7R functions, such as apoptosis/necrosis, triggered by epileptic seizures are greatly facilitated under neuroinflammatory conditions.

2. Materials and Methods

2.1. Preparation of Hippocampal Brain Slices and the Corresponding Organotypic Slice Cultures

Hippocampal brain slices were obtained from C57BL/6J mice (bred in-house) or from mice overexpressing green fluorescent protein (GFP) under the control of the nestin gene (Tg(*nestin/EGFP*); gift from Helmut Kettenmann, Berlin). All animal use procedures were approved by the relevant Committee of Animal Protection (Regierungspraesidium Leipzig, Germany, CGZ216).

Mice pups (postnatal days 4–6; P4–6) were decapitated under CO_2 anesthesia. The preparation and culturing of organotypic slices were similar to those described previously [20,21]. Briefly, the hippocampi were rapidly dissected and were placed in ice-cold preparation solution (minimum essential medium (MEM) supplemented with 2 mM glutamine and 50 μg/mL gentamicin; all from Invitrogen, Carlsbad, CA, USA; the pH was adjusted to 7.3). Subsequently, transverse slices (thickness, 350 μm) were prepared with a McIlwain tissue chopper (Saur Laborbedarf, Reutlingen, Germany), and were stored in Petri dishes filled with the same solution. Then, the slices were placed on moistened translucent membranes (six slices per membrane, 0.4-μm membranes; Millicell-CM, Millipore, Bedford, MO, USA). These membranes were transferred into six-well plates, each filled with 1 mL of incubation medium (50% MEM, 25% Basal Medium Eagle, 25% heat-inactivated horse serum, supplemented with 2 mM glutamine; all from Invitrogen; and 0.625% glucose purchased from Sigma-Aldrich, St. Louis, MO, USA). The slices were stored in an incubator at a constant temperature of 37 °C and an atmosphere of 5% CO_2 in air; the medium was changed three times weekly. Organotypic brain slices were subjected to electrophysiological recordings and immunohistochemistry after 1–3 weeks in culture.

2.2. Whole-Cell Patch-Clamp Recordings

Organotypic cultured slices were superfused in an organ bath with 95% O_2 plus 5% CO_2-saturated artificial cerebrospinal solution (aCSF; 3 mL/min, room temperature). This aCSF had the following composition (in mM): NaCl 126, KCl 2.5, $CaCl_2$ 2.4, $MgCl_2$ 1.3, NaH_2PO_4 1.2, $NaHCO_3$ 25, and glucose 11; the pH was 7.4, adjusted with NaOH. To create a low divalent cation-containing (low X^{2+}) solution, $MgCl_2$ was omitted from the medium and the $CaCl_2$ concentration was decreased to 0.5 mM. Neural progenitor cells and/or astrocytes in the subgranular zone of the hippocampal *dentate gyrus* were visualized with an upright interference contrast microscope and a 40× water-immersion objective (Axioskope FS, Carl Zeiss, Oberkochen, Germany). Patch pipettes were filled with intracellular solution of the following composition (in mM): K-gluconic acid 140, NaCl 10, $MgCl_2$ 1, HEPES 10, EGTA 11, Mg-ATP 1.5, Li-GTP 0.3; the pH was 7.2, adjusted with KOH. Pipettes (4–7 MΩ resistances) were pulled by a micropipette puller (P-97, Sutter Instruments, Novato, CA, USA) from borosilicate capillaries. The resting membrane potential (V_m) of the cells was measured in the current-clamp mode of the patch-clamp amplifier (Multiclamp 700A; Molecular Devices, San Jose, CA, USA) immediately after establishing whole-cell access.

Neural progenitor cells were identified by their green fluorescence under an appropriate filter. Astrocytes (no fluorescence) and NPCs (green fluorescence) were discriminated from neurons by their failure to fire action potentials. For this purpose, hyper- and depolarizing current pulses (−80, −20, 40, 100, and 160 pA) were injected into the respective cells. Then, in the voltage-clamp recording mode of the amplifier, the holding potential of the astrocytes and NPCs were set at −80 mV, near their membrane potentials. Multiclamp and pClamp software (Molecular Devices) were used to store the recorded data to perform offline analysis/filtering and to trigger the application system used.

2.3. Drug Application Protocols

Dibenzoyl-ATP (300 μM) was pressure-ejected locally by means of a computer-controlled DAD-12 superfusion system (ALA Scientific Instruments, Farmingdale, NY, USA). The drug application tip touched the surface of the brain slice and was placed within 100–150 μm of the patched cell. Dibenzoyl-ATP (300 μM) induced a low-X^{2+} medium inward current, whose amplitude was at the quasi-linear part of the semi-logarithmic concentration–response curves generated both in astrocytes [22] and NPCs [18]. Organotypic hippocampal slices were grown in incubation medium for one week before they were subjected to Bz-ATP (300 μM) pulses (for 10 s, every 2 min, three times; the first response was discarded). All substances were present in the culturing medium for 14 h, one day, or one week before using the organotypic slices for patch-clamp recordings. In some cases, the effect of Bz-ATP (300 μM) was compared in a normal and low-X^{2+} medium.

2.4. Multiple Immunofluorescence Labeling Under Confocal Microscopic Observation

After the incubation period of three weeks, the Millicell membranes (Millipore, Bedford, MA, USA) were taken out and the hippocampal cultures were fixed for 2 h in a solution containing 4% paraformaldehyde (Merck, Darmstadt, Germany), 0.1% glutaraldehyde (Serva Electrophoresis, Heidelberg, Germany), and 0.2% picric acid (Sigma-Aldrich) in 0.1 M phosphate buffer (PB; pH 7.4). Afterward, cultures were rinsed intensively with PB and were cut into 50-μm slices using the vibratome (Typ VT 1200S, Leica Biosystems, Wetzlar, Germany).

Following pre-incubation in a blocking solution (0.05 M tris-buffered saline (TBS), pH 7.6, supplemented with 5% fetal calf serum and 0.3% Triton X-100), the slices were incubated in a mixture of primary antibodies diluted in the blocking solution for 48 h at 4°C. The following antibodies were used: anti-glial fibrillary acidic protein (GFAP; mouse, 1:1000; Sigma-Aldrich), anti-Iba1 (goat, 1:100; Abcam, Cambridge, UK), anti-nestin (mouse, 1:50; Millipore), or mouse anti-GFP (1:100; Clontech, Wisconsin, PE, USA), as well as anti-P2X7 (rabbit, 1:600; APR-004, Alomone Labs, Jerusalem, Israel). This incubation period was followed by rinsing in TBS. The simultaneous visualization of different primary antisera was performed with a mixture of secondary antibodies specific for the appropriate species immunoglobulin G (IgG; rabbit, mouse, goat). Carbocyanine (Cy)2- (1:400), Cy3- (1:1000), Cy5- (1:100) conjugated IgGs (all Jackson ImmunoResearch, West Grove, PE, USA) diluted in the blocking solution were applied for 2 h at room temperature. For nuclear staining, the slices were incubated with Hoechst 33342 (Hoe; final concentration 40 µg/mL, Molecular Probes, Eugene, OR, USA) for 5 min in TBS at room temperature. After intensive washing and mounting on glass slides, sections were dehydrated and cover-slipped as described above. Control experiments were performed without primary antibodies or by pre-adsorption of the antibody with the immunizing peptides.

The multiple immunofluorescence was investigated using a confocal laser scanning microscope (LSM 510 Meta, Zeiss) using excitation wavelengths of 488 nm (argon, yellow-green Cy2 immunofluorescence), 543 nm (helium/neon, red Cy3 immunofluorescence), and 633 nm (helium/neon2, blue Cy5 labeling). An ultraviolet laser (362 nm) was used to excite the blue–cyan Hoe 33342 fluorescence.

2.5. Materials

The following drugs were used: interleukin-1β murine (IL-1β; Biomol, Hamburg, Germany), antimycin A, $2'(3')$-O-(4-benzoylbenzoyl)adenosine $5'$-triphosphate triethylammonium salt (Bz-ATP), epidermal growth factor from mouse (EGF), fibroblast growth factor-2 (FGF-2), interleukin-1RA murine (IL-1RA), LPS from *Escherichia coli*, nerve growth factor-β from mouse (NGF), and sodium iodoacetate (Sigma-Aldrich).

2.6. Statistics

Means ± standard errors of the mean (SEM) are given throughout. SigmaPlot 13.0 was used for statistical evaluation (Systat Software Inc., Chicago, IL, USA). We tested for and found that, when using parametric tests, all sampled distributions satisfied the normality and equal variances criteria. Multiple comparisons between data were performed with a one-way analysis of variance (ANOVA) followed by the Holm–Sidak test. Two datasets were compared either using the parametric Student's *t*-test or the non-parametric Mann–Whitney rank sum test, as appropriate. A probability level of 0.05 or less was considered to be statistically significant.

3. Results

3.1. Sensitivity Increase of P2X7Rs at SGZ NPCs in Organotypic Hippocampal Slices Caused by Pre-Incubation with Lipopolysaccharide and Cytokines

Combination of four criteria can verify that Bz-ATP at a submaximal concentration of 300 µM selectively activates the P2X7Rs in SGZ NPCs: (1) the responses to both Bz-ATP and ATP are potentiated in a low-X^{2+} bath medium; (2) Bz-ATP causes comparable inward currents at about 10-times lower concentrations than ATP itself; (3) the Bz-ATP effect is nearly abolished by the highly selective P2X7R antagonist A-438079; and (4) the Bz-ATP current exhibits a reversal potential around 0 mV, characteristic for non-selective cationic channels [18]. All of these criteria held true for SGZ NPCs in a slice preparation [18].

Therefore, we applied, in all subsequent experiments, 300 µM Bz-ATP as a test concentration to investigate changes in P2X7R sensitivity. Furthermore, 4-AP (50 µM; one-week incubation) facilitated the effect of Bz-ATP (300 µM) on NPCs in hippocampal slice cultures [19]. This effect was thought to be due to a lengthening of the half amplitude duration of action potentials in *dentate gyrus* granule neurons increasing the release of glutamate and ATP onto SGZ NPCs [19]. Incubation with LPS (10 ng/mL) for 14 h had an effect similar to that of 4-AP (Figure 1A,B). It is noteworthy that only Bz-ATP-induced current responses measured in a low-X^{2+} medium exhibited potentiation, but not those measured in a normal external medium.

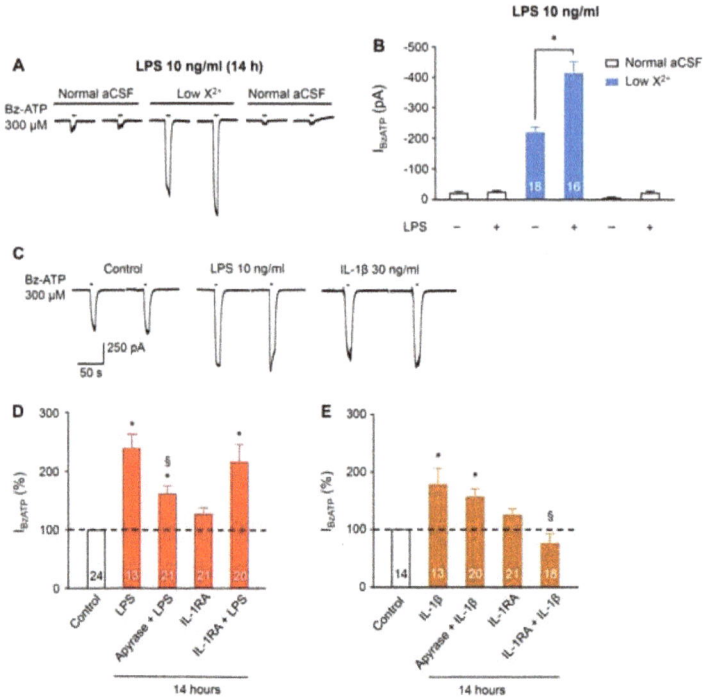

Figure 1. Effects of 4-aminopyridine (4-AP), lipopolysaccharide (LPS), and interleukin-1β (IL-1β) on dibenzoyl-ATP (Bz-ATP)-induced current responses of neural progenitor cells (NPCs) located in organotypic hippocampal slices cultured for one week. Normal artificial cerebrospinal solution (aCSF) or low X^{2+} aCSF has been used. Lipopolysaccharide (10 ng/mL) and IL-1β (30 ng/mL) were added either alone or together with apyrase (30 IU/mL), or interleukin-1RA murine (IL-1RA) (100 ng/mL) for the last 14 h of culturing. (**A**,**B**) Effect of LPS on the Bz-ATP (300 μM)-induced current amplitudes (I_{BzATP}). Dibenzoyl-ATP was applied six times in total, both in the absence and presence of LPS. A normal external medium was changed to one which contained no Mg^{2+} and a low Ca^{2+} concentration (low X^{2+}). Representative current tracings in the presence of LPS (**A**). Mean ± standard error of the mean (SEM) of the indicated number of cells (**B**). Lipopolysaccharide potentiated I_{BzATP} in a low-X^{2+} medium only. The mean of two subsequent responses is shown in (**B**). * $p < 0.05$; statistically significant difference between the respective pairs of currents recorded in the absence and presence of LPS. (**C–E**) Representative tracings show a potentiation of Bz-ATP (300 μM) currents by incubation of hippocampal slices in culturing medium containing LPS or IL-1β (**C**). Dibenzoyl-ATP pulses were applied three times (the first response was discarded). Percentage potentiation of I_{BzATP} by LPS alone, or in the combined presence of LPS plus apyrase, or LPS plus IL-1RA (**D**). Comparison was with I_{BzATP} measured in a drug-free medium (control). Mean ± SEM of the indicated number of cells in both (**D**) and (**E**). Percentage potentiation of I_{BzATP} by IL-1β alone, or in the combined presence of IL-1β plus apyrase or IL-1β plus IL-1RA (**E**). Comparison was with I_{BzATP} measured in a drug-free bath medium (control). The effect of IL-1RA on I_{BzATP} in (**E**) was re-plotted from (**D**). * $p < 0.05$; statistically significant difference from the control values. § $p < 0.05$; statistically significant difference from the effect of LPS (**D**) and IL-1β alone (**E**).

Incubation with ATP (10 μM) for 14 h caused a facilitation of the Bz-ATP-induced current (I_{BzATP}); this effect was abolished by co-incubation of ATP with the ecto-ATPase apyrase (10 IU/mL; [19]) which by itself did not increase I_{BzATP}. Therefore, it was concluded that the effect of ATP is, in fact, mediated by the activation of P2Rs. Apyrase also depressed the effect of co-applied LPS (10 ng/mL; 14 h), indicating that LPS releases endogenous ATP which then supposedly acts at P2X7Rs (Figure 1C,D). By contrast, the IL-1β antagonist, IL-1RA (100 ng/mL; 14 h), failed to influence the LPS effect (Figure 1D). Furthermore, IL-1β (100 ng/mL) facilitated I_{BzATP}, just as ATP and LPS did; however, this was via a different mechanism, because the effect of IL-1β was obliterated by IL-1RA, but not by apyrase (Figure 1C,E). We assume that exogenous ATP, as well as endogenous ATP released by LPS, activates P2X7Rs, thereby potentiating the action of Bz-ATP probably by allowing increased Ca^{2+} entry into the cells. By contrast, IL-1β may directly facilitate cationic fluxes through P2X7Rs apparently contradicting the confirmed permissive role of ATP for the LPS-induced secretion of IL-1β under our experimental conditions.

3.2. Sensitivity Increase of P2X7Rs at SGZ NPCs in Organotypic Hippocampal Slices Caused Pre-Incubation with Growth Factors, but not by Pre-Incubation with Reactive Oxygen Species or Metabolic Inhibitors

Neuroinflammation is mediated not only by cytokines, but also by growth factors, and it follows the neuronal damage caused by metabolic limitation. It is a major condition in stroke pathophysiology and contributes to secondary neuronal damage in both acute and chronic stages of the ischemic injury [23]. Neuroinflammation and epilepsy are also thoroughly interrelated pathological events [13,24,25].

Therefore, we incubated brain slice cultures for one day or one week with NGF (30 ng/mL) which increased I_{BzATP} of NPCs in comparison with controls (Figure 2A,B). The combination of EGF (20 ng/mL) with FGF-2 (10 ng/mL) for one week had a similar effect. Eventually, organotypic hippocampal slice cultures were damaged either by the free oxygen radical, H_2O_2 (10 μM; 14-h incubation), or by the combined application of antimycin (25 nM) and sodium iodoacetate (10 μM) for 14 h to block oxidative phosphorylation and glycolysis, respectively (Figure 1C,D; [26]). Both oxidative and metabolic damage failed to cause a potentiation of Bz-ATP currents at NPCs. We did not measure the effect of H_2O_2 and antimycin plus sodium iodoacetate on I_{BzATP} after longer-lasting incubation of hippocampal slices (e.g., one week); it is quite possible that, under these conditions, a secondary neuroinflammation would cause potentiation of the Bz-ATP-induced current responses.

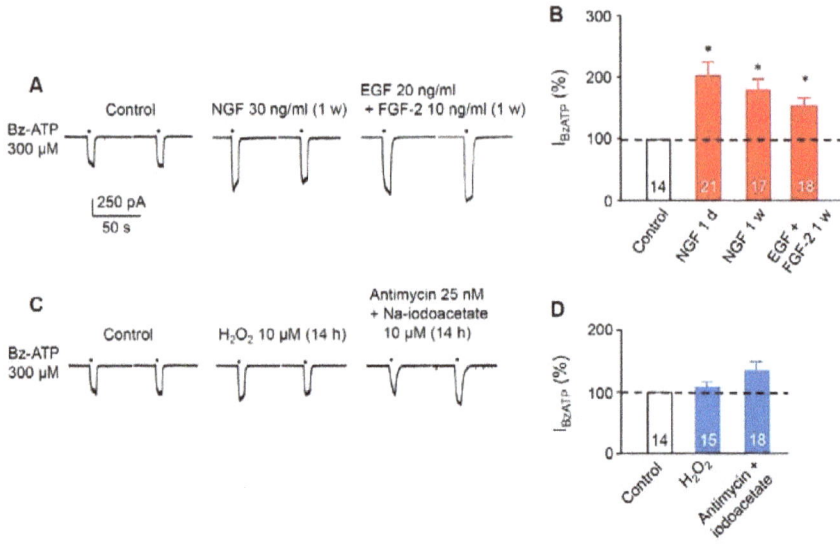

Figure 2. Effects of growth factors or the in vitro modelling of reperfusion injury/metabolic limitation on Bz-ATP-induced current responses of NPCs located in organotypic hippocampal slices cultured for one week. (**A,B**) Nerve growth factor (NGF; 30 ng/mL) or epidermal growth factor (EGF; 20 ng/mL) plus fibroblast growth factor-2 (FGF-2; 10 ng/mL) were present in the external medium for the whole week (1 w). In some experiments, NGF was present only for the last 24 h of cultivation (1 d). Representative tracings show potentiation of the Bz-ATP (300 µM) currents (I_{BzATP}) by NGF or EGF plus FGF-2 (**A**). Dibenzoyl-ATP pulses were applied three times (the first response was discarded). Percentage potentiation of I_{BzATP} by NGF for the time periods indicated, or in the combined presence of EGF plus FGF-2 for one week (**B**). Comparison was with I_{BzATP} measured in a drug-free bath medium (control). Mean ± SEM of the indicated number of cells. (**C,D**) H_2O_2 (10 µM) or antimycin (25 nM) plus Na-iodoacetate (10 µM) were present in the external medium for the last 14 h of culturing only. Representative tracings show no changes of Bz-ATP (300 µM) currents by H_2O_2 or antimycin plus Na-iodoacetate (**C**). Mean ± SEM of the indicated number of cells (**D**). * $p < 0.05$; statistically significant difference from the control value.

3.3. P2X7R Immunoreactivity in Organotypic Hippocampal Slice Cultures

The exemplary structure of the hippocampus in a three-week-old organotypic slice culture shows cell bodies stained with Hoechst 33342 (Hoe) in a black-and-white confocal laser-scanning microscopic picture (Figure 3A). Incubation with a 4-AP (50 µM)-containing medium after the initial two weeks of culturing for a further week did not cause an appreciable change in the gross structural view (not shown). Subsequently, we evaluated the colored images in the SGZ of the hippocampal *dentate gyrus* after mechanical removal of the glial cap, interfering with visibility. For this purpose about 50 µm of the superficial tissue layers were cut away from the slice culture by means of a vibratome (VT1200, Leica Biosystems).

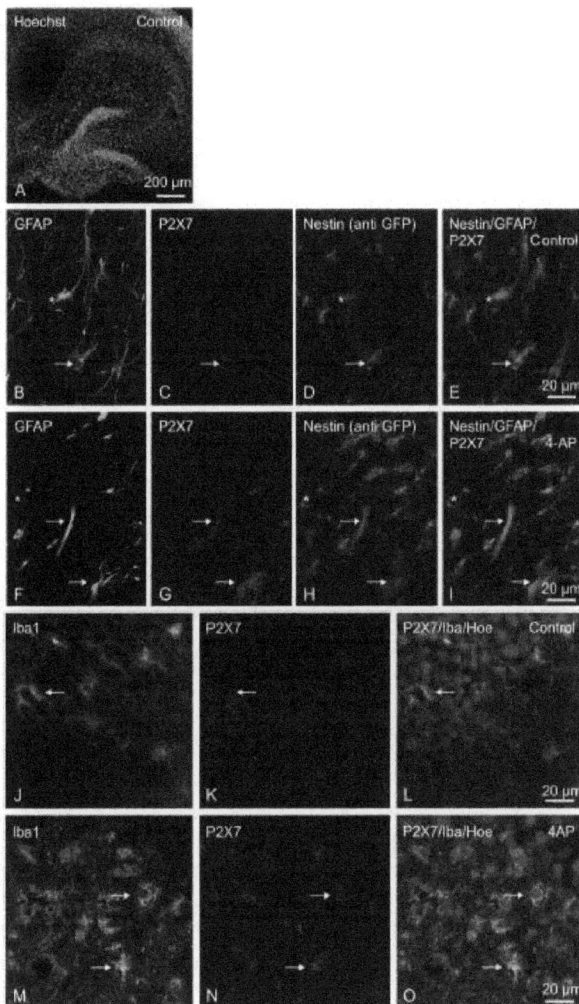

Figure 3. P2X7 receptor (R) immunoreactivity (IR) in three-week-old organotypic hippocampal slice cultures of mice overexpressing green fluorescent protein under the control of the nestin gene (Tg(*nestin-EGFP*)). (**A**) Black-and-white structure of the hippocampus under confocal laser-scanning microscopic observation; the cell nuclei were stained with Hoechst 33342 (Hoe) here and in (**L**) and (**O**). Images show, in the specimens, various immunoreactive (IR) structures in the subgranular zone of the dentate gyrus after labeling with specific antibodies. Arrows mark the overlaying IR structures throughout. Asterisks mark anti-glial fibrillary acidic protein (GFAP)/nestin double IR, with no staining for P2X7 in (**B–E**) and (**F–I**). (**B–E**) Weak GFAP-, nestin-, and P2X7R-IR structures and their overlay. (**F–I**) Stronger GFAP-, nestin-, and P2X7-IR structures and their overlay after incubation with 4-AP (50 μM) for the last week of cultivation. The number of triple IR cells also increased. (**J–L**) Iba- and P2X7R-IR structures are co-localized on microglial cells. (**M–O**) Incubation with 4-AP caused an increase in the number of co-labeled cells and their intensity of staining for Iba/P2X7-IR structures. Scale bars, 200 μm (**A**) and 20 μm (**B–O**). Representative snapshots obtained from three to four animals per group.

Because the specimens were prepared from Tg(*nestin/EGFP*) mice, the staining with anti-EGFP labeled nestin-immunoreactive (IR) NPCs. We observed weak GFAP-, P2X7-, and nestin-IR NPCs in the control SGZ (Figure 3B–E). Incubation of the slices with 4-AP caused upregulation of the nestin/GFAP/P2X7-IR cell number and the appropriate staining intensity (Figure 3F–I). Whereas radial glia-like type 1 NPCs exhibit IRs for both GFAP and nestin, astrocytes are IR for GFAP only. We did not observe P2X7-IR at these astrocytes. However, it should be mentioned that, in spite of the lack of P2X7-IR at astrocytes, functional P2X7Rs can be detected at this cell type, e.g., in the prefrontal cortex, especially in a low-X^{2+} medium [22]. We assume that the density of P2X7Rs at astrocytes is much lower than the density of P2X7Rs at NPCs.

In the hippocampal cell formation and on the surface of the tissue slices, P2X7-IR was observed on activated microglia (marked by anti-Iba1; Figure 3J–L); both IRs increased after incubation with 4-AP (Figure 3M–O).

Hence, in accordance with the potentiation of the Bz-ATP-induced currents of NPCs by a long-lasting treatment with 4-AP, both the number of nestin/GFAP/P2X7 triple-labeled type 1 NPCs and the staining intensity for the investigated antibodies at these cells were upregulated. In other words, the facilitated P2X7R function appears to be due to an enhancement of protein synthesis, and probably also to alleviated post-receptor signaling due to the activation of a calcium/calmodulin binding site at the C-terminus of the P2X7R [27].

4. Discussion

The main findings of this study were the following: (1) incubation with LPS, IL-1β, or growth factors (NGF, EGF, or FGF) facilitated the Bz-ATP sensitivity of NPCs located in the SGZ of organotypic hippocampal slice cultures; (2) incubation with the reactive oxygen species, H_2O_2, or the blockade of oxidative phosphorylation and glycolysis (antimycin plus sodium iodoacetate) had no comparable effect; (3) incubation with 4-AP caused upregulation of the nestin/GFAP/P2X7-IR cell number and the appropriate staining intensity, indicating that a facilitated P2X7R function may be due to enhanced protein synthesis, and probably also to alleviated post-receptor signaling in NPCs.

Experimental evidence in rodents demonstrates that seizures largely increase the levels of inflammatory mediators in brain regions involved in the generation and propagation of epileptic activity [13,24,25]. Prototypic inflammatory cytokines, such as IL-1β, IL-6, and tumor necrosis factor-α (TNF-α), are upregulated in activated microglia and astrocytes, before triggering a cascade of downstream inflammatory events that also involve neurons and endothelial cells of the blood–brain barrier. In models of chronic inflammation, such as transgenic mice systemically overexpressing IL-6 or TNF-α, a reduced seizure threshold was observed, which predisposes the brain to seizure-induced neuronal loss [28]. Furthermore, TNF-α and IL-10 were associated with the regulation of seizure duration in experimental kindling models [29]. On the contrary, mild inflammatory response evoked by LPS during a critical period of development caused a long-lasting increase in hippocampal excitability in vitro, and enhanced seizure susceptibility to the convulsants, pilocarpine, kanic acid, and pentetrazol [30]. It was concluded that cytokine-induced modifications in brain excitability underlying seizure phenomena involve both the rapid post-translational and the long-term transcriptional changes in voltage-gated and ligand-gated ion channels, as well as cytokine-mediated changes in genes involved in neurotransmission and synaptic plasticity [31,32].

In view of the contribution of neuro/glio-inflammation to epileptogenesis, we investigated the effect of LPS on I_{BzATP} of NPCs, which is supposed to release IL-1β, e.g., from microglia/macrophages only in case of the co-stimulation of permissive P2X7Rs [14,15,33]. Experiments in a low-X^{2+} external medium showed an increase in I_{BzATP} by pre-treatment of the organotypic slice cultures with both 4-AP [19] and LPS (present paper). A potentiation by a low divalent cation-containing external medium of the agonist effects at P2X7Rs are most probably due to the removal of an allosteric block exerted by Ca^{2+} [34]. A low extracellular Ca^{2+}/Mg^{2+} concentration may, on the one hand, induce pathological firing in hippocampal CA1 and CA3 pyramidal cells in vitro, and, on the other hand, it corresponds to the ionic constitution of the extracellular microenvironment during seizures in vivo [35].

It was an unexpected finding that LPS facilitated I_{BzATP} via the release of ATP without the involvement of IL-1β receptors; apyrase, but not IL-1RA, depressed the LPS-induced increase of P2X7R currents at NPCs. It was reported recently that a long-lasting stimulation of P2X7Rs by ATP increases the sensitivity of this receptor to Bz-ATP [19]. By contrast, IL-1β itself potentiated I_{BzATP} via activation of an interleukin 1 receptor (IL-1R), because its effect was antagonized by the selective IL-1R antagonist, IL-1RA, but not apyrase. Thus, two different mechanisms appear to result in an increased sensitivity of P2X7Rs toward ATP, one of them via a facilitated ATP release and the other via the direct stimulation of P2X7Rs by inflammatory cytokines. We assume that, in both cases, increased Ca^{2+} entry into the cells occurs, with subsequent occupation of an intracellular Ca^{2+}/calmodulin binding motif at the C-terminus of the P2X7R, leading to a potentiation of I_{BzATP} [27], or to increased trafficking of intracellular P2X7Rs to the plasma membrane. It should be pointed out that IL-1β is mainly released from microglial cells, which thereby take a central position in causing a conductance increase of P2X7Rs at NPCs. Of course it is possible that pre-incubation with 4-AP, ATP, LPS, and IL-1β all potentiate the Bz-ATP-induced current by facilitating a non-P2X7R-mediated component of I_{BzATP} (Reference [19] and present paper). This is, however, unlikely; in previous experiments, we found that the selective P2X7R antagonist, A-438079, almost completely inhibited the 4-AP-potentiated I_{BzATP} [19]. Therefore, it is tentatively suggested that, because the last link in the sequence of events triggered by 4-AP and IL-β is identical (i.e., an elevated intracellular Ca^{2+} concentration), A-438079 could block also the IL-1β-potentiated I_{BzATP}.

Proliferation of reactive astrocytes termed astrogliosis is mediated not only by ATP acting at P2X7Rs, but also by additional nucleotide receptors of the P2X and P2Y types [36,37]. However, ATP is only one of the numerous endogenous factors determining astrogliosis, acting alone or together with cytokines (IL, TNF, or interferons), growth factors (FGF-2 or leukemia inhibitory factor), neurotransmitters (glutamate or noradrenaline), reactive oxygen radicals, nitric oxide, etc. [38]. In order to elucidate a possible role of various growth factors in the increased function of P2X7Rs at hippocampal NPCs, we pre-treated our organotypic brain slices with NGF or EGF plus FGF-2. In fact, all growth factors investigated potentiated I_{BzATP} under the present experimental conditions.

Medial cerebral artery occlusion as a model of focal cerebral ischemia leads to a massive outflow of ATP from damaged CNS cells and upregulates P2X7R-IR in the penumbra of the damaged brain area [39,40]. There is an early microglial response associated with the activation of this cell type followed by a late response restricted to neurons and astrocytes. The blocking of P2X7Rs decreased the infarct size, brain edema, and neurological deficits after cerebral infarction [41,42]. P2X7R antagonists also ameliorated delayed neuronal death after transient global ischemia [43,44]. Because in vitro ischemia in cerebrocortical cell cultures caused supersensitivity of P2X7Rs to their agonists [45], we investigated whether the free oxygen radical, H_2O_2, known to be produced during reperfusion of brain tissue following a temporary stop of blood flow, facilitates I_{BzATP} in SGZ NPCs. Neither H_2O_2 nor the combined application of antimycin and sodium iodoacetate, to block oxidative phosphorylation and glycolysis, respectively, had any effect on the sensitivity of P2X7Rs at NPCs.

In conclusion, our in vitro experiments supported the hypothesis that the increased release of ATP from granule cells onto the hippocampal SGZ during a status epilepticus might foster the proliferation of NPCs [2,18]. Subsequently, proliferating NPCs migrate into ectopic locations, differentiate into mature neurons, and become integrated into pathological neuronal circuits. The activation of P2X7Rs by ATP in combination with the neuroinflammatory stimulation of P2X7Rs by cytokines causes necrosis/apoptosis of NPCs, thereby potentially preventing these deleterious processes. Thus, P2X7Rs could inhibit the transition of a one-time status epilepticus (possibly febrile seizures in childhood/early adolescence [46]) into chronic limbic epilepsy in humans.

Author Contributions: Conceptualization, P.I. Data curation, P.I. and J.L. Formal analysis, Y.T. Funding acquisition, Y.T. Investigation, J.L., M.T.K., and H.F. Methodology, M.T.K. and H.F. Project administration, Y.T. Supervision, P.I., Y.T., and H.F. Validation, J.L. Writing—original draft, P.I.

Funding: This research was funded by the Deutsche Forschungsgemeinschaft (DFG; IL-20/21-1) and the Sino-German Centre for the Promotion of Science (GZ919).

Acknowledgments: The expert technical assistance by Katrin Becker is gratefully acknowledged.

Conflicts of Interest: The authors declare no conflict of interest.

References

1. Jessberger, S.; Gage, F.H. Adult neurogenesis: Bridging the gap between mice and humans. *Trends Cell. Biol.* **2014**, *24*, 558–563. [CrossRef] [PubMed]

2. Tang, Y.; Illes, P. Regulation of adult neural progenitor cell functions by purinergic signaling. *Glia* **2017**, *65*, 213–230. [CrossRef] [PubMed]

3. Oliveira, A.; Illes, P.; Ulrich, H. Purinergic receptors in embryonic and adult neurogenesis. *Neuropharmacology* **2016**, *104*, 272–281. [CrossRef] [PubMed]

4. Braun, S.M.; Jessberger, S. Adult neurogenesis: Mechanisms and functional significance. *Development* **2014**, *141*, 1983–1986. [CrossRef] [PubMed]

5. Aimone, J.B.; Li, Y.; Lee, S.W.; Clemenson, G.D.; Deng, W.; Gage, F.H. Regulation and function of adult neurogenesis: From genes to cognition. *Physiol. Rev.* **2014**, *94*, 991–1026. [CrossRef] [PubMed]

6. Liu, H.; Song, N. Molecular Mechanism of Adult Neurogenesis and its Association with Human Brain Diseases. *J. Cent. Nerv. Syst. Dis.* **2016**, *8*, 5–11. [CrossRef] [PubMed]

7. Parent, J.M.; Yu, T.W.; Leibowitz, R.T.; Geschwind, D.H.; Sloviter, R.S.; Lowenstein, D.H. Dentate granule cell neurogenesis is increased by seizures and contributes to aberrant network reorganization in the adult rat hippocampus. *J. Neurosci.* **1997**, *17*, 3727–3738. [CrossRef] [PubMed]

8. Jessberger, S.; Parent, J.M. Epilepsy and Adult Neurogenesis. *Cold Spring Harb. Perspect. Biol.* **2015**, *7*, a020677. [CrossRef] [PubMed]

9. Sperlagh, B.; Illes, P. P2X7 receptor: An emerging target in central nervous system diseases. *Trends Pharmacol. Sci.* **2014**, *35*, 537–547. [CrossRef] [PubMed]

10. Illes, P.; Khan, T.M.; Rubini, P. Neuronal P2X7 Receptors Revisited: Do They Really Exist? *J. Neurosci.* **2017**, *37*, 7049–7062. [CrossRef] [PubMed]

11. Sim, J.A.; Young, M.T.; Sung, H.Y.; North, R.A.; Surprenant, A. Reanalysis of P2X7 receptor expression in rodent brain. *J. Neurosci.* **2004**, *24*, 6307–6314. [CrossRef] [PubMed]

12. Devinsky, O.; Vezzani, A.; Najjar, S.; De Lanerolle, N.C.; Rogawski, M.A. Glia and epilepsy: Excitability and inflammation. *Trends Neurosci.* **2013**, *36*, 174–184. [CrossRef] [PubMed]

13. Beamer, E.; Goloncser, F.; Horvath, G.; Beko, K.; Otrokocsi, L.; Kovanyi, B.; Sperlagh, B. Purinergic mechanisms in neuroinflammation: An update from molecules to behavior. *Neuropharmacology* **2016**, *104*, 94–104. [CrossRef] [PubMed]

14. Ferrari, D.; Pizzirani, C.; Adinolfi, E.; Lemoli, R.M.; Curti, A.; Idzko, M.; Panther, E.; Di Virgilio, F. The P2X7 receptor: A key player in IL-1 processing and release. *J. Immunol.* **2006**, *176*, 3877–3883. [CrossRef] [PubMed]

15. Giuliani, A.L.; Sarti, A.C.; Falzoni, S.; Di Virgilio, F. The P2X7 Receptor-Interleukin-1 Liaison. *Front. Pharmacol.* **2017**, *8*, 123. [CrossRef] [PubMed]

16. Young, C.N.J.; Gorecki, D.C. P2RX7 Purinoceptor as a Therapeutic Target-The Second Coming? *Front. Chem.* **2018**, *6*, 248. [CrossRef] [PubMed]

17. Di Virgilio, F.; Dal, B.D.; Sarti, A.C.; Giuliani, A.L.; Falzoni, S. The P2X7 Receptor in Infection and Inflammation. *Immunity* **2017**, *47*, 15–31. [CrossRef] [PubMed]

18. Rozmer, K.; Gao, P.; Araujo, M.G.L.; Khan, M.T.; Liu, J.; Rong, W.; Tang, Y.; Franke, H.; Krugel, U.; Fernandes, M.J.S.; et al. Pilocarpine-Induced Status Epilepticus Increases the Sensitivity of P2X7 and P2Y1 Receptors to Nucleotides at Neural Progenitor Cells of the Juvenile Rodent Hippocampus. *Cereb. Cortex* **2017**, *27*, 3568–3585. [CrossRef] [PubMed]

19. Khan, M.T.; Liu, J.; Tang, Y.; Illes, P. Regulation of P2X7 receptor function of neural progenitor cells in the hippocampal subgranular zone by neuronal activity in the *dentate gyrus*. *Neuropharmacology* **2018**, *140*, 139–149. [CrossRef] [PubMed]

20. Dossi, E.; Heine, C.; Servettini, I.; Gullo, F.; Sygnecka, K.; Franke, H.; Illes, P.; Wanke, E. Functional regeneration of the ex-vivo reconstructed mesocorticolimbic dopaminergic system. *Cereb. Cortex* **2013**, *23*, 2905–2922. [CrossRef] [PubMed]

21. Gao, P.; Ding, X.; Khan, T.M.; Rong, W.; Franke, H.; Illes, P. P2X7 receptor-sensitivity of astrocytes and neurons in the *substantia gelatinosa* of organotypic spinal cord slices of the mouse depends on the length of the culture period. *Neuroscience* **2017**, *349*, 195–207. [CrossRef] [PubMed]

22. Oliveira, J.F.; Riedel, T.; Leichsenring, A.; Heine, C.; Franke, H.; Krugel, U.; Norenberg, W.; Illes, P. Rodent cortical astroglia express in situ functional P2X7 receptors sensing pathologically high ATP concentrations. *Cereb. Cortex* **2011**, *21*, 806–820. [CrossRef] [PubMed]

23. Martin, A.; Domercq, M.; Matute, C. Inflammation in stroke: The role of cholinergic, purinergic and glutamatergic signaling. *Ther. Adv. Neurol. Disord.* **2018**, *11*, 1756286418774267. [CrossRef] [PubMed]

24. Vezzani, A. Epilepsy and inflammation in the brain: Overview and pathophysiology. *Epilepsy Curr.* **2014**, *14*, 3–7. [CrossRef] [PubMed]

25. Webster, K.M.; Sun, M.; Crack, P.; O'Brien, T.J.; Shultz, S.R.; Semple, B.D. Inflammation in epileptogenesis after traumatic brain injury. *J. Neuroinflammation* **2017**, *14*, 10. [CrossRef] [PubMed]

26. Leichsenring, A.; Riedel, T.; Qin, Y.; Rubini, P.; Illes, P. Anoxic depolarization of hippocampal astrocytes: Possible modulation by P2X7 receptors. *Neurochem. Int.* **2013**, *62*, 15–22. [CrossRef] [PubMed]

27. Roger, S.; Pelegrin, P.; Surprenant, A. Facilitation of P2X7 receptor currernts and membrane blebbing via constitutive and dynamic calmodulin binding. *J. Neurosci.* **2008**, *28*, 6393–6401. [CrossRef] [PubMed]

28. Probert, L.; Akassoglou, K.; Pasparakis, M.; Kontogeorgos, G.; Kollias, G. Spontaneous inflammatory demyelinating disease in transgenic mice showing central nervous system-specific expression of tumor necrosis factor alpha. *Proc. Natl. Acad. Sci. USA* **1995**, *92*, 11294–11298. [CrossRef] [PubMed]

29. Godukhin, O.V.; Levin, S.G.; Parnyshkova, E.Y. The effects of interleukin-10 on the development of epileptiform activity in the hippocampus induced by transient hypoxia, bicuculline, and electrical kindling. *Neurosci. Behav. Physiol.* **2009**, *39*, 625–631. [CrossRef] [PubMed]

30. Galic, M.A.; Riazi, K.; Heida, J.G.; Mouihate, A.; Fournier, N.M.; Spencer, S.J.; Kalynchuk, L.E.; Teskey, G.C.; Pittman, Q.J. Postnatal inflammation increases seizure susceptibility in adult rats. *J. Neurosci.* **2008**, *28*, 6904–6913. [CrossRef] [PubMed]

31. Harre, E.M.; Galic, M.A.; Mouihate, A.; Noorbakhsh, F.; Pittman, Q.J. Neonatal inflammation produces selective behavioural deficits and alters N-methyl-D-aspartate receptor subunit mRNA in the adult rat brain. *Eur. J. Neurosci.* **2008**, *27*, 644–653. [CrossRef] [PubMed]

32. Vezzani, A.; Viviani, B. Neuromodulatory properties of inflammatory cytokines and their impact on neuronal excitability. *Neuropharmacology* **2015**, *96*, 70–82. [CrossRef] [PubMed]

33. Solle, M.; Labasi, J.; Perregaux, D.G.; Stam, E.; Petrushova, N.; Koller, B.H.; Griffiths, R.J.; Gabel, C.A. Altered cytokine production in mice lacking P2X7 receptors. *J. Biol. Chem.* **2001**, *276*, 125–132. [CrossRef] [PubMed]

34. Yan, Z.; Khadra, A.; Sherman, A.; Stojilkovic, S.S. Calcium-dependent block of P2X7 receptor channel function is allosteric. *J. Gen. Physiol.* **2011**, *138*, 437–452. [CrossRef] [PubMed]

35. Leschinger, A.; Stabel, J.; Igelmund, P.; Heinemann, U. Pharmacological and electrographic properties of epileptiform activity induced by elevated K^+ and lowered Ca^{2+} and Mg^{2+} concentration in rat hippocampal slices. *Exp. Brain. Res.* **1993**, *96*, 230–240. [CrossRef] [PubMed]

36. Franke, H.; Illes, P. Nucleotide signaling in astrogliosis. *Neurosci. Lett.* **2014**, *565*, 14–22. [CrossRef] [PubMed]

37. Franke, H.; Illes, P. Pathological potential of astroglial purinergic receptors. *Adv. Neurobiol.* **2014**, *11*, 213–256. [PubMed]

38. Franke, H.; Verkhratsky, A.; Burnstock, G.; Illes, P. Pathophysiology of astroglial purinergic signalling. *Purinergic Signal.* **2012**, *8*, 629–657. [CrossRef] [PubMed]

39. Franke, H.; Günther, A.; Grosche, J.; Schmidt, R.; Rossner, S.; Reinhardt, R.; Faber-Zuschratter, H.; Schneider, D.; Illes, P. P2X7 receptor expression after ischemia in the cerebral cortex of rats. *J. Neuropathol. Exp. Neurol.* **2004**, *63*, 686–699. [CrossRef] [PubMed]

40. Bai, H.Y.; Li, A.P. P2X7 receptors in cerebral ischemia. *Neurosci. Bull.* **2013**, *29*, 390–398. [CrossRef] [PubMed]

41. Melani, A.; Amadio, S.; Gianfriddo, M.; Vannucchi, M.G.; Volonte, C.; Bernardi, G.; Pedata, F.; Sancesario, G. P2X7 receptor modulation on microglial cells and reduction of brain infarct caused by middle cerebral artery occlusion in rat. *J. Cereb. Blood Flow Metab.* **2006**, *26*, 974–982. [CrossRef] [PubMed]

42. Kaiser, M.; Penk, A.; Franke, H.; Krugel, U.; Norenberg, W.; Huster, D.; Schaefer, M. Lack of functional P2X7 receptor aggravates brain edema development after middle cerebral artery occlusion. *Purinergic Signal.* **2016**, *12*, 453–463. [CrossRef] [PubMed]
43. Yu, Q.; Guo, Z.; Liu, X.; Ouyang, Q.; He, C.; Burnstock, G.; Yuan, H.; Xiang, Z. Block of P2X7 receptors could partly reverse the delayed neuronal death in area CA1 of the hippocampus after transient global cerebral ischemia. *Purinergic Signal.* **2013**, *9*, 663–675. [CrossRef] [PubMed]
44. Chu, K.; Yin, B.; Wang, J.; Peng, G.; Liang, H.; Xu, Z.; Du, Y.; Fang, M.; Xia, Q.; Luo, B. Inhibition of P2X7 receptor ameliorates transient global cerebral ischemia/reperfusion injury via modulating inflammatory responses in the rat hippocampus. *J. Neuroinflammation* **2012**, *9*, 69. [CrossRef] [PubMed]
45. Wirkner, K.; Kofalvi, A.; Fischer, W.; Gunther, A.; Franke, H.; Groger-Arndt, H.; Norenberg, W.; Madarasz, E.; Vizi, E.S.; Schneider, D.; et al. Supersensitivity of P2X receptors in cerebrocortical cell cultures after in vitro ischemia. *J. Neurochem.* **2005**, *95*, 1421–1437. [CrossRef] [PubMed]
46. Dubé, C.M.; Brewster, A.L.; Richichi, C.; Zha, Q.; Baram, T.Z. Fever, febrile seizures and epilepsy. *Trends Neurosci.* **2007**, *30*, 490–496. [CrossRef] [PubMed]

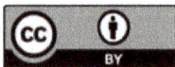

Article

Syncytial Isopotentiality: An Electrical Feature of Spinal Cord Astrocyte Networks

Mi Huang [1,2], Yixing Du [2], Conrad M. Kiyoshi [2], Xiao Wu [2,3], Candice C. Askwith [2], Dana M. McTigue [2] and Min Zhou [2,*]

[1]   Department of Spine Surgery, Wuhan First Hospital, Wuhan 430022, China; huang.3155@osu.edu
[2]   Department of Neuroscience, Ohio State University Wexner Medical Center, Columbus, OH 43210, USA; du.337@osu.edu (Y.D.); kiyoshi.1@osu.edu (C.M.K.); xiao.wu@osumc.edu (X.W.); askwith.1@osu.edu (C.C.A.); mctigue.2@osu.edu (D.M.M.)
[3]   Department of Neurology, Wuhan First Hospital, Wuhan 430022, China
*   Correspondence: zhou.787@osu.edu; Tel.: +1-614-366-9406

Received: 2 August 2018; Accepted: 22 August 2018; Published: 24 August 2018

Abstract: Due to strong electrical coupling, syncytial isopotentiality emerges as a physiological mechanism that coordinates astrocytes into a highly efficient system in brain homeostasis. Although this electrophysiological phenomenon has now been observed in astrocyte networks established by different astrocyte subtypes, the spinal cord remains a brain region that is still unexplored. In ALDH1L1-eGFP transgenic mice, astrocytes can be visualized by confocal microscopy and the spinal cord astrocytes in grey matter are organized in a distinctive pattern. Namely, each astrocyte resides with more directly coupled neighbors at shorter interastrocytic distances compared to protoplasmic astrocytes in the hippocampal CA1 region. In whole-cell patch clamp recording, the spinal cord grey matter astrocytes exhibit passive K^+ conductance and a highly hyperpolarized membrane potential of -80 mV. To answer whether syncytial isopotentiality is a shared feature of astrocyte networks in the spinal cord, the K^+ content in a physiological recording solution was substituted by equimolar Na^+ for whole-cell recording in spinal cord slices. In uncoupled single astrocytes, this substitution of endogenous K^+ with Na^+ is known to depolarize astrocytes to around 0 mV as predicted by Goldman–Hodgkin–Katz (GHK) equation. In contrast, the existence of syncytial isopotentiality is indicated by a disobedience of the GHK predication as the recorded astrocyte's membrane potential remains at a quasi-physiological level that is comparable to its neighbors due to strong electrical coupling. We showed that the strength of syncytial isopotentiality in spinal cord grey matter is significantly stronger than that of astrocyte network in the hippocampal CA1 region. Thus, this study corroborates the notion that syncytial isopotentiality most likely represents a system-wide electrical feature of astrocytic networks throughout the brain.

Keywords: astrocytes; spinal cord; gap junctions; electrical coupling; syncytial isopotentiality

1. Introduction

A distinctive feature of astrocytes lies in the establishment of the largest syncytial networks through gap junction coupling. The syncytial networks run through the entire central nervous system (CNS), including astrocytes in the spinal cord [1,2]. Over several decades, this unique anatomic attribute has sparked the speculation and exploration of the physiological mechanisms that enable astrocytes to indeed function as a system in the brain function [3,4]. One mechanism that was revealed in our recent study shows that strong electrical coupling enables hippocampal astrocytes to constantly equalize their membrane potentials so that a syncytial isopotentiality can be achieved [5]. Functionally, the dependence of syncytial isopotentiality for the operation of the K^+ spatial buffering was speculated over 20 years [6]. Now, our study indeed showed that a sustained and highly efficient K^+ uptake driving force crucially depends on gap junctional coupling, which establishes syncytial isopotentiality [5].

Syncytial isopotentiality was initially identified from hippocampal astrocytes. Thereafter, the syncytial isopotentiality has been further uncovered as a broadly existing electrophysiological phenomenon in other parts of the brain, including protoplasmic astrocytes in the motor, sensory and visual cortical regions; cerebellar Bergman glia; velate astrocytes; and fibrous astrocytes in the *corpus callosum* [7]. The spinal cord constitutes a major portion of CNS, which connects the brain to the peripheral nervous system. However, it remains unknown whether syncytial isopotentiality also operates in astrocyte networks in this critical part of the brain. This question is important because astrocytes in different brain subregions vary in their cell morphology, spatial organization, association with different neuronal circuitries and gene expression [8–13]. Additionally, an early study, which used an elegant fluorescence after photo-bleaching (FRAP) method, showed that the cultured spinal cord astrocytes exhibited poor syncytial coupling compared to other brain regions [2].

To answer this question, we have examined the morphology, spatial organization pattern and syncytial isopotentiality expression in spinal cord grey matter. In doing so, confocal microscopy was used to examine the morphology of astrocytes and their spatial organizations in ALDH1L1-eGFP mice at a high resolution. The existence of syncytial isopotentiality was examined by our newly developed methodology, which involves the use of K^+-free/Na^+-containing recording pipette solutions [5].

We showed that astrocytes in cervical spinal cord grey matter are organized with more directly coupled neighbors at shorter interastrocytic distances compared to hippocampal astrocytes. This is associated with a higher strength of syncytial isopotentiality. This finding reinforces the notion that syncytial isopotentiality represents a general feature of astrocytic networks throughout the brain.

2. Materials and Methods

2.1. Animals

All experimental procedures were performed in accordance with a protocol that was approved by the Institutional Animal Care and Use Committee of The Ohio State University (2011A00000065-R2). All experiments were performed with the use of wild-type C57BL/J6 and BAC ALDH1L1-eGFP transgenic mice of both sexes at postnatal day (P) 15−21 [7,14,15]. Mice were housed in a 12-h light/dark cycle and temperature controlled (22 $\pm$ 2 °C) environment with *ad libitum* access to food and water.

2.2. Preparation of Acute Spinal Cord Slices

Mice were anesthetized with 8% chloral hydrate in 0.9% NaCl saline [16]. Spinal cord slices were prepared as previously described with modifications [17]. After deep anesthesia, the spinal cord was removed and placed into ice-cold oxygenated (95%O_2/5%CO_2) cutting artificial cerebrospinal fluid (aCSF) with reduced Ca^{2+} and increased Mg^{2+} (in mM: 125 NaCl, 3.5 KCl, 25 NaHCO$_3$, 1.25 NaH$_2$PO$_4$, 0.1 CaCl$_2$, 3 MgCl$_2$ and 10 glucose). The spinal cord was then transferred into a solid embedding-mold prepared by adding 4% low melt agar to the cutting aCSF, which was followed by the filling of the mold with liquid 2% agar dissolved in the cutting aCSF at ~35 °C. This mixture quickly solidified on ice. Several 400-μm sections were cut from the cervical regions using a Vibratome (MicroSlicer Zero 1N, Ted Pella, Redding, CA, USA) in ice-cold artificial cerebrospinal fluid (in mM: 125 NaCl, 25 NaHCO$_3$, 1.25 NaH$_2$PO$_4$, 3.5 KCl, 2 CaCl$_2$, 1 MgCl$_2$ and 10 glucose, osmolality, 295 $\pm$ 5 mOsm; pH of 7.3–7.4). The slices were allowed to recover from any damage caused by the preparation for at least 15 min at room temperature (RT) before electrophysiological recording.

2.3. Sulforhodamine 101 Staining

After recovery, spinal cord slices were transferred to a slice-holding basket containing 0.6 μM sulforhodamine 101 (SR101) in aCSF at 34 °C for 30 min. After this, the slices were transferred back to normal aCSF at RT before the experiment [14].

2.4. Confocal Imaging of Spinal Cord Astrocyte Syncytia

Anesthetized mice were cardially perfused with 4% paraformaldehyde (PFA) in 0.1 M phosphate-buffered saline (PBS). The 1-mm spinal cord cervical slices were sectioned and post-fixed in 4% PFA/0.1 M PBS at 4 °C overnight. Slices were incubated in a blocking solution, which consisted of 5% normal donkey serum and 0.1% Triton X-100 in PBS, for 24 h at RT. Images were acquired by confocal microscopy (SP8, Leica, Wetzlar, Germany).

2.5. Imaging Acquisition for Astrocyte Identification In Situ

An infrared differential interference contrast (IR-DIC) video camera was used to visualize the macroscopic structure of the spinal cord and astrocyte cell bodies for electrode placement and whole-cell patch clamp recording.

2.6. Electrophysiology

Individual spinal cord slices were transferred to the recording chamber and mounted on an Olympus BX51WI microscope (Center Valley, PA, USA) with constant oxygenated aCSF (2.0 mL/min) bath perfusion. Whole-cell patch clamp recordings were performed using a MultiClamp 700A amplifier and pClamp 9.2 software (Molecular Devices, Sunnyvale, CA, USA). Borosilicate glass pipettes (Warner Instrument, Hamden, CT, USA) were pulled from a Micropipette Puller (Model P-87, Sutter Instrument, Novato, CA, USA). The recording electrodes had a resistance of 3–5 MΩ when filled with the electrode solution that contained (in mM) 140 KCl (or NaCl), 1.0 MgCl$_2$, 0.5 CaCl$_2$, 10 HEPES, 5 EGTA, 3 Mg-ATP and 0.3 Na-GTP (pH = 7.25–7.30, 280 ± 5 mOsm). The physiological 140 KCl-containing pipette solution is referred to as [K$^+$]$_P$, whereas the K$^+$-free/140 mM NaCl-containing pipette solution is referred as [Na$^+$]$_P$ in this study. For whole-cell recording, the liquid junction potential was compensated prior to all recordings. The membrane potential (V_M) was read in I = 0 mode or continuously recorded under the current clamp mode in PClamp 9.2 program. To ensure the quality of current clamp recording, the input resistance (R_{in}) was periodically measured by "Resistance test" (a 63 pA/600 ms pulse) before and during the recording. Recordings with an initial R_{in} greater than 50 MΩ or R_{in} varied greater than 10% during recording were discarded. All the experiments were conducted at RT.

2.7. Chemical Reagents

All chemicals were purchased from Sigma-Aldrich (St. Louis, MO, USA).

2.8. Data Analyses

The patch clamp recording data were analyzed by Clampfit 9.0 (Molecular Devices). Statistical analysis was performed using Origin 8.0 (OriginLab, Northampton, MA, USA) or IBM SPSS Statistics 25.0 (IBM, Armonk, NY, USA). Results are given as means ± standard error of the mean (SEM).

3. Results

3.1. Spatial Organization of Astrocyte Syncytium in Cervical Spinal Cord

To visualize astrocytes and their spatial organization in spinal cord grey matter, the cervical sections of the spinal cord were prepared from ALDH1L1-eGFP mice (Figure 1). The interastrocytic distance and the number of the nearest neighbors for each individual astrocyte were quantitatively analyzed according to the procedure described in our previous reports [7,18].

For interastrocytic distance analysis, the distance between two astrocytes was measured between the nearest neighbors at the central points of the soma (Figure 1C). The grey matter astrocytes were spaced apart at an average of 30.1 ± 1.4 μm (*n* = 30 measurements from 3 slices). This distance is significantly shorter than the distance between astrocytes in the hippocampal CA1 region, which was found to be 39.5 μm in our recent report [7]. We further explored this by analyzing newly prepared hippocampal

CA1 syncytium. Consistently, astrocytes in hippocampal CA1 exhibited significantly longer interastrocytic distances than spinal cord grey matter as they were found to have an average interastrocytic distance of 41 ± 1.2 (n = 30 measurements from 3 slices, $p < 0.001$, image data not shown).

In the nearest neighbor analysis, a randomly chosen astrocyte is set as the reference cell and astrocytes were considered as the nearest neighbors if there was no intermediate astrocyte or a blood vessel between them (Figure 1D) [18]. Each astrocyte in spinal cord grey matter was directly coupled to 9.9 ± 0.3 astrocytes (n = 9 measurements from 3 slices), which was also significantly higher than the number of nearest neighbors of hippocampal CA1 astrocytes (8.7 ± 0.3; n = 9 measurements from 3 slices, $p < 0.01$).

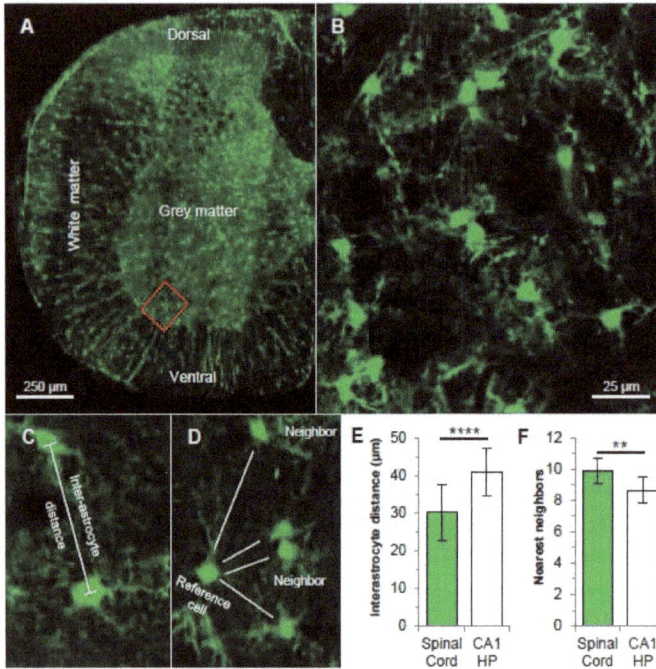

Figure 1. Astrocyte syncytial networks in the cervical spinal cord. (**A**) Confocal image of astrocyte networks in a cervical section of the spinal cord from ALDH1L1-eGFP mouse. (**B**) Astrocytes in a subfield of grey matter marked inside the red rectangle in (**A**) are shown in higher magnification. (**C,D**) Representations of astrocyte syncytium anatomical parameters, which are namely interastrocytic distance and the nearest neighbors as indicated. (**E,F**) In a comparison of the hippocampal CA1 (CA1 HP) region, spinal cord astrocytes show significantly shorter interastrocytic distances (**E**). Furthermore, each spinal cord astrocyte is coupled to ~9 nearest neighbors, which is ~1 more than hippocampal astrocyte. ** $p < 0.01$, **** $p < 0.001$.

Overall, astrocytes in the spinal cord grey matter are organized in a pattern that is distinct from the patterns of astrocytes in hippocampal CA1 and cortical regions. Specifically, each astrocyte is directly coupled to more surrounding neighbors at a shorter interastrocytic distance, which resembles the astrocyte networks that are established by velate astrocytes in the cerebellum [7].

3.2. Electrophysiological Properties of Grey Matter Astrocytes in the Spinal Cord

In acute spinal cord slices, astrocytes in the grey matter could be readily visualized under DIC (Figure 2A,B). Astrocytes can be identified based on the expression of eGFP in ALDH1L1-eGFP transgenic mice or positive staining to astrocytic marker SR101. A representative astrocyte identification based on SR101 staining is shown in Figure 2B,C. Astrocytes in the white matter could hardly be visualized and thus, we have focused on grey matter astrocytes for the following electrophysiological studies.

In whole-cell voltage clamp recording with a K^+-based solution, astrocytes exhibited a characteristic linear current–voltage (I–V) relationship membrane K^+ conductance or passive conductance (Figure 2C,D). This current profile was consistent with the findings of other studies that focused on spinal grey matter [19,20]. Furthermore, these astrocytes exhibit a relatively negative resting membrane potential of -80.8 ± 3.7 mV ($n = 9$) and a low input membrane resistance (R_{in}) of 21.1 ± 7.0 MΩ ($n = 5$). These electrophysiological features also resemble astrocytes in other brain regions, which are namely mature astrocytes in the hippocampus, cortical regions and cerebellum [7,21].

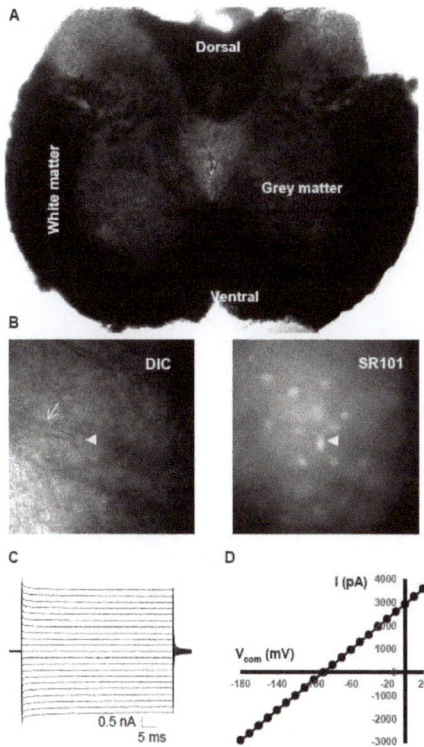

Figure 2. Electrophysiological properties of astrocytes in spinal cord grey matter. (**A**) Differential interference contrast (DIC) image of a cervical spinal cord slice. (**B**) An astrocyte in grey matter identified based on morphology during recording. Arrow and arrowhead point to the recording electrode and a recorded cell, respectively. The astrocytic identity of the recorded cell is confirmed by its sulforhodamine 101 (SR101) positive staining. (**C,D**) Whole-cell recording from an SR101 positively stained astrocyte. For whole-cell membrane current induction, the command voltages, which range from -180 mV to $+20$ mV at increments of 10 mV and duration of 50 ms, were delivered. This induced an ohmic behavioral passive K^+ membrane conductance characterized by a linear current-voltage (I–V) relationship.

3.3. Syncytial Isopotentiality—An Electrical Feature of Spinal Cord Astrocyte Networks

As a result of strong electrical coupling, astrocytes in various brain regions constantly equalize their membrane potential (V_M) so that a syncytial isopotentiality can be achieved [5,7]. Technically, the existence of syncytial isopotentiality can be readily detected by whole-cell membrane potential (V_M) recording with K⁺-free/Na⁺-containing electrode solutions ([Na⁺]ₚ) [5]. Under this condition, dialysis of the recorded cell with [Na⁺]ₚ creates a "K⁺-deficient astrocyte" inside a syncytial network (Figure 3A) and a V_M depolarization to ~0 mV is anticipated in the recorded cell. However, in various brain regions, this V_M depolarization can be largely suppressed by the physiological V_M of astrocytes in the associated syncytium. Consequently, a steady-state quasi-physiological V_M ($V_{M,SS}$) or syncytial isopotentiality remains throughout the recording [5,7]. As shown in Figure 3B, after the rupture of the membrane that switches on the whole-cell mode, the recorded V_M remained at a steady-state level throughout the recording with a $V_{M,SS}$ of -75.2 ± 1.1 ($n = 8$).

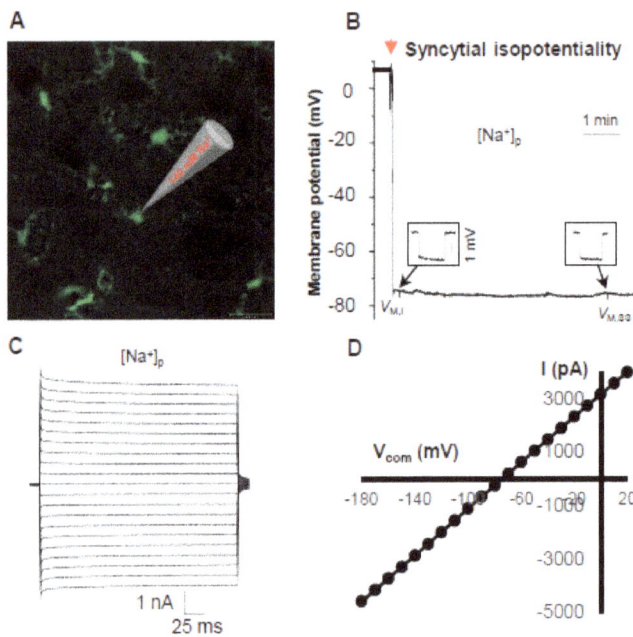

Figure 3. Syncytial isopotentiality in spinal cord grey matter. (**A**) A small field of astrocyte network in grey matter spinal cord revealed from an Aldh1L1-eGFP mouse for illustration of examination of syncytial isopotentiality with K⁺-free/Na⁺-containing electrode solution ([Na⁺]ₚ). (**B**). Membrane potential (V_M) recorded from [Na⁺]ₚ. After reaching a gigaohm formation, the break-in of the membrane, which is indicated by the red arrow, led to a rapid downward deflection of V_M toward the resting V_M. Thereafter, the V_M remained at a steady-state quasi-physiological level ($V_{M,SS}$) at around -75 mV, which indicated a strong electrical coupling of astrocytes that prevents the anticipated depolarization as predicted by Goldman–Hodgkin–Katz (GHK) equation. (**C**) In [Na⁺]ₚ recording, an absence of outward K⁺ conductance is predicted by the GHK equation. However, the "missing" outward K⁺ conductance was fully compensated for by the associated syncytium that resulted in a linear I–V K⁺ conductance (**D**).

In an uncoupled "K⁺-deficient astrocyte", the absence of outward conducting K⁺ ions is anticipated to eliminate the outward K⁺ conductance. In a syncytial coupled "K⁺-deficient astrocyte", this "missing" outward K⁺ conductance can be fully compensated for by its associated syncytium [5]. As shown in Figure 3C,D, in an experimentally created spinal cord "K⁺-deficient astrocyte", the syncytial coupling was indeed able to compensate for the missing outward K^+ conductance to a level so that the resultant linear I–V relationship did not differ from the recordings made with K^+ recording electrode solution (Figure 2D).

In summary, syncytial isopotentiality appears as a shared feature of astrocyte networks in spinal cord grey matter astrocytes. Functionally, a strong gap junction coupling provides spinal cord syncytium with the ability to effectively redistribute K^+ ions throughout the network.

4. Discussion

Now, syncytial isopotentiality has been identified in various brain regions, including the hippocampus, visual, sensory and motor cortex, cerebellar and *corpus callosum* [5,7]. Nevertheless, the spinal cord remains a significant portion of the CNS that has still not been explored. In the present study, this issue was examined using acute slices prepared from the cervical sections of the spinal cord. We showed that syncytial isopotentiality is a shared feature of astrocyte networks in spinal cord grey matter.

4.1. Anatomical Characteristics of Grey Matter Spinal Cord Astrocyte Networks

Astrocytes are known to establish the largest syncytial networks through gap junction coupling in the brain. This distinct anatomic attribute has led to the speculation that astrocytes may act as a system in basic and advanced brain functions [3]. In the search for the mechanisms that enable astrocytes to function at network system levels, syncytial isopotentiality has been revealed as a network physiological mechanism that coordinates astrocytes into a highly efficient system for homeostatic regulation of K^+ concentration in the brain [5].

Now, the study of astrocyte heterogeneity has expanded from early cytoarchitecture to embryonic origins, gene expression and physiological functions [22,23]. In our recent study, we showed that the morphology and spatial organization partners vary from brain region to brain region. However, syncytial isopotentiality is still a general feature of astrocyte syncytial networks [7]. Despite that, a question that is not fully understood is the existence of syncytial isopotentiality in the entire brain and how this is associated with the anatomy of the astrocyte network. An early study from cultured spinal cord astrocytes showed that spinal cord astrocytes exhibited a rather poor gap junction coupling [2]. However, whether this early observation holds true to native spinal cord astrocytes remains unknown.

In our morphological analysis of syncytial organization in the grey matter of the spinal cord, we found that the morphology of individual astrocytes does not differ between the spinal cord and protoplasmic astrocytes in other parts of the brain, such as the hippocampus and visual cortex (data not shown). However, astrocytes in the spinal cord grey matter are characterized by having more surrounding neighbors and a significantly shorter interastrocytic distance compared to those in the hippocampal CA1 region and visual cortex. Interestingly, these features resemble the syncytial network established by velate astrocytes in the cerebellar molecular layer [7].

4.2. Spinal Cord Astrocytes Establish Syncytial Isopotentiality in Their Networks

Extending from our previous studies, the present findings from spinal cord grey matter astrocytes further corroborate the notion that syncytial isopotentiality is a general feature of astrocyte networks. Interestingly, the strength of syncytial isopotentiality in spinal cord astrocytes appears to be stronger than that of hippocampal astrocytes, which was indicated by a more negative $V_{M/SS}$. This is correlated with a shorter interastrocytic distance and one more nearest neighbor. However, although the spinal cord astrocytes share a similar interastrocytic distance and nearest neighbors with velate astrocytes, the latter exhibits a weaker strength of syncytial isopotentiality than the spinal cord. Interestingly, spinal cord astrocytes share a comparable interastrocytic distance and strength of syncytial isopotentiality to astrocytes in layer I motor, sensory and visual cortex, but appear to have one more nearest neighbor.

Previously, we have demonstrated that a minimum of 7–9 directly coupled neighbors is sufficient for establishing syncytial isopotentiality [5]. However, it remains unknown how the fine-tuning of coupling strength is achieved and regulated. From a structural standing point, these observations again stress the importance of the identification of the generic astrocyte-connectome, which underpins syncytial isopotentiality. This could be better answered by electron microscopy (EM) reconstruction of the adjacent astrocytes in conjunction with computational modeling in future studies.

4.3. Pathological Implications Affecting Astrocyte Syncytial Isopotentiality

Astrocytes become reactive in response to neurological injuries and diseases by exhibiting changes in cell morphology, genetic and molecular expression [24]. The expression of gap junction channels and functional dye coupling are reported to be affected in various disease models [25]. A question that yet unknown is how the disease conditions alter syncytial isopotentiality in the spinal cord.

It has been shown that connexin 43 (Cx43), but not connexin 30 (Cx30), plays a critical role in the development of chronic neuropathic pain following spinal cord injury [26]. In compression injuries, Cx43 undergo a marked alteration in localization and expression [27]. These observations suggest that pathological conditions may alter the spatial organization of astrocyte syncytium in the spinal cord, which may subsequently disrupt the physiological syncytial isopotentiality. Nevertheless, no study has yet been carried out to determine a causal relationship between syncytial isopotentiality and the pathogenesis of various types of neurological disorders in the spinal cord.

Author Contributions: M.H. and M.Z.: project conception and design. M.H., Y.D., C.M.K., X.W.: data collection, data analysis, and interpretation. C.C.A.: provided core facility support; M.H., D.M.M., C.C.A., M.Z.: manuscript writing and editing. All authors corrected and approved the manuscript.

Funding: This work is sponsored by grants from the National Institute of Neurological Disorders and Stroke RO1NS062784, R56NS097972 (M.Z.), P30NS104177 (C.C.A.).

Conflicts of Interest: The authors declare no conflict of interest.

References

1. Scemes, E.; Suadicani, S.O.; Spray, D.C. Intercellular communication in spinal cord astrocytes: Fine tuning between gap junctions and P2 nucleotide receptors in calcium wave propagation. *J. Neurosci.* **2000**, *20*, 1435–1445. [CrossRef] [PubMed]
2. Lee, S.H.; Kim, W.T.; Cornell-Bell, A.H.; Sontheimer, H. Astrocytes exhibit regional specificity in gap-junction coupling. *Glia* **1994**, *11*, 315–325. [CrossRef] [PubMed]
3. Nimmerjahn, A.; Bergles, D.E. Large-scale recording of astrocyte activity. *Curr. Opin. Neurobiol.* **2015**, *32*, 95–106. [CrossRef] [PubMed]
4. Verkhratsky, A.; Nedergaard, M. Physiology of Astroglia. *Physiol. Rev.* **2018**, *98*, 239–389. [CrossRef] [PubMed]
5. Ma, B.; Buckalew, R.; Du, Y.; Kiyoshi, C.M.; Alford, C.C.; Wang, W.; McTigue, D.M.; Enyeart, J.J.; Terman, D.; Zhou, M. Gap junction coupling confers isopotentiality on astrocyte syncytium. *Glia* **2016**, *64*, 214–226. [CrossRef] [PubMed]
6. Muller, C.M. Gap-junctional communication in mammalian cortical astrocytes: Development, modifiability and possible functions. In *Gap Junctions in the Nervous System*; Spray, D.C., Ed.; RG Landes Company: Austin, TX, USA, 1996; pp. 203–212.
7. Kiyoshi, C.M.; Du, Y.; Zhong, S.; Wang, W.; Taylor, A.T.; Xiong, B.; Ma, B.; Terman, D.; Zhou, M. Syncytial isopotentiality: A system-wide electrical feature of astrocytic networks in the brain. *Glia* **2018**, in press.
8. Houades, V.; Rouach, N.; Ezan, P.; Kirchhoff, F.; Koulakoff, A.; Giaume, C. Shapes of astrocyte networks in the juvenile brain. *Neuron Glia Biol.* **2006**, *2*, 3–14. [CrossRef] [PubMed]
9. Houades, V.; Koulakoff, A.; Ezan, P.; Seif, I.; Giaume, C. Gap junction-mediated astrocytic networks in the mouse barrel cortex. *J. Neurosci.* **2008**, *28*, 5207–5217. [CrossRef] [PubMed]
10. Roux, L.; Benchenane, K.; Rothstein, J.D.; Bonvento, G.; Giaume, C. Plasticity of astroglial networks in olfactory glomeruli. *Proc. Natl. Acad. Sci. USA* **2011**, *108*, 18442–18446. [CrossRef] [PubMed]

11. Nadarajah, B.; Thomaidou, D.; Evans, W.H.; Parnavelas, J.G. Gap junctions in the adult cerebral cortex: Regional differences in their distribution and cellular expression of connexins. *J. Comp. Neurol.* **1996**, *376*, 326–342. [CrossRef]

12. Morel, L.; Chiang, M.S.R.; Higashimori, H.; Shoneye, T.; Iyer, L.K.; Yelick, J.; Tai, A.; Yang, Y. Molecular and Functional Properties of Regional Astrocytes in the Adult Brain. *J. Neurosci.* **2017**, *37*, 8706–8717. [CrossRef] [PubMed]

13. Zhang, Y.; Barres, B.A. Astrocyte heterogeneity: An underappreciated topic in neurobiology. *Curr. Opin. Neurobiol.* **2010**, *20*, 588–594. [CrossRef] [PubMed]

14. Zhong, S.; Du, Y.; Kiyoshi, C.M.; Ma, B.; Alford, C.C.; Wang, Q.; Yang, Y.; Liu, X.; Zhou, M. Electrophysiological behavior of neonatal astrocytes in hippocampal stratum radiatum. *Mol. Brain* **2016**, *9*, 34. [CrossRef] [PubMed]

15. Yang, Y.; Vidensky, S.; Jin, L.; Jie, C.; Lorenzini, I.; Frankl, M.; Rothstein, J.D. Molecular comparison of GLT1+ and ALDH1L1+ astrocytes in vivo in astroglial reporter mice. *Glia* **2011**, *59*, 200–207. [CrossRef] [PubMed]

16. Wang, W.; Putra, A.; Schools, G.P.; Ma, B.; Chen, H.; Kaczmarek, L.K.; Barhanin, J.; Lesage, F.; Zhou, M. The contribution of TWIK-1 channels to astrocyte K(+) current is limited by retention in intracellular compartments. *Front. Cell. Neurosci.* **2013**, *7*, 246. [CrossRef] [PubMed]

17. Olsen, M.L.; Higashimori, H.; Campbell, S.L.; Hablitz, J.J.; Sontheimer, H. Functional expression of Kir4.1 channels in spinal cord astrocytes. *Glia* **2006**, *53*, 516–528. [CrossRef] [PubMed]

18. Xu, G.; Wang, W.; Kimelberg, H.K.; Zhou, M. Electrical coupling of astrocytes in rat hippocampal slices under physiological and simulated ischemic conditions. *Glia* **2010**, *58*, 481–493. [CrossRef] [PubMed]

19. Ficker, C.; Rozmer, K.; Kato, E.; Ando, R.D.; Schumann, L.; Krugel, U.; Franke, H.; Sperlagh, B.; Riedel, T.; Illes, P. Astrocyte-neuron interaction in the substantia gelatinosa of the spinal cord dorsal horn via P2X7 receptor-mediated release of glutamate and reactive oxygen species. *Glia* **2014**, *62*, 1671–1686. [CrossRef] [PubMed]

20. Minkel, H.R.; Anwer, T.Z.; Arps, K.M.; Brenner, M.; Olsen, M.L. Elevated GFAP induces astrocyte dysfunction in caudal brain regions: A potential mechanism for hindbrain involved symptoms in type II Alexander disease. *Glia* **2015**, *63*, 2285–2297. [CrossRef] [PubMed]

21. Du, Y.; Ma, B.; Kiyoshi, C.M.; Alford, C.C.; Wang, W.; Zhou, M. Freshly dissociated mature hippocampal astrocytes exhibit similar passive membrane conductance and low membrane resistance as syncytial coupled astrocytes. *J. Neurophysiol.* **2015**, *113*, 3744–3750. [CrossRef] [PubMed]

22. Ben Haim, L.; Rowitch, D.H. Functional diversity of astrocytes in neural circuit regulation. *Nat. Rev. Neurosci.* **2017**, *18*, 31–41. [CrossRef] [PubMed]

23. Bayraktar, O.A.; Fuentealba, L.C.; Alvarez-Buylla, A.; Rowitch, D.H. Astrocyte development and heterogeneity. *Cold Spring Harb. Perspect. Biol.* **2014**, *7*, a020362. [CrossRef] [PubMed]

24. Liddelow, S.A.; Barres, B.A. Reactive Astrocytes: Production, Function, and Therapeutic Potential. *Immunity* **2017**, *46*, 957–967. [CrossRef] [PubMed]

25. Giaume, C.; Koulakoff, A.; Roux, L.; Holcman, D.; Rouach, N. Astroglial networks: A step further in neuroglial and gliovascular interactions. *Nat. Rev. Neurosci.* **2010**, *11*, 87–99. [CrossRef] [PubMed]

26. Chen, M.J.; Kress, B.; Han, X.; Moll, K.; Peng, W.; Ji, R.R.; Nedergaard, M. Astrocytic CX43 hemichannels and gap junctions play a crucial role in development of chronic neuropathic pain following spinal cord injury. *Glia* **2012**, *60*, 1660–1670. [CrossRef] [PubMed]

27. Theriault, E.; Frankenstein, U.N.; Hertzberg, E.L.; Nagy, J.I. Connexin43 and astrocytic gap junctions in the rat spinal cord after acute compression injury. *J. Comp. Neurol.* **1997**, *382*, 199–214. [CrossRef]

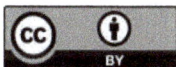

neuroglia

MDPI

Article

Mediation of FoxO1 in Activated Neuroglia Deficient for Nucleoside Diphosphate Kinase B during Vascular Degeneration

Yi Qiu [1,†], Hongpeng Huang [1,†], Anupriya Chatterjee [1], Loïc Dongmo Teuma [1],
Fabienne Suzanne Baumann [1], Hans-Peter Hammes [2], Thomas Wieland [1] and Yuxi Feng [1,*]

1 Experimental Pharmacology, European Center of Angioscience, Medical Faculty Mannheim, Heidelberg
   University, 68167 Mannheim, Germany; yiqiu@hotmail.de (Y.Q.);
   hongpeng.huang@medma.uni-heidelberg.de (H.H.); anupriya.chatterjee@medma.uni-heidelberg.de (A.C.);
   teuma@stud.uni-heidelberg.de (L.D.T.); f.s.baumann@web.de (F.S.B.);
   thomas.wieland@medma.uni-heidelberg.de (T.W.)
2 5th Med, Medical Faculty Mannheim, Heidelberg University, 68167 Mannheim, Germany;
   hans-peter.hammes@medma.uni-heidelberg.de
* Correspondence: yuxi.feng@medma.uni-heidelberg.de; Tel.: +49-621-383-71762
† Y.Q. and H.H. share first authorship.

Received: 4 July 2018; Accepted: 3 September 2018; Published: 7 September 2018

Abstract: The pathogenesis of diabetic retinopathy is closely associated with the breakdown of the neurovascular unit including the glial cells. Deficiency of nucleoside diphosphate kinase B (NDPK-B) results in retinal vasoregression mimicking diabetic retinopathy. Increased retinal expression of Angiopoietin-2 (Ang-2) initiates vasoregression. In this study, Müller cell activation, glial Ang-2 expression, and the underlying mechanisms were investigated in streptozotocin-induced diabetic NDPK-B deficient (KO) retinas and Müller cells isolated from the NDPK-B KO retinas. Müller cells were activated and Ang-2 expression was predominantly increased in Müller cells in normoglycemic NDPK-B KO retinas, similar to diabetic wild type (WT) retinas. Diabetes induction in the NDPK-B KO mice did not further increase its activation. Additionally, cultured NDPK-B KO Müller cells were more activated and showed higher Ang-2 expression than WT cells. Müller cell activation and Ang-2 elevation were observed upon high glucose treatment in WT, but not in NDPK-B KO cells. Moreover, increased levels of the transcription factor forkhead box protein O1 (FoxO1) were detected in non-diabetic NDPK-B KO Müller cells. The siRNA-mediated knockdown of FoxO1 in NDPK-B deficient cells interfered with Ang-2 upregulation. These data suggest that FoxO1 mediates Ang-2 upregulation induced by NDPK-B deficiency in the Müller cells and thus contributes to the onset of retinal vascular degeneration.

Keywords: angiopoietin-2; FoxO1; NDPK-B; neuroglia

1. Introduction

The pathogenesis of diabetic retinopathy (DR) is closely associated with the disturbance in the interplay between the retinal microvasculature, neurons, and glial cells [1]. Diabetic retinopathy is a common complication of diabetes and one of the leading causes of blindness in working-age adults [2]. The first morphological sign of DR is the loss of pericyte coverage in the microvasculature and the formation of acellular capillaries [1]. Several lines of evidence have indicated a pivotal role of angiopoietin-2 (Ang-2) in initiating the loss of pericytes [3–5].

Among the retinal neuroglia, i.e., astrocytes and Müller cells, Müller cells are the principal glial cells of the retina and play an important role in the maintenance of the retinal microenvironment [6]. Müller cells are now considered crucial players in the development of DR. For instance, Müller cells become activated during diabetes, which is indicated by the strong upregulation of the intermediate filament protein glial fibrillary acidic protein (GFAP) [6–8]. They also contribute to the neurotoxicity of glutamate during diabetes [9,10]. Furthermore, Müller cell-derived vascular endothelial growth factor (VEGF) stimulates retinal neovascularization [11]. Müller cells are also connected to DR because they are, besides endothelial cells, an important source of Ang-2 [12,13].

Nucleoside diphosphate kinase B (NDPK-B) is a ubiquitously expressed enzyme required for the synthesis of nucleoside triphosphates [14,15]. It is, besides NDPK-A, the second of the two major isoforms of the NDPK family [16]. NDPK-B has been reported to play multiple roles in cellular functions, including cell proliferation, migration, apoptosis [17–19], and signal transduction [20–22]. NDPK-B also plays a role in retinopathies [23,24]. Our previous data showed that the deficiency of NDPK-B resulted in increased level of Ang-2 in the retina and cultured endothelial cells, which is likely the cause of pericyte loss in NDPK-B deficient mice [24]. As the observed pathology in the eye is similar to DR, NDPK-B deficiency apparently mimics the effects of hyperglycemia at normoglycemic conditions.

In this study, we therefore investigated the role of Müller cells, glial Ang-2 expression, and the underlying mechanisms in the regulation of Ang-2 in the NDPK-B deficient retina. We found that NDPK-B deficiency induced an activation of retinal neuroglia during vascular degeneration, and Ang-2 expression was strongly upregulated in the activated Müller cells. Using Müller cells isolated from NDPK-B deficient retinas, we demonstrated that the transcription factor FoxO1 mediates the Ang-2 upregulation in the NDPK-B deficient retinas.

2. Materials and Methods

2.1. Animals

All animal studies were approved by the local ethics committee (Regierungspraesidium Karlsruhe, Germany), approval number 35-9185.81/G-203/10, date of approval 7 April 2011. The care and experimental use of animals were in accordance with institutional guidelines and in compliance with the Association for Research in Vision and Ophthalmology statement. The generation of NDPK-B$^{-/-}$ mice were as described previously [25]. Diabetes induction was achieved by intraperitoneal (i.p.) injection of streptozotocin (STZ, 145 mg/kg body weight; Roche, Mannheim, Germany) dissolved in citrate buffer (pH 4.5) in 2-month-old male mice. Age-matched mice injected with citrate buffer served as non-diabetic controls. Successful induction of diabetes was confirmed by blood glucose measurements over 250 mg/dL at one week after STZ treatment. Postnatal mice were killed at one week for Müller cell isolation or at three months after diabetes induction for the analysis of retinas.

2.2. Immunofluorescence and Quantification

The eyes were fixed with 4% formalin for 48 h at 4 °C and were dehydrated, paraffinized, and subsequently embedded in paraffin blocks. Sections of 6 μm were made and collected on silanized glass object slides. The sections were initially deparaffinized with incubation at 60 °C. The slides were then cooled and further de-paraffinized with Roti-Histol (Roth, Karlsruhe, Germany) and hydrated with ethanol solution of decreasing concentrations. Antigen retrieval treatment was performed by heating the slides in citrate buffer. After cooling down, the sections were washed and then blocked/permeabilized with 2.5% bovine serum albumin (BSA) and 0.3% Triton for 1 h at room temperature. Afterwards, the sections were incubated in primary antibodies at 4 °C overnight, then with corresponding secondary antibodies conjugated with fluorescein isothyocyanate (FITC) or tetramethylrhodamine (TRITC) for 1 h. Nuclear staining was done with 4′,6-diamidino-2-phenylindole (DAPI) for 15 min at room temperature. The sections were mounted with Roti-Mount FluorCare (Roth, Karlsruhe, Germany). The primary antibodies were rabbit-anti-GFAP (Dako, Glostrup, Denmark), rabbit-anti-Ang-2 (Acris, Herford, Germany), mouse-anti-Cellular retinaldehyde binding protein (CRALBP) (Abcam, Cambridge, UK), and mouse-anti-glutamine synthetase (GS) (Merck Millipore,

Darmstaft, Germany). The secondary antibodies were swine-anti-rabbit FITC (Dako, Glostrup, Denmark), swine-anti-rabbit TRITC (Dako, Glostrup, Denmark), and goat-anti-mouse FITC (Sigma-Aldrich, Saint Louis, MO, USA). Images were taken with a confocal laser scanning microscope (Leica Microsystems, Wetzlar, Germany). Immunofluorescence staining of the paraffin sections was quantified by measuring the mean gray value of images. The expression pattern for GFAP and Ang-2 were measured using Image J software (NIH, Bethesda, MD, USA).

For Müller cell characterization, the cells were fixed in 4% paraformaldehyde for 10 min at room temperature. After washing steps, the cells were incubated in blocking/permeabilization buffer with 2.5% BSA and 0.3% Triton for 1 h. Then, the cells were stained with primary antibodies against GFAP, CRALBP, or GS overnight and corresponding secondary antibodies were used on the second day. Nuclei were counterstained with DAPI. Finally, photos were taken with a fluorescence microscope (Olympus, BX-51, Hamburg, Germany).

2.3. Cell Culture and High Glucose Stimulation

Müller cells were isolated from 8–10-day-old NDPK-B deficient and wild type (WT) mice as previously described [26,27]. The cells were cultured at 37 °C, 5% CO_2 in a humidified incubator in DMEM containing 10% FCS, 200 mM Glutamine, which was replenished every 3–4 days. Cells until passage 4 were used in the experiments. The cells were seeded onto 6-well plates and serum-starved (0.5% FCS) overnight followed by stimulation with 30 mM D-glucose (high glucose, HG) or 5.5 mM D-glucose (normal glucose, NG) for 24 h as described [24].

2.4. siRNA Mediated FoxO1 Knockdown in Müller Cells

siRNA transfection was performed using lipofectamine RNAiMax (Life Technologies, Darmstadt, Germany) according to the manufacturer's protocol. FoxO1-specific siRNA (GGU UCU AAU UUC CAG AUA ATT) and control siRNA (Qiagen, Hilden, Germany) were used. Forty-eight hours after transfection, the cells were collected and used for Western blot analysis.

2.5. Western Blot

Western blot was performed using Müller cell proteins extracted with the radioimmunoprecipitation assay buffer (RIPA buffer) as previously described [23]. The proteins were separated by SDS-PAGE and transferred onto nitrocellulose membranes. After blocking with Roti-block (Roth), the membranes were incubated with primary antibodies overnight and then with corresponding secondary antibodies and visualized using a chemiluminescent peroxidase substrate (Roche; or Thermo Scientific, Rockford, IL, USA). Protein expression was quantified using Image J (NIH, USA). Specific primary antibodies were mouse-anti-NDPK-B (Kamiya Biomedical, Seattle, WA, USA), rabbit-anti-Ang-2 (Acris, Herford, Germany), rabbit-anti-FoxO1 (Cell Signaling Technology, Beverly, MA, USA), rabbit-anti-GFAP (Dako, Glostrup, Denmark), and mouse-anti-Tubulin (Sigma-Aldrich, Munich, Germany). The secondary antibodies were rabbit-anti-mouse, goat-anti-rabbit or rabbit-anti-goat from Sigma-Aldrich.

2.6. Quantitative Real Time PCR

Quantitative real time PCR was performed as described previously [5]. In brief, RNA was isolated from Müller cells homogenized in 1 mL Trizol reagent (Invitrogen, Karlsruhe, Germany) at 4 °C according to the manufacturer's instructions. RNA was then reverse transcribed with Superscript VILO cDNA synthesis kit (Thermo Fischer Scientific, Darmstadt, Germany) and subjected to Taqman analysis using the Taqman 2 × PCR master Mix (Applied Biosystems, Weiterstadt, Germany). The expression of genes was analysed by the 2−ΔΔCT method using β-Actin as housekeeping control. All primers and probes labeled with MGB-FAM for amplification were purchased from Thermo Fisher Scientific, β-Actin: Mm00607939_s1; Ang-2: Mm00545822_m1.

2.7. Statistical Analysis

Data are represented as mean ± standard error of the mean (SEM). One-way ANOVA with Bonferroni post-test was performed using GraphPad Prism 5 (GraphPad Software, La Jolla, CA, USA). *p*-values < 0.05 were considered significant.

3. Results

3.1. Müller Cells Are Activated in NDPK-B Deficient Retinas

Müller cell activation is an important process in the development of diabetic retinopathy [6]. Vascular degeneration occurring in NDPK-B deficient retinas without hyperglycemia mimics vascular pathology in DR [24]. Therefore, we investigated firstly, if glial cells were activated in the NDPK-B knockout (KO) retinas by detecting the expression of GFAP using immunoblotting and immunofluorescence. As shown in Figure 1A,B, in NDPK-B KO non-diabetic (NC) retinas, the expression of GFAP increased significantly in comparison with WT non-diabetic retinas (WT NC) (*p* < 0.01 vs. WT NC). Diabetes (DC) significantly enhanced GFAP expression in WT retinas as expected (*p* < 0.05, WT DC vs. WT NC). GFAP expression in diabetic NDPK-B KO (KO DC) retinas were also significantly enhanced compared to WT NC (*p* < 0.001), but diabetes induction in KO animals did not further enhance GFAP expression as compared to WT DC and KO NC retinas.

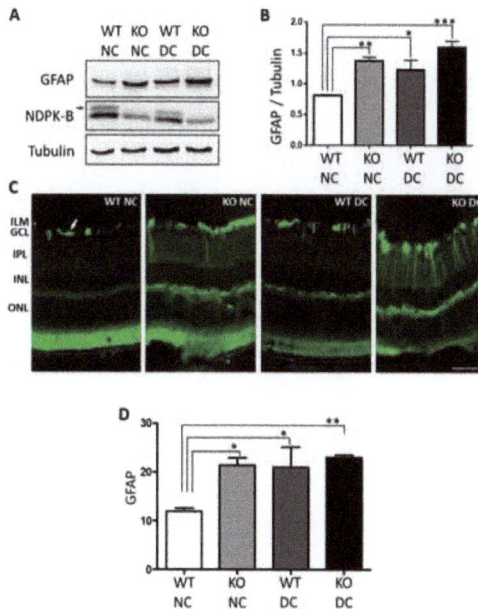

Figure 1. Müller cells are activated in NDPK-B deficient retinas. (**A,B**): representative Western blot and quantification of GFAP (glial fibrillary acidic protein) expression in the retina. In both KO NC and WT DC retina, GFAP levels significantly increased compared to WT NC retinas; GFAP level in KO DC retinas is similar to KO NC and WT DC retinas. (**C,D**): Immunofluorescence staining and quantification of GFAP in the retina. GFAP localized in astrocytes in WT NC retinas (arrow). Diabetes increased a radial expression pattern of GFAP immunoreactivity similar to Müller cells. NDPK-B deficiency induced a staining pattern similar to WT DC. KO: NDPK-B knockout; DC: diabetic; NC: non-diabetic; WT: wild type; ILM: inner limiting membrane; GCL: ganglion cell layer; IPL: inner plexiform layer; INL: inner nuclear layer; ONL: outer nuclear layer. Scale bar: 50 μm. * *p* < 0.05, ** *p* < 0.01, *n* = 3–4 in each group.

Additionally, we assessed the localization of elevated GFAP expression in the NDPK-B deficient retinas by staining the retinal paraffin sections with GFAP. As shown in Figure 1C, GFAP in WT NC retinas was predominantly localized in the astrocytes. Diabetes induced increased GFAP expression not only in the astrocytes but also a fiber-like staining pattern across the entire WT retina, indicating an enhanced expression of GFAP in the Müller cells. NDPK-B deficient retinas showed GFAP staining pattern similar to WT DC retinas, exhibiting markedly enhanced GFAP expression in astrocytes and Müller cells. There was significant increase in GFAP expression in KO NC/DC and WT DC compared to WT NC, but no difference between WT/KO DC as well as KO NC/DC. In the negative control staining, no signal was detected in the astrocytes or in the Müller cells (data not shown). GFAP expression by astrocytes in WT NC and by astrocyte and Müller cells in WT DC and KO retinas were confirmed by co-staining GFAP with the Müller cell marker GS (Supplementary Figure S1). Taken together, the elevated levels of GFAP in both the NDPK-B deficient and diabetic retinas verify the activation of retinal astrocytes/Müller cells, confirming the similarity between these two models [24].

3.2. Ang-2 Is Preferentially Upregulated in Müller Cells in the Retina during Vascular Degeneration

Our previous data have shown that diabetes as well as the loss of NDPK-B caused a significant increase in Ang-2 levels in the retina [24]. To identify the source of upregulated Ang-2 in the NDPK-B retinas, we stained Ang-2 in retinal paraffin sections and investigated its localization. As shown in Figure 2, Ang-2 prominently localized in fiber-like structure spanning across the entire thickness of the retina, mostly in the inner retina. When the sections were co-stained against CRALBP, a Müller cell marker, the majority of Ang-2 co-localized with CRALBP, identifying retinal Müller cells as the major source of retinal Ang-2. In WT NC retinas Ang-2 was only detected at modest levels, whereas under NDPK-B deficient and diabetic conditions, Ang-2 was expressed abundantly in Müller cells. The Ang-2 staining intensity in diabetic NDPK-B KO retinas was similar to NDPK-B KO NC and WT DC retinas. Ang-2 levels were significantly enhanced in KO NC, WT DC, and KO DC groups compared to WT NC. These results confirm our previously published data showing that Ang-2 levels are elevated in hyperglycemia and in NDPK-B deficient retinas [24]. The main source of the upregulated Ang-2 in hyperglycemia and NDPK-B deficient retinas appears to be the Müller cells.

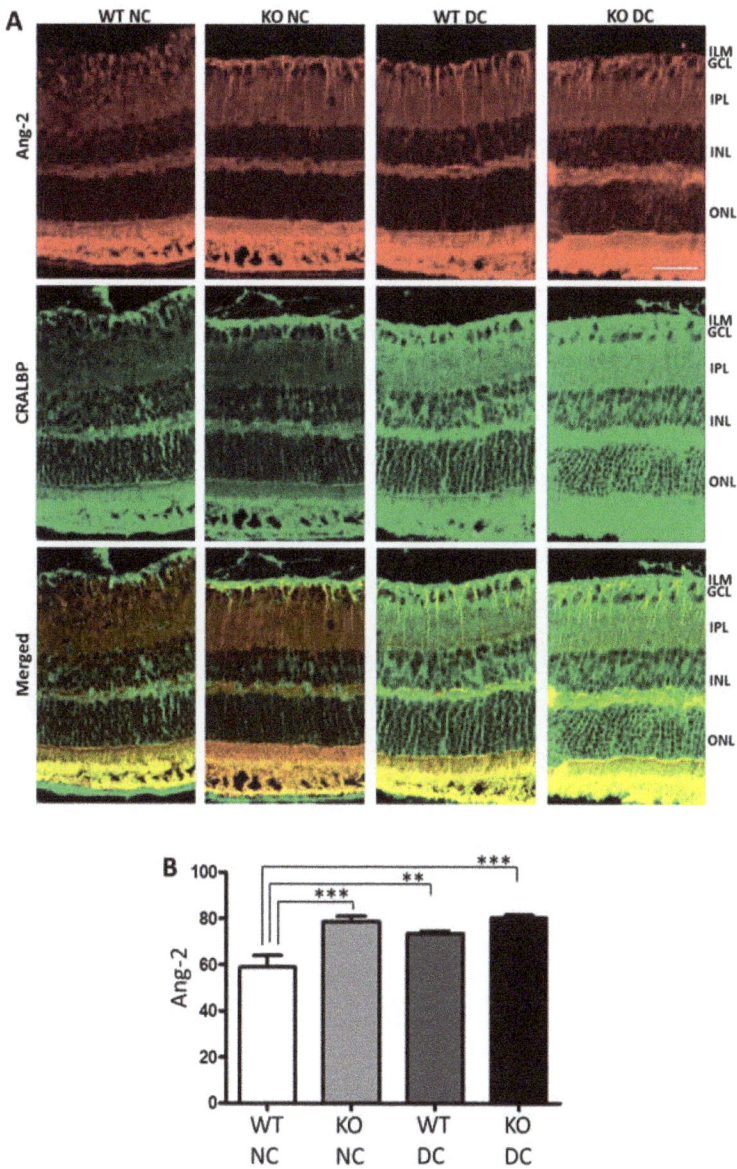

Figure 2. Ang-2 is upregulated in Müller cells in the retina. Immunofluorescence staining (**A**) and quantification (**B**) of Ang-2. Ang-2 (red) and the Müller cell marker CRALBP (green) were stained in the retina. Significantly enhanced levels of Ang-2 were detected in KO NC, WT DC, and KO DC conditions compared to WT NC. As shown the merged images, the majority of Ang-2 was detected in the CRALBP positive Müller cells. ILM: inner limiting membrane; GCL: ganglion cell layer; IPL: inner plexiform layer; INL: inner nuclear layer; ONL: outer nuclear layer. Scale bar: 50 μm. ** $p < 0.01$, *** $p < 0.001$, n = 4–5 in each group.

3.3. NDPK-B Deficiency Caused Enhancement of Ang-2 in Isolated Müller Cells

To verify Müller cells as a source of Ang-2 expression in NDPK B-deficient retinas and to further investigate the underlying mechanisms, we isolated Müller cells from NDPK-B KO and WT mice. The Müller cells were characterized by the positive staining for GFAP, GS, and CRALBP (Supplementary Figure S2). Firstly, we examined the GFAP levels of the WT and KO cells using Western blotting to determine the activation status of the isolated cells. As shown in Figure 3A,B, a basal GFAP expression was detectable in WT cells incubated in NG condition. In WT cells stimulated with HG, GFAP levels increased significantly compared with WT NG cells ($p < 0.05$). In NDPK-B deficiency GFAP levels were even higher ($p < 0.001$ vs. WT NG). GFAP levels in NDPK-B KO NG are higher than WT HG cells, indicating KO NG Müller cells are more active than the WT HG cells. In KO cells stimulated with HG, GFAP levels were significantly higher compared with WT cells stimulated with HG ($p < 0.05$), but were not further increased compared to KO NG cells. The deficiency of NDPK-B in the KO cells was confirmed by immunoblotting. These data confirm the previously stated results from the retinal immunofluorescence and demonstrate that NDPK-B deficiency induces the Müller cell activation, thereby mimicking the effect of hyperglycemia/high glucose.

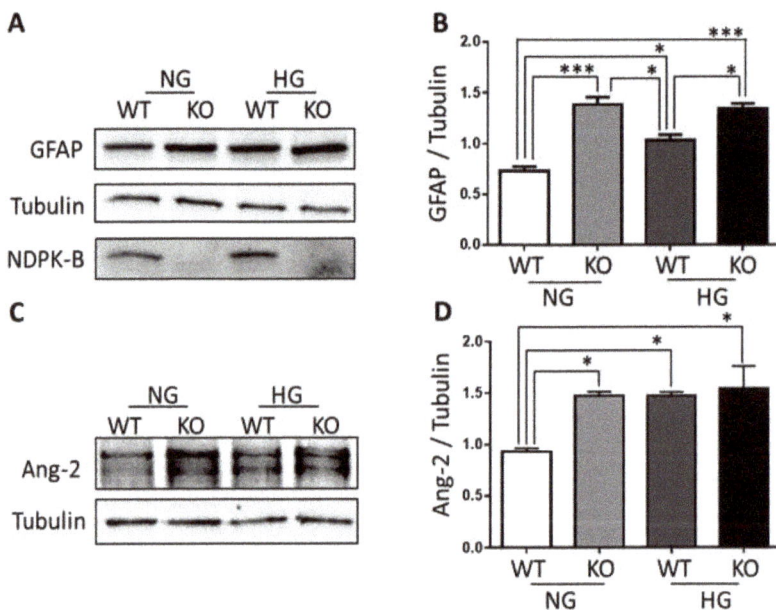

Figure 3. NDPK-B deficiency enhanced Ang-2 content in isolated Müller cells. (**A,B**): Representative Western blot and quantification of GFAP expression in the Müller cells, respectively. In both KO normal glucose (NG) cells and WT high glucose (HG) cells, the level of GFAP increased significantly compared to WT NG cells. GFAP in KO HG cells is significantly higher than in WT HG cells. * $p < 0.05$, *** $p < 0.001$, $n = 4$. (**C,D**): Representative Western blot and quantification of Ang-2 expression in the isolated NDPK-B KO Müller cells. Both NDPK-B deficiency and HG induced a significant increase in Ang-2 levels in the Müller cells. The level of Ang-2 in KO HG cells was similar as in KO NG cells and WT HG cells. * $p < 0.05$, $n = 4$.

Subsequently, we examined Ang-2 expression in the isolated Müller cells by Western blotting (Figure 3C,D). HG treatment significantly increased the Ang-2 expression ($p < 0.05$ vs. WT NG), which is in agreement with previously published data [28]. Similar to the whole retina lysates, NDPK-B deficiency increased the Ang-2 content in cultured Müller cells to a similar level observed in

WT cells stimulated with HG ($p < 0.05$ vs. WT NG). However, when NDPK-B KO cells were treated with HG, no further elevation of Ang-2 was detected. There was no difference in Ang-2 levels between KO NG, WT HG and KO HG. The data are in agreement with those on Ang-2 regulation in the diabetic NDPK-B deficient retinas we published before [24]. To assess the transcriptional regulation of Ang-2, we performed quantitative PCR in Müller cells isolated from KO and WT retinas with and without HG stimulation. Neither NDPK-B deficiency nor high glucose stimulation regulated Ang-2 expression in Müller cells (Supplementary Figure S3).

3.4. FoxO1 Is Required for NDPK-B Deficiency Induced Ang-2 Upregulation in Müller Cells

The transcription factor FoxO1 has been shown to regulate Ang-2 expression [29,30]. To examine whether FoxO1 is involved in the NDPK-B deficiency-induced Ang-2 upregulation, we estimated the level of FoxO1 in isolated NDPK-B KO Müller cells. As shown in Figure 4A,B, in NDPK-B KO cells, FoxO1 expression increased significantly compared to WT Müller cells under NG condition ($p < 0.05$); FoxO1 level did not further increase when KO Müller cells were stimulated with HG. In WT Müller cells stimulated with HG, a similar increase in the FoxO1 level was observed, which however did not reach statistical significance. Nevertheless, the data imply a possible role for FoxO1 in the regulation of Ang-2 in NDPK-B deficient Müller cells.

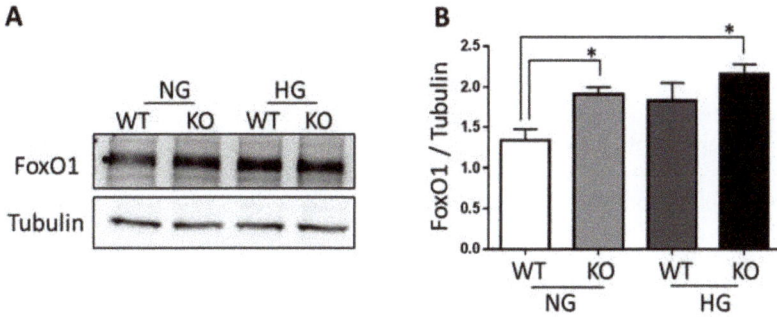

Figure 4. FoxO1 is increased in NDPK-B KO Müller cells. (**A,B**): Representative Western blot and quantification of FoxO1 content in the Müller cells, respectively. NDPK-B deficiency significantly increased FoxO1 in the Müller cells compared to WT NG cells. The FoxO1 level in KO HG cells is similar to KO NG cells. * $p < 0.05$, $n = 5$.

To examine whether FoxO1 controls the enhancement of Ang-2 induced by NDPK-B deficiency in Müller cells, we performed siRNA-mediated knockdown of FoxO1 and quantified the expression of Ang-2. As shown in Figure 5, FoxO1 depletion was successfully achieved by siRNA-mediated gene knockdown. In WT Müller cells, FoxO1 knockdown resulted in a decrease in Ang-2 levels (WT siControl vs. WT siFoxO1: $p < 0.05$). In KO Müller cells, NDPK-B deficiency significantly enhanced Ang-2 (KO siControl vs. WT siControl: $p < 0.001$). This increase of Ang-2 in NDPK-B KO Müller cells was suppressed by FoxO1 knockdown (KO siFoxO1 vs. KO siControl: $p < 0.001$). Taken together, these data argue for FoxO1 as an important mediator in NDPK-B deficiency-induced Ang-2 upregulation in Müller cells during vascular degeneration.

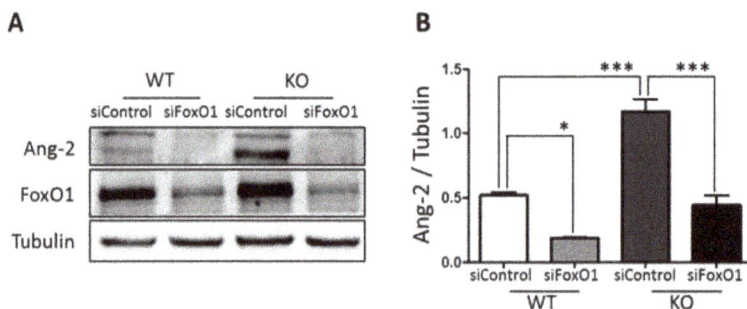

Figure 5. FoxO1 is required for Ang-2 upregulation induced by NDPK-B deficiency in Müller cells. (**A,B**): Representative Western blot and quantification of Ang-2 expression in Müller cells isolated from WT and NDPK-B deficient mice 48 h after siRNA transfection. FoxO1 knockdown suppressed the inhibited basal as well as NDPK-B deficiency induced Ang-2 content. siControl: control siRNA, siFoxO1: FoxO1 siRNA. * $p < 0.05$, *** $p < 0.001$, $n = 4$.

4. Discussion

In this study, we demonstrated that NDPK-B deficiency led to an activation of neuroglia in the retina during vascular degeneration, and that Ang-2 expression was strongly and preferentially upregulated in cells stained by the retinal Müller cell marker CRALBP. We confirmed, by isolation and culture of Müller cells, that enhanced Ang-2 expression due to NDPK-B deficiency indeed occurred in Müller cells and required the transcription factor FoxO1 as mediator for the Ang-2 upregulation. Importantly, hyperglycemia or HG treatment of WT Müller cells caused a similar activation of Müller cells and upregulation of Ang-2 expression upon NDPK-B deficiency.

We have previously demonstrated that NDPK-B deficiency is a risk factor for development of DR and showed that the retinal level of Ang-2 is elevated in NDPK-B deficiency-related vascular degeneration in the eyes [24]. Ang-2 is normally produced and released by endothelial cells [31,32]. In the retina, however, Müller cells are considered to be another important source for Ang-2 [11,12]. Although in our previous study, a similar upregulation of Ang-2 was found in endothelial cells [24], the immunofluorescence staining of Ang-2 in the retina performed herein fully supports that Müller cells are a major source of Ang-2 in the retina thus at least partially responsible for driving the vasoregressive pathology. In accordance with this, transgenic mOpsinhAng-2 mice with overexpression of human Ang-2 in the photoreceptor cells exhibited reduced pericyte coverage [33] and intravitreal injection of recombinant Ang-2 led to pericyte dropout [5]. These data show that Ang-2 secretion in the retina leads to pericyte loss independent of the source of Ang-2. As Müller cells and endothelial cells synergistically overproduce Ang-2 in the retina, both cell types are likely responsible for the DR-like pathology occurring under NDPK-B deficiency. How NDPK-B regulates Ang-2 remains elusive. Berberich et al. reported that NDPK-B may regulate gene transcriptional elements through the NDPK-B/PuF binding site [34]. Our data demonstrated that NDPK-B likely regulates Ang-2 through translational but not transcriptional levels, although NDPK-B may act as a co-transcriptional regulator. Ang-2 might be regulated by NDPK-B in an indirect manner.

We found that the presence and expression level of the transcription factor FoxO1 is important for the NDPK-B deficiency-induced Ang-2 in activated Müller cells isolated from NDPK-B deficient and littermate WT retinas. Whether the observed increase in FoxO1 content occurs also in other cells of the retina is currently not known. Due to lack of antibodies detecting FoxO1 in retinal paraffin sections and cryosections, we were not able to address this question directly. Nevertheless, we recently found that siRNA-mediated depletion of NDPK-B in endothelial cells increased the FoxO1 content, and like HG treatment, induced the upregulation of Ang-2 [24]. These data indicate that FoxO1 might be associated with the upregulation of Ang-2 in retinal endothelial cells as well as Müller cells.

Interestingly, FoxO1 might also be the regulatory factor where the effects of NDPK-B deficiency and hyperglycemia/HG treatment converge. Levels of FoxO1 tended to be increased in HG treated Müller cells, and the NDPK-B deficiency-induced upregulation of Ang-2 was attenuated by FoxO1 depletion. Indeed, a transcriptional regulation of Ang-2 by FoxO1 has been reported previously [29,30]. FoxO1 plays an important role in the insulin pathway [35,36], and is an apoptotic factor in retinal endothelial cells and pericytes [37,38]. The activity of FoxO1 can be regulated by multiple pathways, such as the insulin pathway though IRS-1 and Akt, the ROS through c-Jun N-terminal kinase (JNK) signaling [35]. Furthermore, O-GlcNAc modification of FoxO1 increases its activity in hepatocytes [39,40]. How NDPK-B deficiency upregulates FoxO1 in Müller cells remains unclear, but taking into account that high glucose levels also enhance protein O-GlcNAcylation of proteins, this might be an interesting hypothesis. On the other hand, HG also upregulates Ang-2 through enhanced O-GlcNAc and methylglyoxal modification of the transcription factors Sp3 [28]. Thus, other possibilities have to be considered as well. Therefore, more work is needed to identify how NDPK-B-deficiency and hyperglycemia regulate the activity and content of FoxO1 in endothelial and Müller cells.

Supplementary Materials: The following are available online at http://www.mdpi.com/2571-6980/1/1/19/s1, Figure S1: GFAP is expressed in astrocytes and Müller cells in the retina, Figure S2: Characterization of Müller cells in vitro, Figure S3: Ang-2 RNA expression is unaltered in NDPK-B KO NG/HG and WT NG/HG Müller cells.

Author Contributions: Conceptualization, H.-P.H., T.W., and Y.F.; Formal analysis, Y.Q., H.H., and A.C.; Funding acquisition, Y.F.; Investigation, Y.Q., H.H., L.D.T., F.S.B., and A.C.; Methodology, Y.Q., H.H., L.D.T., F.S.B., and A.C.; Project administration, T.W. and Y.F.; Supervision, H.-P.H., T.W., and Y.F.; Validation, H.H.; Writing—original draft, Y.Q. and Y.F.; Writing—review & editing, H.H., A.C., H.-P.H., T.W., and Y.F.

Funding: This research was funded by the European Foundation for the Study of Diabetes (EFSD, Novartis-2014, Y.F.), the Deutsche Forschungsgemeinschaft (DFG, FE 969/2-1) and the Deutsche Diabetes Gesellschaft (DDG, A.C.).

Acknowledgments: The authors thank Heike Rauscher for her excellent technical assistance. We are grateful to Michael Potente from Max Planck Institute for Heart and Lung Research, Bad Nauheim, for his support.

Conflicts of Interest: The authors declare no conflict of interest. The funders had no role in the design of the study; in the collection, analyses, or interpretation of data; in the writing of the manuscript, and in the decision to publish the results.

References

1. Hammes, H.P.; Feng, Y.; Pfister, F.; Brownlee, M. Diabetic retinopathy: Targeting vasoregression. *Diabetes* **2011**, *60*, 9–16. [CrossRef] [PubMed]
2. Frank, R.N. Diabetic retinopathy. *N. Engl. J. Med.* **2004**, *350*, 48–58. [CrossRef] [PubMed]
3. Feng, Y.; Vom Hagen, F.; Wang, Y.; Beck, S.; Schreiter, K.; Pfister, F.; Hoffmann, S.; Wagner, P.; Seeliger, M.; Molema, G. The absence of angiopoietin-2 leads to abnormal vascular maturation and persistent proliferative retinopathy. *Thromb. Haemost.* **2009**, *102*, 120–130. [CrossRef] [PubMed]
4. Hammes, H.-P.; Lin, J.; Wagner, P.; Feng, Y.; Vom Hagen, F.; Krzizok, T.; Renner, O.; Breier, G.; Brownlee, M.; Deutsch, U. Angiopoietin-2 causes pericyte dropout in the normal retina: Evidence for involvement in diabetic retinopathy. *Diabetes* **2004**, *53*, 1104–1110. [CrossRef] [PubMed]
5. Pfister, F.; Wang, Y.; Schreiter, K.; Vom Hagen, F.; Altvater, K.; Hoffmann, S.; Deutsch, U.; Hammes, H.-P.; Feng, Y. Retinal overexpression of angiopoietin-2 mimics diabetic retinopathy and enhances vascular damages in hyperglycemia. *Acta Diabetol.* **2010**, *47*, 59–64. [CrossRef] [PubMed]
6. Bringmann, A.; Pannicke, T.; Grosche, J.; Francke, M.; Wiedemann, P.; Skatchkov, S.N.; Osborne, N.N.; Reichenbach, A. Müller cells in the healthy and diseased retina. *Prog. Retin. Eye Res.* **2006**, *25*, 397–424. [CrossRef] [PubMed]
7. Bringmann, A.; Iandiev, I.; Pannicke, T.; Wurm, A.; Hollborn, M.; Wiedemann, P.; Osborne, N.N.; Reichenbach, A. Cellular signaling and factors involved in Müller cell gliosis: Neuroprotective and detrimental effects. *Prog. Retin. Eye Res.* **2009**, *28*, 423–451. [CrossRef] [PubMed]

8. Zong, H.; Ward, M.; Madden, A.; Yong, P.; Limb, G.; Curtis, T.; Stitt, A. Hyperglycaemia-induced pro-inflammatory responses by retinal Müller glia are regulated by the receptor for advanced glycation end-products (rage). *Diabetologia* **2010**, *53*, 2656–2666. [CrossRef] [PubMed]

9. Bringmann, A.; Pannicke, T.; Biedermann, B.; Francke, M.; Iandiev, I.; Grosche, J.; Wiedemann, P.; Albrecht, J.; Reichenbach, A. Role of retinal glial cells in neurotransmitter uptake and metabolism. *Neurochem. Int.* **2009**, *54*, 143–160. [CrossRef] [PubMed]

10. Reichelt, W.; Stabel-Burow, J.; Pannicke, T.; Weichert, H.; Heinemann, U. The glutathione level of retinal Müller glial cells is dependent on the high-affinity sodium-dependent uptake of glutamate. *Neuroscience* **1997**, *77*, 1213–1224. [CrossRef]

11. Bai, Y.; Ma, J.X.; Guo, J.; Wang, J.; Zhu, M.; Chen, Y.; Le, Y.Z. Müller cell-derived VEGF is a significant contributor to retinal neovascularization. *J. Pathol.* **2009**, *219*, 446–454. [CrossRef] [PubMed]

12. Hammes, H.-P.; Porta, M. Subject Index. In *Experimental Approaches to Diabetic Retinopathy*; Karger Publishers: Basel, Switzerland, 2010; Volume 20, pp. 229–232.

13. Matsumura, T.; Hammes, H.-P.; Thornalley, P.J.; Edelstein, D.; Brownlee, M. Hyperglycemia increases angiopoietin-2 expression in retinal muller cells through superoxide-induced overproduction of [Alpha]-Oxoaldehyde age precursors. *Diabetes* **2000**, *49*, A55.

14. Gilles, A.-M.; Presecan, E.; Vonica, A.; Lascu, I. Nucleoside diphosphate kinase from human erythrocytes. Structural characterization of the two polypeptide chains responsible for heterogeneity of the hexameric enzyme. *J. Biol. Chem.* **1991**, *266*, 8784–8789. [PubMed]

15. Lascu, I.; Gonin, P. The catalytic mechanism of nucleoside diphosphate kinases. *J. Bioenerg. Biomembr.* **2000**, *32*, 237–246. [CrossRef] [PubMed]

16. Janin, J.; Dumas, C.; Moréra, S.; Xu, Y.; Meyer, P.; Chiadmi, M.; Cherfils, J. Three-dimensional structure of nucleoside diphosphate kinase. *J. Bioenerg. Biomembr.* **2000**, *32*, 215–225. [CrossRef] [PubMed]

17. Fancsalszky, L.; Monostori, E.; Farkas, Z.; Pourkarimi, E.; Masoudi, N.; Hargitai, B.; Bosnar, M.H.; Deželjin, M.; Zsákai, A.; Vellai, T. NDK-1, the homolog of NM23-H1/H2 regulates cell migration and apoptotic engulfment in C. Elegans. *PLoS ONE* **2014**, *9*, e92687. [CrossRef] [PubMed]

18. Fournier, H.-N.; Albigès-Rizo, C.; Block, M.R. New insights into NM23 control of cell adhesion and migration. *J. Bioenerg. Biomembr.* **2003**, *35*, 81–87. [CrossRef] [PubMed]

19. Snider, N.T.; Altshuler, P.J.; Omary, M.B. Modulation of cytoskeletal dynamics by mammalian nucleoside diphosphate kinase (NDPK) proteins. *Naunyn-Schmiedeberg's Arch. Pharmacol.* **2015**, *388*, 189–197. [CrossRef] [PubMed]

20. Hippe, H.-J.; Luedde, M.; Lutz, S.; Koehler, H.; Eschenhagen, T.; Frey, N.; Katus, H.A.; Wieland, T.; Niroomand, F. Regulation of cardiac camp synthesis and contractility by nucleoside diphosphate kinase b/g protein $\beta\gamma$ dimer complexes. *Circ. Res.* **2007**, *100*, 1191–1199. [CrossRef] [PubMed]

21. Hippe, H.-J.; Lutz, S.; Cuello, F.; Knorr, K.; Vogt, A.; Jakobs, K.H.; Wieland, T.; Niroomand, F. Activation of heterotrimeric G proteins by a high energy phosphate transfer via nucleoside diphosphate kinase (NDPK) B and Gβ subunits specific activation of G$_s\alpha$ by an NDPK B·G$\beta\gamma$ complex in H10 cells. *J. Biol. Chem.* **2003**, *278*, 7227–7233. [CrossRef] [PubMed]

22. Hippe, H.-J.; Wolf, N.M.; Abu-Taha, H.I.; Lutz, S.; Le Lay, S.; Just, S.; Rottbauer, W.; Katus, H.A.; Wieland, T. Nucleoside diphosphate kinase B is required for the formation of heterotrimeric G protein containing caveolae. *Naunyn-Schmiedeberg's Arch. Pharmacol.* **2011**, *384*, 461–472. [CrossRef] [PubMed]

23. Feng, Y.; Gross, S.; Wolf, N.M.; Butenschön, V.M.; Qiu, Y.; Devraj, K.; Liebner, S.; Kroll, J.; Skolnik, E.Y.; Hammes, H.-P. Nucleoside diphosphate kinase B regulates angiogenesis through modulation of vascular endothelial growth factor receptor type 2 and endothelial adherens junction proteins. *Arterioscler. Throm. Vasc. Biol.* **2014**, *34*, 2292–2300. [CrossRef] [PubMed]

24. Qiu, Y.; Zhao, D.; Butenschön, V.-M.; Bauer, A.T.; Schneider, S.W.; Skolnik, E.Y.; Hammes, H.-P.; Wieland, T.; Feng, Y. Nucleoside diphosphate kinase B deficiency causes a diabetes-like vascular pathology via up-regulation of endothelial angiopoietin-2 in the retina. *Acta Diabetol.* **2016**, *53*, 81–89. [CrossRef] [PubMed]

25. Di, L.; Srivastava, S.; Zhdanova, O.; Sun, Y.; Li, Z.; Skolnik, E.Y. Nucleoside diphosphate kinase B knock-out mice have impaired activation of the k$^+$ channel KCa3. 1, resulting in defective T cell activation. *J. Biol. Chem.* **2010**, *285*, 38765–38771. [CrossRef] [PubMed]

26. Hicks, D.; Courtois, Y. The growth and behaviour of rat retinal Müller cells in vitro 1. An improved method for isolation and culture. *Exp. Eye Res.* **1990**, *51*, 119–129. [CrossRef]

27. Hu, J.; Popp, R.; Frömel, T.; Ehling, M.; Awwad, K.; Adams, R.H.; Hammes, H.-P.; Fleming, I. Müller glia cells regulate Notch signaling and retinal angiogenesis via the generation of 19,20-dihydroxydocosapentaenoic acid. *J. Exp. Med.* **2014**, *211*, 281–295. [CrossRef] [PubMed]

28. Yao, D.; Taguchi, T.; Matsumura, T.; Pestell, R.; Edelstein, D.; Giardino, I.; Suske, G.; Rabbani, N.; Thornalley, P.J.; Sarthy, V.P. High glucose increases angiopoietin-2 transcription in microvascular endothelial cells through methylglyoxal modification of mSin3A. *J. Biol. Chem.* **2007**, *282*, 31038–31045. [CrossRef] [PubMed]

29. Daly, C.; Wong, V.; Burova, E.; Wei, Y.; Zabski, S.; Griffiths, J.; Lai, K.-M.; Lin, H.C.; Ioffe, E.; Yancopoulos, G.D. Angiopoietin-1 modulates endothelial cell function and gene expression via the transcription factor FKHR (FOXO1). *Genes Dev.* **2004**, *18*, 1060–1071. [CrossRef] [PubMed]

30. Potente, M.; Urbich, C.; Sasaki, K.-I.; Hofmann, W.K.; Heeschen, C.; Aicher, A.; Kollipara, R.; DePinho, R.A.; Zeiher, A.M.; Dimmeler, S. Involvement of Foxo transcription factors in angiogenesis and postnatal neovascularization. *J. Clin. Investig.* **2005**, *115*, 2382–2392. [CrossRef] [PubMed]

31. Augustin, H.G.; Koh, G.Y.; Thurston, G.; Alitalo, K. Control of vascular morphogenesis and homeostasis through the angiopoietin-Tie system. *Nat. Rev. Mol. Cell Biol.* **2009**, *10*, 165–177. [CrossRef] [PubMed]

32. Hanahan, D. Signaling vascular morphogenesis and maintenance. *Science* **1997**, *277*, 48–50. [CrossRef] [PubMed]

33. Feng, Y.; Vom, H.F.; Pfister, F.; Djokic, S.; Hoffmann, S.; Back, W.; Wagner, P.; Lin, J.; Deutsch, U.; Hammes, H.P. Impaired pericyte recruitment and abnormal retinal angiogenesis as a result of angiopoietin-2 overexpression. *Thromb. Haemost.* **2007**, *97*, 99–108. [CrossRef] [PubMed]

34. Berberich, S.; Postel, E. PuF/NM23-H2/NDPK-B transactivates a human c-myc promoter-CAT gene via a functional nuclease hypersensitive element. *Oncogene* **1995**, *10*, 2343–2347. [PubMed]

35. Eijkelenboom, A.; Burgering, B.M.T. Foxos: Signalling integrators for homeostasis maintenance. *Nat. Rev. Mol. Cell Biol.* **2013**, *14*, 83–97. [CrossRef] [PubMed]

36. Nakae, J.; Kitamura, T.; Silver, D.L.; Accili, D. The forkhead transcription factor Foxo1 (Fkhr) confers insulin sensitivity onto glucose-6-phosphatase expression. *J. Clin. Investig.* **2001**, *108*, 1359–1367. [CrossRef] [PubMed]

37. Alikhani, M.; Roy, S.; Graves, D.T. FoxO1 plays an essential role in apoptosis of retinal pericytes. *Mol. Vis.* **2010**, *16*, 408–415. [PubMed]

38. Behl, Y.; Krothapalli, P.; Desta, T.; Roy, S.; Graves, D.T. FoxO1 plays an important role in enhanced microvascular cell apoptosis and microvascular cell loss in type 1 and type 2 diabetic rats. *Diabetes* **2009**, *58*, 917–925. [CrossRef] [PubMed]

39. Housley, M.P.; Rodgers, J.T.; Udeshi, N.D.; Kelly, T.J.; Shabanowitz, J.; Hunt, D.F.; Puigserver, P.; Hart, G.W. O-GlcNAc regulates FoxO activation in response to glucose. *J. Biol. Chem.* **2008**, *283*, 16283–16292. [CrossRef] [PubMed]

40. Kuo, M.; Zilberfarb, V.; Gangneux, N.; Christeff, N.; Issad, T. O-glycosylation of FoxO1 increases its transcriptional activity towards the glucose 6-phosphatase gene. *FEBS Lett.* **2008**, *582*, 829–834. [CrossRef] [PubMed]

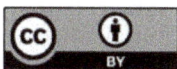

![neuroglia]

neuroglia

MDPI

Review

In Search of a Breakthrough Therapy for Glioblastoma Multiforme

Alex Vasilev [1,†], Roba Sofi [2,†], Li Tong [2], Anja G. Teschemacher [2] and Sergey Kasparov [2,*]

[1] Institute of Living Systems, Immanuel Kant Baltic Federal University, Universitetskaya str, 2, Kaliningrad 236041, Russia; otherlife@bk.ru

[2] School of Physiology, Pharmacology and Neuroscience, University of Bristol, University Walk, Bristol BS8 1TD, UK; roba.sofi@bristol.ac.uk (R.S.); lt17408@my.bristol.ac.uk (L.T.); anja.teschemacher@bristol.ac.uk (A.G.T.)

* Correspondence: sergey.kasparov@bristol.ac.uk; Tel.: +44-117-331-2275

† Those authors make equal contributions to this work.

Received: 21 August 2018; Accepted: 20 September 2018; Published: 26 September 2018

Abstract: Glioblastoma multiforme (GBM) is an extremely malignant type of brain cancer which originates from astrocytes or their precursors. Glioblastoma multiforme cells share some features with astrocytes but are characterized by highly unstable genomes with multiple driver mutations and aberrations. Effective therapies for GBM are lacking and hardly any progress has been made in the last 15 years in terms of improving the outcomes for patients. The lack of new especially targeted anti-GBM medications has prompted scientists in academia around the world to test whether any of the currently approved drugs might be used to fight this devastating disease. This approach is known as repurposing. Dozens of drugs have been reported to have anti-GBM properties in vitro but there is no solid evidence for the clinical efficacy of any of them. Perhaps the most interesting group of those repurposed are tricyclic antidepressants but the mechanism of their action on GBM cells remains obscure. In this brief review we consider various approaches to repurpose drugs for therapy of GBM and highlight their limitations. We also pay special attention to the mitochondria, which appear to be intimately involved in the process of apoptosis and could be a focus of future developments in search of a better treatment for patients suffering from GBM.

Keywords: glioblastoma multiforme; repurposing; tricyclic antidepressants; mitochondria

1. Introduction

Glial cells are an essential component of the mammalian brain and are primarily responsible for its homeostasis. In contrast to neurons, which are terminally differentiated cells where genes responsible for cell division are methylated and essentially inactive, glial cells are much more plastic and even in the human brain they probably can divide, albeit seldomly. This can be seen particularly clearly in case of a mechanical brain trauma, leading to the formation of the so-called glial scars, areas densely populated by astrocytes which show signs of "reactivity". This implies that the parts of the genome required for cell division are accessible in astrocytes, which makes oncogenic transformation of these cells fundamentally possible. Stochastic mutations in genes which control replication eventually trigger uncontrollable division of these cells and formation of a tumor. These tumors can be more or less malignant. The least malignant are low-grade astrocytomas, which in many cases can be treated surgically. Unfortunately, in many patients, multiple mutations and chromosomal aberrations combine, creating increasingly aggressive pools of cells and transformation into glioblastoma multiforme (GBM).

Glioblastoma multiforme is the most common central nervous system (CNS) tumor [1]. There are around 2200 people diagnosed with GBM every year in England, accounting for 55% of malignant brain tumors [2]. According to World Health Organization (WHO) Classification of Tumors of the Central Nervous System, GBM is categorized as grade IV glioma, the most malignant one [1]. Glioblastoma multiforme either appears as de novo (primary GBM), or through progression of a lower grade glioma, leading to a secondary GBM [1]. Despite the dramatic advances in understanding the molecular basis of malignant glioma, this type of cancer is very aggressive and still incurable. The median survival after diagnosis is 10–11 months with standard treatment [3], and the overall 5-year survival is less than 5% [4]. Burnet et al. reported that GBM is the cause of the greatest average loss of life-years among all cancers [5].

Standard treatment of GBM involves surgical resection with radiotherapy and chemotherapy. However, recurrence seems to be inevitable [6]. Complete surgical resection of GMB is hardly ever possible because the boundaries of GBM are diffuse. The tumor sends "streaks" along nervous tracts and blood vessels, and often surgeons have no choice but to leave certain areas untouched because of the risk of causing severe disabilities in the patients [7].

In 2005, protocols consisting of surgery followed by radiotherapy alone were supplemented by a lipophilic alkylating agent, temozolomide (TMZ), approved by the Food and Drug Administration (FDA). Concurrent and adjuvant chemotherapy with TMZ was found to improve median survival by 2.5 months compared to radiotherapy alone in a large 5-year phase III randomized trial [8]. This so-called "Stupp Protocol" is, to this day, the universally accepted standard of care.

Strikingly, despite the desperate need for new treatments, there have been no other major advances for many years now. This is partially due to the complexity of the problem but also reflects the lack of interest of the pharmaceutical companies in this relatively rare form of cancer. From 2005 to 2015, 216 phase-II or III clinical trials on glioblastoma treatment were registered at clinicaltrial.gov database, some of which are still ongoing [9]. Clinical trials are testing different therapeutic approaches including molecular targeted drugs, immunotherapy, viral vector-based gene therapy, electrotherapy and novel strategies to increase tumor sensitivity to radiotherapy [10]. In addition to the traditional strategies based on the research into the mechanisms of oncogenesis, cell division, and tumor resistance, multiple attempts have been made to improve the outcomes in GBM patients by "repurposing" drugs which are already available in clinics. Quite a few various drugs have been claimed to have anti-GBM effects. The problem with most of these studies is that they were carried out on either in vitro or, at best, on mouse models with transplanted GBM and there is very little solid evidence for any of these strategies to be beneficial clinically.

In this review, we summarize some of the available information on repurposed drugs suggested for therapy of GBM. We specifically focus on two key issues. First, how strong is the evidence that any suggested drug is actually more harmful to GBM than to the healthy cells, are the concentrations used to demonstrate the anti-GBM effects physiologically and clinically relevant? Second, is there any common potential cellular mechanism or target for such drugs, something what might be a point of convergence for the action for at least some of them. We believe that GBM mitochondria could be such a "weak spot" of GBM.

2. Repurposing of Drugs for Glioblastoma Multiforme

Fairly low output of new and effective therapies stimulates efforts directed towards finding any possible new treatments among existent medicines. Table 1 illustrates the plethora of drugs suggested for repurposing against GBM, but the list of such studies is actually significantly longer. Specific anticancer drugs developed for other types of tumors and tested against GBM are not included.

Table 1. Some of the drugs suggested for repurposing as glioblastoma multiforme (GBM) therapeutics and their proposed mechanisms of action.

Agent	Proposed Anti-GBM Mechanism	Existing Indication and Main Mechanism (If Known)	Reference
Nelfinavir	PI3K-Akt signaling inhibition	HIV protease inhibitor	[11]
Cimetidine	Immunomodulation	Peptic ulcers (Histamine H2 blocker)	[12]
Diclofenac	Prostaglandin synthesis inhibition	Inflammation and pain (COX-2 inhibitor)	[13]
Nitroglycerin	Nitric oxide donor	Angina	[14]
Thioridazine	Induces autophagy and upregulates AMPK activity	Antipsychotic psychosis (blocks D_2, $5\text{-}HT_{2A}$ and other receptors)	[15]
Pimozide	Serotonin receptor-7 inhibition	Antipsychotic (blocks D_2, $5\text{-}HT_{2A}$ receptors, has relatively high affinity to $5\text{-}HT_7$ receptors)	[16]
Risperidone	Serotonin receptor-7 inhibition	Schizophrenia, bipolar disorder, and irritability	[16]
Paliperidone	Serotonin receptor-7 inhibition	Antipsychotic (blocks D_2, $5\text{-}HT_{2A}$ receptors, has relatively high affinity to $5\text{-}HT_7$ receptors)	[16]
Apomorphine	Mitochondrial metabolic gene downregulation	Emetic, sometimes used in Parkinson disease. Agonist of DA_2, DA_1, $5\text{-}HT_2$ and $\alpha\text{-}AR$	[17]
Flupenthixol	Dopamine receptor modulation	Antipsychotic (typical anti-D_2-agent)	[18]
Mebendazole	Tubulin polymerization inhibition	Nematode infestations	[19]
Disulfiram	Proteasome and alcohol dehydrogenase inhibition	Alcoholism	[20]
Valproic acid	Histone deacetylase inhibition	Epilepsy	[21]
Levetiracetam	MGMT activity inhibition	Epilepsy	[22]
Methadone	cAMP reduction	Severe pain, opioid agonist	[23]
Sulfasalazine	NF-κB activity suppression	Inflammatory bowel disease	[24]
Captopril	Angiotensin-converting enzyme inhibitor	Hypertension	[25]
Nicardipine	EGF and calcium channel antagonism	Hypertension and angina	[26]
Mibefradil	T-type calcium channel inhibition	Hypertension and angina	[27]
Prazosin	AKT pathway inhibition	Hypertension	[28]
Nimodipine	Calcium channel antagonism	Hypertension and angina	[29]
Minocycline	Apoptosis and autophagy	Antibiotic has multiple known central side effects	[30]
Quinidine	Ornithine decarboxylase activity inhibition	Heart arrhythmia	[31]
Accutane	Reduction of EGFR activity	Acne (13-*cis*-retinoic acid. Has known central side effects)	[32]
Thalidomide	Angiogenesis inhibition	Multiple myeloma, leprosy.	[33]
Dichloroacetate	Inhibition of anaerobic metabolism	Topically: warts removal. Congenital lactic acidosis. Inhibits pyruvate dehydrogenase kinase, which increase mitochondrial consumption of pyruvate.	[34]
Hydroxy-chloroquine	Autophagy inhibition	Malaria	[35]
Chloroquine	Oxidative stress enhancement	Malaria	[36]

PI3K-Akt: phosphoinositide 3-kinase-protein kinase B, HIV: human immunodeficiency virus, COX-2: cyclooxygenase 2, AMPK: adenosine monophosphate activated protein kinase, EGFR: epidermal growth factor receptor, DA: Dopamine, 5-HT: Serotonin, cAMP: Cyclic adenosine monophosphate, NFκB: Nuclear factor kappa-light-chain-enhancer of activated B cells. Table 1 has been compiled based on the literature searches at the time of writing using standard keywords, data from clinical trials database and recent reviews. Conventional anti-cancer therapies are not included, since cancer is their main indication.

Already a quick look at Table 1 suggests that there is very little commonality between the proposed drugs or their suggested mechanisms of action. Moreover, for all these drugs, evidence for their clinical anti-GBM efficacy is weak or lacking altogether. Often anti-GBM effects are reported based on in vitro tests on cultured GBM cells, which in many cases are commercially available lines, which have been in vitro for decades and therefore perhaps are hardly representative of the real biology and genetics of the GBM. It is also noticeable that many of the drugs proposed for therapy of GBM have not been shown to cross the blood-brain barrier (GBM core might have leaky barrier but it the periphery it is probably still sufficiently tight). Importantly, many studies used drugs in vitro without much regard to what is known about the biologically relevant concentrations in humans, or the effect of these chemicals on normal cells at the same concentrations at which they had a negative effect on the GBM. An example of these issues is the reported antiproliferative effect of quinidine which was demonstrated using C6 cell line and a high concentration of the drug, half maximal effective concentration (EC_{50}) = 112 μM [31]. For reference, an average therapeutic plasma concentration of quinidine is 1.68 μg/mL [37], which equals to 2.5 μM when converted to molar concentration. This is just one of many studies with the same limitation. It seems logic that even if an anti-GBM effect of a drug can be demonstrated, one would expect the malignant cells to be more sensitive to such an effect, than the healthy ones. However, studies where accurate comparisons have been made are extremely rare.

Some scientists believe that combination of many repurposed drugs can be advantageous. Kast et al. [38] developed the Coordinated Undermining of Survival Paths protocol, known as CUSP9, based on a combination of nine repurposed drugs which are to be combined with continuous low dose TMZ administration. It was expected to augment the clinical efficacy and tolerability of TMZ. Patients in Belgium are currently being recruited to take part in a phase I clinical trial of this CUSP9 protocol. The primary completion date of this study is March 2019. In theory, combinations of drugs could improve their efficacy but equally their side effects could combine. It remains to be seen whether CUSP9 will be any more successful that previous attempts.

Below we further discuss some commonly used drugs in clinical practice that have been tested on GBM for possible repurposing and try to illustrate some of the limitations of this research.

3. Biguanides: Metformin and Phenformin

Metformin is one of the most commonly prescribed drugs in clinical practice. It is used to treat type II diabetes, polycystic ovary disease, and metabolic syndrome [39]. The use of phenformin has been discontinued because of its side effects.

Biguanides are known to inhibit gluconeogenesis in the liver and stimulate glycolysis by altering the activity of different enzymes involved in these pathways [39]. They also improve the sensitivity of insulin receptors in skeletal muscle cells and enhance insulin-mediated glucose uptake through enhanced activity and translocation of glucose transporters, such as glucose transporter type-4 [39]. Moreover, biguanides increase circulating levels of glucagon-like peptide-1 (GLP-1) and stimulate expression of GLP-1 receptor in the pancreas. GLP-1 increases insulin secretion and decreases glucagon secretion [39]. All these effects are either directly or indirectly related to biguanides' inhibitory effect on complex I of the mitochondrial electron transport chain, reducing ATP and increasing adenosine monophosphate (AMP) production and AMP-activated kinase activity [39]. This effect is stronger with phenformin, thus the higher incidence of side effects, i.e., lactic acidosis [39].

Anti-cancer properties of biguanides were first demonstrated with metformin on pancreatic, breast, and lung cancer [40–43]. Metformin was also found to inhibit proliferation, induce apoptosis, and reduce cell adhesion and invasion of GBM [44–48]. Likewise, phenformin was found to inhibit proliferation of glioma stem cells (GSCs), impair sphere formation, decrease stemness, and induce apoptosis [49].

Some of the proposed mechanisms for the antitumor effect of biguanides include: (1) activation of AMPK which leads to blockade of Rheb (Ras homolog enriched in brain)-mTOR (mammalian target of rapamycin) pathways of protein synthesis and cellular growth and activation of tumor suppressor gene p53 [39], (2) reduction of available insulin which reduces the activity of insulin-like growth factor-1 (IGF-1) anabolic pathway [39], (3) suppression of Febulin-3 and Matrix Metalloproteinase-2 expression [44], (4) stimulation of the expression of tumor suppressor micro RNA (miRNA) Lethal-7 [49].

Anticancer effects of metformin described above were achieved using millimolar concentrations of the drug. Lower concentrations either failed to show statistical significance or did only affect a few (1 of 5) glioma cell lines tested [46,47]. The commonly used concentrations are much higher than average plasma concentration for diabetes treatment; 0.86 mg/L (6.6 μM) [50]. In fact, plasma concentrations exceeding 2.5 mg/L (20 μM) are associated with the risk of lactic acidosis [50].

4. Statins: Atorvastatin, Lovastatin, Simvastatin, and Pravastatin

Statins are 3-hydroxy-3-methyl-glutaryl-coenzyme A reductase (HMG-CoA-R) inhibitors, which are prescribed for their lipid-lowering effect. They inhibit the rate limiting step in the mevalonate pathway in hepatocytes, leading to decreased de novo cholesterol synthesis, intracellular lipid stores, and circulating low-density lipoproteins [51].

The reduction in availability of downstream products of the mevalonate pathway is thought to be a key mechanism for the observed growth inhibiting effect of different statins on different cancer cell types including glioma cells [51–58]. Downstream products of the mevalonate pathway are important for prenylation (activation) of cellular proteins Ras, Rho, and Rac, which are small GTPases critical for regulation of cell growth and survival [51]. Other proposed mechanisms include induction of apoptosis and inhibition of cell migration: Apoptosis may be induced by altering the cellular response to stress through the Jun N-terminal kinase (JNK)-dependent cell death pathway [59], by indirectly activating Caspase-3 [56,57], or by decreasing the expression of antiapoptotic proteins such as Bcl-2 and upregulating the expression of proapoptotic proteins such as Bax and Bim [52]. Cellular migration and invasion may be inhibited through inactivation of focal adhesion kinase (FAK) [60], or decreasing the amount of extracellular matrix-degrading enzymes and matrix metalloproteinases released from microglia into the glioma environment [61]. Atorvastatin was also suggested to decrease the expression of proinflammatory proteins and interleukins (IL) [57].

Therapeutic lipid-lowering doses of statins range between 5–80 mg/day and produce plasma concentrations that range from approximately 2 to 15 nM [62]. However, statin concentrations employed in the above-mentioned in vitro experiments commonly ranged between 1–10 μM. The lower end of this range is already 100-fold higher than the average therapeutic plasma concentration of statins in human. One may also wonder why, if these drugs under realistic in vivo conditions inhibit Ras, Rho and Rac signaling, they do not lead to general toxicity, which would have prevented their wide-spread use.

5. Antimicrobial Agents: Dapsone and Nitroxoline

Dapsone is one of three antibiotics used as first line treatment for leprosy [63]. It is also used to treat dermatitis herpetiformis, malaria, and as a disease-modifying anti-rheumatoid drug [64]. Dapsone is bactericidal and bacteriostatic. It works by inhibiting folic acid synthesis in bacteria [63]. For noninfectious indications, dapsone is used for its ability to inhibit synthesis or function of immune chemotactic factors which impairs functions of neutrophils and limits neutrophil-induced tissue destruction [63].

A recent study has shown that dapsone and dapsone derivatives inhibit glioma cells' anchorage-independent growth (colony formation) and impair glioma cell migration [65]. The authors hypothesized that the antineoplastic effect of dapsone is mediated by inhibition of IL-8. Interleukin-8 is well recognized as growth-promoting and pro-angiogenic factor in many cancer types [64]. By inhibiting IL-8, dapsone impairs neutrophil chemotaxis and migration, and interferes with neutrophil-dependent delivery of vascular endothelial growth factor to glioma cells [65]. In vitro antineoplastic effects of dapsone were achieved using concentrations ranging from 10 to 50 μM, which are slightly higher than average therapeutic molar plasma concentration of dapsone (2–20 μM, calculated from the reported concentration range of 0.5 to 5 mg/L) [66].

Nitroxoline (5-nitro-8-hydroxy-quinoline) is a quinoline-based antibiotic that is FDA approved for treatment of urinary tract infection [67]. Nitroxoline is bactericidal and/or bacteriostatic depending on the type of microorganism [68]. Generally, its mode of action depends on its ability to chelate divalent cations and disrupt the organization of the bacterial cell wall [69]. Nitroxoline has been tested against different types of neoplasia, including bladder, gastrointestinal, lung and breast cancers [67,70,71].

Nitroxoline has been shown to have anti-angiogenic properties. A screen of a library of 175,000 compounds has identified nitroxoline as an inhibitor of methionine aminopeptidase 2 (MetAP-2), which it inhibited in a dose-dependent fashion, with half maximal inhibitory concentration (IC_{50}) = 54.8 nM [71]. Inhibiting MetAP-2 suppresses endothelial cell proliferation. Nitroxoline was also found to inhibit non-cancerous Human Umbilical Vein Endothelial Cells proliferation dose-dependently with IC_{50} = 1.9 μM [71]. In vivo, 60 mg/(kg·day) of nitroxoline was able to inhibit neovascularization in breast cancer [71] and bladder cancer xenografts [67]. This dose for mice is equivalent to the common antimicrobial dose used in human (750 mg/day) [67].

Another mechanistic theory explains the anti-cancer effect of nitroxoline through its inhibitory effect on cathepsin B. Cathepsin B is an enzyme which degrades extracellular matrix enabling invasion, migration, and metastasis of tumor cells. Cathepsin B is found in higher concentrations in invading edges of tumors including glioma tumors [72]. Nitroxoline at concentrations ranging from 0.1–100 μM was shown to reversibly inhibit cathepsin B [73].

In relation to GBM, nitroxoline inhibited growth of U251 and U87 glioma cell lines, induced cell cycle arrest at G_0/G_1, induced apoptosis and decreased invasion in vitro in a dose-dependent manner [74]. Toxic concentrations ranged from 5 to 100 μg/mL (≈26 to 520 μM) [74]. In vivo, a specific strain of genetically engineered mouse (PTEN/KRAS mouse, where PTEN is deleted in astrocytes and human Kirsten rat sarcoma viral oncogene homolog KRAS is overexpressed) which spontaneously develops grade III glioblastomas were injected intraperitonially with 80 mg/(kg·day) nitroxoline. Magnetic Resonance Imaging taken on days 0, 7, and 14 after treatment showed a significant decrease in tumor sizes in treatment group compared to controls [74]. Immunohistochemical staining of brain slices for TUNEL (terminal deoxynucleotidyl transferase dUTP nick end labeling assay of apoptosis), revealed significantly more apoptotic cells in treated mice than control mice [74]. It is important to remember that this study used "long term" GBM cell lines which are in many ways different to the cellular populations found in human GBM patients. There is also no good evidence for nitroxoline to accumulate in the brain.

6. Quinolines: Chloroquine and Quinidine

Since 1947, chloroquine has been used to treat malaria infection. It is also used to treat symptoms of some connective tissue disorders, such as systemic lupus erythematosus and rheumatoid arthritis [75].

Quinolines are widely investigated as adjuvant therapy in cancer treatment [76]. They are believed to inhibit lysosome-dependent autophagy and improve chemo and radio sensitivity [76]. Some of the most recent publications on this matter included breast cancer [77], pancreatic cancer [78,79], lung cancer [80], colon cancer [81], and bladder cancer [82].

Chloroquine was found to increase GBM cells' sensitivity to TMZ by inhibiting autophagy and increasing the production of reactive oxygen species induced by TMZ [83–86]. Golden et al. have demonstrated this effect in vivo in mice bearing human glioma xenografts, with concentrations similar to therapeutic concentrations used for the original indication of the drug (10 mg/kg of chloroquine) [83]. Chloroquine was also reported to potentiate radiation induced apoptosis in GBM cells [87–89]. It seems that the anti-GBM effect of chloroquine deserves more focus, especially as a supplement to TMZ.

7. Antidepressants

Antidepressants often receive special attention as putative anti-GBM agents. Serendipity played a part in their appearance in this field because many cancer and GBM patients are prescribed antidepressants against depression which is a common comorbidity. Depression is not only a result of the psychological burden of the diagnosis but is a consequence of the standard treatment procedures. Interest to the anti-GBM potential has been motivated by findings from retrospective studies such as the large-scale epidemiology study conducted by Walker et al. [90], who found an inverse association between treatment with tricyclic antidepressants (TCA) and the incidence of GBM. Antidepressants have several features which are expected for drugs which could be potentially retargeted towards GBM. They are small and lipid soluble molecules which cross the blood-brain barrier and sequester in the brain in relatively high concentrations. In addition, these drugs are relatively nontoxic and induce few serious side effects.

Many studies investigated the possibility of repurposing antidepressants for GBM treatment. Levkovitz et al. [91] studied the effect of several different antidepressants on apoptotic markers in both glioma C6 and neuroblastoma SH-SY5Y cell lines. They reported that paroxetine and fluoxetine, two serotonin selective reuptake inhibitors (SSRIs), and clomipramine, a TCA, caused apoptosis in both cell lines. Interestingly, the toxic effect of clomipramine on C6 cells developed in almost all-or-nothing manner. At 12 μM there was hardly any toxicity while at 25 μM the effect was already maximal. Similarly, with fluoxetine there was little toxicity at 25 μM but 50 μM had a strong negative effect on viability. This is consistent with the results from a much earlier study in the C6 cell line, showing that fluoxetine caused DNA fragmentation, which is a major known step in apoptosis [92]. Similarly, Liu et al. [93] reported that fluoxetine suppressed the growth of GMB cell lines. The effective concentration of fluoxetine in that study was 25–30 μM in vitro. The authors explained this effect by activation of the intrinsic apoptotic pathway (see below). In vivo, fluoxetine strongly suppressed growth of tumors from U87 implants in the brains of Nu/Nu mice when administered daily at 10 mg/kg orally. Its effect was comparable to that of TMZ at 5 mg/kg intraperitonially. This study illustrates a stark contrast between the available models of GBM and clinic, where fluoxetine has never shown such potency against GMB. Fluvoxamine, another SSRI, at 40 μM was able to suppress migration and invasion of human GBM cell lines (A172, U87-MG, and U251-MG) [94]. This effect was accompanied by inhibition of FAK/Akt mTOR pathway activity. Regarding the feasibility of the concentrations of fluoxetine and other TCA used in anti-GBM studies, human data suggest that they do accumulate in the brain, reaching remarkably high concentrations, up to 10 μg/ml, which converts to approximately 20–30 μM [95,96]. Bielecka-Wajdman et al. [97] examined the influence of six different antidepressants on the phenotypic signature and viability of GSCs isolated from a human GBM cell line. In that study only imipramine and amitriptyline significantly altered cell viability. Imipramine and amitriptyline were most effective in reducing quantity and expression of various stem cell markers, thus silencing the GSC profile. Jeon et al. [98] also used two different GBM cell lines (U87 and C6) and reported that 40 and 60 μM of imipramine-induced cell death in GBM models but, remarkably, not normal primary rat astrocytes. The authors explain the effects of imipramine by activation of autophagy and implicate protein Beclin-1 in this process, because short hairpin RNA (sh-RNA) mediated knock-down of this protein conferred resistance to imipramine-induced cell death. Again, limitations of this study are the use of very old and hypermutated cell lines, and the use of very high concentrations of the antidepressant [98]. In yet another study, Shchors et al. [99] reported that imipramine treatment prolonged the overall survival of glioma-bearing mice by 18 days compared to that of a control cohort. These authors also concluded that TCAs induce autophagic cell death. Their explanation for this effect, however, was different to the previous two studies. The authors proposed that TCAs activate the G-protein αs subunit which, in turn, activates adenylyl cyclase resulting in an elevation of cellular cyclic adenosine monophosphate (cAMP). This was thought to induce autophagy associated cell death in glioma cells via the EPAC branch of the cAMP signaling cascade. This hypothesis was supported by an additional finding that inhibition of the purinergic receptor P2Y$_{12}$, activation of which inhibits adenylyl cyclase, potentiated the effects of imipramine, making the combination of drugs particularly effective [99]. The problem with this explanation is that it relies on the monoamine theory for the mechanism of action of TCA which is the canonical explanation of the antidepressant effect of TCA. It poses that TCA act by inhibiting reuptake of noradrenaline and serotonin into the monoaminergic terminals from which they are released in the brain. Meanwhile in the in vitro experiments on GBM cultures there are neither monoamines, nor the terminals which could release and then reuptake them and therefore the very substrate for the "classic" monoamine-dependent action is lacking. In addition, TCAs block re-uptake of monoamines in nanomolar concentrations, which is orders of magnitude lower than what is commonly used in GBM experiments. Therefore, the effects reported in that paper require a different explanation.

The studies listed above illustrate the issues common to the literature on anti-GBM effects of TCAs (and, in fact, other repurposed drugs). These issues include: (a) use of the GBM cell lines such as C6, which have been in vitro for decades and accumulated mutations and acquired qualities which make them very different to the real tumors in human brain, (b) the use of unrealistically high concentrations of antidepressants, and (c) lack of coherency in terms of the proposed molecular targets for these drugs between different studies. Another major general limitation is the lack of an adequate model for studying toxic effects of these drugs on healthy human cells. Typically, researchers use either primary rodent astrocytes or human embryonic astrocytes. Neither of these are a close replica of mature human astrocytes or a good match for the GBM cells found in the human brain in the second half of life. Therefore, we do not know whether high concentrations of antidepressants used in GMB studies can be tolerated by healthy adult human brain cells or we are dealing with some un-specific cellular toxicity.

8. Are Mitochondria a Possible "Weak Spot" of Glioblastoma Multiforme?

Of many different explanations for the anti-GBM effects of repurposed drugs, one mechanism stands out. Quite a few studies by unconnected groups of researchers eventually implicate mitochondria in anti-tumor and pro-apoptotic effects, registered under different conditions (Figure 1). Abnormalities in mitochondrial gene regulation and metabolism in GBM are well known and have been reviewed elsewhere [100]. From the analysis presented in that review, it appears that multiple mutations of mitochondrial genes reported in various studies do not directly drive onco-transformation into the GBM but may significantly affect the properties of the individual lines or subclones of GBM cells within the same tumor. It is also important to remember that most mitochondrial proteins are encoded by nuclear DNA and it is the changes in the nuclear DNA which result in onco-transformation. Chaotization of gene expression caused by genomic instability may have an impact on the fine tuning of the reactions mediated by these nucleus-encoded proteins in the mitochondria, which depend on the supply of these proteins, possibly making GBM mitochondria more vulnerable. On the other hand, the principle of clonal selection which takes place in tumors, can lead to elimination of the GBM cells with severely dysregulated mitochondrial function. It is worth notice, that there is a paucity of information, concerning differences between mitochondria in "regular" GBM cells and GSCs [100].

Although mitochondria have been suggested to be the key organelle to target in GBM, different studies approach this idea from completely different angles. Some authors believe that it is possible to use the ability of mitochondria to initiate apoptosis by acting on the GBM mitochondria directly with some of the repurposed drugs [101,102]. It has also been proposed that mitochondrially induced apoptosis can be induced indirectly, via Ca^{2+} overload [93] or proteasome inhibition [103]. Finally, there is evidence that mitochondrial biogenesis induced by activation of cAMP-mediated signaling can reduce malignancy of GBM cells [104].

In normal glial cells, cellular energy is mainly produced in mitochondria through aerobic respiration [105]. Yet, metabolism starts with glycolysis, whereby glucose is converted into pyruvate with production of ATP in the cytosol. Pyruvate is then transported into the mitochondria where it is oxidized to acetyl-CoA and then used in the citric acid cycle. Unlike normal cells,

GBM has a lower number of mitochondria, indicating high mitochondrial degradation activity [106]. Glioblastoma multiforme, as well as other cancer cells, are known to have active aerobic glycolysis despite the presence of normal oxygen concentrations, and rely on it, rather than on oxidative phosphorylation as the main source of energy [107,108]. Early studies have found that this metabolic shift, known as Warburg effect, is due to mitochondrial dysfunction in many tumor cell types including glioma [109,110]. The Warburg effect seems to be an essential feature of GBM, but to this day the exact reason for high glycolytic activity of tumor cells is unknown [111]. Possibly, cancer cells cannot fully use pyruvate due to decreased pyruvate transporter activity [106], which transports pyruvate inside the mitochondrial matrix. Pyruvate transporters isolated from mitochondria of tumor cells are slower and have lower affinity to pyruvate than transporters isolated from normal cells' mitochondria [112], limiting pyruvate uptake. In addition, pyruvate in mitochondria of tumor cells undergoes decarboxylation into acetaldehyde instead of oxidation [113]. Two acetaldehydes condense to form acetoin which inhibits pyruvate dehydrogenase complex so that pyruvate cannot be converted into acetyl-CoA [113]. In any case, active glycolysis is a landmark of tumors including GBM and seems to confer to them some important survival advantages, possibly by supplying actively dividing cells with new building blocks for lipids, nucleotides and proteins [111].

9. Mitochondria Are the Central Hub of the "Intrinsic" Apoptotic Pathway

Apoptosis is a cascade of events that leads to programmed cell death which can be triggered by both extrinsic and intrinsic pathways (Figure 1). The extrinsic pathway, also known as the death receptor pathway, is initiated when specific ligands bind and stimulate death receptors on the cell surface, initiating a signaling pathway eventually leading to activation of proteases, called caspases [114]. First, procaspases 8 and 10 are cleaved and activated. Next, they cleave and activate the executioner caspases 3 and 7, which start the apoptotic cascade [114]. The intrinsic pathway of apoptosis is activated by direct damage to the cell, such as metabolic failures, hypoxia, radiotherapy, and chemotherapy. In case of direct damage to DNA, upregulation of proapoptotic and downregulation of prosurvival proteins trigger the opening of the mitochondrial permeability transition pore [114]. This pore allows the release of cytochrome C. Cytochrome C binds to apoptotic peptidase activating factor-1 (Apaf-1) eventually leading to the activation of caspase 9 which, similarly to what was described above for the extrinsic pathway, leads to cleavage of the procaspases into the executioner caspases 3, 6 and 7 and triggers fatal apoptotic events [114–116]. Another factor released by mitochondria into the cytoplasm is Smac, which blocks the function of inhibitor of apoptosis proteins, thus facilitating activation of the executioner caspases [114].

Abnormalities in both apoptotic pathways are usually found in GBM. The extrinsic pathway is inhibited by developing resistance to TRAIL apoptosis cascade (apoptosis triggered by Tumor necrosis factor-Related Apoptosis-Inducing Ligands) in glioma [117]. This apoptotic resistance may result from suppression by mammalian target of rapamycin (mTOR), which is closely associated with cell proliferation and growth [118].

In the intrinsic pathway, inhibitors of apoptosis proteins are overexpressed in human malignant glioma cells [119]. Immunostaining of the mitochondria in human glioma cell lines showed that the prosurvival Bcl-2 protein is upregulated. This pathway may suppress apoptosis in GBM cells after DNA damage [120]. It has been also reported that more than 90% of human GBM samples exhibit elevated levels of pro-survival Bcl-2 such as 12 (BCL2L12) protein which suppresses the executioner caspases 3 and 7 directly [121]. Other studies show elevated levels of prosurvival Bcl-2 family members but also proapoptotic proteins in GBM compared to normal astrocytes [122,123] However, a significant upregulation of prosurvival Bcl-2 and Bcl-X$_L$ and downregulation of proapoptotic Bcl-2 associated X protein (Bax) are shown in GBM recurrences after treatment [124]. Therefore, GBM cells appear to actively counteract the proapoptotic events initiated via mitochondria. Nevertheless, several studies indicate that GBM mitochondria can be affected by drugs leading to the anti-tumor effects.

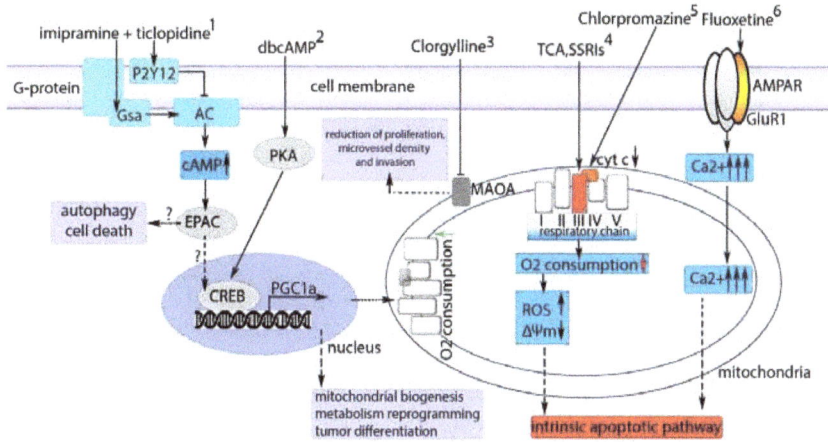

Figure 1. Some of the drugs which could be acting via mitochondria in GBM [107]. Involvement of mitochondria in the mechanism of action of some of the drugs suggested for therapy of GBM. (**1**) Effect of imipramine and P2Y12 purinergic receptor blocker ticlopidine (TIC) on GBM cells, as described by Shchors et al. [99]. Imipramine and TIC together act synergistically. Imipramine activates Gsα protein-coupled monoamine receptors, which in turn activate adenylate cyclase. Ticlopidine blocks P2Y12 receptor, a Gi protein-coupled purinergic receptor that normally inhibits adenylyl cyclase. eventually, activity of adenylate cyclase increases and cAMP level rises leading to -via EPAC pathway- autophagy and cell death. (**2**) Dibutyryl-cAMP (dbcAMP) activates phosphoprotein kinase A and across cAMP response element-binding protein (CREB protein) activates the synthesis of Peroxisome proliferator-activated receptor γ (PPARγ) coactivator 1α (PGC-1α) protein. It finally leads to mitochondrial biogenesis, metabolic reprogramming, and tumor cell differentiation [104]. (**3**) Clorgyline alone or with TMZ acts as monoamine oxidase A inhibitor and reduces tumor growth [125]. (**4**) TCA clomipramine and SSRIs directly interact with complex III of respiratory chain, decreasing O_2 consumption and stimulating reactive oxygen species generation. Mitochondrial membrane potential is reduced finally resulting in apoptosis [101]. (**5**) Chlorpromazine interacts with cytochrome c oxidase and reduces its activity, this leads to cell cycle arrest and inhibition of proliferation of GBM cells [126]. (**6**) Fluoxetine interacts with GluR1 subunit of AMPA receptors, leading to an increase in intracellular Ca^{2+}, mitochondrial calcium overload and activation of the intrinsic apoptotic pathway [93].

10. Antidepressants and Glioblastoma Multiforme Mitochondria

Antidepressants appear to be one group where the involvement of mitochondria has been considered by many studies (Figure 1). Daley et al. [101] demonstrated that the TCA clomipramine can cause cell death of human glioma cells without affecting human fetal astrocytes. A toxic effect of clomipramine on GBM cells was evident within 2 hours of exposure, by which time fetal astrocytes exhibited no clear signs of toxicity. However, this effect only became significant with 114 µM of clomipramine, which is improbable in vivo. In that study, clomipramine concentration-dependently decreased oxygen consumption of glioma cells but, again, the lowest concentration used was 140 µM. This was accompanied by a decrease in mitochondrial membrane potential, which is a direct indicator of the activity of oxidative phosphorylation mechanisms. To explain these effects, the authors measured the effect of clomipramine on the activity of mitochondrial complexes I, II, III and IV, isolated from the mitochondria from various organs. The most consistent effect was the inhibition by 25 µM of clomipramine of complex III activity which was approximately the same in mitochondria from different organs (Figure 1). Importantly, mitochondria were not from GBM cells but were isolated from normal rat tissues. The study also reported activation of caspases which was explained by the insult to the mitochondria caused by clomipramine and the consequent recruitment of the intrinsic pathway mentioned above. On balance, while the study highlights the mitochondria as the direct target for clomipramine, the effective concentrations of the drug appear to be very high and human fetal astrocytes cannot be seen as an adequate model of postnatal human astrocytes, raising the possibility that such high concentrations of clomipramine could be equally toxic to malignant and healthy cells in living brain. At least the study offers no answer as to why mitochondria in GBM could be more sensitive to clomipramine. It is also not entirely clear why the focus was on the short-term effects (1–3 h) while it could be more relevant to look for the effects of lower concentrations developing over longer time scale. For further discussion of this topic see [102].

Mitochondria appear to be the ultimate target for the effect of fluoxetine in the study mentioned previously [93]. That study used glioma cell lines C6 (rat) and U87, GBM8401, Hs683 (human). Fluoxetine had a highly non-linear effect on glioma cell lines, decreasing their viability at concentrations 25–30 µM while at 15–20 µM the effect was hardly visible. Fluoxetine evoked strong elevations in intracellular Ca^{2+} in GBM cell lines, which was attributed to its ability to directly bind to the R1 subunit of glutamate receptors (GluR1) and activate the receptor. Remarkably, normal rat primary astrocytes in that study were fairly resistant to fluoxetine, which the authors explain by high expression of GluR1 on the cell membrane in GBM but not normal astrocytes. It is unclear, though, why GluR1 expression should lead to a strong Ca^{2+} influx because normally Ca^{2+} permeability of AMPA receptors which are formed with GluR1 is low. Nevertheless, the study concludes that Ca^{2+} overload eventually led to mitochondrial damage and activation of the intrinsic apoptotic cascade.

Interestingly, in another study where the effect of fluoxetine was studied on non-GBM cancer cell lines, mitochondrial calcium overload and cell death were explained by a completely different mechanism [127]. The effects were observed after exposure to 100 µM of fluoxetine, a clearly supra-pharmacologic concentration. Fluoxetine is known to enter and accumulate in the mitochondria and seems to be able to inhibit the respiratory chain directly at these concentrations. This could reduce ATP production, which is required for maintenance of the low intracellular Ca^{2+} concentration. Eventually the increased Ca^{2+} load was causing direct damage to the mitochondria and release of pro-apoptotic molecules [127].

Overall, it seems that antidepressants can affect mitochondria in GBM when administered at high concentrations but the explanations for this effect put forward by different groups are inconsistent. It is also worth noting that cytochromes residing in mitochondria are involved in oxidation of numerous molecules and drugs, including antidepressants. One might then ask whether this additional chemical activity, caused by extensive oxidation of xenobiotics, is not the reason these molecules become cytotoxic at sufficiently high concentrations, especially if GBM mitochondria are, indeed, somewhat vulnerable.

11. Can Differences in Glioblastoma Multiforme Mitochondria Be Used for Targeted Therapy?

Typically, GBM mitochondria produce rather high quantities of reactive oxygen species (ROS) which is a consequence of inefficient coupling and oxidative phosphorylation. As mentioned above, one possible reason for this is the loss of fine tuning between mitochondrial and nuclear genomes which is required for perfect functioning of these semi-autonomous organelles. Temozolomide is a typical alkylating agent which primarily disrupts nuclear DNA making cell vulnerable to all kinds of damaging factors including ROS. Interestingly, however, in TMZ-resistant lines mitochondrial coupling is improved compared to the susceptible lines and ROS production is reduced, which is probably a result of the clonal selection mentioned above. It is likely that any treatment targeted at mitochondria in GBM mitochondria can make tumors more susceptible to TMZ chemotherapy [128]. An example of realization of this concept is the development of cytochrome C oxidase inhibitors with tropism to chemo-resistant GBM cells [129,130].

Another interesting idea is based on the high activity of one of the isoforms of monoamine oxidases (MAO), MAO-B in GBM [131]. Monoamine oxidase-B is located on the outer mitochondrial membrane, it is normally highly expressed by astrocytes and oxidizes various amines and other molecules. Activity of MAO-B is also particularly high in glial tumors. The authors generated a pro-drug called *"MP-MUS"* which can be activated by MAO-B and found that this new molecule was selective to primary human glioma cells but, remarkably, had very little toxicity against normal human astrocytes for which the study used commercially available embryonic cells. Encouraging as they are, these results suffer from the same limitation as many other studies mentioned above, because embryonic astrocytes may not be a close match to the astrocytes and other brain cells which populate the brain in the second half of life.

12. Summary

In this brief review we have illustrated some of the current ideas for possible re-targeting of currently available drugs to improve the outcomes for the patients suffering from GBM. Glioblastoma Multiforme represents one of the most difficult cancers to attack not only because of its location and the issues of drug penetration through the blood-brain barrier, but also because of the specific molecular and cellular features of this tumor. Unfortunately, being a relatively small market, GBM does not attract enough interest from the pharmaceutical industry. This puts additional pressure on basic researchers to find new, possibly unconventional, approaches which could help offer a better prognosis to the patients. We have also noted, that within the plethora of suggested mechanisms of action for re-targeted drugs and new developments, mitochondria seem to occupy a particularly prominent place. Potentially mitochondria are the weak spot of GBM which could be exploited to find new therapeutic opportunities.

Author Contributions: Conceptualization, S.K. and A.G.T., Writing—Original Draft, A.V., R.S., L.T., S.K., Writing—Review & Editing, S.K., A.G.T.

Funding: A.V. was supported by 5/100 programme (Russian Federation). R.S. is in receipt of fellowship from King Abdulaziz University (Kingdom of Saudi Arabia). S.K. and A.G.T. were supported by M.R.C. (MR/L020661/1) and BBSRC (BB/L019396/1).

Conflicts of Interest: The authors declare no conflict of interest.

References

1. Adamson, C.; Kanu, O.O.; Mehta, A.I.; Di, C.; Lin, N.; Mattox, A.K.; Bigner, D.D. Glioblastoma multiforme: A review of where we have been and where we are going. *Expert Opin. Investig. Drugs* **2009**, *18*, 1061–1083. [CrossRef] [PubMed]
2. Brodbelt, A.; Greenberg, D.; Winters, T.; Williams, M.; Vernon, S.; Collins, V.P. Glioblastoma in England: 2007–2011. *Eur. J. Cancer* **2015**, *51*, 533–542. [CrossRef] [PubMed]
3. Rick, J.; Chandra, A.; Aghi, M.K. Tumor treating fields: A new approach to glioblastoma therapy. *J. Neurooncol.* **2018**, *137*, 447–453. [CrossRef] [PubMed]
4. Li, Q.J.; Cai, J.Q.; Liu, C.Y. Evolving Molecular Genetics of Glioblastoma. *Chin. Med. J.* **2016**, *129*, 464–471. [CrossRef] [PubMed]
5. Burnet, N.G.; Jefferies, S.J.; Benson, R.J.; Hunt, D.P.; Treasure, F.P. Years of life lost (YLL) from cancer is an important measure of population burden—and should be considered when allocating research funds. *Br. J. Cancer* **2005**, *92*, 241–245. [CrossRef] [PubMed]
6. Alifieris, C.; Trafalis, D.T. Glioblastoma multiforme: Pathogenesis and treatment. *Pharmacol. Ther.* **2015**, *152*, 63–82. [CrossRef] [PubMed]
7. Krivosheya, D.; Prabhu, S.S.; Weinberg, J.S.; Sawaya, R. Technical principles in glioma surgery and preoperative considerations. *J. Neurooncol.* **2016**, *130*, 243–252. [CrossRef] [PubMed]
8. Stupp, R.; Hegi, M.E.; Mason, W.P.; van den Bent, M.J.; Taphoorn, M.J.; Janzer, R.C.; Ludwin, S.K.; Allgeier, A.; Fisher, B.; Belanger, K.; et al. Effects of radiotherapy with concomitant and adjuvant temozolomide versus radiotherapy alone on survival in glioblastoma in a randomised phase III study: 5-Year analysis of the EORTC-NCIC trial. *Lancet Oncol.* **2009**, *10*, 459–466. [CrossRef]

9. Cihoric, N.; Tsikkinis, A.; Minniti, G.; Lagerwaard, F.J.; Herrlinger, U.; Mathier, E.; Soldatovic, I.; Jeremic, B.; Ghadjar, P.; Elicin, O.; et al. Current status and perspectives of interventional clinical trials for glioblastoma—analysis of ClinicalTrials.gov. *Radiat. Oncol.* **2017**, *12*, 1. [CrossRef] [PubMed]

10. Lieberman, F. Glioblastoma update: Molecular biology, diagnosis, treatment, response assessment, and translational clinical trials. *F1000Research* **2017**, *6*, 1892. [CrossRef] [PubMed]

11. Alonso-Basanta, M.; Fang, P.; Maity, A.; Hahn, S.M.; Lustig, R.A.; Dorsey, J.F. A phase I study of nelfinavir concurrent with temozolomide and radiotherapy in patients with glioblastoma multiforme. *J. Neurooncol.* **2014**, *116*, 365–372. [CrossRef] [PubMed]

12. Lefranc, F.; Yeaton, P.; Brotchi, J.; Kiss, R. Cimetidine, an unexpected anti-tumor agent, and its potential for the treatment of glioblastoma (review). *Int. J. Oncol.* **2006**, *28*, 1021–1030. [CrossRef] [PubMed]

13. Pantziarka, P.; Sukhatme, V.; Bouche, G.; Meheus, L.; Sukhatme, V.P. Repurposing Drugs in Oncology (ReDO)-diclofenac as an anti-cancer agent. *Ecancermedicalscience* **2016**, *10*, 610. [CrossRef] [PubMed]

14. Sukhatme, V.; Bouche, G.; Meheus, L.; Sukhatme, V.P.; Pantziarka, P. Repurposing Drugs in Oncology (ReDO)-nitroglycerin as an anti-cancer agent. *Ecancermedicalscience* **2015**, *9*, 568. [CrossRef] [PubMed]

15. Cheng, H.W.; Liang, Y.H.; Kuo, Y.L.; Chuu, C.P.; Lin, C.Y.; Lee, M.H.; Wu, A.T.; Yeh, C.T.; Chen, E.I.; Whang-Peng, J.; et al. Identification of thioridazine, an antipsychotic drug, as an antiglioblastoma and anticancer stem cell agent using public gene expression data. *Cell Death Dis.* **2015**, *6*, e1753. [CrossRef] [PubMed]

16. Kast, R.E. Glioblastoma chemotherapy adjunct via potent serotonin receptor-7 inhibition using currently marketed high-affinity antipsychotic medicines. *Br. J. Pharmacol.* **2010**, *161*, 481–487. [CrossRef] [PubMed]

17. Lee, H.; Kang, S.; Kim, W. Drug Repositioning for Cancer Therapy Based on Large-Scale Drug-Induced Transcriptional Signatures. *PLoS ONE* **2016**, *11*, e0150460. [CrossRef] [PubMed]

18. Lee, J.K.; Nam, D.H.; Lee, J. Repurposing antipsychotics as glioblastoma therapeutics: Potentials and challenges. *Oncol. Lett.* **2016**, *11*, 1281–1286. [CrossRef] [PubMed]

19. Pantziarka, P.; Bouche, G.; Meheus, L.; Sukhatme, V.; Sukhatme, V.P. Repurposing Drugs in Oncology (ReDO)-mebendazole as an anti-cancer agent. *Ecancermedicalscience* **2014**, *8*, 443. [CrossRef] [PubMed]

20. Hothi, P.; Martins, T.J.; Chen, L.; Deleyrolle, L.; Yoon, J.G.; Reynolds, B.; Foltz, G. High-throughput chemical screens identify disulfiram as an inhibitor of human glioblastoma stem cells. *Oncotarget* **2012**, *3*, 1124–1136. [CrossRef] [PubMed]

21. Krauze, A.V.; Myrehaug, S.D.; Chang, M.G.; Holdford, D.J.; Smith, S.; Shih, J.; Tofilon, P.J.; Fine, H.A.; Camphausen, K. A Phase 2 Study of Concurrent Radiation Therapy, Temozolomide, and the Histone Deacetylase Inhibitor Valproic Acid for Patients With Glioblastoma. *Int. J. Radiat. Oncol. Biol. Phys.* **2015**, *92*, 986–992. [CrossRef] [PubMed]

22. Kim, Y.H.; Kim, T.; Joo, J.D.; Han, J.H.; Kim, Y.J.; Kim, I.A.; Yun, C.H.; Kim, C.Y. Survival benefit of levetiracetam in patients treated with concomitant chemoradiotherapy and adjuvant chemotherapy with temozolomide for glioblastoma multiforme. *Cancer* **2015**, *121*, 2926–2932. [CrossRef] [PubMed]

23. Friesen, C.; Hormann, I.; Roscher, M.; Fichtner, I.; Alt, A.; Hilger, R.; Debatin, K.M.; Miltner, E. Opioid receptor activation triggering downregulation of cAMP improves effectiveness of anti-cancer drugs in treatment of glioblastoma. *Cell Cycle* **2014**, *13*, 1560–1570. [CrossRef] [PubMed]

24. Robe, P.A.; Bentires-Alj, M.; Bonif, M.; Rogister, B.; Deprez, M.; Haddada, H.; Khac, M.T.; Jolois, O.; Erkmen, K.; Merville, M.P.; et al. In vitro and in vivo activity of the nuclear factor-κB inhibitor sulfasalazine in human glioblastomas. *Clin Cancer Res.* **2004**, *10*, 5595–5603. [CrossRef] [PubMed]

25. Arrieta, O.; Guevara, P.; Escobar, E.; García-Navarrete, R.; Pineda, B.; Sotelo, J. Blockage of angiotensin II type I receptor decreases the synthesis of growth factors and induces apoptosis in C6 cultured cells and C6 rat glioma. *Br. J. Cancer* **2005**, *92*, 1247–1252. [CrossRef] [PubMed]

26. Huang, C.; Hu, S.; Chen, B. Growth inhibition of epidermal growth factor-stimulated human glioblastoma cells by nicardipine in vitro. *J. Neurosurg. Sci.* **2001**, *45*, 151–155. [PubMed]

27. Zhang, Y.; Cruickshanks, N.; Yuan, F.; Wang, B.; Pahuski, M.; Wulfkuhle, J.; Gallagher, I.; Koeppel, A.F.; Hatef, S.; Papanicolas, C.; et al. Targetable T-type Calcium Channels Drive Glioblastoma. *Cancer Res.* **2017**, *77*, 3479–3490. [CrossRef] [PubMed]

28. Assad Kahn, S.; Costa, S.L.; Gholamin, S.; Nitta, R.T.; Dubois, L.G.; Fève, M.; Zeniou, M.; Coelho, P.L.; El-Habr, E.; Cadusseau, J.; et al. The anti-hypertensive drug prazosin inhibits glioblastoma growth via the PKCδ-dependent inhibition of the AKT pathway. *EMBO Mol. Med.* **2016**, *8*, 511–526. [CrossRef] [PubMed]

29. Durmaz, R.; Deliorman, S.; Uyar, R.; Işiksoy, S.; Erol, K.; Tel, E. The effects of anticancer drugs in combination with nimodipine and verapamil on cultured cells of glioblastoma multiforme. *Clin. Neurol. Neurosurg.* **1999**, *101*, 238–244. [CrossRef]

30. Liu, W.T.; Huang, C.Y.; Lu, I.C.; Gean, P.W. Inhibition of glioma growth by minocycline is mediated through endoplasmic reticulum stress-induced apoptosis and autophagic cell death. *Neuro-Oncoloy* **2013**, *15*, 1127–1141. [CrossRef] [PubMed]

31. Weiger, T.M.; Colombatto, S.; Kainz, V.; Heidegger, W.; Grillo, M.A.; Hermann, A. Potassium channel blockers quinidine and caesium halt cell proliferation in C6 glioma cells via a polyamine-dependent mechanism. *Biochem. Soc. Trans.* **2007**, *35*, 391–395. [CrossRef] [PubMed]

32. Yung, W.K.; Kyritsis, A.P.; Gleason, M.J.; Levin, V.A. Treatment of recurrent malignant gliomas with high-dose 13-*cis*-retinoic acid. *Clin. Cancer Res.* **1996**, *2*, 1931–1935. [PubMed]

33. Baumann, F.; Bjeljac, M.; Kollias, S.S.; Baumert, B.G.; Brandner, S.; Rousson, V.; Yonekawa, Y.; Bernays, R.L. Combined thalidomide and temozolomide treatment in patients with glioblastoma multiforme. *J. Neurooncol.* **2004**, *67*, 191–200. [CrossRef] [PubMed]

34. Michelakis, E.D.; Sutendra, G.; Dromparis, P.; Webster, L.; Haromy, A.; Niven, E.; Maguire, C.; Gammer, T.L.; Mackey, J.R.; Fulton, D.; et al. Metabolic modulation of glioblastoma with dichloroacetate. *Sci. Transl. Med.* **2010**, *2*, 31–34. [CrossRef] [PubMed]

35. Rosenfeld, M.R.; Ye, X.; Supko, J.G.; Desideri, S.; Grossman, S.A.; Brem, S.; Mikkelson, T.; Wang, D.; Chang, Y.C.; Hu, J.; et al. A phase I/II trial of hydroxychloroquine in conjunction with radiation therapy and concurrent and adjuvant temozolomide in patients with newly diagnosed glioblastoma multiforme. *Autophagy* **2014**, *10*, 1359–1368. [CrossRef] [PubMed]

36. Toler, S.M.; Noe, D.; Sharma, A. Selective enhancement of cellular oxidative stress by chloroquine: Implications for the treatment of glioblastoma multiforme. *Neurosurg. Focus* **2006**, *21*, E10. [CrossRef] [PubMed]

37. Gey, G.O.; Levy, R.H.; Pettet, G.; Fisher, L. Quinidine plasma concentration and exertional arrhythmia. *Am. Heart J.* **1975**, *90*, 19–24. [CrossRef]

38. Kast, R.E.; Boockvar, J.A.; Brüning, A.; Cappello, F.; Chang, W.W.; Cvek, B.; Dou, Q.P.; Duenas-Gonzalez, A.; Efferth, T.; Focosi, D.; et al. A conceptually new treatment approach for relapsed glioblastoma: Coordinated undermining of survival paths with nine repurposed drugs (CUSP9) by the International Initiative for Accelerated Improvement of Glioblastoma Care. *Oncotarget* **2013**, *4*, 502–530. [CrossRef] [PubMed]

39. Pernicova, I.; Korbonits, M. Metformin—mode of action and clinical implications for diabetes and cancer. *Nat. Rev. Endocrinol.* **2014**, *10*, 143–156. [CrossRef] [PubMed]

40. Antonoff, M.B.; D'Cunha, J. Teaching an old drug new tricks: Metformin as a targeted therapy for lung cancer. *Semin. Thorac. Cardiovasc. Surg.* **2010**, *22*, 195–196. [CrossRef] [PubMed]

41. Memmott, R.M.; Mercado, J.R.; Maier, C.R.; Kawabata, S.; Fox, S.D.; Dennis, P.A. Metformin prevents tobacco carcinogen—induced lung tumorigenesis. *Cancer Prev. Res.* **2010**, *3*, 1066–1076. [CrossRef] [PubMed]

42. Schneider, M.B.; Matsuzaki, H.; Haorah, J.; Ulrich, A.; Standop, J.; Ding, X.Z.; Adrian, T.E.; Pour, P.M. Prevention of pancreatic cancer induction in hamsters by metformin. *Gastroenterology* **2001**, *120*, 1263–1270. [CrossRef] [PubMed]

43. Zakikhani, M.; Dowling, R.; Fantus, I.G.; Sonenberg, N.; Pollak, M. Metformin is an AMP kinase-dependent growth inhibitor for breast cancer cells. *Cancer Res.* **2006**, *66*, 10269–10273. [CrossRef] [PubMed]

44. Gao, L.B.; Tian, S.; Gao, H.H.; Xu, Y.Y. Metformin inhibits glioma cell U251 invasion by downregulation of fibulin-3. *Neuroreport* **2013**, *24*, 504–508. [CrossRef] [PubMed]

45. Gritti, M.; Würth, R.; Angelini, M.; Barbieri, F.; Peretti, M.; Pizzi, E.; Pattarozzi, A.; Carra, E.; Sirito, R.; Daga, A.; et al. Metformin repositioning as antitumoral agent: Selective antiproliferative effects in human glioblastoma stem cells, via inhibition of CLIC1-mediated ion current. *Oncotarget* **2014**, *5*, 11252–11268. [CrossRef] [PubMed]

46. Isakovic, A.; Harhaji, L.; Stevanovic, D.; Markovic, Z.; Sumarac-Dumanovic, M.; Starcevic, V.; Micic, D.; Trajkovic, V. Dual antiglioma action of metformin: Cell cycle arrest and mitochondria-dependent apoptosis. *Cell. Mol. Life Sci.* **2007**, *64*, 1290–1302. [CrossRef] [PubMed]

47. Seliger, C.; Meyer, A.L.; Renner, K.; Leidgens, V.; Moeckel, S.; Jachnik, B.; Dettmer, K.; Tischler, U.; Gerthofer, V.; Rauer, L.; et al. Metformin inhibits proliferation and migration of glioblastoma cells independently of TGF-β2. *Cell Cycle* **2016**, *15*, 1755–1766. [CrossRef] [PubMed]

48. Yu, Z.; Zhao, G.; Xie, G.; Zhao, L.; Chen, Y.; Yu, H.; Zhang, Z.; Li, C.; Li, Y. Metformin and temozolomide act synergistically to inhibit growth of glioma cells and glioma stem cells in vitro and in vivo. *Oncotarget* **2015**, *6*, 32930–32943. [CrossRef] [PubMed]

49. Jiang, W.; Finniss, S.; Cazacu, S.; Xiang, C.; Brodie, Z.; Mikkelsen, T.; Poisson, L.; Shackelford, D.B.; Brodie, C. Repurposing phenformin for the targeting of glioma stem cells and the treatment of glioblastoma. *Oncotarget* **2016**, *7*, 56456–56470. [CrossRef] [PubMed]

50. Graham, G.G.; Punt, J.; Arora, M.; Day, R.O.; Doogue, M.P.; Duong, J.K.; Furlong, T.J.; Greenfield, J.R.; Greenup, L.C.; Kirkpatrick, C.M.; et al. Clinical pharmacokinetics of metformin. *Clin. Pharmacokinet.* **2011**, *50*, 81–98. [CrossRef] [PubMed]

51. Davies, J.T.; Delfino, S.F.; Feinberg, C.E.; Johnson, M.F.; Nappi, V.L.; Olinger, J.T.; Schwab, A.P.; Swanson, H.I. Current and Emerging Uses of Statins in Clinical Therapeutics: A Review. *Lipid Insights* **2016**, *9*, 13–29. [CrossRef] [PubMed]

52. Bayat, N.; Ebrahimi-Barough, S.; Norouzi-Javidan, A.; Saberi, H.; Tajerian, R.; Ardakan, M.M.M.; Shirian, S.; Ai, A.; Ai, J. Apoptotic effect of atorvastatin in glioblastoma spheroids tumor cultured in fibrin gel. *Biomed. Pharmacother.* **2016**, *84*, 1959–1966. [CrossRef] [PubMed]

53. May, M.B.; Glode, A. Novel Uses for Lipid-Lowering Agents. *J. Adv. Pract. Oncol.* **2016**, *7*, 181–187. [PubMed]

54. Oliveira, K.A.; Dal-Cim, T.; Lopes, F.G.; Ludka, F.K.; Nedel, C.B.; Tasca, C.I. Atorvastatin Promotes Cytotoxicity and Reduces Migration and Proliferation of Human A172 Glioma Cells. *Mol. Neurobiol.* **2018**, *55*, 1509–1523. [CrossRef] [PubMed]

55. Tapia-Perez, J.H.; Kirches, E.; Mawrin, C.; Firsching, R.; Schneider, T. Cytotoxic effect of different statins and thiazolidinediones on malignant glioma cells. *Cancer Chemother. Pharmacol.* **2011**, *67*, 1193–1201. [CrossRef] [PubMed]

56. Yanae, M.; Tsubaki, M.; Satou, T.; Itoh, T.; Imano, M.; Yamazoe, Y.; Nishida, S. Statin-induced apoptosis via the suppression of ERK1/2 and Akt activation by inhibition of the geranylgeranyl-pyrophosphate biosynthesis in glioblastoma. *J. Exp. Clin. Cancer Res.* **2011**, *30*, 74. [CrossRef] [PubMed]

57. Bayat, N.; Ebrahimi-Barough, S.; Norouzi-Javidan, A.; Saberi, H.; Ardakan, M.M.M.; Ai, A.; Soleimannejad, M.; Ai, J. Anti-inflammatory Effects of Atorvastatin by Suppressing TRAF3IP2 and IL-17RA in Human Glioblastoma Spheroids Cultured in a Three-dimensional Model: Possible Relevance to Glioblastoma Treatment. *Mol. Neurobiol.* **2018**, *55*, 2102–2110. [CrossRef] [PubMed]

58. Girgert, R.; Vogt, Y.; Becke, D.; Bruchelt, G.; Schweizer, P. Growth inhibition of neuroblastoma cells by lovastatin and L-ascorbic acid is based on different mechanisms. *Cancer Lett.* **1999**, *137*, 167–172. [CrossRef]

59. Koyuturk, M.; Ersoz, M.; Altiok, N. Simvastatin induces proliferation inhibition and apoptosis in C6 glioma cells via c-jun N-terminal kinase. *Neurosci. Lett.* **2004**, *370*, 212–217. [CrossRef] [PubMed]

60. Obara, S.; Nakata, M.; Takeshima, H.; Kuratsu, J.; Maruyama, I.; Kitajima, I. Inhibition of migration of human glioblastoma cells by cerivastatin in association with focal adhesion kinase (FAK). *Cancer Lett.* **2002**, *185*, 153–161. [CrossRef]

61. Yongjun, Y.; Shuyun, H.; Lei, C.; Xiangrong, C.; Zhilin, Y.; Yiquan, K. Atorvastatin suppresses glioma invasion and migration by reducing microglial MT1-MMP expression. *J. Neuroimmunol.* **2013**, *260*, 1–8. [CrossRef] [PubMed]

62. Björkhem-Bergman, L.; Lindh, J.D.; Bergman, P. What is a relevant statin concentration in cell experiments claiming pleiotropic effects? *Br. J. Clin. Pharmacol.* **2011**, *72*, 164–165. [CrossRef] [PubMed]

63. Kurien, G.; Pellegrini, M.V. Dapsone. In *StatPearls*; StatPearls Publishing LLC.: Treasure Island, FL, USA, 2018.

64. Kast, R.E.; Lefranc, F.; Karpel-Massler, G.; Halatsch, M.E. Why dapsone stops seizures and may stop neutrophils' delivery of VEGF to glioblastoma. *Br. J. Neurosurg.* **2012**, *26*, 813–817. [CrossRef] [PubMed]

65. Karpel-Massler, G.; Kast, R.E.; Siegelin, M.D.; Dwucet, A.; Schneider, E.; Westhoff, M.A.; Wirtz, C.R.; Chen, X.Y.; Halatsch, M.E.; Bolm, C. Anti-glioma Activity of Dapsone and Its Enhancement by Synthetic Chemical Modification. *Neurochem. Res.* **2017**, *42*, 3382–3389. [CrossRef] [PubMed]

66. Zuidema, J.; Hilbers-Modderman, E.S.; Merkus, F.W. Clinical pharmacokinetics of dapsone. *Clin. Pharmacokinet.* **1986**, *11*, 299–315. [CrossRef] [PubMed]

67. Zhang, Q.I.; Wang, S.; Yang, D.; Pan, K.; Li, L.; Yuan, S. Preclinical pharmacodynamic evaluation of antibiotic nitroxoline for anticancer drug repurposing. *Oncol. Lett.* **2016**, *11*, 3265–3272. [CrossRef] [PubMed]
68. Pelletier, C.; Prognon, P.; Bourlioux, P. Roles of divalent cations and pH in mechanism of action of nitroxoline against *Escherichia coli* strains. *Antimicrob. Agents Chemother.* **1995**, *39*, 707–713. [CrossRef] [PubMed]
69. Wagenlehner, F.M.E.; Münch, F.; Pilatz, A.; Bärmann, B.; Weidner, W.; Wagenlehner, C.M.; Straubinger, M.; Blenk, H.; Pfister, W.; Kresken, M.; et al. Urinary Concentrations and Antibacterial Activities of Nitroxoline at 250 Milligrams versus Trimethoprim at 200 Milligrams against Uropathogens in Healthy Volunteers. *Antimicrob. Agents Chemother.* **2014**, *58*, 713–721. [CrossRef] [PubMed]
70. Chan-on, W.; Huyen, N.T.B.; Songtawee, N.; Suwanjang, W.; Prachayasittikul, S.; Prachayasittikul, V. Quinoline-based clioquinol and nitroxoline exhibit anticancer activity inducing FoxM1 inhibition in cholangiocarcinoma cells. *Drug Des. Dev. Ther.* **2015**, *9*, 2033–2047.
71. Shim, J.S.; Matsui, Y.; Bhat, S.; Nacev, B.A.; Xu, J.; Bhang, H.E.; Dhara, S.; Han, K.C.; Chong, C.R.; Pomper, M.G.; et al. Effect of nitroxoline on angiogenesis and growth of human bladder cancer. *J. Natl. Cancer Inst.* **2010**, *102*, 1855–1873. [CrossRef] [PubMed]
72. Mai, J.; Sameni, M.; Mikkelsen, T.; Sloane, B.F. Degradation of extracellular matrix protein tenascin-C by cathepsin B: An interaction involved in the progression of gliomas. *Biol. Chem.* **2002**, *383*, 1407–1413. [CrossRef] [PubMed]
73. Mirkovic, B.; Renko, M.; Turk, S.; Sosic, I.; Jevnikar, Z.; Obermajer, N.; Turk, D.; Gobec, S.; Kos, J. Novel mechanism of cathepsin B inhibition by antibiotic nitroxoline and related compounds. *ChemMedChem* **2011**, *6*, 1351–1356. [CrossRef] [PubMed]
74. Lazovic, J.; Guo, L.; Nakashima, J.; Mirsadraei, L.; Yong, W.; Kim, H.J.; Ellingson, B.; Wu, H.; Pope, W.B. Nitroxoline induces apoptosis and slows glioma growth in vivo. *Neuro-Oncoloy* **2015**, *17*, 53–62. [CrossRef] [PubMed]
75. Mushtaque, M.; Shahjahan. Reemergence of chloroquine (CQ) analogs as multi-targeting antimalarial agents: A review. *Eur. J. Med. Chem.* **2015**, *90*, 280–295. [CrossRef] [PubMed]
76. Manic, G.; Obrist, F.; Kroemer, G.; Vitale, I.; Galluzzi, L. Chloroquine and hydroxychloroquine for cancer therapy. *Mol. Cell. Oncol.* **2014**, *1*, e29911. [CrossRef] [PubMed]
77. Guan, Y.D.; Jiang, S.L.; Yu, P.; Wen, M.; Zhang, Y.; Xiao, S.S.; Xu, X.J.; Cheng, Y. Suppression of eEF-2K-mediated autophagy enhances the cytotoxicity of Raddeanin A against human breast cancer cells in vitro. *Acta Pharmacol. Sin.* **2017**. [CrossRef] [PubMed]
78. Fu, Z.; Xi, C.; Kuang, J.; Feng, H.; Chen, L.; Liang, J.; Shen, X.; Yuen, S.; Chenghong, P.; Baiyong, S.; et al. CQ sensitizes human pancreatic cancer cells to gemcitabine through the lysosomal apoptotic pathway via reactive oxygen species. *Mol. Oncol.* **2018**, *12*, 529–544. [CrossRef] [PubMed]
79. Monma, H.; Iida, Y.; Moritani, T.; Okimoto, T.; Tanino, R.; Tajima, Y.; Harada, M. Chloroquine augments TRAIL-induced apoptosis and induces G2/M phase arrest in human pancreatic cancer cells. *PLoS ONE* **2018**, *13*, e0193990. [CrossRef] [PubMed]
80. Wang, H.; Wang, L.; Cao, L.; Zhang, Q.; Song, Q.; Meng, Z.; Wu, X.; Xu, K. Inhibition of autophagy potentiates the anti-metastasis effect of phenethyl isothiocyanate through JAK2/STAT3 pathway in lung cancer cells. *Mol. Carcinog.* **2018**, *57*, 522–535. [CrossRef] [PubMed]
81. Ouyang, G.; Xiong, L.; Liu, Z.; Lam, B.; Bui, B.; Ma, L.; Chen, X.; Zhou, P.; Wang, K.; Zhang, Z.; et al. Inhibition of autophagy potentiates the apoptosis-inducing effects of photodynamic therapy on human colon cancer cells. *Photodiagn. Photodyn. Ther.* **2018**, *21*, 396–403. [CrossRef] [PubMed]
82. Wang, F.; Tang, J.; Li, P.; Si, S.; Yu, H.; Yang, X.; Tao, J.; Lv, Q.; Gu, M.; Yang, H.; et al. Chloroquine Enhances the Radiosensitivity of Bladder Cancer Cells by Inhibiting Autophagy and Activating Apoptosis. *Cell. Physiol. Biochem.* **2018**, *45*, 54–66. [CrossRef] [PubMed]
83. Golden, E.B.; Cho, H.Y.; Jahanian, A.; Hofman, F.M.; Louie, S.G.; Schonthal, A.H.; Chen, T.C. Chloroquine enhances temozolomide cytotoxicity in malignant gliomas by blocking autophagy. *Neurosurg. Focus* **2014**, *37*, E12. [CrossRef] [PubMed]
84. Hori, Y.S.; Hosoda, R.; Akiyama, Y.; Sebori, R.; Wanibuchi, M.; Mikami, T.; Sugino, T.; Suzuki, K.; Maruyama, M.; Tsukamoto, M.; et al. Chloroquine potentiates temozolomide cytotoxicity by inhibiting mitochondrial autophagy in glioma cells. *J. Neurooncol.* **2015**, *122*, 11–20. [CrossRef] [PubMed]

85. Lee, S.W.; Kim, H.K.; Lee, N.H.; Yi, H.Y.; Kim, H.S.; Hong, S.H.; Hong, Y.K.; Joe, Y.A. The synergistic effect of combination temozolomide and chloroquine treatment is dependent on autophagy formation and p53 status in glioma cells. *Cancer Lett.* **2015**, *360*, 195–204. [CrossRef] [PubMed]

86. Yan, Y.; Xu, Z.; Dai, S.; Qian, L.; Sun, L.; Gong, Z. Targeting autophagy to sensitive glioma to temozolomide treatment. *J. Exp. Clin. Cancer Res.* **2016**, *35*, 23. [CrossRef] [PubMed]

87. Firat, E.; Weyerbrock, A.; Gaedicke, S.; Grosu, A.L.; Niedermann, G. Chloroquine or chloroquine-PI3K/Akt pathway inhibitor combinations strongly promote gamma-irradiation-induced cell death in primary stem-like glioma cells. *PLoS ONE* **2012**, *7*, e47357. [CrossRef] [PubMed]

88. Ye, H.; Chen, M.; Cao, F.; Huang, H.; Zhan, R.; Zheng, X. Chloroquine, an autophagy inhibitor, potentiates the radiosensitivity of glioma initiating cells by inhibiting autophagy and activating apoptosis. *BMC Neurol.* **2016**, *16*, 178. [CrossRef] [PubMed]

89. Zhuang, W.; Qin, Z.; Liang, Z. The role of autophagy in sensitizing malignant glioma cells to radiation therapy. *Acta Biochim. Biophys. Sin.* **2009**, *41*, 341–351. [CrossRef] [PubMed]

90. Walker, A.J.; Card, T.; Bates, T.E.; Muir, K. Tricyclic antidepressants and the incidence of certain cancers: A study using the GPRD. *Br. J. Cancer* **2011**, *104*, 193–197. [CrossRef] [PubMed]

91. Levkovitz, Y.; Gil-Ad, I.; Zeldich, E.; Dayag, M.; Weizman, A. Differential induction of apoptosis by antidepressants in glioma and neuroblastoma cell lines: Evidence for p-c-Jun, cytochrome c, and caspase-3 involvement. *J. Mol. Neurosci.* **2005**, *27*, 29–42. [CrossRef]

92. Spanová, A.; Kovářů, H.; Lisá, V.; Lukásová, E.; Rittich, B. Estimation of apoptosis in C6 glioma cells treated with antidepressants. *Physiol. Res.* **1997**, *46*, 161–164. [PubMed]

93. Liu, K.H.; Yang, S.T.; Lin, Y.K.; Lin, J.W.; Lee, Y.H.; Wang, J.Y.; Hu, C.J.; Lin, E.Y.; Chen, S.M.; Then, C.K.; et al. Fluoxetine, an antidepressant, suppresses glioblastoma by evoking AMPAR-mediated calcium-dependent apoptosis. *Oncotarget* **2015**, *6*, 5088–5101. [CrossRef] [PubMed]

94. Hayashi, K.; Michiue, H.; Yamada, H.; Takata, K.; Nakayama, H.; Wei, F.Y.; Fujimura, A.; Tazawa, H.; Asai, A.; Ogo, N.; et al. Fluvoxamine, an anti-depressant, inhibits human glioblastoma invasion by disrupting actin polymerization. *Sci. Rep.* **2016**, *6*, 23372. [CrossRef] [PubMed]

95. Johnson, R.D.; Lewis, R.J.; Angier, M.K. The distribution of fluoxetine in human fluids and tissues. *J. Anal. Toxicol.* **2007**, *31*, 409–414. [CrossRef] [PubMed]

96. Karson, C.N.; Newton, J.E.; Livingston, R.; Jolly, J.B.; Cooper, T.B.; Sprigg, J.; Komoroski, R.A. Human brain fluoxetine concentrations. *J. Neuropsychiatry Clin. Neurosci.* **1993**, *5*, 322–329. [PubMed]

97. Bielecka-Wajdman, A.M.; Lesiak, M.; Ludyga, T.; Sieron, A.; Obuchowicz, E. Reversing glioma malignancy: A new look at the role of antidepressant drugs as adjuvant therapy for glioblastoma multiforme. *Cancer Chemother. Pharmacol.* **2017**, *79*, 1249–1256. [CrossRef] [PubMed]

98. Jeon, S.H.; Kim, S.H.; Kim, Y.; Kim, Y.S.; Lim, Y.; Lee, Y.H.; Shin, S.Y. The tricyclic antidepressant imipramine induces autophagic cell death in U-87MG glioma cells. *Biochem. Biophys. Res. Commun.* **2011**, *413*, 311–317. [CrossRef] [PubMed]

99. Shchors, K.; Massaras, A.; Hanahan, D. Dual Targeting of the Autophagic Regulatory Circuitry in Gliomas with Repurposed Drugs Elicits Cell-Lethal Autophagy and Therapeutic Benefit. *Cancer Cell* **2015**, *28*, 456–471. [CrossRef] [PubMed]

100. Nagy, A.; Eder, K.; Selak, M.A.; Kalman, B. Mitochondrial energy metabolism and apoptosis regulation in glioblastoma. *Brain Res.* **2015**, *1595*, 127–142. [CrossRef] [PubMed]

101. Daley, E.; Wilkie, D.; Loesch, A.; Hargreaves, I.P.; Kendall, D.A.; Pilkington, G.J.; Bates, T.E. Chlorimipramine: A novel anticancer agent with a mitochondrial target. *Biochem. Biophys. Res. Commun.* **2005**, *328*, 623–632. [CrossRef] [PubMed]

102. Pilkington, G.J.; Parker, K.; Murray, S.A. Approaches to mitochondrially mediated cancer therapy. *Semin. Cancer Biol.* **2008**, *18*, 226–235. [CrossRef] [PubMed]

103. Zanotto-Filho, A.; Braganhol, E.; Battastini, A.M.; Moreira, J.C. Proteasome inhibitor MG132 induces selective apoptosis in glioblastoma cells through inhibition of PI3K/Akt and NFκB pathways, mitochondrial dysfunction, and activation of p38-JNK1/2 signaling. *Investig. New Drugs* **2012**, *30*, 2252–2262. [CrossRef] [PubMed]

104. Xing, F.; Luan, Y.; Cai, J.; Wu, S.; Mai, J.; Gu, J.; Zhang, H.; Li, K.; Lin, Y.; Xiao, X.; et al. The Anti-Warburg Effect Elicited by the cAMP-PGC1α Pathway Drives Differentiation of Glioblastoma Cells into Astrocytes. *Cell Rep.* **2017**, *18*, 468–481. [CrossRef] [PubMed]

105. Hertz, L.; Peng, L.; Dienel, G.A. Energy metabolism in astrocytes: High rate of oxidative metabolism and spatiotemporal dependence on glycolysis/glycogenolysis. *J. Cereb. Blood Flow MeTable* **2007**, *27*, 219–249. [CrossRef] [PubMed]

106. Moreno-Sanchez, R.; Rodriguez-Enriquez, S.; Marin-Hernandez, A.; Saavedra, E. Energy metabolism in tumor cells. *FEBS J.* **2007**, *274*, 1393–1418. [CrossRef] [PubMed]

107. Ordys, B.B.; Launay, S.; Deighton, R.F.; McCulloch, J.; Whittle, I.R. The role of mitochondria in glioma pathophysiology. *Mol. Neurobiol.* **2010**, *42*, 64–75. [CrossRef] [PubMed]

108. Marie, S.K.N.; Shinjo, S.M.O. Metabolism and Brain Cancer. *Clinics* **2011**, *66*, 33–43. [CrossRef] [PubMed]

109. Warburg, O. On the origin of cancer cells. *Science* **1956**, *123*, 309–314. [CrossRef] [PubMed]

110. Galarraga, J.; Loreck, D.J.; Graham, J.F.; DeLaPaz, R.L.; Smith, B.H.; Hallgren, D.; Cummins, C.J. Glucose metabolism in human gliomas: Correspondence of in situ and in vitro metabolic rates and altered energy metabolism. *Metab. Brain Dis.* **1986**, *1*, 279–291. [CrossRef] [PubMed]

111. Liberti, M.V.; Locasale, J.W. The Warburg Effect: How Does it Benefit Cancer Cells? *Trends Biochem. Sci.* **2016**, *41*, 211–218. [CrossRef] [PubMed]

112. Paradies, G.; Capuano, F.; Palombini, G.; Galeotti, T.; Papa, S. Transport of Pyruvate in Mitochondria from Different Tumor Cells. *Cancer Res.* **1983**, *43*, 5068–5071. [PubMed]

113. Baggetto, L.G.; Lehninger, A.L. Formation and utilization of acetoin, an unusual product of pyruvate metabolism by Ehrlich and AS30-D tumor mitochondria. *J. Biol. Chem.* **1987**, *262*, 9535–9541. [PubMed]

114. Degterev, A.; Boyce, M.; Yuan, J. A decade of caspases. *Oncogene* **2003**, *22*, 8543–8567. [CrossRef] [PubMed]

115. Klein, S.; McCormick, F.; Levitzki, A. Killing time for cancer cells. *Nat. Rev. Cancer* **2005**, *5*, 573–580. [CrossRef] [PubMed]

116. O'Neill, J.; Manion, M.; Schwartz, P.; Hockenbery, D.M. Promises and challenges of targeting Bcl-2 anti-apoptotic proteins for cancer therapy. *Biochim. Biophys. Acta* **2004**, *1705*, 43–51. [CrossRef] [PubMed]

117. Frank, S.; Kohler, U.; Schackert, G.; Schackert, H.K. Expression of TRAIL and its receptors in human brain tumors. *Biochem. Biophys. Res. Commun.* **1999**, *257*, 454–459. [CrossRef] [PubMed]

118. Vignot, S.; Faivre, S.; Aguirre, D.; Raymond, E. mTOR-targeted therapy of cancer with rapamycin derivatives. *Ann. Oncol.* **2005**, *16*, 525–537. [CrossRef] [PubMed]

119. Wagenknecht, B.; Glaser, T.; Naumann, U.; Kugler, S.; Isenmann, S.; Bahr, M.; Korneluk, R.; Liston, P.; Weller, M. Expression and biological activity of X-linked inhibitor of apoptosis (XIAP) in human malignant glioma. *Cell Death Differ.* **1999**, *6*, 370–376. [CrossRef] [PubMed]

120. Weller, M.; Malipiero, U.; Aguzzi, A.; Reed, J.C.; Fontana, A. Protooncogene bcl-2 gene transfer abrogates Fas/APO-1 antibody-mediated apoptosis of human malignant glioma cells and confers resistance to chemotherapeutic drugs and therapeutic irradiation. *J. Clin. Investig.* **1995**, *95*, 2633–2643. [CrossRef] [PubMed]

121. Stegh, A.H.; Kim, H.; Bachoo, R.M.; Forloney, K.L.; Zhang, J.; Schulze, H.; Park, K.; Hannon, G.J.; Yuan, J.; Louis, D.N.; et al. Bcl2L12 inhibits post-mitochondrial apoptosis signaling in glioblastoma. *Genes Dev.* **2007**, *21*, 98–111. [CrossRef] [PubMed]

122. Krajewska, M.; Krajewski, S.; Epstein, J.I.; Shabaik, A.; Sauvageot, J.; Song, K.; Kitada, S.; Reed, J.C. Immunohistochemical analysis of bcl-2, bax, bcl-X, and mcl-1 expression in prostate cancers. *Am. J. Pathol.* **1996**, *148*, 1567–1576. [PubMed]

123. Nakasu, S.; Nakasu, Y.; Nioka, H.; Nakajima, M.; Handa, J. bcl-2 protein expression in tumors of the central nervous system. *Acta Neuropathol.* **1994**, *88*, 520–526. [CrossRef] [PubMed]

124. Krakstad, C.; Chekenya, M. Survival signalling and apoptosis resistance in glioblastomas: Opportunities for targeted therapeutics. *Mol. Cancer* **2010**, *9*, 135. [CrossRef] [PubMed]

125. Kushal, S.; Wang, W.; Vaikari, V.P.; Kota, R.; Chen, K.; Yeh, T.S.; Jhaveri, N.; Groshen, S.L.; Olenyuk, B.Z.; Chen, T.C.; et al. Monoamine oxidase A (MAO A) inhibitors decrease glioma progression. *Oncotarget* **2016**, *7*, 13842–13853. [CrossRef] [PubMed]

126. Oliva, C.R.; Zhang, W.; Langford, C.; Suto, M.J.; Griguer, C.E. Repositioning chlorpromazine for treating chemoresistant glioma through the inhibition of cytochrome c oxidase bearing the COX4-1 regulatory subunit. *Oncotarget* **2017**, *8*, 37568–37583. [CrossRef] [PubMed]

127. Charles, E.; Hammadi, M.; Kischel, P.; Delcroix, V.; Demaurex, N.; Castelbou, C.; Vacher, A.M.; Devin, A.; Ducret, T.; Nunes, P.; et al. The antidepressant fluoxetine induces necrosis by energy depletion and mitochondrial calcium overload. *Oncotarget* **2017**, *8*, 3181–3196. [CrossRef] [PubMed]

128. Oliva, C.R.; Moellering, D.R.; Gillespie, G.Y.; Griguer, C.E. Acquisition of chemoresistance in gliomas is associated with increased mitochondrial coupling and decreased ROS production. *PLoS ONE* **2011**, *6*, e24665. [CrossRef] [PubMed]

129. Oliva, C.R.; Markert, T.; Gillespie, G.Y.; Griguer, C.E. Nuclear-encoded cytochrome c oxidase subunit 4 regulates BMI1 expression and determines proliferative capacity of high-grade gliomas. *Oncotarget* **2015**, *6*, 4330–4344. [CrossRef] [PubMed]

130. Oliva, C.R.; Markert, T.; Ross, L.J.; White, E.L.; Rasmussen, L.; Zhang, W.; Everts, M.; Moellering, D.R.; Bailey, S.M.; Suto, M.J.; et al. Identification of Small Molecule Inhibitors of Human Cytochrome C Oxidase That Target Chemoresistant Glioma Cells. *J. Biol. Chem.* **2016**, *291*, 24188–24199. [CrossRef] [PubMed]

131. Sharpe, M.A.; Han, J.; Baskin, A.M.; Baskin, D.S. Design and synthesis of a MAO-B-selectively activated prodrug based on MPTP: A mitochondria-targeting chemotherapeutic agent for treatment of human malignant gliomas. *ChemMedChem* **2015**, *10*, 621–628. [CrossRef] [PubMed]

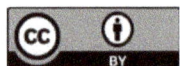

neuroglia

MDPI

Article

Ultrastructural Remodeling of the Neurovascular Unit in the Female Diabetic db/db Model–Part II: Microglia and Mitochondria

Melvin R. Hayden [1,2,*], DeAna G Grant [3], Annayya R. Aroor [1,2,4] and Vincent G. DeMarco [1,2,4,5]

[1] Diabetes and Cardiovascular Center, University of Missouri School of Medicine, Columbia, MO 65212, USA; aroora@health.missouri.edu (A.R.A.); demarcov@missouri.edu (V.G.D.)
[2] Division of Endocrinology and Metabolism, Department of Medicine, University of Missouri, Columbia, MO 65211, USA
[3] Electron Microscopy Core Facility, University of Missouri, Columbia, MO 65211, USA; GrantDe@missouri.edu
[4] Research Service, Harry S. Truman Memorial Veterans Hospital, Columbia, MO 65291, USA
[5] Department of Medical Pharmacology and Physiology, University of Missouri, Columbia, MO 65211, USA
* Correspondence: mrh29pete@gmail.com; Tel.: +1-573-346-3019

Received: 27 August 2018; Accepted: 27 September 2018; Published: 7 October 2018

Abstract: Obesity, insulin resistance, and type 2 diabetes mellitus are associated with diabetic cognopathy. This study tested the hypothesis that neurovascular unit(s) (NVU) within cerebral cortical gray matter regions may depict abnormal cellular remodeling. The monogenic ($Lepr^{db}$) female diabetic db/db [BKS.Cg$Dock7^m$ +/+$Lepr^{db}$/J] (DBC) mouse model was utilized for this ultrastructural study. Upon sacrifice (20 weeks), left-brain hemispheres of the DBC and age-matched nondiabetic control C57BL/KsJ (CKC) mice were immediately immersion-fixed. We observed an attenuation/loss of endothelial blood–brain barrier tight/adherens junctions and pericytes, thickened basement membranes, adherent red and white blood cells, neurovascular unit microbleeds and pathologic remodeling of protoplasmic astrocytes. In this second of a three-part series, we focus on the observational ultrastructural remodeling of microglia and mitochondria in relation to the NVU in leptin receptor deficient DBC models. This study identified novel ultrastructural core signature remodeling changes, which consisted of invasive activated microglia, microglial aberrant mitochondria with nuclear chromatin condensation and adhesion of white blood cells to an activated endothelium of the NVU. In conclusion, the results implicate activated microglia in NVU uncoupling and the resulting ischemic neuronal and synaptic damage, which may be related to impaired cognition and diabetic cognopathy.

Keywords: astrocyte; db/db mouse model; microglia; mitochondria; neuroglia; neurovascular unit; type 2 diabetes

1. Introduction

Previously, we have overviewed the background, and documented the observations of the 20-week old female db/db [BKS.Cg$Dock7^m$ +/+$Lepr^{db}$/J] (DBC) and its comparison to the age-matched control (CKC) model with a focus on ultrastructure protoplasmic astrocyte remodeling in relation to the neurovascular unit (NVU) [1]. We demonstrated marked multicellular ultrastructure remodeling comprised by the following: (i) attenuation and/or loss of blood–brain barrier tight and adherens junctions (TJ/AJ); (iia) adherent red blood cells to endothelial cell(s) (EC) of the NVU; (iib) microbleeds of the NVU; (iic) endothelial cell thinning and activation with white blood cell adherence to

ECs; (iii) maladaptive pericyte attenuation and/or loss; (iv) NVU basement membrane thickening; (v) detachment and retraction of protoplasmic astrocytes from the NUV [1]. In this second of a three-part series our focus will be on the microglia, mitochondria and white blood cell adhesion to the neurovascular unit endothelial cell in the diabetic DBC as compared to the nondiabetic control CKC models. The identifying ultrastructure characteristics of microglia have been described in our previous article [1] and are illustrated (Figure 1). Additional supplemental videos are also provided.

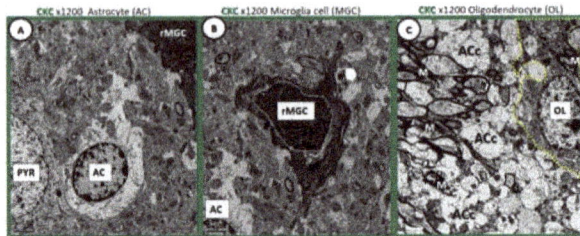

Figure 1. Comparison of ramified microglia to glia and pyramidal cells in cortical grey matter layer III to supplement the extracted description from Table 1 [1]. (**A**) Depicts an astrocyte (AC) with electron lucent cytoplasm with a neuronal pyramidal (PYR) cell immediately adjacent. (**B**) Depicts a ramified microglial cell (rMGC) with its highly electron-dense cytoplasm and nucleus outlined by white dashed line. (**C**) Depicts just a partial image of an oligodendrocyte (OL) in the transition zone between the cortical grey matter and white matter. Note the ramified cytoplasmic extensions. Microglia are the smallest of the glia cells and their cytoplasm is the most electron-dense of the neurovascular unit (NVU) cells and brain cortical grey matter. In their nonactivated phenotypic state, they have elongated cytoplasmic process in ramified form. They have an extensive endoplasmic reticulum, Golgi body system and contain multiple mitochondria. Their cytoplasmic processes are known to be capable of extending and contracting. They have a unique morphology of their nuclei with an outer stippled chromatin at its neurolemma and a more stippled diffuse chromatin electron-dense appearance of the central nuclei. Magnification 1200×; bar = 2 µm.

Microglial cells are the resident innate immune cells of the brain, which represent approximately 5–20% of the brain neuroglial population and have a large number of membranous and intracellular microglial markers; a large number of signaling molecules, which include numerous microglial cytokines and chemokines [2]. Microglia contribute to the regulation of brain development, shaping synaptic connectivity within neuronal networks and are of major importance in brain defense injury [2–4]. In the healthy brain, ramified microglia are constantly surveilling their regional environment and provide the necessary housekeeping-cleaning-gatekeeping functions to maintain brain tissue homeostasis (Figure S1, Figure S2 and Video S1). Microglia are capable of producing numerous free radicals (superoxide, reduced nicotinamide adenine dinucleotide phosphate (NADPH Ox), inducible nitric oxide and mitochondrial-derived reactive oxygen/nitrogen (mtROS)) and are the major killing and phagocytic cell in the brain if bacterial, viral or parasitic infections become invasive. Importantly, microglia are able to return to return to their surveilling-ramified phenotype once the invaders or danger–damage signals have been eradicated and assume their normal cellular debris housekeeping role [2–12].

Mesoderm (yolk sac)-derived microglia cells are the first and main form of active immune defense in the brain [2–12]. Microglia are unique from bone marrow derived peripheral monocyte-macrophage cells in that they are not dependent on recruitment from the peripheral systemic circulation but are capable of undergoing proliferation mechanisms if needed [13]. Microglia may play both a protective role of surveillance for injury to the NVU unit (Figure S2, Figure S3 and Video S2) as well as a possible damaging role to the NVU in the DBC models due to microglia invasiveness with resulting detachment and separation of protoplasmic astrocytes from the BM of the endothelial cells and pericytes of the NVU [1].

We originally hypothesized that microglia might demonstrate some of their reactive changes similar to our previous observations in the diet-induced obesity and insulin resistant Western models with impaired intermittent glucose elevation [14].

Microglia in CKC animals display distinct phenotypes in transmission electron microscopy (TEM) (Joel 1400-EX TEM JOEL (JOEL, Peabody, MA, USA) images and these cells will be referred to as ramified microglial cells (rMGC). These cells survey their surrounding milieu of endothelial cells, pericytes, astrocytes of the NVU and neurons. They maintain this ramified phenotype and function in association with intact tight and adherence junctions of the ECs blood–brain barrier and the intact adherent protoplasmic astrocytes to the basement membrane of the NVU. Ramified microglia cells are constantly prepared to undergo a rapid diverse phenotypic remodeling change to what we will reference as the activated-amoeboid microglial cell phenotype (aMGC). These changes may be due to morphological remodeling and/or the expressions of their cell surface receptors in response to danger or damage signals such as pathogen associated molecular patterns (PAMPs) or damage associated molecular patterns (DAMPS) due to oxidized/glycated proteins/polypeptides, lipids, and nucleic acids from their diabetic hyperglycemic microenvironment [2–13]. The phenotypic remodeling changes need to be qualified by the model (i.e., control CKC or diabetic DBC), the region of the brain (as in our gray matter cortical layer III), the disease state (obesity, insulin resistance and type 2 diabetes mellitus (T2DM)) and their age (20 weeks) [2–13]. Activated microglial phenotypes have been classified by some to be similar to peripheral macrophages, i.e., M1 (classically activated macrophages) and M2 (alternatively activated macrophages) cells [7,8]; however, the possibly more preferred method of identification of MGCs relies on individual cell surface markers or their response to inducible cytokines [9–11]. We have chosen to utilize only rMGC or aMGC when referring to our morphofunctional–pathomorphologic phenotypic polarization in TEM observations (Figure 2).

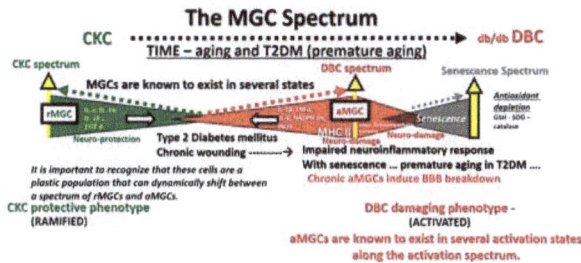

Figure 2. Microglia spectrum phenotypes in type 2 diabetes mellitus (T2DM). The microglia cell(s) (MGC) are very unique and capable of undergoing a marked diversity of morphological and functional phenotypic remodeling change as they pass along a spectrum of phenotypes from the ramified MGC (rMGC) (green colorization) on the far left-hand side of this cartoon to the chronically activated-amoeboid microglia cells (aMGC) (red colorization) on the right hand in addition to some microglia progressing to a senescent type of MGC on the far right (grey colorization), which may implicate advanced aging. Note the various cytokines profiles associated with each of the rMGC and the aMGC phenotypes. In our age-matched nondiabetic control C57BL/KsJ (CKC) models, the predominate MGC would be rMGC and in the DBC models the predominant microglia would be aMGC since we are only studying the ultrastructural phenotypic ultrastructural remodeling changes. Note that in health or homeostasis we demonstrate that the MGC may be in a flux or spectral change between rMGCs and more activated/amoeboid MGCs. The regions between open arrows may even represent a range of homeostasis between rMGCs and versatile aMGCs phenotypes, while the dashed lines suggest multiple spectral morphologic phenotypes. IL-1β: interleukin 1 beta; IL-14: interleukin 14; IL-10: interleukin 10; TGF-β: Transforming growth factor beta; TNFα: tumor necrosis factor alpha; IL-6: interleukin 6; NADPH Ox: reduced nicotinamide adenine dinucleotide phosphate; Inos: inducible nitric oxide synthase; GSH: glutathione; SOD: superoxide dismutase.

2. Materials and Methods

2.1. Sample Preparation for Serial Block Face Imaging: Focused Ion Beam/Scanning Electron Microscopy for Supplemental Video 3

Samples were prepared following a modified version of NCMIR (National Center for Microscopy and Imaging Research) methods for three-dimensional (3D) EM. Unless otherwise stated, all reagents wefre purchased from Electron Microscopy Sciences and all specimen preparation was performed at the Electron Microscopy Core Facility, University of Missouri. Tissues were fixed in 2% paraformaldehyde, 2% glutaraldehyde in 100 mM sodium cacodylate buffer pH = 7.35. Next, fixed tissues were rinsed with 100 mM sodium cacodylate buffer, pH = 7.35 containing 130 mM sucrose. Secondary fixation was performed using equal parts 4% osmium tetroxide and 3% potassium ferrocyanide in cacodylate buffer and incubated on ice for 1 h, then rinsed with cacodylate buffer and further with distilled water. En block staining was performed for one hour in a 1% thiocarbohydrazide solution followed by distilled water rinses. Rinsed tissues were incubated in an additional 2% aqueous osmium tetroxide solution for 30 min at room temperature, then rinsed with distilled water. Additional en bloc staining was performed using 1% aqueous uranyl acetate and incubated at 4 °C overnight, then rinsed with distilled water. A final en bloc staining was performed using Walton's Lead Nitrate solution (Lawrence Livermore Laboratory University of California, Livermore, CA, USA) for 30 min at 60 °C. Tissues were rinsed and dehydrated using ethanol, transitioned into acetone, and then infiltrated with Durcapan resin and polymerized at 60 °C overnight. Block faces were prepared using an ultramicrotome (Ultracut UCT, Leica Microsystems, Germany) and a diamond knife (Diatome, Hatfield, PA, USA) and mounted on an SEM stub and coated with 20 nm of platinum using the EMS 150T-ES Sputter Coater (Leica Microsystems Inc. Buffalo Grove, IL USA). Serial block face data was acquired on a Thermo Fisher Scientific Scios Analytical Dualbeam (Hillsboro, OR, USA). The region of interest was identified using established landmarks and protected with a 1-μm layer of platinum using the ion column. Trenches were rough cut to the side and the front of the block face using a high ion beam current (30 kV 5 nA) to expose the desired block face. Next, the block face was polished using an ion beam current of 50 pA prior to collecting serial images using the Slice &View automated software package. Serial sections were cut at a thickness of 20 nm (30 kV 1 nA) and SEM images were acquired at 2 keV and 25 pA using the T1-BSE detector and reverse contrast. Image segmentation was performed using ThermoScientific Amira 6 Software (Thermo Fisher Scientific). Approximately 250 slices were obtained to create the video for Supplementary Video S3.

2.2. Microglia Ultrastructure Examination and Observation

Three models per group were studied by TEM (n = 3 in control CKC and in diabetic DBC models). Regions of interest were selected based on the presence of NVU capillaries in gray matter cortical layer III. A total of 60 microglia were eventually studied for all models with 10 from each model providing 30 microglia from CKC and 30 from DBC models. Age-matched nondiabetic control C57BL/KsJ microglia demonstrated 28 of 30 with ramified cytoplasmic projections, 5 of 30 microglia with aMt of 5–6 or more and 3 of 30 with some degree of nuclear chromatin condensation, while in DBC 9 of 30 microglia demonstrated ramifications, 25 of 30 microglia demonstrated aberrant Mt (aMt) with 6–14 aMt and 24 of 30 depicted marked chromatin condensation. Herein, we depict representative ultrastructural remodeling changes in aMGC of the diabetic DBC compared to the rMGC in control CKC models.

3. Results

3.1. Microglial Cell of the Neurovascular Unit in Control CKC Model

Microglial cells reside throughout the brain parenchyma and are frequently adjacent to the endothelial cell, pericytes, mural cells and astrocytes of the NVU in the cortical grey matter of layer III.

The normal ultrastructure morphology of ramified microglial cells in control models (CKC) in relation to the NVU and other interstitial regions are depicted (Figures 3 and 4).

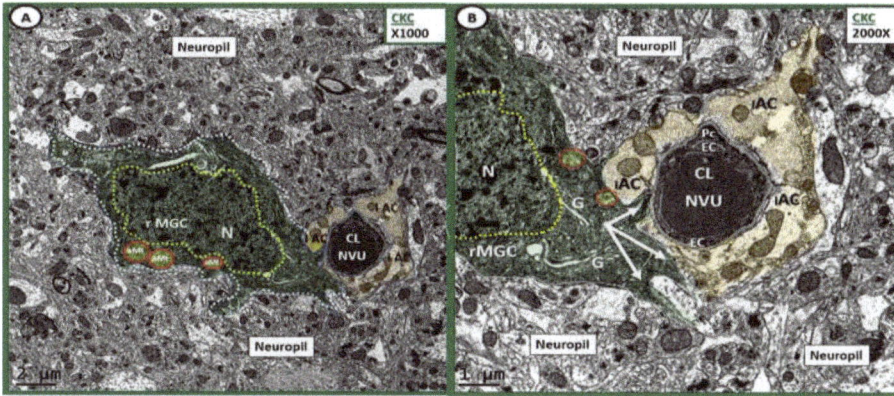

Figure 3. Ramified microglia as a part of the neurovascular unit in control CKC models. (**A,B**) Depict the normal ultrastructure of the ramified microglia cells in the control CKC models at different magnifications. (**A**) Depicts a ramified microglia cell (rMGC) phenotype surveilling the NVU. Note how the rMGC cytoplasmic processes (pseudo-colored green) appear to slide in between the intact astrocytes (pseudo-colored golden iAC) in panel (**A,B**) as if surveilling or probing the NVU (arrows in panel (**B**) for danger or damage signals. Ramified MGCs are known to have a stippled outer chromatin electron density and also a diffuse inner stippled chromatin arrangement. Also, note the aberrant Mt (aMt) numbering 3 in panel (**A**) and two in panel (**B**) (pseudo-colored yellow with red outline), which are in contrast to the multiple aMt in the DBC depicted later. (**A**) Magnification ×1000; scale bar = 2 μm; (**B**) Magnification ×2000; scale bar = 1 μm. Cl: capillary lumen; EC: endothelial cell; G: Golgi body; iAC: intact astrocyte; N: nucleus: Pc: pericyte.

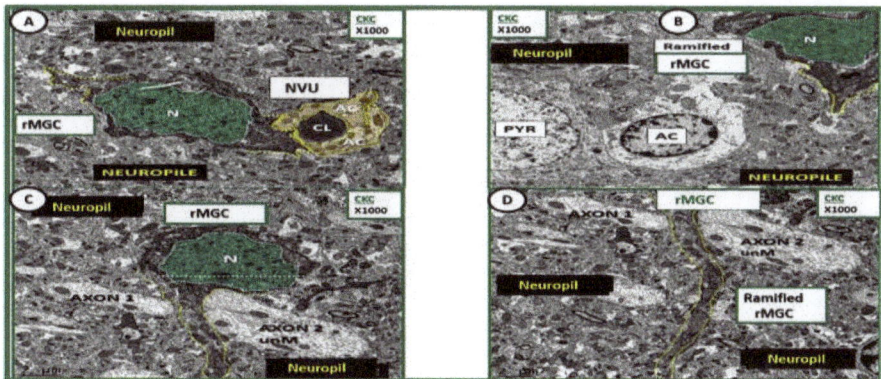

Figure 4. Ultrastructure of ramified microglia in control CKC models. (**A–D**) Depict the normal ultrastructure of the ramified microglia (rMGC) in nondiabetic control CKC models. Ramified microglia typically have elongated cytoplasmic processes (yellow-dashed lines) and they typically have a large prominent nucleus (N) (pseudo-colored green and outlined with white-dashed line). Note the diffuse electron-dense chromatin pattern that will undergo extensive chromatin condensation-clumping in activated microglia of diabetic DBC models depicted later. Magnification ×1000; scale bar = 2 μm. AC: astrocyte; CL: capillary lumen; NVU: neurovascular unit; PYR: pyramidal cell.

We have previously demonstrated how the ramified microglia with their elongated processes are very responsive and mobile in cleaning Layer III of the cortical grey matter in the diet-induced Western models (Figure S1, Figure S2 and Video S1). Interestingly, the more proximal somal regions of microglia appear linearly and are observed to be attached to one another similar to box cars of a train between layer III and layer IV and thus, we refer to them as 'trains of microglia' (Video S2). We also observed microglia interrogating the NVU; however, in Western models they appear to back away and do not invade the NVU (as in diabetic DBC models discussed later) since they do not detect any danger or damage signals and do not invade the NVU and appear to back away from the NVU (Video S2).

3.2. Microglia Remodeling in Diabetic DBC Models

The aMGC in DBC models were observed to invade the endothelial cells of the NVU and were associated with the detachment and separation / retraction of the astrocyte from the NVU, attenuation and/or loss of the TJ/AJ in the blood brain barrier (BBB) of the NVU and have aberrant mitochondria and chromatin condensation (Figures 5 and 6)

Ramified MGC CKC

1. Have long extended cytoplasmic processes for normal housekeeping functions in healthy brain

2. Chromatin is diffusely dispersed within the nucleus

3. Few aberrant Mt. (numbering 4-6)

4. Cytokines: L IL-4, IL-10 TGF-β

Activated MGC DBC

1. LOSS OF LONG CYTOPLASMIC PROCESSES: amoeboid phenotype once damage or danger signals have been detected.

> activation marker MHC II in activated microglia

2. Chromatin is highly condensed

3. Aberrant Mt are markedly increased (12-15)

4. Cytokines: IL-1β, TNFα, Glutamate, * ROS-RNS, NAD(P)H Oxidase, iNOS.

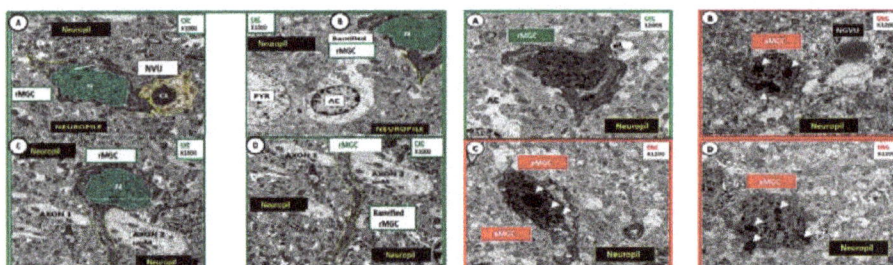

Figure 5. Comparison of ramified MGC to an activated MGC in control CKC and diabetic DBC models. (**A–D**) Depict the ramified (rMGC) (colorized with green nucleus) to demonstrate at low magnification the different morphology of the rMGC as compared to the activated aMGC DBC model (**B–D**). One notes the aMGC assumes a more amoeboid morphology in the DBC model (**B–D**) on the right outlined in red as compared to the CKC models on the left with CKC with ramified cytoplasmic extensions (outlined with yellow dashed lines). Also note that the nuclear chromatin is condensed, aggregated/clumped in the DBC models on right when compared to the diffuse nuclear chromatin in the CKC on the left. Importantly, note the major differences between the CKC and DBC in the upper 1–4 numbered major differences between CKC rMGC and DBC aMGC. The low magnification in these images is unable to demonstrate or appreciate the differences in mitochondria in these images. Magnification ×1000 (**A–D** in CKC) and ×1200 (**A–D** in DBC); Scale bar = 2 μm.

Microglial cells undergo ultrastructural maladaptive remodeling changes to the cytoplasmic and nuclear components including cytoplasmic aMt that are characterized by markedly swollen mitochondria with loss of electron-dense mitochondrial matrix proteins and crista in the cytoplasm and nuclear chromatin condensation in addition to becoming invasive of the NVU (Figure 7) (Figure S4 and Video S3).

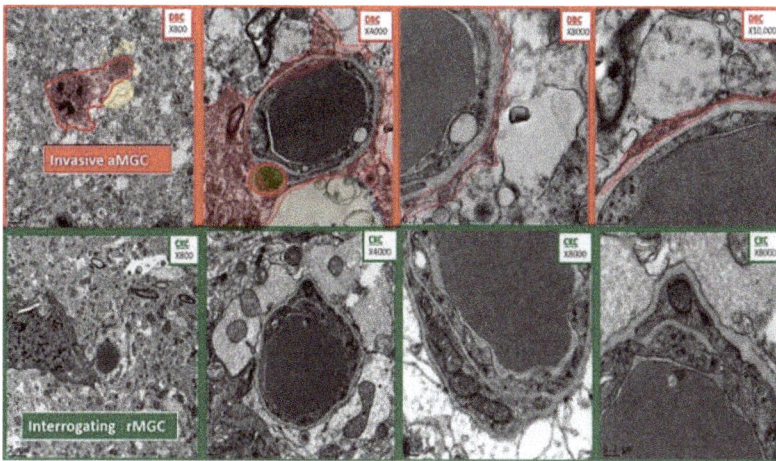

Figure 6. Comparison of microglia invasion in the diabetic DBC and interrogation in control CKC models. The top four panels depict the invasiveness of an activated microglial cell (aMGC) (pseudo-colored red) with marked chromatin clumping–aggregation invading a NUV with capillary lumen in progressively increased magnifications from left to right. Note the thin rim of the aMGC cytoplasmic extensions as it approaches the NVU and begins to encircle the enclosed endothelial and pericyte basement membrane with early detachment of the normally adherent intact astrocyte. In some images they will result in the complete astrocyte detachment and retraction from the NVU. Magnifications at the top right of each image and scale bars are indicated in the lower left of each panel. In the lower four panels of comparable magnifications note how the rMGC is only undergoing an interrogating function and does not invade the NVU.

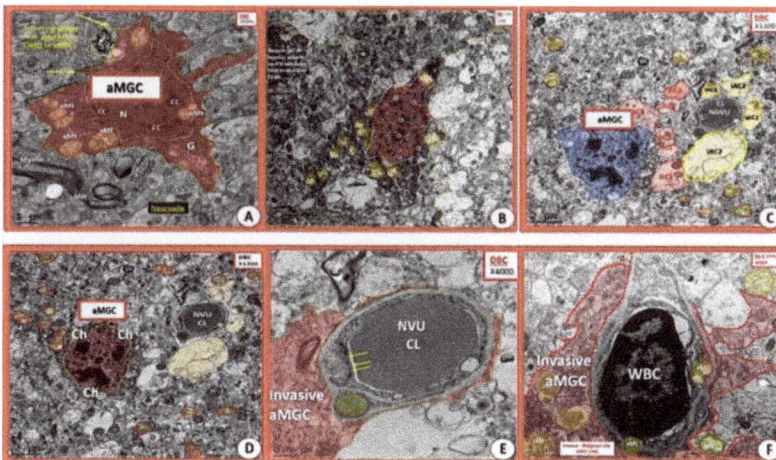

Figure 7. Activated microglia become invasive of the neurovascular unit in diabetic DBC models. Panels (**C–F**) depict how activated MGCs (aMGCs) become invasive to the NVU in DBC models. In contrast to the CKC ramified MGC (rMGC), which are surveilling, aMGC (pseudo-colored red except for the 'frown-faced' aMGC (pseudo-colored blue)) nucleus in (**C**). Panel F depicts a mononuclear white blood cell (lymphocyte) (WBC) adherent to the luminal NVU endothelial cell. Magnification ×2000 (**A**); ×1200 (**B–D**); ×4000 (**E**); ×3000 (**F**) with varying scale bars lower left of each panel.

Activated-amoeboid microglia have a marked increase in cytoplasmic aMt and also demonstrate extensive nuclear chromatin condensation in contrast to a diffuse stippled chromatin pattern in CKC and contain increased numbers of aberrant mitochondria within the cytoplasm, as compared to the ramified microglia in controls Figures 8–12.

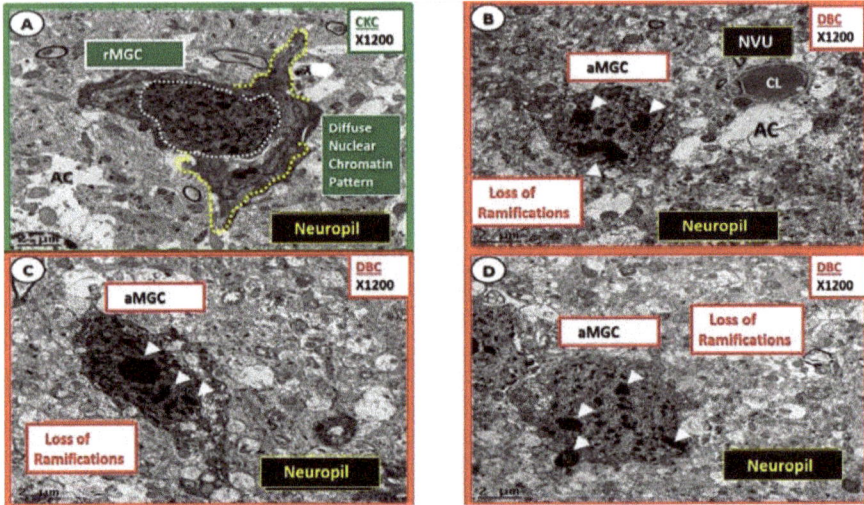

Figure 8. Nuclear chromatin condensation of activated microglia in diabetic DBC models. (**A**) Depicts the appearance of the nucleus with diffuse nuclear chromatin pattern (outlined in white dashed lines) and ramified cytoplasmic extensions (yellow dashed lines). Panels (**B–D**) demonstrate a distinct phenotypic nuclear chromatin condensation (arrowheads) within the nuclei of the activated microglia cells (aMGC) in the diabetic DBC as compared to the ramified microglia cells (rMGC) in control nondiabetic CKC models. Specifically, note the unusual 'frown-faced' nuclei in panel **B** due to nuclear chromatin condensation. Magnification ×1200; scale bar = 2 µm. CL: capillary lumen; NVU: neurovascular unit.

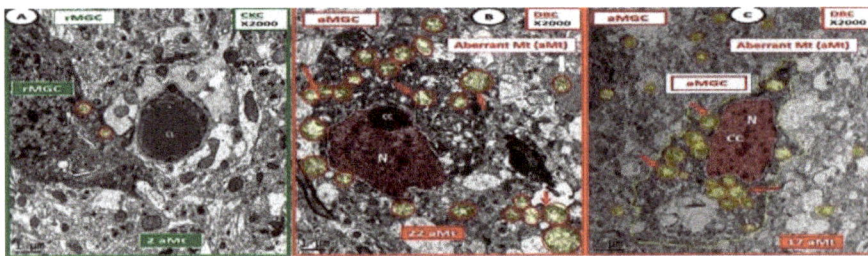

Figure 9. Activated microglia cells depict aberrant mitochondria in diabetic DBC models. Panels (**B,C**) illustrate the pseudo-colored red nuclei of activated microglia cells (aMGC) and the aberrant mitochondria (aMt) (pseudo-colored yellow with encircling red lines) (arrows) that are markedly increased in number and demonstrate marked mitochondrial (Mt) swelling with loss of electron-dense Mt matrix and crista as compared to control CKC model (**Panel A**) in diabetic DBC. Aberrant Mt will also be observed in other neurovascular unit cells and neurons in later images. Also, some aMGCs were extremely dark as in panel (**B**). However, all MGC are dark when compared to other glia and neurons. Magnification ×2000; bar = 1 µm in panels (**A,B**) and bar = 2 µm in panel (**C**). CC: chromatin condensation; CL: capillary lumen; N: nucleus.

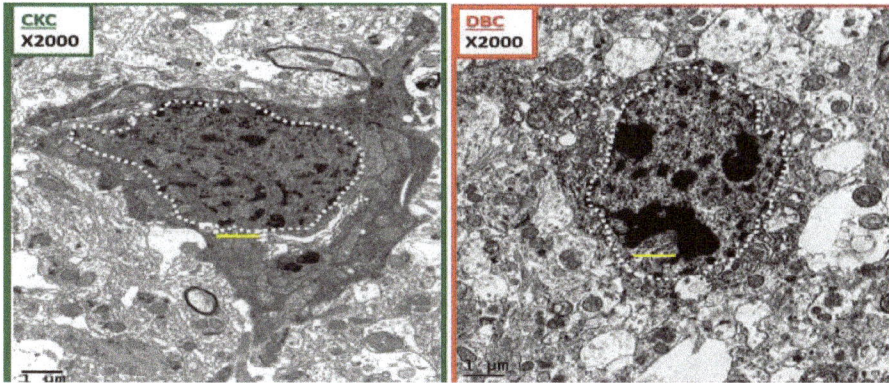

Figure 10. Chromatin condensation in the diabetic DBC. The above images depict ramified and amoeboid-activated microglia in a side-by-side comparison. A ramified microglia (rMGC) on the left with a stippled outer chromatin at the neurolemma and a diffuse stippling of chromatin within the core of the nucleus in the control CKC. In contrast, the amoeboid-activated microglia (aMGC) on the right depicts marked nuclear chromatin condensation in the DBC. Note that in the aMGC of the diabetic DBC the nuclear chromatin condensation–compaction volume is markedly greater than in the nondiabetic control rMGC CKC models. Magnification ×2000; scale bar = 1 μm and was copied and placed within the nuclei to appreciate the sizes of the chromatin.

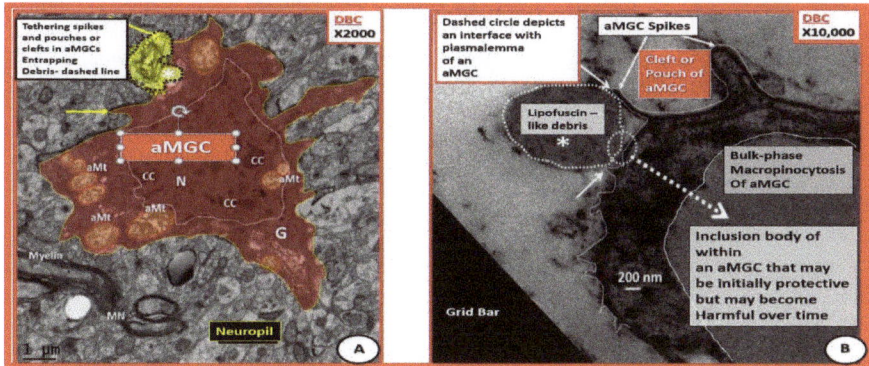

Figure 11. Activated microglia with aberrant mitochondria and tethering spikes and pouches in diabetic DBC. (**A**) Depicts a pseudo-colored red aMGC. (**B**) Depicts a high magnification of a portion of an outer cytoplasmic MGC phagocytosing lipofuscin-like debris. In (**A**), the plasma membrane appears to be taking up a residual body (dashed line with yellow color) and uptake of lipofuscin-like debris (white dashed line) in (**B**). Panel (**A**) depicts spikes (arrows) and pouches or clefts and aberrant mitochondria (aMt) (pseudo-colored yellow with red outer lines). Panel B illustrates bulk phase macropinocytosis of lipofuscin-like debris across the plasma membrane and appears to be being deposited within the cytoplasm of an aMGC. These two aMGCs are different cells but both are within the cerebral cortical grey matter in layer III and demonstrate the important process of phagocytosis. Note the prominent chromatin condensation (CC) within the nucleus. Panel A magnification ×2000; bar = 1μm. Panel B magnification ×10,000; bar = 200 nm. G = Golgi apparatus; MN = myelinated neuron.

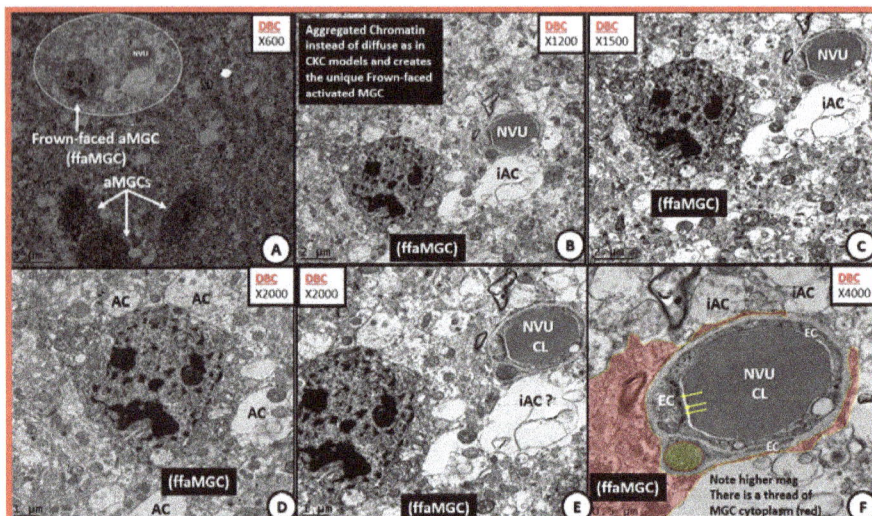

Figure 12. Activated microglia cells are associated with chromatin condensation and invasiveness of the neurovascular unit in the diabetic DBC Models. Panels (**A**–**F**) depict an activated 'frown-faced' activated/amoeboid microglia cell (aMGC) and follows it through progressively increased magnifications to demonstrate how the aMGC invades the NVU and associates with early astrocyte (AC) detachment. Additionally, note how the blood brain barrier (BBB) tight and adherent junctions (TJ/AJ) are attenuated via interruption of the normally continuous TJ/AJ of the BBB in panel (**F**). Also note in panel (**F**) that the aMGC of the 'frown-faced' microglia with marked chromatin condensation appears to not only invade but may also lift and promote the early separation of the intact AC from the basement membrane of the NVU inferiorly and superiorly. CL: capillary lumen.

The observation of aMt in aMGCs may set the stage for redox injuries not only to the microglia itself and their organelles but also the surrounding cells of the NVU.

In summary, aMGCs in the diabetic DBC may be characterized by four ultrastructure remodeling core signature changes: (i) Loss of ramified cytoplasmic extensions with amoeboid phenotypes; (ii) invasive phenotypes of the NVU; (iii) aberrant mitochondria with swelling, loss of electron-dense matrix, and loss or fragmented crista; (iv) nuclear chromatin condensation when compared to nondiabetic CKC models.

We have included the newer technology of Focused Ion Beam/Scanning Electron Microscopy (FIB/SEM) videos of the aMGC in the DBC models, which demonstrate not only the nuclear chromatin condensation but also help to better understand the 3D motion of the aM) as they come into and out of view within the cytoplasm of the DBC aMGC (Figure S4 and Video S3).

3.3. Aberrant Mitochondria in the Diabetic DBC Models

Mitochondria play a vital and essential role in nutrient metabolism of brain cells including the vascular mural cells, glia, dendritic synapses and neurons [13,15–17]. Aberrant mitochondria were primarily found to be observed in the cytoplasm of aMGCs; however, these similar aMt remodeling changes also were found in some EC, pericyte (Pc) and Pc foot processes, AC, myelinated and unmyelinated neurons within the neuropil (Figure 13).

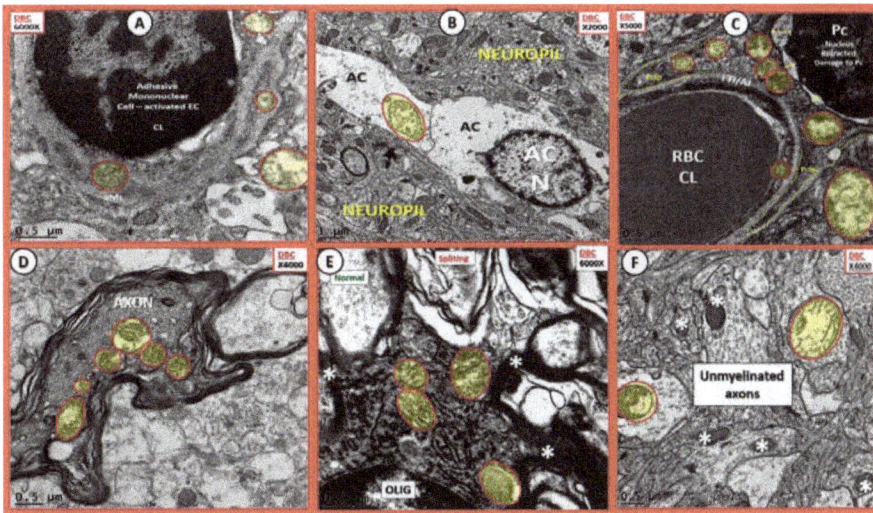

Figure 13. Aberrant mitochondria in endothelial cells, pericytes and foot processes, astrocytes, oligodendrocytes, myelinated and unmyelinated neurons. Panels (**A–F**) demonstrate that aberrant mitochondria (aMt) are found to be present in multiple cells in addition to activated microglia cells (aMGCs). The aMt are pseudo-colored in each of these panels (yellow outlined in red lines) in order to allow rapid recognition. Panels (**B,F**) are especially important since they demonstrate the aMt characterized by swollen mitochondria (Mt), loss of electron-dense Mt matrix and crista. Panel (**A**) illustrates the aMt within the endothelial cells and surrounding aMGC. Panel (**B**) depicts aMt in ACs. Panel (**C**) demonstrates aMt in pericytes and foot processes (Pc and Pcfp). Panel (**D**) depicts aMt in a dysmyelinated neuronal axon. Panel (**E**) depicts aMt in an oligodendrocyte and Panel (**F**) illustrates aMt in an AC to the left and an unmyelinated axon on the right within the neuropil. Magnifications are noted in the upper part of each panel and scale bars are located at the lower left-hand side of all panels. Scale bars = 0.5 μm in all images except for panel (**B**) with scale bar = 1 μm.

3.4. Implications of White Blood Cell (Mononuclear) Lymphocyte Adherence in DBC Models

Adherence of the mononuclear white blood cell (WBC) (lymphocyte) in some NUVs of the diabetic DBC models have allowed not only the concept of an activated endothelium in DBC to be strongly considered as compared to CKC but also have stimulated the question as to the possibility that the aMGC may also be playing a role in signaling the WBC to come in contact with the EC and adhere to an activated endothelium (Figure 13).

Previously, we had to include images of WBC adherence in Part I because there is such widespread multicellular remodeling that it is difficult to just examine one aspect of cellular remodeling in one image without including other cellular remodeling changes that concurrently occur in DBC models [1]. Also, these glial remodeling changes are associated with hyperglycemia and it is important to understand how hyperglycemia may drive the chronic neuroinflammation and the associated compromise of BBB TJ/AJ, which promote an increase in permeability and leads to memory loss and impaired cognition in T2DM mouse models in the diabetic DBC [18]. Activated microglia are known not only to contain certain cell surface receptors but also are responsible for the secretion of a specialized group of signaling cytokines and chemokines, which include monocyte chemoattractant protein 1 (MCP-1) chemokine also known as CCL2. Monocyte chemoattractant protein and other inflammatory signaling molecules are thought to signal peripheral monocytes, neutrophils and lymphocytes to adhere to the NVU endothelial cell and eventually undergo chemotaxis into the brain and migrate to regions of injury (Figure 14) [19].

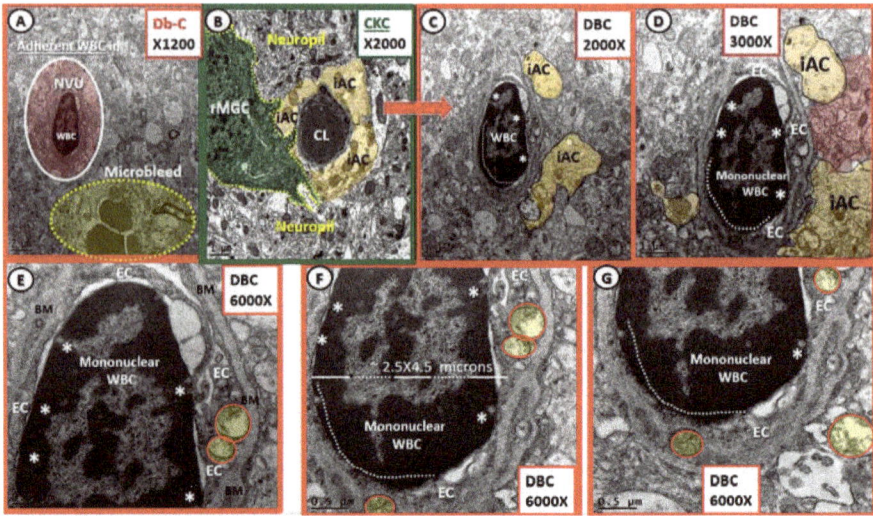

Figure 14. Compilation of white blood cell adherence in diabetic DBC models. Panels (**A,C–G**) depict multiple increasing magnifications of a white blood cell (WBC) adhering to the luminal activated endothelial cell (EC). Panel B demonstrates a surveilling ramified microglia (rMGC) and note how it is only surveilling the NVU for danger or damage signals. Also note the intact golden halo of astrocyte end feet surrounding the NVU. This is in contrast to the reactive-activated (aMGC), which appears to be invading the NVU. Note that in higher magnified images in panels (**E–G**) that the ECs also have aberrant mitochondria (depicted as yellow cores with encircling red lines). Also, note in (**C,D**) that there are some remaining intact astrocytes (iAC) to the right of the NVU (pseudo-colored golden); however to the left, note the absence of iACs adjacent to the outer basement membrane (BM) of the EC and pericyte of the NVU. Panel A depicts not only the adherence of a WBC to the activated EC but also depicts a region of microbleeds (encircled pseudo-colored yellow with yellow dashed line and the abnormal NVU with adherent WBC enclosed in a white line oval with pseudo-colored red interior. Panels (**C–G**) depict adhesion sites (asterisks) with a dashed line where the adherence appears to be continuous. The adherent mononuclear WBC cell is too small (2.5×4.5 µm) to be a monocyte and because of the thinned nearly absent cytoplasm is morphologically considered to represent a lymphocyte. Varying magnifications are present in the identifying boxes and the scale bars are present in the lower left of each image. 2;1;1;1 µm (panels (**A–D**) respectively) and 0.5 µm (panels (**E,G**) respectively).

4. Discussion

Previously, we have presented the data supporting concurrent multicellular maladaptive remodeling in the cells comprising the NVU structures I [1]. In the present paper we describe ultrastructural remodeling of activated microglia, which also contain aberrant mitochondria and NVU adherent WBCs to the activated luminal endothelial cell of the diabetic. Previously, we have posited that activated microglia may be related to accelerated aging and the increased risk of developing age-related neurodegeneration associated with T2DM (1). Furthermore, the ultrastructural changes noted in the DBC models may possibly contribute to the increased risk of developing age-related neurodegenerative disease and dementia such as sporadic Alzheimer's disease (AD) and Parkinson's disease (PD) [1].

Mitochondrial dynamics are of critical importance in T2DM [20] and it has previously been documented that there is an increase in dynamin-1-like protein (Drp1) fission protein and increased activity of the glycogen synthase kinase 3 beta (GSK3β) proteins, while fusion proteins mitofusin-2 (Mfn2) and optic atrophy 1 (OPA-1) remain similar in T2DM as healthy controls [21,22]. Subsequently, the aberrant mitochondria are locked into a state of fission/fusion imbalance with mitochondrial fission being predominate. Further, these aberrant mitochondria may result in damage not only to the inner membranes but also the outer mitochondrial membranes that may allow for herniation and loss of the mitochondrial matrix proteins and sometimes result in mitochondria swelling (Figure 15) [23].

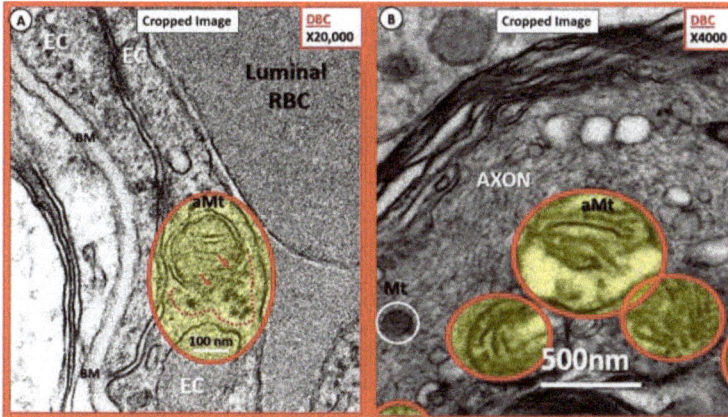

Figure 15. Possible mechanisms for the development of aberrant mitochondria (aMt) in the diabetic DBC models. (**A,B**) Illustrate possible Mt herniation with loss of Mt matrix proteins and crista with intact scale bars. Panel (**A**) original magnification ×20,000 with intact scale bar = 100 nm. Panel (**B**) original magnification ×4000 with intact scale bar = 500 nm. (**A**) depicts the loss of Mt matrix proteins and crista with protein aggregation into the surrounding EC cytoplasm in the aMt possibly via herniation (pseudo-colored yellow with encircling red line). Note that the outer Mt and inner Mt membranes appear to be disrupted allowing it contents to herniate outward or leak into the surrounding EC cytoplasm (arrows and red dashed lines). Interestingly, note the interruption of tight junction/adherens junction (TJ/AJ electron-dense staining where there are overlapping ECs in (**A**). Panel (**B**) also demonstrates three aMt with the superior aMt demonstrating possible herniation in a dysmyelinated neuronal axon (pseudo-colored yellow with encircling red line). Importantly, note the adjacent normal electron-dense Mt (encircled white) with electron-dense matrix and smaller size as compared to the aMt in this myelinated axon. aMt: Aberrant mitochondria; BM: Basement membrane; EC: endothelial cell; Mt: mitochondria; RBC: red blood cell.

Recently, there has been an interest in hyperglycemia-driven neuroinflammation, which may compromise the integrity of BBB with increased permeability that leads to memory loss and impaired cognition [18]. This, along with the increasing interest in the vascular contributions to cognitive impairment and dementia, wherein scientific experts convened to discuss the research gaps in our understanding of how vascular factors contribute to Alzheimer's disease and related dementia has been discussed. [24,25]. These contributions to cognitive impairment and dementia could be considered inclusive of our current findings of the NVU remodeling including the glia ultrastructural remodeling in the diabetic DBC models. We propose that this terminology would be even more inclusive and put forth the title of microvascular contributions to cognitive impairment and dementia (Figure 16). The clinical importance of which, may be discussed over the coming years and could possibly remain a constant when discussing the microvascular and glia remodeling of the brain as an end-organ in T2DM and diabetic cognopathy. The process of neuroinflammation including the activated microglia remodeling abnormalities in the DBC are also now candidates to be included in this microvascular contribution to cognitive impairment and dementia scenario. Importantly, a recent publication regarding the virtual kaleidoscopic presentation of identifying core gene microglial phenotypes and disease-specific microglial signatures has been shared, which aid in our trek into the future along with the concept of metabolic shifts and reprogramming of microglia [12,26].

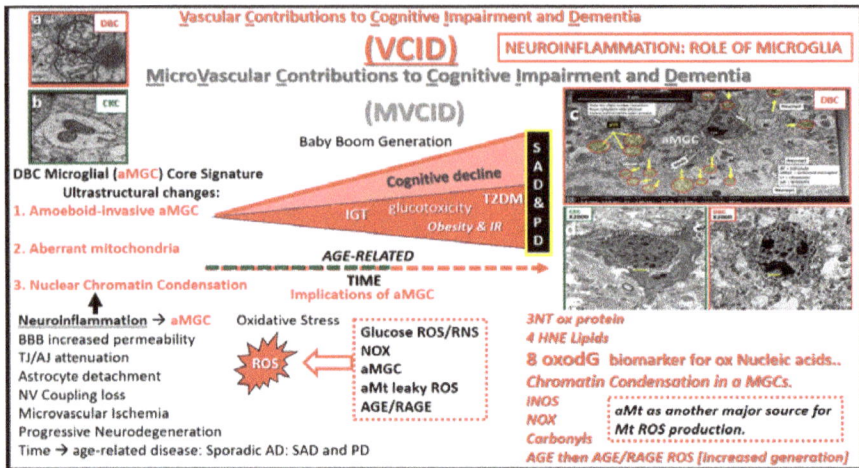

Figure 16. Microvascular contribution to cognitive impairment and dementia. This cartoon image with transmission electron microscopic image inserts (**a–d**) depict impaired glucose tolerance (IGT), obesity and insulin resistance (IR) in diet-induced obesity (DIO) as the disease process progresses to increased glucotoxicity to overt type 2 diabetes mellitus (T2DM) in humans and our DBC models and may be associated with increasing cognitive impairment and dementia. As previously discussed, this is associated with a plethora of morphological ultrastructural multicellular remodeling changes and abnormalities, which include activated-amoeboid microglia cells (aMGC) (insert **c**) that may be associated with increased synthesis and secretion of functional toxic cytokines and chemokines in the DBC models. These abnormalities may contribute to neurodegeneration in addition to aMGC nuclear chromatin condensation (insert **d**) and leaky aberrant Mt (aMt) (insert **a**). These aMGCs may be associated and contribute to neuroinflammation, which may lead to the development of microvascular contributions to cognitive impairment and dementia (MVCID) and furthermore, may contribute to the development of sporadic Alzheimer's disease (SAD) and sporadic Parkinson's disease (PD). AGE = advanced glycation end products; BBB: Blood brain barrier; DIO: Diet-induced obesity; Inos: Inducible nitric oxide synthase; NOX = NADPH Ox (reduced nicotinamide adenine dinucleotide phosphate); NV: Neurovascular; RAGE: Receptor for advanced glycation endproducts; ROS: Reactive oxygen species; TJ/AJ: Tight junctions/adherens junctions; 3NT: 3 nitrotyrosine; 4HNE: 4 hydroxynonenal; 8oxodG: 8-Oxo-2′-deoxyguanosine, which are biomarkers of oxidative stress for proteins, lipids, nucleic acids respectively.

Indeed, these are exciting times having identified microglial core ultrastructural phenotype signatures consisting of amoeboid phenotypes, invasive NVU phenotypes, aberrant mitochondria and chromatin condensation-compaction as described by utilizing the established technique of TEM and the newer techniques of FIB/SEM. These established and newer techniques have allowed us to further explore some of the hidden secrets as put forth in part I and now this part II series of the microglia and mitochondria.

On October 2nd, 2018, we found the following paper updating the role of microglia and feel that our readers should supplement our ultrastructural remodeling changes with a summary of the functional microglia changes put forth by Hammond T.R., Robinson D. and Stevens B. in their published preprint [27]. In the past few years there has been an explosion of functional information regarding microglia receptors and secreted proteins for surveillance and immune responses to better understand

their multiple roles. It is now very clear amongst microglia researchers that microglia may assume a myriad of activation states or spectrum changes of activation (Figure 2) from their development to their roles in forming ramified microglia to their spectrums of activated states, which includes synaptic pruning in health and disease and their supportive role of synaptic maintenance [6,27], Hammond T.R. et al. [27] state the following: "First, we must better understand the states that microglia assume in both development and disease. It is widely agreed that the term activation, or the bimodal M1/M2 scheme, does not sufficiently describe the multitude of ways in which these cells can respond to changes in their environment or the diversity of their functional states." Because of these evolving current concepts, we only discussed our observational ultrastructural remodeling changes of the microglia in relation to the neurovascular unit and other glial cells found in the female diabetic db/db models (DBC) and did not go into any depth regarding their functional changes as we were only performing ultrastructural remodeling changes. Indeed, these are exciting times to study the brain and microglial cells and reflect on the secret (the tissues [1]) to see how they undergo ultrastructural remodeling changes.

Supplementary Materials: The following are available online at http://www.mdpi.com/2571-6980/1/2/21/s1, Figure S1: Cubed image pyramidal layer III region of interest, Figure S2: Region of Interest, Figure S3: Neurovascular Unit with intact astrocytes, Figure S4: Activated microglia with aberrant mitochondria and chromatin condensation, Video S1: Microglia actively cleaning pyramidal layer III, Video S2: Ramified microglia surveilling the Neurovascular Unit, Video S3: Activated microglia with aberrant mitochondria and chromatin.

Author Contributions: M.R.H. and V.G.D. conceptualized the study; M.R.H. performed the image collection and interpretation; D.G.G. prepared the tissue specimens for transmission electron microscopic studies and assisted M.R.H.; M.R.H. prepared the manuscript; A.R.A. collected tissue specimens; V.G.D., A.R.A., and D.G.G. assisted in editing.

Funding: This study was supported by an internal grant entitled: Excellence in Electron Microscopy grant and issued by the University of Missouri Electron Microscopy Core and Office of Research. No external funding was available.

Acknowledgments: Authors wish to thank Tommi White of the University of Missouri Electron Microscopy Core Facility. Authors also wish to thank our mentor James R. Sowers, who inspired us to interrogate, characterize, and understand the secrets that the tissues behold.

Conflicts of Interest: The authors declare no conflicts of interest.

References

1. Hayden, M.R.; Grant, D.; Aroor, A.; Demarco, V.G. Ultrastructural remodeling of the neurovascular unit in the female diabetic db/db Model—Part I: Astrocyte. *Neuroglia* **2018**, *1*, 15. [CrossRef]
2. Tambuyzer, B.R.; Ponsaerts, P.; Nouwen, E.J. Microglia: Gatekeepers of the central nervous system immunology. *J. Leukoc. Biol.* **2009**, *85*, 352–370. [CrossRef] [PubMed]
3. Pósfai, B.; Cserép, C.; Orsolits, B.; Dénes, Á. New Insights into microglia-neuron interactions: A neuron's perspective. *Neuroscience* **2018**. [CrossRef] [PubMed]
4. Liu, Y.; Li, M.; Zhang, Z.; Ye, Y.; Zhou, J. Role of microglia-neuron interactions in diabetic encephalopathy. *Ageing Res. Rev.* **2017**, *42*, 28–39. [CrossRef] [PubMed]
5. Glass, C.K.; Saijo, K.; Winner, B.; Marchetto, M.C.; Gage, F.H. Mechanisms underlying inflammation in neurodegeneration. *Cell* **2010**, *140*, 918–934. [CrossRef] [PubMed]
6. Koellhoffer, E.C.; McCullough, L.D.; Ritzel, R.M. Old maids: Aging and its impact on microglia function. *Int. J. Mol. Sci.* **2017**, *18*, 769. [CrossRef] [PubMed]
7. Tang, Y. Editorial: microglial polarization in the pathogenesis and therapeutics of neurodegenerative diseases. *Front. Aging Neurosci.* **2018**, *10*, 154. [CrossRef] [PubMed]
8. Tang, Y.; Le, W. Differential roles of M1 and M2 microglia in neurodegenerative diseases. *Mol. Neurobiol.* **2016**, *53*, 1181–1194. [CrossRef] [PubMed]
9. Crotti, A.; Ransohoff, R.M. Microglial physiology and pathophysiology: Insights from genome-wide transcriptional profiling. *Immunity* **2016**, *44*, 505–515. [CrossRef] [PubMed]
10. Ransohoff, R.M.; Perry, V.H. Microglial physiology: Unique stimuli, specialized responses. *Annu. Rev. Immunol.* **2009**, *27*, 119–145. [CrossRef] [PubMed]

11. Ransohoff, R.M. A polarizing question: Do M1 and M2 microglia exist? *Nat. Neurosci.* **2016**, *19*, 987–991. [CrossRef] [PubMed]
12. Orihuela, R.; McPherson, C.A.; Harry, G.J. Microglial M1/M2 polarization and metabolic states. *Br. J. Pharmacol.* **2016**, *173*, 649–665. [CrossRef] [PubMed]
13. Sousa, C.; Biber, K.; Micheluccie, A. Cellular and molecular characterization of microglia: A unique immune cell population. *Front. Immunol.* **2017**, *8*, 198. [CrossRef] [PubMed]
14. Hayden, M.R.; Banks, W.A.; Shah, G.N.; Gu, Z.; Sowers, J.R. Cardiorenal metabolic syndrome and diabetic cognopathy. *Cardiorenal Med.* **2013**, *3*, 265–282. [CrossRef] [PubMed]
15. Abdul-Ghani, M.A.; DeFronzo, R.A. Mitochondrial dysfunction, insulin resistance, and type 2 diabetes mellitus. *Curr. Diabetes Rep.* **2008**, *8*, 173–178. [CrossRef]
16. Yu, L.; Fink, B.D.; Herlein, J.A.; Sivitz, W.I. Mitochondrial function in diabetes: Novel methodology and new insight. *Diabetes* **2013**, *62*, 1833–1842. [CrossRef] [PubMed]
17. Sivitz, W.I.; Yorek, M.A. Mitochondrial dysfunction in diabetes: From molecular mechanisms to functional significance and therapeutic opportunities. *Antioxid. Redox Signal.* **2010**, *12*, 537–577. [CrossRef] [PubMed]
18. Rom, S.; Zuluaga-Ramirez, V.; Gajghate, S.; Seliga, A.; Winfield, M.; Heldt, N.A.; Kolpakov, M.A.; Bashkirova, Y.V.; Sabri, A.K.; Persidsky, Y. Hyperglycemia-driven neuroinflammation compromises BBB leading to memory loss in both diabetes mellitus (DM) type 1 and type 2 mouse models. *Mol. Neurobiol.* **2018**, 1–14. [CrossRef] [PubMed]
19. Deshmane, S.L.; Kremlev, S.; Amini, S.; Sawaya, B.E. Monocyte chemoattractant protein-1 (MCP-1): An overview. *J. Interferon Cytokine Res.* **2009**, *29*, 313–326. [CrossRef] [PubMed]
20. Rovira-Llopis, S.; Bañuls, C.; Diaz-Morales, N.; Hernandez-Mijares, A.; Rocha, M.; Victor, V.M. Mitochondrial dynamics in type 2 diabetes: Pathophysiological implications. *Redox Biol.* **2017**, *11*, 637–645. [CrossRef] [PubMed]
21. Huang, S.; Wang, Y.; Gan, X.; Fang, D.; Zhong, C.; Wu, L.; Hu, G.; Sosunov, A.A.; McKhann, G.M.; Yu, H.; et al. Drp1-mediated mitochondrial abnormalities link to synaptic injury in diabetes model. *Diabetes* **2015**, *64*, 1728–1742. [CrossRef] [PubMed]
22. Gottlieb, R.A.; Daniel Bernstein, D. Mitochondrial remodeling: Rearranging, recycling, and reprogramming. *Cell Calcium* **2016**, *60*, 88–101. [CrossRef] [PubMed]
23. Sesso, A.; Belizário, J.E.; Marques, M.M.; Higuchi, M.L.; Schumacher, R.I.; Colquhoun, A.; Ito, E.; Kawakami, J. Mitochondrial swelling and incipient outer membrane rupture in preapoptotic and apoptotic cells. *Anat. Rec. (Hoboken)* **2012**, *295*, 1647–1659. [CrossRef] [PubMed]
24. Snyder, H.M.; Corriveau, R.A.; Craft, S.; Faber, J.E.; Greenberg, S.M.; Knopman, D.; Lamb, B.T.; Montine, T.J.; Nedergaard, M.; Schaffer, C.B.; et al. Vascular contributions to cognitive impairment and dementia including Alzheimer's disease. *Alzheimer's Dement.* **2015**, *11*, 710–717. [CrossRef] [PubMed]
25. Corriveau, R.A.; Bosetti, F.; Emr, M.; Gladman, J.T.; Koenig, J.I.; Moy, C.S.; Pahigiannis, K.; Waddy, S.P.; Koroshetz, W. the science of vascular contributions to cognitive impairment and dementia (VCID): A framework for advancing research priorities in the cerebrovascular biology of cognitive decline. *Cell Mol. Neurobiol.* **2016**, *36*, 281–288. [CrossRef] [PubMed]
26. Dubbelaar, M.L.; Kracht, L.; Eggen, B.J.L.; Boddeke, E. The kaleidoscope of microglial phenotypes. *Front. Immunol.* **2018**. [CrossRef] [PubMed]
27. Hammond, T.R.; Robinton, D.; Stevens, B. Microglia and the brain: complementary partners in development and disease. *Annu. Rev. Cell Dev. Biol.* **2018**, 34. [CrossRef] [PubMed]

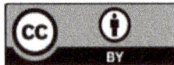

neuroglia

MDPI

Article

Effects of Chemically-Functionalized Single-Walled Carbon Nanotubes on the Morphology and Vitality of D54MG Human Glioblastoma Cells

Seantel Hopkins [1,2,†], **Manoj K. Gottipati** [2,3,4,†], **Vedrana Montana** [2], **Elena Bekyarova** [5,6],
Robert C. Haddon [5,‡] **and Vladimir Parpura** [2,*]

1   Department of Biology, The University of Alabama at Birmingham, Birmingham, AL 35294, USA;
     seantelhopkins@gmail.com
2   Department of Neurobiology, The University of Alabama at Birmingham, Birmingham, AL 35294, USA;
     vedranam@uab.edu
3   Department of Biomedical Engineering and Center for Biotechnology and Interdisciplinary Studies,
     Rensselaer Polytechnic Institute, Troy, NY 12180, USA; gottim2@rpi.edu
4   Department of Neuroscience, Center for Brain and Spinal Cord Repair and Wexner Medical Center,
     The Ohio State University, Columbus, OH 43210, USA
5   Departments of Chemistry and Chemical Engineering and Center for Nanoscale Science and Engineering,
     University of California, Riverside, CA 92521, USA; elena.bekyarova@ucr.edu
6   Carbon Solutions, Inc., Riverside, CA 92507, USA
*   Correspondence: vlad@uab.edu; Tel.: +1-205-996-7369
†   These authors contributed equally to this work.
‡   Deceased on 21 April 2016.

Received: 30 August 2018; Accepted: 8 October 2018; Published: 16 October 2018

Abstract: The unique properties of single-walled carbon nanotubes (SWCNTs) have made them interesting candidates for applications in biomedicine. There are diverse chemical groups that can be attached to SWCNTs in order for these tiny tubes to gain various functionalities, for example, water solubility. Due to the availability of these "functionalization" approaches, SWCNTs are seen as agents for a potential anti-cancer therapy. In this context, we tested different chemically-functionalized forms of SWCNTs to determine which modifications make them better combatants against glioblastoma (astrocytoma grade IV), the deadliest brain cancer. We investigated the effects that two types of water soluble SWCNTs, functionalized with polyethylene glycol (SWCNT-PEG) or tetrahydrofurfuryl-terminated polyethylene glycol (SWCNT-PEG-THFF), have on the morphology and vitality, that is, cell adhesion, proliferation and death rate, of the D54MG human glioblastoma cells in culture. We found that SWCNT-PEG-THFF solute, when added to culture media, makes D54MG cells less round (measured as a significant decrease, by ~23%, in the form factor). This morphological change was induced by the PEG-THFF functional group, but not the SWCNT backbone itself. We also found that SWCNT-PEG-THFF solute reduces the proliferation rate of D54MG cells while increasing the rate of cell death. The functional groups PEG and PEG-THFF, on the other hand, reduce the cell death rate of D54MG human glioma cells. These data indicate that the process of functionalization of SWCNTs for potential use as glioma therapeutics may affect their biological effects.

Keywords: glioblastoma multiforme; carbon nanotubes; morphology; cell adhesion; cell proliferation; cell death rate

---

1. Introduction

Gliomas comprise the large majority of malignant brain tumors and are one of the deadliest cancers, with a median survival of 14 months. The most aggressive glioma type is classified, based on its cell origin, as astrocytoma (high) grade IV, traditionally referred to as a glioblastoma multiforme (GBM), which is the subject of this work. High grade gliomas are characterized by extensive dispersal throughout the brain, indicative of their highly invasive nature [1]. Glioma cells have to adjust their morphology, that is, become less round, during their invasion through the narrow and tortuous extracellular space of the brain [2]. Aside from their invasive nature, their adhesion and proliferative capabilities are factors contributing to their malignancy [3,4]. Finding new treatments that would stop/attenuate the spread of GBMs would be a milestone; this requires a detailed analysis of GBM biology.

The unique properties of single-walled carbon nanotubes (SWCNTs) have made them interesting candidates for applications in biotechnology and biomedicine [5,6]. In the context of glioma nanotechnology and translational therapeutics, functionalized SWCNTs have been used as carriers in advanced drug delivery systems [7–9] or as agents for photothermal therapy [10–13] in variety of human GBM and murine models, capitalizing on the availability of diverse and well established chemistries for the functionalization of SWCNTs [5,6] (i.e., attachment of various chemicals to the SWCNTs in order for tubes to gain a functionality, e.g., water solubility) and their properties to produce heat when exposed to non-ionizing near-infrared radiation [14]. These investigations have driven the development of functionalized SWCNTs as a carrier/delivery agent to cancer tissue; a variety of functionalizations of SWCNTs with molecules rendering their water solubility, a prerequisite for bio applications, have been developed. However, there has been a void in understating the effect of the components of such conjugate nanomaterials on GBM cells. For instance, possible effects of the functionalization group(s) of the conjugate SWCNT nanomaterial are not well described in the literature. Similarly, basic cell biology measurements, such as cell morphology, adhesion, proliferation and death rate, caused by the conjugate SWCNTs vs. their solubilization functional groups, have not been well described. In the present work we set to investigate these issues.

Our present work logically sprouts from our previous studies of the effect that SWCNTs have on primary astrocytes, as reviewed elsewhere [15]. Briefly, to investigate the effects of SWCNTs on primary mouse astrocytes in culture, we used graft copolymers/conjugates of SWCNTs chemically functionalized with polyethylene glycol (PEG) or poly-m-aminobenzene sulfonic acid (PABS) making SWCNTs water soluble (wsSWCNTs) [16,17]. When added to the culturing medium, wsSWCNTs were able to make astrocytes larger and less round compared to the untreated astrocytes, but these nanomaterials did not affect astrocyte vitality, that is, cell adhesion, proliferation and death rate [17]. Generally, the data indicated the necessity of the SWCNT backbone for the changes induced by the water-soluble graft copolymers, while some subtle differences in the effects that SWCNTs had on astrocytes (for clarity details omitted here, but summarized and reviewed in [15] and Table 1 of [17]; also see discussion) were due to the various functional groups attached to the SWCNTs.

In the present study, we aim to investigate the effects that two types of wsSWCNTs, SWCNTs functionalized with polyethylene glycol (SWCNT-PEG) [16,17] and SWCNTs functionalized with tetrahydrofurfuryl-terminated polyethylene glycol (SWCNT-PEG-THFF) [18], have on the morphology and vitality of the D54MG human glioma cell line. We found that SWCNT-PEG-THFF solute induces morphological changes in D54MG human glioma cells. These changes were induced by the functional group, and not the SWCNT backbone itself. Other findings show that, SWCNT-PEG-THFF solute reduces the proliferation potential of D54MG human glioma along with increasing the relative cell death rate, while the functional groups PEG and PEG-THFF reduce the cell death rate of D54MG human glioma cells. Taken together, our present work indicates that additional care should be taken in the process of functionalization of SWCNTs for potential use as glioma therapeutics, as SWCNT conjugates may cause differential biological effects pending on the functional group rendering their water solubility.

2. Materials and Methods

2.1. Water-Soluble Single-Walled Carbon Nanotubes

Single-walled carbon nanotubes were rendered water soluble by covalent attachment of PEG (molecular mass 600 g/mol) or PEG-THFF (molecular mass 200 g/mol) to their walls. These graft copolymers were synthesized and characterized as described in detail elsewhere [16,18]. Single-walled carbon nanotubes- polyethylene glycol used in this study contained, 23 wt% PEG, while the SWCNT-PEG-THFF contained 21 wt% PEG-THFF. Both the SWCNT graft co-polymers were used as colloidal aqueous solutes in cell culture media (see below) at a concentration of 5 µg/mL, chosen based on our previous work [16,17,19]. The functional groups, PEG or PEG-THFF, were used at a concentration of 1 µg/mL, corresponding to 20 wt% of the functionalized wsSWCNTs.

2.2. Human Glioblastoma Multiforme Cell Culture

The human glioma cell line D54MG (classified as a glioblastoma multiforme, GBM, also known as grade IV astrocytoma) modified to stably express enhanced green fluorescent protein (EGFP), as previously described [20,21], was provided by Dr. Harald Sontheimer (at that time at The University of Alabama at Birmingham). From here, we refer to these cells as D54MG-EGFP cells, which were used in all the experiments with the exception of the immunocytochemistry data in Supplementary information, where we used unmodified D54MG cells, also provided by Dr. Harald Sontheimer [20], which originate from Dr. Darrell D. Bigner (Duke University, Durham, NC, USA). We maintained these cells in tissue culture dishes at 37 °C in a 90% air/10% CO_2 atmosphere incubator in cell culture media containing Dulbecco's Modified Eagle Medium/Nutrient Mixture F-12 (DMEM/F-12, Life Technologies, Carlsbad, CA, USA) supplemented with 2 mM L-glutamine and 7% Fetal Bovine Serum (Hyclone™, ThermoFisher Scientific, Waltham, MA, USA) and used them in the experiments within 20 passages. For the experiments, glioma cells propagating in the dishes were washed with Hank's balanced salt solution (ThermoFisher Scientific, Waltham, MA, USA) and treated with 0.25% trypsin-EDTA (ThermoFisher Scientific, Waltham, MA, USA) for 2 mins to detach the cells. The resulting cell suspension was pelleted by centrifugation for 7 mins at $100\times g$. The pellet was resuspended in fresh culture media and plated onto round glass coverslips (12 mm in diameter) pre-cleaned with RBS™ 35 (ThermoFisher Scientific, Waltham, MA, USA) [22]. To allow cells to settle, coverslips were returned to the incubator for 1 h, after which the cell suspension was replaced with fresh cell culture media. At this point, a subset of the cells on coverslips received treatments of SWCNT-PEG or SWCNT-PEG-THFF, or the functional groups, PEG or PEG-THFF, added to the culture media and returned to the incubator until used in the experiments.

2.3. Live Cell Imaging

The coverslips with D54MG-EGFP cells were mounted onto an imaging chamber filled with external solution (pH 7.4), consisting of sodium chloride (140 mM), potassium chloride (5 mM), calcium chloride (2 mM), magnesium chloride (2 mM), D-glucose (5 mM) and HEPES (10 mM), at room temperature (22–25 °C) and standard atmospheric conditions. An inverted microscope (Nikon TE300; Nikon, Inc., Melville, NY, USA) equipped with differential interference contrast (DIC) and wide-field epifluorescence illumination (100 W halogen and 75 W metal halide lamps, respectively) was used with a standard fluorescein isothiocyanate (FITC) filter set to visualize the D54MG-EGFP cells. Images were acquired using a CoolSNAP®-HQ cooled charge coupled device camera (Photometrics, Tucson, AZ, USA) driven by MetaMorph® 6.1 imaging software (Molecular Devices, Chicago, IL, USA).

2.4. Morphometric Analysis

To assess the cellular morphology, solitary D54MG-EGFP cells were imaged, 1-day post-plating, using the above described microscope and a 60× Plan Apochromatic oil-immersion objective. The images were analyzed using a previously described algorithm [16] to measure the area and perimeter of the individual cells, except that here we used the EGFP fluorescence instead of the previously used calcein fluorescence to obtain the outline of the cell. The area and perimeter values were further used to calculate the form factor (FF; defined as $[4\pi \times (\text{Area})/(\text{Perimeter})^2]$) which is a measure of the roundness of an object/cell; a perfectly round/circular object has a FF = 1, while FF $\approx$ 0 describes a line.

2.5. Vitality Assay

To assess the vitality characteristics of SWCNT-treated D54MG-EGFP cells, that is, cell adhesion, proliferation and death rate, coverslips with cells were imaged 2 h and 2 days post-plating. The 2-h time point was used to establish initial plating density, that is, cell adhesion, while the 2-day time point was used to assess the proliferation of cells, under each condition. Prior to imaging, all the cells were incubated for 10 min in external solution containing 1 μg/mL of the cell permeable nuclear dye Hoechst 33342 (2′-[4-ethoxyphenyl]-5-[4-methyl-1-piperazinyl]-2,5′-bi-1H-benzimidazole trihydrochloride trihydrate; ThermoFisher Scientific, Waltham, MA, USA) to label the nuclei. After rinsing, the cells were then imaged using the above described microscope and a 20× Plan Fluor objective. The fluorescence of Hoechst 33342 was visualized using a standard 4′,6-diamidino-2-phenylindole (DAPI) filter set, while a FITC filter set was used to image the cytosol of cells, containing EGFP, with their plasma membranes intact. The FITC and DAPI images where then merged, using ImageJ software (National Institutes of Health, Bethesda, MD, USA), to visualize the cells and their corresponding nuclei. The cells positive for EGFP and Hoechst were considered live, while positively stained nuclei with Hoechst lacking surrounding EGFP stain were considered to represent dead cells. The number of nuclei per total viewed area (0.75 mm^2) was counted, as we described in detail elsewhere [23]; cell density was expressed as number of cells per cm^2.

2.6. Statistics

Statistical analysis was done using GB-STAT version 6.5 software (Dynamic Microsystems, Inc., Silver Spring, MD, USA) and SAS Software, version 9.2 of the SAS software for Windows (SAS Institute Inc., Cary, NC, USA). The number of subjects (cells or coverslips) required for comparison was estimated using power analysis (set 80% and α = 0.05) and guided by our previously published work [16,17,19,23]. Some groups deviated from normality based on Shapiro-Wilk or D'Agostino-Pearson tests for normality. Consequently, all the data are reported as median with interquartile range (IQR) and nonparametric statistics were used. To test the difference between the 2-h and 2-day time points in the vitality assay, the two groups were compared using Mann-Whitney U-test. For all the other experiments, the multiple independent groups were analyzed using Kruskal-Wallis One-Way ANOVA followed by Dunn's test (significance established at $p < 0.05$).

3. Results

3.1. Effect of wsSWCNTs on the Morphology of D54MG-EGFP Glioma Cells

During their invasion through the extracellular space of the brain, glioma cells have to adjust their morphology and become less round [2]. Thus, we assessed the effects of wsSWCNTs on the morphological parameters of D54MG-EGFP human glioma cell line (Figure 1). To accomplish this, D54MG-EGFP cells were plated onto glass coverslips and incubated for 24 h in the absence or the presence of 5 μg/mL SWCNT-PEG or 5 μg/mL SWCNT-PEG-THFF, and then imaged using a standard FITC filter set and a 60× objective (Figure 1A). Images of solitary cells, that is, cells devoid of contact with other cells, were analyzed to obtain the area and perimeter values of the cells (Figure 1B). These values were further used to calculate the form factor, a measure of cell roundness (Figure 1B). We found that D54MG-EGFP cells, when treated with SWCNT-PEG, did not show any differences in the morphological parameters compared to the untreated cells (Figure 1B). D54MG-EGFP cells treated with SWCNT-PEG-THFF also showed no significant changes in the area and perimeter of the cells compared to the untreated cells. However, they showed a significant decrease (by ~23%) in the form factor compared to the untreated cells implying that the SWCNT-PEG-THFF causes a change in the cell shape (cells were less rounded), but not the size of D54MG-EGFP cells.

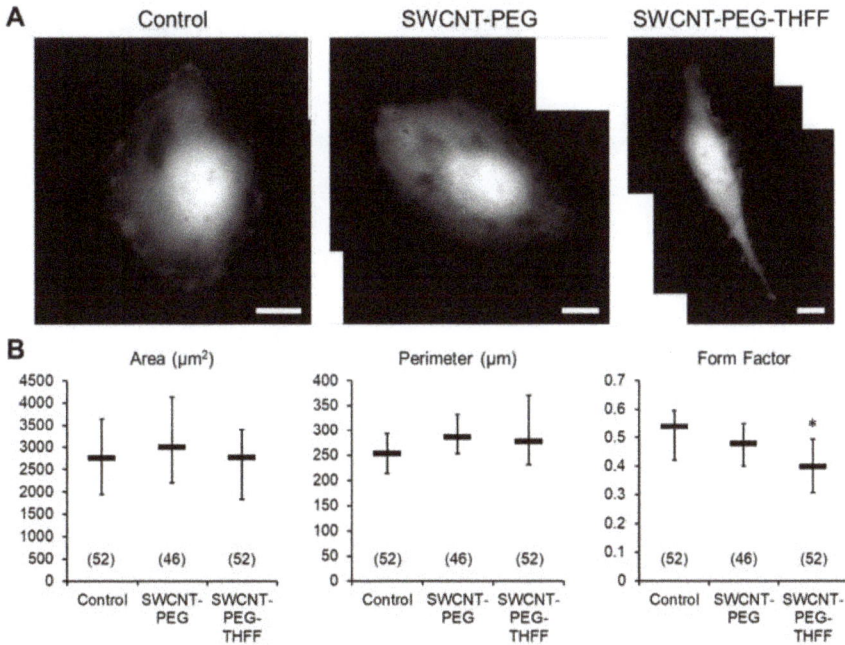

Figure 1. Single-walled carbon nanotubes functionalized with tetrahydrofurfuryl-terminated polyethylene glycol (SWCNT-PEG-THFF) solute induces morphological changes in D54MG- enhanced green fluorescent protein (EGFP) human glioma cells. (**A**) Images of solitary control, SWCNT-PEG-treated and SWCNT-PEG-THFF-treated D54MG-EGFP glioma cells in culture plated onto glass coverslips. Scale bars, 20 μm. (**B**) Summary graphs showing the effects of SWCNT-PEG and SWCNT-PEG-THFF on the morphology of D54MG-EGFP human glioma cells. Number of D54MG-EGFP cells studied in each condition is given in parentheses. The boxes represent medians with interquartile range (IQR). Asterisk indicates a statistical difference when compared to the control group. Kruskal-Wallis one-way ANOVA followed by Dunn's test. *: $p < 0.05$.

Since the SWCNTs have been chemically functionalized to render aqueous solubility, the question arose if the functional groups by themselves could cause any changes in the morphology of D54MG-EGFP cells. To assess this, D54MG-EGFP cells were treated with the functional groups PEG (1 μg/mL) or PEG-THFF (1 μg/mL), imaged (Figure 2A) and the morphological parameters of the cells were quantified (Figure 2B); the rationale for choosing the concentration of functional groups used is provided in Material and Methods. We found similar results to those obtained when cells were treated with wsSWCNTs, that is, the cells treated with PEG showed no significant differences in all the morphological parameters assessed and PEG-THFF-treated cells showed no significant differences in the area and the perimeter compared to the untreated cells (Figure 2B). However, there was a significant decrease (by ~24%) in the form factor of cells treated with the functional group PEG-THFF compared to the untreated cells as well to that of cells treated with PEG alone (Figure 2B). As the magnitude of this decrease in the form factor was comparable to that seen in cells treated with SWCNT-PEG-THFF (24% vs. 23%, compare Figures 1B and 2B, respectively), morphological changes observed in D54MG-EGFP cells treated with SWCNT-PEG-THFF appear to be caused by the functional group, likely its THFF moiety (as per additional comparison to SWCNT-PEG data), and not the SWCNT backbone itself.

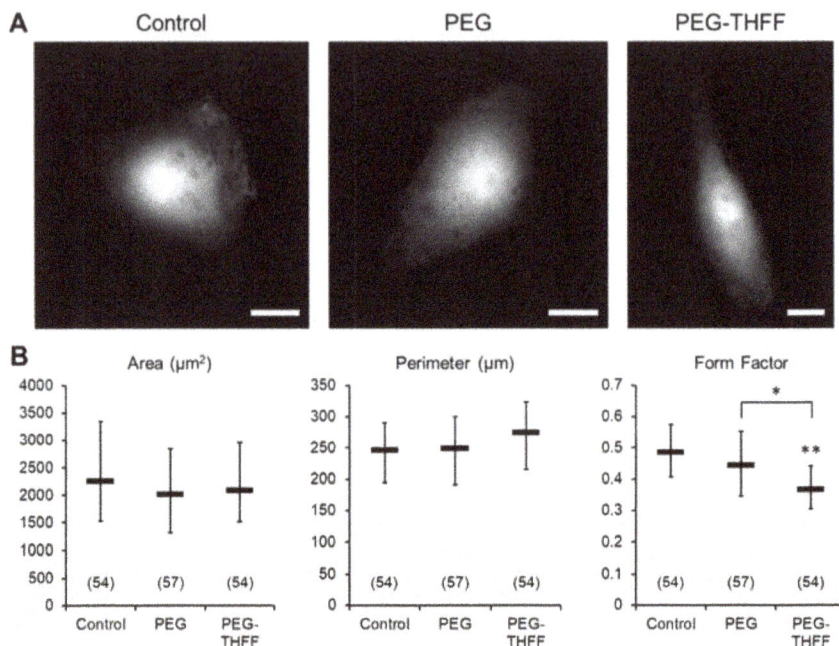

Figure 2. The functional group PEG-THFF induces morphological changes in D54MG-EGFP human glioma cells. (**A**) Images of solitary control, PEG-treated and PEG-THFF-treated D54MG-EGFP glioma cells in culture plated onto glass coverslips. Scale bars, 20 µm. (**B**) Summary graphs showing the effects of the functional groups PEG and PEG-THFF on the morphology of D54MG-EGFP human glioma cells. Asterisks indicate a statistical difference when compared to the control group. The other difference is marked with a bracket. Other annotations as in Figure 1. *: $p < 0.05$; **: $p < 0.01$.

3.2. Effect of wsSWCNTs on the Vitality of D54MG-EGFP Cells

Cell adhesion and proliferation are the factors contributing to malignancy of GBM [3,4]. Thus, we studied whether wsSWCNTs cause changes in the vitality of D54MG-EGFP cells, by assessing adhesion, proliferation and death rate of these glioma cells (Figure 3). We plated D54MG-EGFP cells onto glass coverslips and incubated them for 2 h or 2 days in the absence, or the presence of 5 µg/mL SWCNT-PEG or 5 µg/mL SWCNT-PEG-THFF. The 2-h time point was used to establish the initial plating density reporting on cell adhesion, while the 2-day time point was used to assess the proliferation capability of the cells. The nuclei of the cells were labeled with a cell permeant dye Hoechst 33342. The cells were imaged using standard FITC (for cytosolic EGFP) and DAPI (nuclear Hoechst stain) filter sets and a 20× objective (Figure 3A). We quantified and reported the number of live D54MG-EGFP in each of the conditions along with the percentage of dead cells (Figure 3B,C). We found that the number of live D54MG-EGFP cells, at the 2-h time point, did not show any significant differences between the groups assessed, implying that the initial seeding density was similar across all the groups (Figure 3B). We also found that the number of live cells at the 2-day time point were significantly higher in all the groups compared to their corresponding 2-h time point implying that the cells undergo proliferation in all the conditions (Figure 3B); the proliferation rate (ratio of counts of live cells at 2-day vs. 2-h time points) was 2.1 in control, 1.6 in SWCNT-PEG-treated and 1.3 in SWCT-PEG-THFF-treated groups. However, we found that the cells treated with SWCNT-PEG-THFF show a significant decrease in the number of live cells compared to the untreated cells at the 2-day time point indicating that SWCNT-PEG-THFF reduces the proliferation rate of D54MG-EGFP cells. The percentage of dead D54MG-EGFP cells, however, did not show any significant differences between the groups at each of the time points (Figure 3C). We also did not find any significant differences between the two time points in the control and SWCNT-PEG-treated groups. However, the cells treated with SWCNT-PEG-THFF showed a significant relative increase (~35%) of dead cells at the 2-day as compared to 2-h time point (Figure 3C). Taken together, these results imply that the SWCNT-PEG-THFF solute causes a reduction in the proliferation rate of D54MG-EGFP cells along with an increase in their cell death rate.

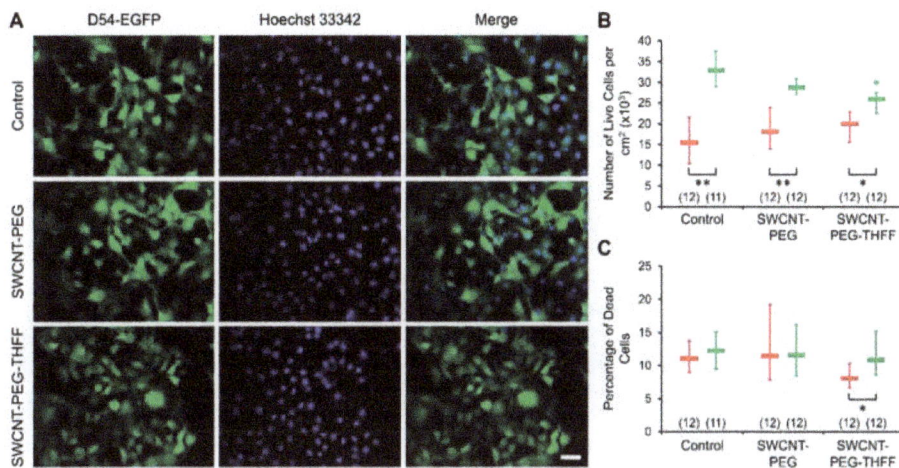

Figure 3. SWCNT-PEG-THFF solute reduces the proliferation rate of D54MG-EGFP human glioma cells. (**A**) Images of D54MG-EGFP glioma cells (left column) and their corresponding nuclei labeled with the cell permeable nuclear dye Hoechst 33342 (middle column); right column shows the merge of the images. Rows (top-bottom) show images of the control, SWCNT-PEG-treated and SWCNT-PEG-THFF-treated D54MG-EGFP glioma cells, 2 days post-plating. Scale bar, 50 μm. (**B**) Summary graph showing the median and IQR numbers of live cells per cm^2 of the control, SWCNT-PEG-treated and SWCNT-PEG-THFF-treated coverslips, 2 h (red) and 2 days (green) post-plating. (**C**) Summary graph showing the median and IQR percentages of dead cells in the above setting. The numbers in parentheses represent the number of coverslips imaged in each group. Asterisks indicate a statistical difference compared to the control group. The other differences are marked by the brackets. Mann-Whitney U-test was used for the comparison between the time points and Kruskal-Wallis one-way ANOVA followed by Dunn's test was used for the comparison between the different conditions at each time point; *: $p < 0.05$; **: $p < 0.01$.

As in the morphology study, we assessed whether the functional groups by themselves could cause any change in the vitality of D54MG-EGFP cells (Figure 4). D54MG-EGFP cells were plated onto glass coverslips and incubated for 2 h or 2 days without or with the addition of the functional groups PEG (1 μg/mL) or PEG-THFF (1 μg/mL). We imaged and quantified the number of live cells in each of the conditions and time points and found that the number of live cells were not significantly different between the groups at each of the time points (Figure 4A,B). The numbers of live D54MG-EGFP cells in all the groups were significantly higher at the 2-day time point compared to the corresponding 2-h time point confirming that the cells are proliferating in all the conditions. The proliferation rates were 2.1 in control group and 1.6 in PEG-treated D54MG-EGFP cells, matching those rates obtained in SWCNT-PEG-treated cells and their controls (compare Figures 3B and 4B). The sole mismatch was a proliferation rate of 1.5 in the PEG-THFF-treated group (Figure 4B) as compared to that of 1.3 seen in SWCT-PEG-THFF-treated D54MG-EGFP cells (Figure 3B). This indicates that the effect of SWCNT-PEG-THFF on D54MG-EGFP proliferation rate seem to be mainly caused by the SWCNT backbone.

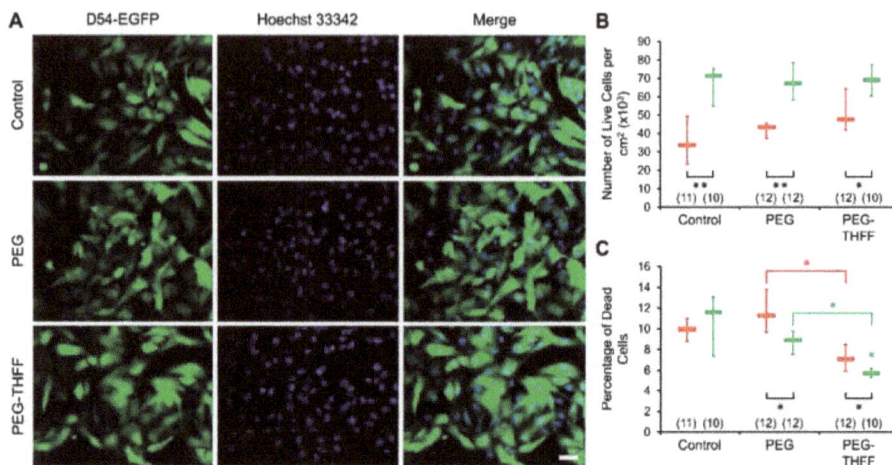

Figure 4. The functional groups PEG and PEG-THFF reduce the cell death rate of D54MG-EGFP human glioma cells. (**A**) Images of D54MG-EGFP glioma cells (left column) and their corresponding nuclei labeled with the cell permeable nuclear dye Hoechst 33342 (middle column); right column shows the merge of the images. Rows (top-bottom) show the control, PEG-treated and PEG-THFF-treated D54MG-EGFP glioma cells, 2 days post-plating. Scale bar, 50 μm. (**B**) Summary graph showing the median and IQR numbers of live cells per cm^2 of the control, PEG-treated and PEG-THFF-treated coverslips, 2 h (red) and 2 days (green) post-plating. (**C**) Summary graph showing the median and IQR percentages of dead cells in the above setting. Other annotations as in Figure 3.

We then analyzed the percentage of dead cells and found that the cells treated with PEG or PEG-THFF did not show any significant difference in the percentage of dead cells at the 2-h time point compared to the untreated cells (Figure 4C). However, the cells treated with PEG-THFF showed significantly lower percentage of dead cells at the 2-h time point compared to the cells treated with PEG. We also found that the percentage of dead cells was significantly lower at the 2-day time point compared to the corresponding 2 h time point for the cells treated with PEG and PEG-THFF; the untreated cells did not show any difference between the two time points. In addition, we found that the cells treated with PEG-THFF showed a significantly lower percentage of dead cells compared to the untreated cells, as well as the cells treated with PEG, at the 2-day time point. Taken together, it appears that both the functional groups, PEG-THFF in particular, have a protective effect on D54MG-EGFP human glioma cells survival (Figure 4C), and that the increase death rate seen in cells treated with SWCNT-PEG-THFF is mediated by the SWCNT backbone (Figure 3C).

4. Discussion

In the present study, the application of SWCNT-PEG to D54MG-EGFP cells didn't cause a change in the morphological characteristics of these malignant human astrocytes. This is in stark contrast with the results we previously obtained using primary cultures of mouse cortical astrocytes, which exhibited a reduction in the form factor upon exposure to SWCNT-PEG [16,17]. That effect, associated with an increase in glial fibrillary acidic protein (GFAP) immunoreactivity [16,17], was taken as a sign of astrocyte maturation and was ascribed to the SWCNT backbone, because PEG alone had no effect on the form factor [17]. However, SWCNT-PEG failed to induce changes in the form factor of astrocytes isolated from knock-out mice lacking GFAP expression [17], pointing to a GFAP-dependent process. Interestingly, D54MG glioblastoma cells lack expression of GFAP (Supplementary Information, Figure S1), as expected for a high malignancy grade glioma [20,24]. Whether GFAP absence in D54MG cells render their irresponsiveness to the SWCNT-PEG in terms of form factor dynamics, observed in the present work, could be experimentally addressed in future by transfection of these cells to express GFAP. Similarly, the differences between the effects that SWCNT-PEG-THFF has on glioma cells, obtained here, as opposed to those it might have on primary astrocytes await further experimentation. It should be noted, however, that in the previous work on astrocytes, we plated astrocytes onto polyethyleneimine-coated coverslips, while in the present work the same kind of glass coverslips have been used plain/uncoated for the plating of D54 glioblastoma cells. As earlier studies suggested that substrate qualities play a role in neuronal [25,26] and astrocytic morphology [23], it is possible that the differential effects of SWCNT-PEG on astrocytes and D54MG-EGFP glioblastoma cells have arisen from the use of different, plain vs. coated, glass coverslips for cell plating.

The vitality assay shows that the D54MG-EGFP cells treated with SWCNT-PEG have similar adhesion, proliferation and death rate as control, untreated cells. These findings are in agreement with the results we previously obtained using wild-type GFAP-expressing astrocytes exposed to this nanomaterial (Figure 4 of [17]). However, based on that previous work, we would predict SWCNT-PEG to promote cell death rate in GFAP-negative D54MG cells. Namely, unlike their control (wild-type GFAP-expressing astrocytes), GFAP knock-out astrocytes exposed to SWCNT-PEG had a significantly increased cell death rate (Figure 4B of [17]). At the time, that finding led us to speculate that GFAP in wild-type astrocytes might have a protective role against hitherto unacknowledged harmful effects of SWCNT-PEG. The present results showing unaffected percentage of dead D54MG-EGFP cells when treated with SWCNT-PEG indicates that the very notion cannot be extended to malignant astrocytes.

In the present work, we find that PEG itself reduced the number of dead D54MG-EGFP cells (Figure 4C). This finding is at odds with our previous data collected from wild-type astrocytes showing the opposite effect, that is, increased astrocyte cell death rate in presence of PEG (Figure S2 of [17]). Thus, it appears that PEG itself is harmful to normal astrocytes, while protective of D54MG-EGFP glioma cells. These disparate finding warrants future investigation regarding the underlying molecular mechanisms that might mediate the differential effect of PEG on normal vs. malignant astrocytes. More importantly, our findings raise concerns in regard to the use of PEG itself for therapeutics in gliomas [27–29].

At present, we are unaware of a study using SWCNT-PEG-THFF on astrocytes, and hence we cannot attempt any comparison on the effects of this nanomaterial on primary astrocytes vs. their malignant counterparts. However, we compare the effects exerted by SWCNT-PEG and SWCNT-PEG-THFF on D54MG-EGFP glioma cells. The reduction of form factor seen in D54MG-EGFP cells treated with SWCNT-PEG-THFF appears to be caused by the THFF moiety of the functional group. Albeit we have not directly tested this idea, the lack of the effect on D54MG-EGFP cells form factor by PEG and SWCNT-PEG supports this inference. Whether presumed direct THFF effect on D54MG-EGFP morphology, as these malignant astrocytes become less round, is an expression of an increase in their invasiveness [2], or perhaps it represents their re-differentiation, similar to stellation/maturation in normal astrocytes [16], remains to be investigated. Vitality assay using D54MG-EGFP cells indicates that SWCNT-PEG-THFF also reduces cell proliferation and increases the cell death rate, both of which were unaffected by SWCNT-PEG (Figure 3B,C); this intuitively points again towards THFF as a mediator of the co-polymer effect on D54MG-EGFP cells. However, this idea is not supported by the effects of functional groups alone (Figure 4C), and the possible explanation is rather more complex. Namely, both functional PEG and PEG-THFF groups, without affecting cell proliferation, reduce the cell death rate (Figure 4C), an effect that is more pronounced in D54MG-EGFP cells treated with PEG-THFF. Taken together, it appears that the functional groups we use are protective for D54MG-EGFP cells, while the SWCNT backbone seems detrimental to these malignant human astrocytes. It is tempting to speculate that the differential effect of SWCNT-PEG and SWCNT-PEG-THFF is due to an increase in the bioactivity of SWCNT-PEG-THFF, likely due to the utilization of THFF, which is known to prevent possible PEG cross-linking between SWCNT-PEG [18] and thus increases water solubility of SWCNT-PEG-THFF and its bioactivity. Consequently, any use of SWCNT co-polymers in therapeutic approaches for gliomas will need to be preceded by the synthesis and characterization of SWCNT copolymers utilizing some functionalization group(s) that would not oppose the SWCNT harmful effect. Given the multitude of chemistries and functional groups available for carbon nanotubes [5], this task seems doable, albeit time-consuming. Moreover, our data raise concerns over the use of THFF groups to enhance bioavailability of variety of compounds (e.g., thiamine) in the brain for in vivo clinical translational applications [30,31].

Interestingly, Santos et al. [10] used carboxylated SWCNTs (SWCNT-COOH) on human U251 glioma cell line. They found that U251 cells had reduced proliferation rate by ~20% upon a 3-day treatment with SWCNT-COOH at the concentration of 3 µg/mL. Furthermore, they observed an increased cell death rate (~36% for apoptotic death rate and ~170% for necrotic death rate; estimated from their Figure 1A) at the concentration of 10 µg/mL [10]. These findings are similar to those we observe when treating D54MG-EGFP cells with SWCNT-PEG-THFF, with the proliferation rate reduced by ~21% (control vs. SWCNT-PEG-THFF; Figure 3B) and the cell death rate percentage increase by ~35% (2-h vs. 2-day time period for SWCNT-PEG-THFF group; Figure 4C). It should be noted that we use SWCNT-COOH (albeit from a different source than those used in Santos et al.) as an initial reactant, which gets completely consumed, in the synthesis of both SWCNT-PEG and SWCNT-PEG-THFF (details available in [16,18]). As the treatment of U251 glioma cells with the COOH functional group was not reported [10], we cannot make further comparisons to our data. Also, the comparison made above is based on two different glioma cell lines grown on two different strata and under different culturing conditions; U251 cells were grown on a plastic stratum [10], while here D54MG-EGFP cells grew on plain glass coverslips. However, these technicalities should not distract from the emerging picture that, depending on conditions and cells treated with SWCNT conjugates, it appears as both the SWCNT backbone and/or functionalized groups, albeit the latter only meant to increase water solubility of SWCNT conjugate, can exert a biological effect.

In the context of glioma SWCNT therapeutics, our present work indicates that additional care should be taken in the selection of functional groups, as SWCNT conjugates may cause differential biological effects mediated by the SWCNT backbone and/or functional group.

Supplementary Materials: The following are available online at http://www.mdpi.com/2571-6980/1/2/22/s1, Figure S1: GFAP expression in primary mouse astrocytes and lack thereof in D54MG human glioma cells.

Author Contributions: Conceptualization, V.M., R.C.H. and V.P.; Data curation, S.H. and V.P.; Formal analysis, S.H., M.K.G., E.B. and V.P.; Funding acquisition, R.C.H. and V.P.; Investigation, S.H. and M.K.G.; Methodology, M.K.G., V.M. and E.B.; Project administration, V.P.; Resources, E.B., R.C.H. and V.P.; Supervision, M.K.G., V.M., R.C.H. and V.P.; Validation, S.H. and M.K.G.; Visualization, S.H. and M.K.G.; Writing—original draft, M.K.G. and V.P.; Writing—review & editing, M.K.G., V.M., E.B. and V.P.

Funding: This work was supported by the National Institutes of Health (The Eunice Kennedy Shriver National Institute of Child Health and Human Development award HD078678 to V.P.) and by the Civitan International McNulty Award (V.P.).

Acknowledgments: We thank Prof.Harald Sontheimer for providing us with an initial stock of the D54MG and D54MG-EGFP glioma cell lines.

Conflicts of Interest: The authors declare no conflict of interest.

References

1. Zagzag, D.; Esencay, M.; Mendez, O.; Yee, H.; Smirnova, I.; Huang, Y.; Chiriboga, L.; Lukyanov, E.; Liu, M.; Newcomb, E.W. Hypoxia- and vascular endothelial growth factor-induced stromal cell-derived factor-1α/CXCR$_4$ expression in glioblastomas. *Am. J. Pathol.* **2008**, *173*, 545–560. [CrossRef] [PubMed]

2.   Sontheimer, H. Role of Ion Channels and Amino-Acid Transporters in the Biology of Astrocytic Tumors. In *Astrocytes in (Patho)Physiology of the Nervous System*; Parpura, V., Haydon, P.G., Eds.; Springer: New York, NY, USA, 2009; pp. 527–546.

3.   Nakada, M.; Niska, J.A.; Tran, N.L.; McDonough, W.S.; Berens, M.E. EphB2/R-Ras signaling regulates glioma cell adhesion, growth, and invasion. *Am. J. Pathol.* **2005**, *167*, 565–576. [CrossRef]

4.   Wang, S.D.; Rath, P.; Lal, B.; Richard, J.P.; Li, Y.; Goodwin, C.R.; Laterra, J.; Xia, S. EphB2 receptor controls proliferation/migration dichotomy of glioblastoma by interacting with focal adhesion kinase. *Oncogene* **2012**, *31*, 5132–5143. [CrossRef] [PubMed]

5.   Bekyarova, E.; Ni, Y.; Malarkey, E.B.; Montana, V.; McWilliams, J.L.; Haddon, R.C.; Parpura, V. Applications of carbon nanotubes in biotechnology and biomedicine. *J. Biomed. Nanotechnol.* **2005**, *1*, 3–17. [CrossRef] [PubMed]

6.   Bekyarova, E.; Haddon, R.C.; Parpura, V. Biofunctionalization of Carbon Nanotubes. In *Nanotechnologies for the Life Sciences*; Wiley-VCH Verlag GmbH & Co. KGaA: Weinheim, Germany, 2007.

7.   Zhao, D.; Alizadeh, D.; Zhang, L.; Liu, W.; Farrukh, O.; Manuel, E.; Diamond, D.J.; Badie, B. Carbon nanotubes enhance CpG uptake and potentiate antiglioma immunity. *Clin. Cancer Res.* **2010**, *17*, 771–782. [CrossRef] [PubMed]

8.   Alizadeh, D.; White, E.E.; Sanchez, T.C.; Liu, S.; Zhang, L.; Badie, B.; Berlin, J.M. Immunostimulatory CpG on carbon nanotubes selectively inhibits migration of brain tumor cells. *Bioconjug. Chem.* **2018**, *29*, 1659–1668. [CrossRef] [PubMed]

9.   Liu, Z.; Cai, W.; He, L.; Nakayama, N.; Chen, K.; Sun, X.; Chen, X.; Dai, H. In vivo biodistribution and highly efficient tumour targeting of carbon nanotubes in mice. *Nat. Nanotechnol.* **2006**, *2*, 47–52. [CrossRef] [PubMed]

10.   Santos, T.; Fang, X.; Chen, M.-T.; Wang, W.; Ferreira, R.; Jhaveri, N.; Gundersen, M.; Zhou, C.; Pagnini, P.; Hofman, F.M.; et al. Sequential administration of carbon nanotubes and near-infrared radiation for the treatment of gliomas. *Front. Oncol.* **2014**, *4*. [CrossRef] [PubMed]

11.   Ou, Z.; Wu, B.; Xing, D.; Zhou, F.; Wang, H.; Tang, Y. Functional single-walled carbon nanotubes based on an integrin $\alpha_v\beta_3$ monoclonal antibody for highly efficient cancer cell targeting. *Nanotechnology* **2009**, *20*, 105102. [CrossRef] [PubMed]

12.   Markovic, Z.M.; Harhaji-Trajkovic, L.M.; Todorovic-Markovic, B.M.; Kepić, D.P.; Arsikin, K.M.; Jovanović, S.P.; Pantovic, A.C.; Dramićanin, M.D.; Trajkovic, V.S. In vitro comparison of the photothermal anticancer activity of graphene nanoparticles and carbon nanotubes. *Biomaterials* **2011**, *32*, 1121–1129. [CrossRef] [PubMed]

13.   Liang, C.; Diao, S.; Wang, C.; Gong, H.; Liu, T.; Hong, G.; Shi, X.; Dai, H.; Liu, Z. Tumor metastasis inhibition by imaging-guided photothermal therapy with single-walled carbon nanotubes. *Adv. Mater.* **2014**, *26*, 5646–5652. [CrossRef] [PubMed]

14.   Itkis, M.E.; Borondics, F.; Yu, A.; Haddon, R.C. Bolometric infrared photoresponse of suspended single-walled carbon nanotube films. *Science* **2006**, *312*, 413–416. [CrossRef] [PubMed]

15.   Gottipati, M.K.; Verkhratsky, A.; Parpura, V. Probing astroglia with carbon nanotubes: Modulation of form and function. *Philos. Trans. R. Soc. B Boil. Sci.* **2014**, *369*, 20130598. [CrossRef] [PubMed]

16.   Gottipati, M.K.; Kalinina, I.; Bekyarova, E.; Haddon, R.C.; Parpura, V. Chemically functionalized water-soluble single-walled carbon nanotubes modulate morpho-functional characteristics of astrocytes. *Nano Lett.* **2012**, *12*, 4742–4747. [CrossRef] [PubMed]

17.   Gottipati, M.K.; Bekyarova, E.; Brenner, M.; Haddon, R.C.; Parpura, V. Changes in the morphology and proliferation of astrocytes induced by two modalities of chemically functionalized single-walled carbon nanotubes are differentially mediated by glial fibrillary acidic protein. *Nano Lett.* **2014**, *14*, 3720–3727. [CrossRef] [PubMed]

18.   Kalinina, I.; Worsley, K.; Lugo, C.; Mandal, S.; Bekyarova, E.; Haddon, R.C. Synthesis, dispersion, and viscosity of Poly(ethylene glycol)-functionalized water-soluble single-walled carbon nanotubes. *Chem. Mater.* **2011**, *23*, 1246–1253. [CrossRef]

19.   Gottipati, M.K.; Bekyarova, E.; Haddon, R.C.; Parpura, V. Chemically functionalized single-walled carbon nanotubes enhance the glutamate uptake characteristics of mouse cortical astrocytes. *Amino Acids* **2015**, *47*, 1379–1388. [CrossRef] [PubMed]

20. Montana, V.; Sontheimer, H. Bradykinin promotes the chemotactic invasion of primary brain tumors. *J. Neurosci.* **2011**, *31*, 4858–4867. [CrossRef] [PubMed]
21. Habela, C.W.; Ernest, N.J.; Swindall, A.F.; Sontheimer, H. Chloride accumulation drives volume dynamics underlying cell proliferation and migration. *J. Neurophysiol.* **2009**, *101*, 750–757. [CrossRef] [PubMed]
22. Lee, W.; Parpura, V. Dissociated Cell Culture for Testing Effects of Carbon Nanotubes on Neuronal Growth. In *Neurotrophic Factors*; Humana Press: Totowa, NJ, USA, 2012; pp. 261–276.
23. Gottipati, M.K.; Samuelson, J.J.; Kalinina, I.; Bekyarova, E.; Haddon, R.C.; Parpura, V. Chemically functionalized single-walled carbon nanotube films modulate the morpho-functional and proliferative characteristics of astrocytes. *Nano Lett.* **2013**, *13*, 4387–4392. [CrossRef] [PubMed]
24. Wilhelmsson, U.; Eliasson, C.; Bjerkvig, R.; Pekny, M. Loss of GFAP expression in high-grade astrocytomas does not contribute to tumor development or progression. *Oncogene* **2003**, *22*, 3407–3411. [CrossRef] [PubMed]
25. Lustgarten, J.H.; Proctor, M.; Haroun, R.I.; Avellino, A.M.; Pindzola, A.A.; Kliot, M. Semipermeable polymer tubes provide a microenvironment for in vivo analysis of dorsal root regeneration. *J. Biomech. Eng.* **1991**, *113*, 184–188. [CrossRef] [PubMed]
26. Mattson, M.P.; Haddon, R.C.; Rao, A.M. Molecular functionalization of carbon nanotubes and use as substrates for neuronal growth. *J. Mol. Neurosci.* **2000**, *14*, 175–182. [CrossRef]
27. Guo, W.; Li, A.; Jia, Z.; Yuan, Y.; Dai, H.; Li, H. Transferrin modified PEG-PLA-resveratrol conjugates: In vitro and in vivo studies for glioma. *Eur. J. Pharmacol.* **2013**, *718*, 41–47. [CrossRef] [PubMed]
28. Gu, G.; Hu, Q.; Feng, X.; Gao, X.; Menglin, J.; Kang, T.; Jiang, D.; Song, Q.; Chen, H.; Chen, J. PEG-PLA nanoparticles modified with APTEDB peptide for enhanced anti-angiogenic and anti-glioma therapy. *Biomaterials* **2014**, *35*, 8215–8226. [CrossRef] [PubMed]
29. Chi, Y.; Zhu, S.; Wang, C.; Zhou, L.; Zhang, L.; Li, Z.; Dai, Y. Glioma homing peptide-modified PEG-PCL nanoparticles for enhanced anti-glioma therapy. *J. Drug Target.* **2015**, *24*, 224–232. [CrossRef] [PubMed]
30. Saiki, M.; Matsui, T.; Soya, M.; Kashibe, T.; Shima, T.; Shimizu, T.; Naruto, T.; Kitayoshi, T.; Akimoto, K.; Ninomiya, S.; et al. Thiamine tetrahydrofurfuryl disulfide promotes voluntary activity through dopaminergic activation in the medial prefrontal cortex. *Sci. Rep.* **2018**, *8*. [CrossRef] [PubMed]
31. Huang, W.-C.; Huang, H.-Y.; Hsu, Y.-J.; Su, W.-H.; Shen, S.-Y.; Lee, M.-C.; Lin, C.-L.; Huang, C.-C. The effects of thiamine tetrahydrofurfuryl disulfide on physiological adaption and exercise performance improvement. *Nutrients* **2018**, *10*, 851. [CrossRef] [PubMed]

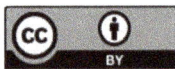

![neuroglia logo] *neuroglia*

MDPI

Review

Understanding the Relevance of Aging-Related Tau Astrogliopathy (ARTAG)

Gabor G. Kovacs[ORCID]

Institute of Neurology, Medical University Vienna, AKH 4J, A-1090 Vienna, Austria;
gabor.kovacs@meduniwien.ac.at; Tel.: +43-1-40400-55070; Fax: +43-1-40400-55110

Received: 9 October 2018; Accepted: 22 October 2018; Published: 29 October 2018

Abstract: Aging-related tau astrogliopathy (ARTAG) is an umbrella term that encompasses a spectrum of morphological abnormalities seen in astrocytes of the aging brain using immunostaining for pathological forms of the microtubule-associated protein tau. Morphologies of ARTAG include thorn-shaped astrocytes (TSA), and additionally granular/fuzzy astrocytes (GFA) characterized by fine granular tau immunoreactivity extending into the astrocytic processes. Thorn-shaped astrocytes can be present in the same brain in subpial, subependymal, perivascular, and white and gray matter locations together with GFAs, which are seen in the gray matter. Primary tauopathies show ARTAG-related morphologies as well, moreover, GFA has been proposed to present a conceptual link between brain ageing and primary tauopathies. Sequential distribution patterns have been recognized for subpial, white and gray matter ARTAG. This either suggests the involvement of astrocytes in the propagation of tau pathology or reflects the consequence of a long-term pathogenic process such as barrier dysfunction, local mechanical impact, or early response to neuronal degeneration. The concept of ARTAG facilitated communication among neuropathologists and researchers, informed biomarker researchers with focus on tau-related indicators and motivated further exploration of the significance of astrocytic lesions in various neurodegenerative conditions.

Keywords: aging-related tau astrogliopathy (ARTAG); aging-related tau astrogliopathy; astroglia; barrier; neurodegenerative disease; protein-astrogliopathy; protein astrogliopathy (PAG); tau

1. Introduction: What Is ARTAG?

Aging-related tau astrogliopathy (ARTAG) is an umbrella term that encompasses a spectrum of morphological abnormalities seen in astrocytes using immunostaining for pathological forms of the microtubule-associated protein tau, mainly in the aging brain [1]. This term was introduced to harmonize the nomenclature and evaluation strategies for the different morphological forms of tau immunoreactive astrocytes previously described by several authors. ARTAG includes morphologies described originally as thorn-shaped astrocytes (TSA) as well as fine granular tau immunoreactivity extending into the astrocytic processes in the gray matter, now called granular/fuzzy astrocytes (GFA) [1].

Ikeda and colleagues were the first to describe TSAs in the subpial or subependymal regions of the gray and white matter, and frequently in the depths of the gyri, as well as in the basal forebrain and brainstem, in aged individuals [2–4]. This was followed by a study from Schultz et al. reporting a high prevalence of TSAs in the aged human medial temporal lobe, particularly at the level of the amygdala [5]. Interestingly, TSA-like morphologies have been described in aged gorillas, and particularly in baboons, but not in other primates [6–9]. This is possibly due to differences in the tau sequence or the lack of sufficient neuropathological studies focusing on tau pathologies in animals [10]. Diffuse granular tau immunoreactivity in astrocytic processes has been described in the context of a study on a peculiar constellation of tau pathology in aged demented individuals [11]. However, the term GFA was introduced only in the consensus paper on ARTAG [1].

In TSAs, tau immunoreactivity is localized in the astrocytic perikarya with extension into the proximal parts of the astrocytic processes, with inclusions also in the astrocytic end feet at the glia limitans around blood vessels and at the pial surface [1]. The processes are thick and short and thus reminiscent of thorns. In contrast, GFAs exhibit fine granular immunoreactivity of branching processes with a few dilations, and the perinuclear soma is densely immunoreactive in most of these astrocytes [1]. These two types of tau immunoreactive astrocytes can both be present in the same brain. Thorn-shaped astrocytes are seen mostly in subpial, subependymal, or perivascular areas, as well as in the white, and less so, in the gray matter. Granular/fuzzy astrocytes are observed in the gray matter. In both the white and gray matter, TSAs and GFAs may build clusters.

For the evaluation of ARTAG a simple strategy has been proposed [1]:

1. Identify the morphologic and distribution types of ARTAG based on parenchymal localization of TSA and GFA: i.e., subpial, subependymal, perivascular, white matter, and gray matter.
2. Identify involvement of gross anatomical regions such as the medial temporal lobe, further lobes of the brain, subcortical structures, and the brainstem.
3. Document the severity of ARTAG pathology; in particular, whether this is seen in occasional or in numerous astrocytes and whether clusters or widespread distribution is noted.
4. Finally, particularly for scientific discovery studies, detailed anatomical mapping is recommended.

In a consecutive study, digital images were evaluated by a group of researchers to evaluate whether these strategies are reproducible [12]. This study revealed the challenging issues of always being able to readily differentiate and clearly classify tau-positive astrocytic lesions. Still, this motivates further exploration of the significance of astrocytic lesions in neurodegenerative disorders and further consensus meetings to reach high agreement. Otherwise, the comparability of research studies will be questionable.

2. ARTAG and Primary Tauopathies

Morphologies of ARTAG may be seen in so-called primary tauopathies as well. Indeed TSA as described by Ikeda et al. [2–4] were similar in morphology to the tau-positive astrocytes described by Nishimura et al. in progressive supranuclear palsy (PSP) [13]. The concept of GFAs has only recently been added to the spectrum of primary tauopathy-related astroglial tau pathologies [14]. Primary tauopathies are biochemically, genetically, clinically and neuropathologically heterogeneous neurodegenerative disorders characterized by the abnormal deposition of tau protein in different cell types of the central nervous system, including neurons and neuroglia. Tauopathies are classified based on the distribution and spectrum of cell types involved and also on a biochemical level. In spite of showing a wide spectrum of biochemical modifications, currently the most widely accepted classification focuses on the predominance of four-repeat (4R) or three-repeat (3R) isoforms of the tau protein, or the presence of both [15].

Importantly, TSAs and GFA-like astrocyte morphologies are common, but not the distinguishing astrocytic morphologies seen in primary tauopathies. The most characteristic astrocytic tau pathologies in primary tauopathies comprise tufted astrocytes in PSP, astrocytic plaques in corticobasal degeneration (CBD), globular glial inclusions in globular glial tauopathies (GGT), and ramified astrocytes in Pick's disease (PiD) [15]. 4R-tauopathies comprise PSP, CBD and GGT, while PiD is a 3R-predominant tauopathy [15]. A further disease affecting the limbic system showing characteristic grains in the neuronal dendrites, hence called argyrophilic grain disease (AGD) also exhibits tau immunoreactive astrocytes in the medial temporal lobe often termed bushy astrocytes in the literature [16,17]. However, these are now also called GFAs due to their similarity to gray matter ARTAG [1]. Finally, the mixed 3R + 4R disease primary tauopathy (PART), which shows neurofibrillary tangles as in Alzheimer's disease (AD), but without significant amyloid-β plaques, does not show the specific tau pathology of astrocytes, but can be associated with ARTAG [14,18]. FTDP-17, or hereditary frontotemporal dementia associated with mutations in the *MAPT* gene, shows a wide variety of tau pathologies and various constellations of tau isoforms [19]. Although astrocytic tau pathology has been readily recognized in several hereditary conditions [9,20], the descriptions vary considerably making comparisons difficult. Tau pathologies resembling ARTAG are also recognized [20]. Interestingly, subpial ARTAG was prominently seen in a recently reported 49-year old demented individual with *MAPT* gene duplication [21,22], suggesting that an imbalance of tau homeostasis may contribute to the early development of an otherwise age-related pathology.

Since GFA-like morphologies are seen in primary tauopathies, we introduced the concept that, analogously to the pretangles, which might be a preceding form of neurofibrillary tangles, the first step of astrocytic pathology might be the fine granular accumulation in astrocytic processes [14,20]. These tau deposits are then potentially redistributed to distal or proximal segments of the astrocytic cytoskeleton and eventually aggregate and become detectable using silver-stainings or anti-ubiquitin antibodies [14,23]. This concept allows the speculation that pure detection of single astrocytes with fine granular phospho-tau immunoreactivity in the human brain might represent an early preclinical form of primary tauopathy or ARTAG, or eventually the first moment of a response to a neurodegenerative event [14,20].

Ferrer et al. [24,25] showed that the biochemical signature of astroglial tau pathology in the elderly in both white and gray matter (i.e., representing ARTAG) differs in some aspects from that of other astrocytic tau pathologies in primary tauopathies. For example, astroglial tau pathologies in the white matter and gray matter in aging brains were not consistently detectable using tau truncated at aspartic acid 421 (tau-C3), or conformational tau modifications at amino acids 312 to 322 (antibody MC1), or phospho-specific anti-tau antibody Ser262 [24,25].

3. ARTAG and Various Disorders Including Chronic Traumatic Encephalopathy

A peculiar aspect of ARTAG is its relation to chronic traumatic encephalopathy (CTE). Astrocytic tau pathology that resembles TSAs (although usually termed astrocytic tangles), is an important component of the morphological alterations reported in CTE, a disorder associated with mild repetitive brain trauma and progressive neurological deterioration [26,27]. Examples of overlapping aspects of CTE and ARTAG include accumulation of subpial, perivascular and gray matter astrocytes in basal brain regions, but also in dorsolateral lobar areas, overrepresentation of males, or association with ventricular enlargement [14,26,28–30]. Importantly, the definition of CTE-associated lesions emphasizes the presence of neuronal tau pathology [26]. Hence, the presence of pure subpial or cortical clusters of astrocytic tau immunoreactivities such as seen in ARTAG should not be at once interpreted as CTE. A study on potential sequential distribution of ARTAG (see below) [31], however, raises an interesting point. Can it be that, at least in some cases, these represent the earliest stage, preceding neuronal tau accumulation, of CTE type pathology? Further studies on CTE cases with early stage tau pathology [30] might be able to address this point.

A wide range of disorders can associate with ARTAG, which could suggest that it is a non-specific condition. Indeed, gray matter ARTAG has been reported in prion diseases, Lewy body disorders, psychiatric conditions (i.e., here mostly restricted to the amygdala), multiple system atrophy, and amyotrophic lateral sclerosis (i.e., here also in the spinal cord) [14,28,32]. However, it might also reflect a response to early neuronal degeneration irrespective of the predominating proteinopathy. Since it is not seen in all cases with some form of neuronal degeneration, a yet unidentified driving force or additional factor need to be considered.

4. Sequential Distribution of ARTAG

In the human brain, hierarchical or stereotypical involvement of anatomical regions (i.e., stages or phases) have been described for several neurodegeneration-related protein pathologies [33]. These focus only on neuronal (tau, α-synuclein, TDP-43) or extracellular (amyloid-β) protein depositions. A recent study evaluated frequencies and hierarchical clustering of anatomical involvement and used conditional probability and logistic regression to model the sequential distribution of ARTAG and astroglial tau pathologies across different brain regions [31]. It has been emphasized that ARTAG does not show such clear stages as neuronal protein pathologies, or in other words not all cases can be put in one box. Therefore, first patterns have to be recognized and then the sequential distribution becomes more visible. Except for subependymal ARTAG, the following sequential patterns have been described for different ARTAG types [31].

4.1. Subpial ARTAG (Thorn-Shaped Astrocytes Morphology)

Pattern 1 (Figure 1): Basal brain regions show subpial ARTAG first (stage 1) followed by a bidirectional sequence rostral (lobar, stage 2a) or caudal (brainstem, stage 2b), which, however, are usually affected together (stage 3).

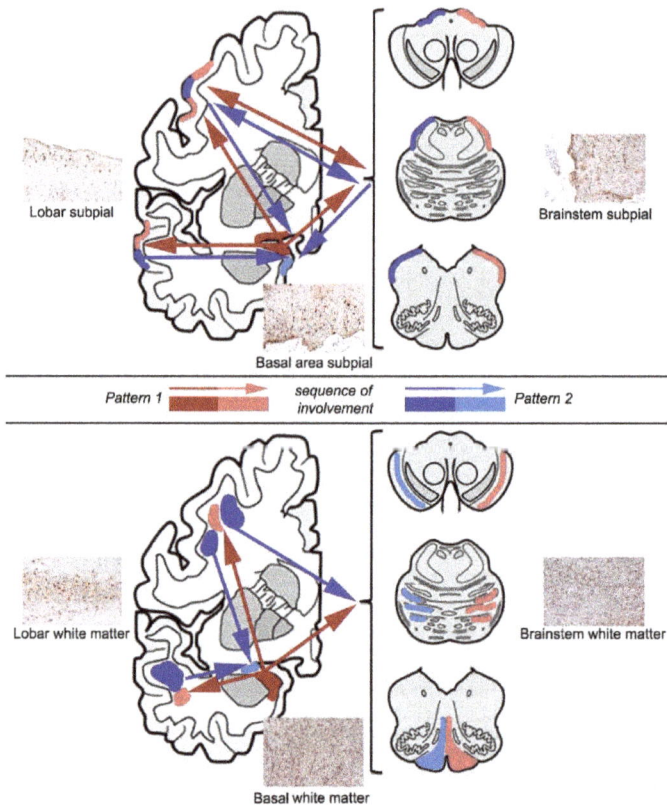

Figure 1. Representative images and sequential distribution patterns of subpial (upper panel) and white matter (lower panel) types of aging-related tau astrogliopathy (ARTAG) in the human brain. For both, two major patterns are seen; one beginning in the basal brain areas, in particular the amygdala (indicated by red arrows), and a second initiated in lobar areas and/or the brainstem (indicated by blue arrows). The arrowheads point towards the direction of sequential involvement and a deeper color represents an earlier stage of involvement. A double-headed arrow means both regions can be involved together as a specific stage of sequential involvement. The deeper color represents the first stage.

Pattern 2 (Figure 1): Subpial ARTAG is initiated in lobar regions (stage 1a) or in the brainstem (stage 1b) followed by the involvement of both (stage 2) preceding basal brain regions (stage 3).

Pattern 3 (Figure 1): This is seen only in CBD, since the morphology of subpial tau accumulation is different. One form, characterized by the immunoreactivity of astrocytic end-feets but not the cell body, is seen regularly in CBD. However, typical TSA morphology can be recognized as well in some CBD cases. Thus, in CBD subpial tau immunoreactivity of astrocytic feet in lobar areas is the predominant pathology independently of subpial ARTAG in basal brain regions (together representing stage 1) and both are followed by the involvement of the brainstem, representing stage 2. We termed this a "masked" bidirectional sequence [31]. This means that pattern 1 as described above, seen in non-CBD cases with the typical subpial TSA morphologies is masked by the predominant end-feet tau immunoreactivity appearing in the lobar subpial location in CBD.

4.2. White Matter ARTAG (Thorn-Shaped Astrocytes Morphology)

Pattern 1 (Figure 1): This is similar to pattern 1 of subpial ARTAG; thus, basal brain regions (stage 1) are followed by the involvement of lobar regions (stage 2a), or brainstem (stage 2b), and then all regions are involved (stage 3).

Pattern 2 (Figure 1): Lobar white matter ARTAG seems to be independent from involvement of the basal brain region. In this case lobar involvement (*stage 1*) is followed by the involvement of the basal brain regions (*stage 2a*) or occasionally the brainstem (*stage 2b*) and then all regions are involved (*stage 3*).

4.3. Gray Matter ARTAG (Granular/Fuzzy Astrocytes Morphology)

Pattern 1, Figure 2 (striatum first): The striatal pathway (stage 1) proceeds either towards the amygdala (stage 2a), cortex (stage 2b), or rarely to the brainstem (stage 2c), followed by stage 3a (striatum + amygdala + cortex), or stage 3b (striatum + amygdala + brainstem), and eventually involves all regions (stage 4). The constellation of striatum + cortex + brainstem has not been observed, hence there is no stage 3c.

Pattern 2, Figure 2 (amygdala first): The amygdala (stage 1) precedes the involvement of the striatum (stage 2a), the cortex (stage 2b) or the brainstem (stage 2c). This is followed by three combinations of stage 3 (a: amygdala + striatum + cortex; b: amygdala + striatum + brainstem; c: amygdala +cortex + brainstem) and is eventually followed by the involvement of all regions (stage 4).

A sequential pattern of astrocytic tau pathology can be better recognized for CBD and PSP [31]. This included the combined evaluation of both GFAs and astrocytic plaques CBD, and GFAs and tufted astrocytes (PSP). In CBD a four-stage sequence was proposed: frontal (including premotor) and parietal cortex (stage 1) is followed by temporal and occipital cortex (stage 2), with parallel movement into subcortical areas, including either, or both, the striatum and the amygdala (stage 3), followed by the brainstem (stage 4) including the substantia nigra followed by the pons and medulla oblongata. In PSP striatum (stage 1) to cortical (frontal-parietal to temporal to occipital) areas (stage 2a and b, respectively) to the amygdala (stage 3) and to the brainstem (stage 4), including the substantia nigra followed by the pons and medulla oblongata, sequence was recognized. Interestingly, the striatal pattern as summarized above for gray matter ARTAG is reminiscent of the combined pattern of tufted astrocytes and GFAs seen in PSP. Therefore, theoretically some cases with gray matter ARTAG in these regions could represent a preclinical form of PSP. Some of these cases might even not proceed to the full-blown neuropathological phenotype either due to a yet unidentified host response that does not allow this, or due to the presence of another predominating neurodegenerative condition.

That study addressed also whether in the same region any type of ARTAG precedes another type or neuronal tau pathology [31]. It has been suggested that in the amygdala, subpial, white matter, and perivascular areas, ARTAG appear together and precede the appearance of subependymal ARTAG. On the other hand, gray matter ARTAG is independent from these. Interestingly, based on the conditional probability values, gray matter ARTAG might precede the presence of dendritic tau-positive grains. This observation would be in line with those showing that in certain regions astrocytic tau pathology may come before neuronal tau pathology (see below) [14,31,34].

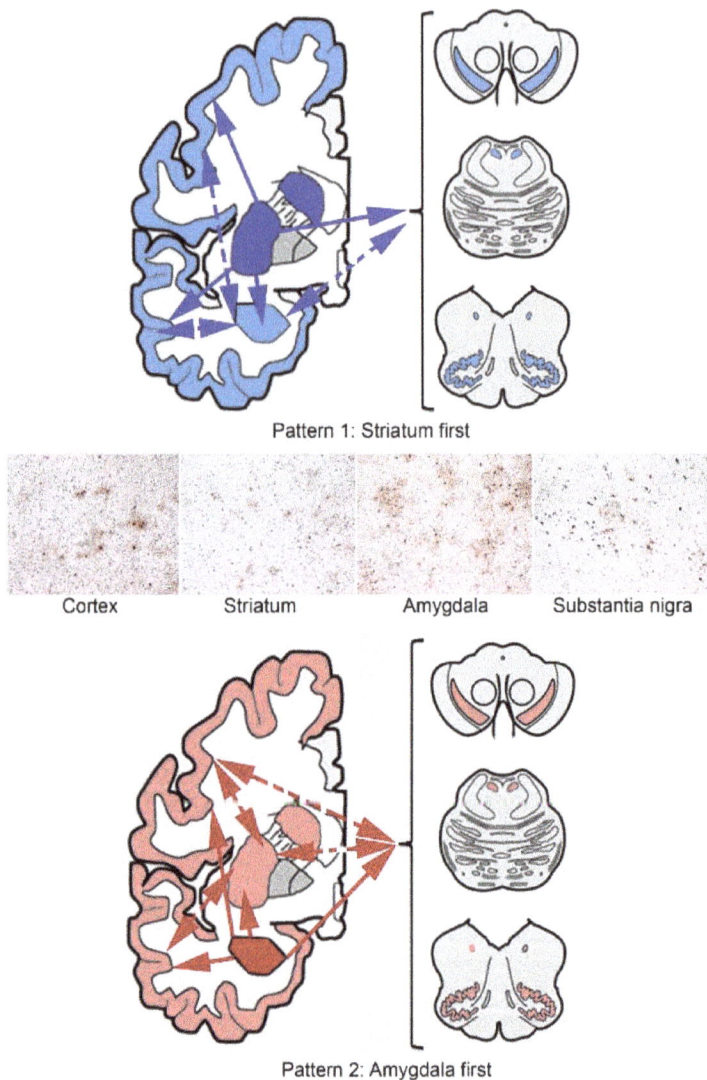

Figure 2. Representative images and sequential distribution patterns of gray matter ARTAG in the human brain. One of these begins in the striatum (upper panel), and another in the amygdala (lower panel), followed by the cortical and brainstem regions. A double-headed arrow with a dashed line means both regions can be involved together as a specific stage of sequential involvement. The deeper color represents the first stage.

5. Considerations on Pathogenesis

Historical studies have identified neuroglia as highly important for barrier function [35]. Importantly, specific types of ARTAG tend to develop at interface regions. Interestingly, tufted astrocytes in PSP and astrocytic plaques in CBD are also often located near the blood vessels [36]; moreover, in a familial disorder with astrocyte-predominant tauopathy, perivascular accumulations are noted as well [37]. Furthermore, tau-containing astrocytes do not always match the distribution of tau-containing neurons in tauopathies [9].

A recent study evaluated the astrocytic markers connexin-43 (Cx43) and aquaporin-4 (AQP4) in relation to ARTAG [38]. A dramatic increase of Cx43 density of immunoreactivity was seen in ARTAG cases and types correlating strongly with tau positive astrocytes, irrespective of the presence of neuronal tau pathology or reactive gliosis measured by glial fibrillar acidic protein (GFAP) density. This could suggest a response to blood-brain barrier dysfunction. However, since this was seen also in the gray matter, it might be that Cx43 expression may promote neuronal survival, for example, by sensing and reducing elevated levels of extracellular glutamate. Therefore, it can be theorized that gray matter ARTAG reflects the efforts of astroglia perceiving early neurodegeneration and leading to tau accumulation in astrocytes as a response of an overwhelming pathogenic process. On the other hand, ARTAG can reflect effective take-up of locally produced and released neuronal tau, thus preventing its accumulation in neurons. Indeed, astrocytes have been found to highly express an array of phagocytic receptors and can phagocytize synapses [39] or axonal mitochondria [40] in the brain.

Aquaporin-4 density of immunoreactivity was increased only in the white and gray matter, and was associated with increased ARTAG density only in white matter and perivascular areas [38]. Aquaporin-4 is a member of the water-channel proteins expressed in the foot processes of glial cells surrounding capillaries, and it is associated with water transfer into and out of the brain parenchyma [41]. Thus, the presence of ARTAG associated with increased AQP4 density in the white matter further supports the notion that pathogenic events are associated with the blood-brain barrier.

And what can we learn about pathogenesis from the sequential distribution patterns? In two studies we reported that GFA-like morphologies appear in cortical areas without local neuronal tau pathology and without obvious clinical symptoms related to this region in primary tauopathies [14,31]. Indeed, this may reach up to 30% of PSP and PiD cases in the occipital lobe [31], which is usually less affected by neuronal tau pathology. The concept that astroglial pathology precedes neuronal tau pathology has also been discussed in presymptomatic cases showing CBD–type pathology [34]. Thus, these tau positive astrocytes might phagocytize pathological tau derived from the endings of projecting neurons, or this may simply represent local astroglial upregulation of tau as a response to a yet unidentified event. We can speculate that GFA astrocytes have the role of scouts in regions not yet affected by neuronal tau pathology. These concepts seem to be supported by animal inoculation studies as well. By injecting pathological tau extracted from post-mortem brains of AD, PSP, and CBD patients into different brain regions of non-transgenic mice, differences in tau strain potency between disorders have been identified [42]. This study found a significant inverse correlation between neuronal and astrocytic tau pathology, supporting the notion of transmission of pathological tau seeding from neurons to neighboring astrocytes. As an alternative mechanism, they proposed that astrocytic tau pathology might spread from one astrocyte to another, possibly through astrocytic gap junction networks [42]. A recent study using tau-enriched fractions of brain homogenates from pure ARTAG (with no associated tauopathy) inoculated into wild-type mice generated intracytoplasmic hyper-phosphorylated tau inclusions in astrocytes, oligodendrocytes and neurons [43]. It has been proposed that ARTAG-related tau might have a cardinal role in seeding tau to neurons and glial cells [43]. Further aspects are highlighted by observations in a tau transgenic mouse model of astrocytic tau pathologies, suggesting its contribution to glial degeneration [44]. As a functional consequence of astrocytic tau pathology, neuronal degeneration can occur in the absence of neuronal tau inclusions [45].

Does the sequential pattern always mean cell-cell-spreading of tau pathology? It might be feasible for gray matter ARTAG, although this needs to be clarified. For subpial, subependymal, white matter, and perivascular ARTAG, however, sequential involvement of regions might reflect consequences of a permanent (or repeated) pathogenic process. For example, subpial ARTAG initiated in basal regions proceeding towards the convexity of the brain (lobar areas), or dorsolateral parts of the brainstem, might indicate a pathogenesis related to the circulation of the cerebrospinal fluid [31]. In contrast, the existence of a second pattern of subpial ARTAG initiated in the dorsolateral lobar areas and dorsolateral parts of the brainstem, suggests a local mechanical inducing factor such as the role of mild traumatic brain injury in some cases [31].

6. What Is the Clinical Relevance of ARTAG?

To understand this, it is crucial to recognize the different ARTAG types. The possibility that TSA may have clinical significance was first discussed by Munoz and colleagues [46]. In a cohort of patients with a non-fluent variant of primary progressive aphasia associated with AD pathology, they detected "argyrophilic thorny astrocyte clusters (ATACs)" and observed them in the frontal, temporal, and parietal cortices and in subcortical white matter in [46]. Further reports also linked TSAs to symptomatology; however, not all found an association between ATACs and focal syndromes [47,48]. Recent studies however, have shown that white matter ARTAG in lobar regions is frequently associated with AD-related pathology [14]. This suggests that a subset of AD cases have additional pathogenic components; for example, hypoperfusion in the white matter, which can eventually be associated with focal symptoms. These concepts merit further confirmation.

A peculiar constellation of tau pathology was reported in elderly patients with dementia with or without parkinsonism [11]. Diffuse granular tau immunoreactivity in astrocytic processes (retrospectively these could be called GFAs) was described as the most characteristic feature [11]. The study emphasized additional neuronal pathologies, including threads and diffuse neuronal cytoplasmic tau immunoreactivity (pretangle-like). A subsequent study found these pathologies and suggested four different patterns based on the anatomical distribution of the tau astrogliopathy and its combination with neuronal tau pathology [49]: (1) medial temporal lobe type; (2) amygdala type; (3) limbic-basal ganglia-nigral type with neuronal tauopathy; and (4) hippocampus-dentate gyrus-amygdala type with neuronal tauopathy. It has been suspected that these might represent stages of the same process whereas other might be distinct conditions. Accumulation of TSAs in the dentate gyrus of the hippocampus were recognized by others as well [49,50]. Mathematical modeling of hippocampal tau immunolabeling patterns suggested that some forms of tau astrogliopathy in the elderly involve hippocampal subregions in a different pattern from that of primary tauopathies [51].

A recent study highlighted an interesting aspect of ARTAG. A study on individuals 90 years or older found an association with cortical but not limbic or brainstem ARTAG, independent of AD pathology, with cognitive decline [52]. Thus, the non-AD dementia group showed more hippocampal sclerosis, cortical ARTAG, TDP-43 and Lewy body pathology, while the cognitive resilient group had less of these [52]. Moreover, the authors found that cortical ARTAG independent of both limbic and brainstem ARTAGs is very rare (4%, 7/185). They speculated on an outward spread of ARTAG from limbic to the brainstem areas and then to the neocortical areas, and that neuronal tau pathology and astrocytic tau pathology are related in the oldest-old [52].

In summary, ARTAG most likely reflects the various impacts that individuals suffer during life, be it barrier dysfunction, mechanical impact, perfusion disturbance or a yet unidentified neurodegenerative event including propagation of pathological tau. Depending on the type and location of ARTAG it might be a sign of a reduced threshold that might lead to, or be associated with, decompensation of cognitive functions. And, especially when combined with other pathologies, perhaps with different pathogenesis, an additive effect might be seen, and individuals reach this threshold for cognitive decompensation more easily.

7. Perspectives

The accumulation of neurodegeneration-related proteins in astrocytes is not unique for tauopathies. Therefore, the term protein astrogliopathy (PAG) has been introduced to encompass different protein accumulations in astroglia in distinct neurodegenerative conditions. This emphasizes the yet unidentified role of astrocytes in the protein pathology of neurodegenerative diseases. Indeed, the variability of astrocytes associated with specific roles is being recognized [53]. Markers are developed [9,54–56] that still need to be linked to the involvement of specific glial cell populations affected by protein pathology. Eventually, these markers can be translated into bodily fluid biomarkers or probes for neuroimaging. These will help to understand the dynamics of astrocytic responses in various neurodegenerative conditions. The role of astrocytes in the processing and propagation, and the exact cytopathological mechanism of neurodegeneration-related proteins, are still not understood across the full spectrum. All these aspects position astrocytes in the center of current research on neurodegenerative conditions. Harmonizing the nomenclature of astrocytic tau pathologies leading to the definition of ARTAG enhanced these studies and further motivated researchers.

Funding: This research received no external funding.

Conflicts of Interest: The author declares no conflict of interest.

References

1. Kovacs, G.G.; Ferrer, I.; Grinberg, L.T.; Alafuzoff, I.; Attems, J.; Budka, H.; Cairns, N.J.; Crary, J.F.; Duyckaerts, C.; Ghetti, B.; et al. Aging-related tau astrogliopathy (ARTAG): Harmonized evaluation strategy. *Acta Neuropathol.* **2016**, *131*, 87–102. [CrossRef] [PubMed]
2. Ikeda, K. Glial fibrillary tangles and argyrophilic threads: Classification and disease specificity. *Neuropathology* **1996**, *16*, 71–77. [CrossRef]
3. Ikeda, K.; Akiyama, H.; Arai, T.; Nishimura, T. Glial tau pathology in neurodegenerative diseases: Their nature and comparison with neuronal tangles. *Neurobiol. Aging* **1998**, *19*, S85–S91. [CrossRef]
4. Ikeda, K.; Akiyama, H.; Kondo, H.; Haga, C.; Tanno, E.; Tokuda, T.; Ikeda, S. Thorn-shaped astrocytes: Possibly secondarily induced tau-positive glial fibrillary tangles. *Acta Neuropathol.* **1995**, *90*, 620–625. [CrossRef] [PubMed]
5. Schultz, C.; Ghebremedhin, E.; Del Tredici, K.; Rub, U.; Braak, H. High prevalence of thorn-shaped astrocytes in the aged human medial temporal lobe. *Neurobiol. Aging* **2004**, *25*, 397–405. [CrossRef]
6. Schultz, C.; Dehghani, F.; Hubbard, G.B.; Thal, D.R.; Struckhoff, G.; Braak, E.; Braak, H. Filamentous tau pathology in nerve cells, astrocytes, and oligodendrocytes of aged baboons. *J. Neuropathol. Exp. Neurol.* **2000**, *59*, 39–52. [CrossRef] [PubMed]
7. Schultz, C.; Hubbard, G.B.; Rub, U.; Braak, E.; Braak, H. Age-related progression of tau pathology in brains of baboons. *Neurobiol. Aging* **2000**, *21*, 905–912. [CrossRef]
8. Perez, S.E.; Raghanti, M.A.; Hof, P.R.; Kramer, L.; Ikonomovic, M.D.; Lacor, P.N.; Erwin, J.M.; Sherwood, C.C.; Mufson, E.J. Alzheimer's disease pathology in the neocortex and hippocampus of the western lowland gorilla (*Gorilla gorilla gorilla*). *J. Comp. Neurol.* **2013**, *521*, 4318–4338. [CrossRef] [PubMed]
9. Ferrer, I. Astrogliopathy in Tauopathies. *Neuroglia* **2018**, *1*, 126–150. [CrossRef]
10. Holzer, M.; Craxton, M.; Jakes, R.; Arendt, T.; Goedert, M. Tau gene (*MAPT*) sequence variation among primates. *Gene* **2004**, *341*, 313–322. [CrossRef] [PubMed]
11. Kovacs, G.G.; Molnar, K.; Laszlo, L.; Strobel, T.; Botond, G.; Honigschnabl, S.; Reiner-Concin, A.; Palkovits, M.; Fischer, P.; Budka, H. A peculiar constellation of tau pathology defines a subset of dementia in the elderly. *Acta Neuropathol.* **2011**, *122*, 205–222. [CrossRef] [PubMed]
12. Kovacs, G.G.; Xie, S.X.; Lee, E.B.; Robinson, J.L.; Caswell, C.; Irwin, D.J.; Toledo, J.B.; Johnson, V.E.; Smith, D.H.; Alafuzoff, I.; et al. Multisite Assessment of Aging-Related Tau Astrogliopathy (ARTAG). *J. Neuropathol. Exp. Neurol.* **2017**, *76*, 605–619. [CrossRef] [PubMed]
13. Nishimura, M.; Namba, Y.; Ikeda, K.; Oda, M. Glial fibrillary tangles with straight tubules in the brains of patients with progressive supranuclear palsy. *Neurosci. Lett.* **1992**, *143*, 35–38. [CrossRef]
14. Kovacs, G.G.; Robinson, J.L.; Xie, S.X.; Lee, E.B.; Grossman, M.; Wolk, D.A.; Irwin, D.J.; Weintraub, D.; Kim, C.F.; Schuck, T.; et al. Evaluating the Patterns of Aging-Related Tau Astrogliopathy Unravels Novel Insights into Brain Aging and Neurodegenerative Diseases. *J. Neuropathol. Exp. Neurol.* **2017**, *76*, 270–288. [CrossRef] [PubMed]
15. Kovacs, G.G. Invited review: Neuropathology of tauopathies: Principles and practice. *Neuropathol. Appl. Neurobiol.* **2015**, *41*, 3–23. [CrossRef] [PubMed]
16. Botez, G.; Probst, A.; Ipsen, S.; Tolnay, M. Astrocytes expressing hyperphosphorylated tau protein without glial fibrillary tangles in argyrophilic grain disease. *Acta Neuropathol.* **1999**, *98*, 251–256. [CrossRef] [PubMed]
17. Tolnay, M.; Clavaguera, F. Argyrophilic grain disease: A late-onset dementia with distinctive features among tauopathies. *Neuropathology* **2004**, *24*, 269–283. [CrossRef] [PubMed]

18. Crary, J.F.; Trojanowski, J.Q.; Schneider, J.A.; Abisambra, J.F.; Abner, E.L.; Alafuzoff, I.; Arnold, S.E.; Attems, J.; Beach, T.G.; Bigio, E.H.; et al. Primary age-related tauopathy (PART): A common pathology associated with human aging. *Acta Neuropathol.* **2014**, *128*, 755–766. [CrossRef] [PubMed]

19. Ghetti, B.; Oblak, A.L.; Boeve, B.F.; Johnson, K.A.; Dickerson, B.C.; Goedert, M. Invited review: Frontotemporal dementia caused by microtubule-associated protein tau gene (*MAPT*) mutations: A chameleon for neuropathology and neuroimaging. *Neuropathol. Appl. Neurobiol.* **2015**, *41*, 24–46. [CrossRef] [PubMed]

20. Kovacs, G.G.; Lee, V.M.; Trojanowski, J. Protein astrogliopathies in human neurodegenerative diseases and aging. *Brain Pathol.* **2017**, *27*, 675–690. [CrossRef] [PubMed]

21. Alexander, J.; Kalev, O.; Mehrabian, S.; Traykov, L.; Raycheva, M.; Kanakis, D.; Drineas, P.; Lutz, M.I.; Strobel, T.; Penz, T.; et al. Familial early-onset dementia with complex neuropathologic phenotype and genomic background. *Neurobiol. Aging* **2016**, *42*, 199–204. [CrossRef] [PubMed]

22. Le Guennec, K.; Quenez, O.; Nicolas, G.; Wallon, D.; Rousseau, S.; Richard, A.C.; Alexander, J.; Paschou, P.; Charbonnier, C.; Bellenguez, C.; et al. 17q21.31 duplication causes prominent tau-related dementia with increased MAPT expression. *Mol. Psychiatry* **2017**, *22*, 1119–1125. [CrossRef] [PubMed]

23. Ikeda, C.; Yokota, O.; Nagao, S.; Ishizu, H.; Oshima, E.; Hasegawa, M.; Okahisa, Y.; Terada, S.; Yamada, N. The Relationship Between Development of Neuronal and Astrocytic Tau Pathologies in Subcortical Nuclei and Progression of Argyrophilic Grain Disease. *Brain Pathol.* **2016**, *26*, 488–505. [CrossRef] [PubMed]

24. Ferrer, I.; Lopez-Gonzalez, I.; Carmona, M.; Arregui, L.; Dalfo, E.; Torrejon-Escribano, B.; Diehl, R.; Kovacs, G.G. Glial and neuronal tau pathology in tauopathies: Characterization of disease-specific phenotypes and tau pathology progression. *J. Neuropathol. Exp. Neurol.* **2014**, *73*, 81–97. [CrossRef] [PubMed]

25. Lopez-Gonzalez, I.; Carmona, M.; Blanco, R.; Luna-Munoz, J.; Martinez-Mandonado, A.; Mena, R.; Ferrer, I. Characterization of thorn-shaped astrocytes in white matter of temporal lobe in Alzheimer's disease brains. *Brain Pathol.* **2013**, *23*, 144–153. [CrossRef] [PubMed]

26. McKee, A.C.; Cairns, N.J.; Dickson, D.W.; Folkerth, R.D.; Keene, C.D.; Litvan, I.; Perl, D.P.; Stein, T.D.; Vonsattel, J.P.; Stewart, W.; et al. The first NINDS/NIBIB consensus meeting to define neuropathological criteria for the diagnosis of chronic traumatic encephalopathy. *Acta Neuropathol.* **2016**, *131*, 75–86. [CrossRef] [PubMed]

27. McKee, A.C.; Daneshvar, D.H. The neuropathology of traumatic brain injury. *Handb. Clin. Neurol.* **2015**, *127*, 45–66. [PubMed]

28. Liu, A.K.; Goldfinger, M.H.; Questari, H.E.; Pearce, R.K.; Gentleman, S.M. ARTAG in the basal forebrain: Widening the constellation of astrocytic tau pathology. *Acta Neuropathol. Commun.* **2016**, *4*, 59. [CrossRef] [PubMed]

29. McKee, A.C.; Stein, T.D.; Kiernan, P.T.; Alvarez, V.E. The neuropathology of chronic traumatic encephalopathy. *Brain Pathol.* **2015**, *25*, 350–364. [CrossRef] [PubMed]

30. McKee, A.C.; Stern, R.A.; Nowinski, C.J.; Stein, T.D.; Alvarez, V.E.; Daneshvar, D.H.; Lee, H.S.; Wojtowicz, S.M.; Hall, G.; Baugh, C.M.; et al. The spectrum of disease in chronic traumatic encephalopathy. *Brain* **2013**, *136*, 43–64. [CrossRef] [PubMed]

31. Kovacs, G.G.; Xie, S.X.; Robinson, J.L.; Lee, E.B.; Smith, D.H.; Schuck, T.; Lee, V.M.; Trojanowski, J.Q. Sequential stages and distribution patterns of aging-related tau astrogliopathy (ARTAG) in the human brain. *Acta Neuropathol. Commun.* **2018**, *6*, 50. [CrossRef] [PubMed]

32. Kovacs, G.G.; Rahimi, J.; Strobel, T.; Lutz, M.I.; Regelsberger, G.; Streichenberger, N.; Perret-Liaudet, A.; Hoftberger, R.; Liberski, P.P.; Budka, H.; et al. Tau pathology in Creutzfeldt-Jakob disease revisited. *Brain Pathol.* **2017**, *27*, 332–344. [CrossRef] [PubMed]

33. Brettschneider, J.; Del Tredici, K.; Lee, V.M.; Trojanowski, J.Q. Spreading of pathology in neurodegenerative diseases: A focus on human studies. *Nat. Rev. Neurosci.* **2015**, *16*, 109–120. [CrossRef] [PubMed]

34. Ling, H.; Kovacs, G.G.; Vonsattel, J.P.; Davey, K.; Mok, K.Y.; Hardy, J.; Morris, H.R.; Warner, T.T.; Holton, J.L.; Revesz, T. Astrogliopathy predominates the earliest stage of corticobasal degeneration pathology. *Brain* **2016**, *139*, 3237–3252. [CrossRef] [PubMed]

35. Chvátal, A.; Verkhratsky, A. An Early History of Neuroglial Research: Personalities. *Neuroglia* **2018**, *1*, 245–281. [CrossRef]

36. Shibuya, K.; Yagishita, S.; Nakamura, A.; Uchihara, T. Perivascular orientation of astrocytic plaques and tuft-shaped astrocytes. *Brain Res.* **2011**, *1404*, 50–54. [CrossRef] [PubMed]

37. Ferrer, I.; Legati, A.; Garcia-Monco, J.C.; Gomez-Beldarrain, M.; Carmona, M.; Blanco, R.; Seeley, W.W.; Coppola, G. Familial behavioral variant frontotemporal dementia associated with astrocyte-predominant tauopathy. *J. Neuropathol. Exp. Neurol.* **2015**, *74*, 370–379. [CrossRef] [PubMed]

38. Kovacs, G.G.; Yousef, A.; Kaindl, S.; Lee, V.M.; Trojanowski, J.Q. Connexin-43 and Aquaporin-4 are markers of ARTAG-related astroglial response. *Neuropathol. Appl. Neurobiol.* **2017**. [CrossRef]

39. Chung, W.S.; Clarke, L.E.; Wang, G.X.; Stafford, B.K.; Sher, A.; Chakraborty, C.; Joung, J.; Foo, L.C.; Thompson, A.; Chen, C.; et al. Astrocytes mediate synapse elimination through MEGF10 and MERTK pathways. *Nature* **2013**, *504*, 394–400. [CrossRef] [PubMed]

40. Davis, C.H.; Kim, K.Y.; Bushong, E.A.; Mills, E.A.; Boassa, D.; Shih, T.; Kinebuchi, M.; Phan, S.; Zhou, Y.; Bihlmeyer, N.A.; et al. Transcellular degradation of axonal mitochondria. *Proc. Natl. Acad. Sci. USA* **2014**, *111*, 9633–9638. [CrossRef] [PubMed]

41. Tang, G.; Yang, G.Y. Aquaporin-4: A Potential Therapeutic Target for Cerebral Edema. *Int. J. Mol. Sci.* **2016**, *17*, 1413. [CrossRef] [PubMed]

42. Narasimhan, S.; Guo, J.L.; Changolkar, L.; Stieber, A.; McBride, J.D.; Silva, L.V.; He, Z.; Zhang, B.; Gathagan, R.J.; Trojanowski, J.Q.; et al. Pathological Tau Strains from Human Brains Recapitulate the Diversity of Tauopathies in Nontransgenic Mouse Brain. *J. Neurosci.* **2017**, *37*, 11406–11423. [CrossRef] [PubMed]

43. Ferrer, I.; Garcia, M.A.; Gonzalez, I.L.; Lucena, D.D.; Villalonga, A.R.; Tech, M.C.; Llorens, F.; Garcia-Esparcia, P.; Martinez-Maldonado, A.; Mendez, M.F.; et al. Aging-related tau astrogliopathy (ARTAG): Not only tau phosphorylation in astrocytes. *Brain Pathol.* **2018**. [CrossRef] [PubMed]

44. Higuchi, M.; Ishihara, T.; Zhang, B.; Hong, M.; Andreadis, A.; Trojanowski, J.; Lee, V.M. Transgenic mouse model of tauopathies with glial pathology and nervous system degeneration. *Neuron* **2002**, *35*, 433–446. [CrossRef]

45. Forman, M.S.; Lal, D.; Zhang, B.; Dabir, D.V.; Swanson, E.; Lee, V.M.; Trojanowski, J.Q. Transgenic mouse model of tau pathology in astrocytes leading to nervous system degeneration. *J. Neurosci.* **2005**, *25*, 3539–3550. [CrossRef] [PubMed]

46. Munoz, D.G.; Woulfe, J.; Kertesz, A. Argyrophilic thorny astrocyte clusters in association with Alzheimer's disease pathology in possible primary progressive aphasia. *Acta Neuropathol.* **2007**, *114*, 347–357. [CrossRef] [PubMed]

47. Bigio, E.H.; Mishra, M.; Hatanpaa, K.J.; White, C.L., 3rd; Johnson, N.; Rademaker, A.; Weitner, B.B.; Deng, H.X.; Dubner, S.D.; Weintraub, S.; et al. TDP-43 pathology in primary progressive aphasia and frontotemporal dementia with pathologic Alzheimer disease. *Acta Neuropathol.* **2010**, *120*, 43–54. [CrossRef] [PubMed]

48. Mesulam, M.; Wicklund, A.; Johnson, N.; Rogalski, E.; Leger, G.C.; Rademaker, A.; Weintraub, S.; Bigio, E.H. Alzheimer and frontotemporal pathology in subsets of primary progressive aphasia. *Ann. Neurol.* **2008**, *63*, 709–719. [CrossRef] [PubMed]

49. Kovacs, G.G.; Milenkovic, I.; Wohrer, A.; Hoftberger, R.; Gelpi, E.; Haberler, C.; Honigschnabl, S.; Reiner-Concin, A.; Heinzl, H.; Jungwirth, S.; et al. Non-Alzheimer neurodegenerative pathologies and their combinations are more frequent than commonly believed in the elderly brain: A community-based autopsy series. *Acta Neuropathol.* **2013**, *126*, 365–384. [CrossRef] [PubMed]

50. Lace, G.; Ince, P.G.; Brayne, C.; Savva, G.M.; Matthews, F.E.; de Silva, R.; Simpson, J.E.; Wharton, S.B. Mesial temporal astrocyte tau pathology in the MRC-CFAS ageing brain cohort. *Dement. Geriatr. Cogn. Disord.* **2012**, *34*, 15–24. [CrossRef] [PubMed]

51. Milenkovic, I.; Petrov, T.; Kovacs, G.G. Patterns of hippocampal tau pathology differentiate neurodegenerative dementias. *Dement. Geriatr. Cogn. Disord.* **2014**, *38*, 375–388. [CrossRef] [PubMed]

52. Robinson, J.L.; Corrada, M.M.; Kovacs, G.G.; Dominique, M.; Caswell, C.; Xie, S.X.; Lee, V.M.; Kawas, C.H.; Trojanowski, J.Q. Non-Alzheimer's contributions to dementia and cognitive resilience in the 90+ Study. *Acta Neuropathol.* **2018**. [CrossRef] [PubMed]

53. Verkhratsky, A.; Oberheim Bush, N.A.; Nedergaard, M.; Butt, A. The Special Case of Human Astrocytes. *Neuroglia* **2018**, *1*, 21–29. [CrossRef]

54. Herculano-Houzel, S.; Dos Santos, S.E. You Do Not Mess with the Glia. *Neuroglia* **2018**, *1*, 193–219. [CrossRef]

55. Ferrer, I. Diversity of astroglial responses across human neurodegenerative disorders and brain aging. *Brain Pathol.* **2017**, *27*, 645–674. [CrossRef] [PubMed]
56. Verkhratsky, A.; Zorec, R.; Parpura, V. Stratification of astrocytes in healthy and diseased brain. *Brain Pathol.* **2017**, *27*, 629–644. [CrossRef] [PubMed]

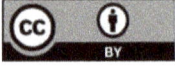

Article

Ultrastructural Remodeling of the Neurovascular Unit in the Female Diabetic db/db Model—Part III: Oligodendrocyte and Myelin

Melvin R. Hayden [1,2,*], Deana G. Grant [3], Aranyra Aroor [1,2,4] and Vincent G. DeMarco [1,2,4,5]

[1] Diabetes and Cardiovascular Center, University of Missouri School of Medicine, Columbia, MO 65212, USA; aroora@health.missouri.edu (A.A.); demarcov@missouri.edu (V.G.D.)

[2] Division of Endocrinology and Metabolism, Department of Medicine, University of Missouri, Columbia, MO 63212, USA

[3] Electron Microscopy Core Facility, University of Missouri, Columbia, MO 65211, USA; GrantDe@missouri.edu

[4] Research Service, Harry S. Truman Memorial Veterans Hospital, Columbia, MO 65212, USA

[5] Department of Medical Pharmacology and Physiology, University of Missouri, Columbia, MO 65212, USA

[*] Correspondence: mrh29pete@gmail.com; Tel.: +1-573-346-3019

Received: 9 October 2018; Accepted: 5 November 2018; Published: 8 November 2018

Abstract: Obesity, insulin resistance, and type 2 diabetes mellitus are associated with diabetic cognopathy. In this study, we tested the hypothesis that neurovascular unit(s) (NVU), oligodendrocytes, and myelin within cerebral cortical grey matter and deeper transitional zone regions between the cortical grey matter and white matter may be abnormal. The monogenic (*Lepr^{db}*) female diabetic db/db [BKS.CgDock7^m +/+ *Lepr^{db}*/J] (DBC) mouse model was utilized for this ultrastructural study. Upon sacrifice (20 weeks of age), left-brain hemispheres of the DBC and age-matched non-diabetic wild type control C57BL/KsJ (CKC) mice were immediately immersion-fixed. We found prominent remodeling of oligodendrocytes with increased nuclear chromatin condensation and volume and increased numbers of active myelination sites of the cytoplasm in transition zones. Marked dysmyelination with outer myelin lamellae sheath splitting, separation, and ballooning with aberrant mitochondria in grey matter and similar myelin remodeling changes with marked disarray with additional axonal collapse in transitional zones in DBC as compared to CKC models.

Keywords: db/db mouse model; myelin; neurovascular unit; oligodendrocyte; subcortical white matter; type 2 diabetes

1. Introduction

Myelin is a multilayered lamellar sheath that enwraps axons in the grey and white matter in the brain and is synthesized in the brain by the oligodendroglia. The myelin sheath provides axonal protection and allows the saltatory conduction of the action potential. Oligodendrocytes (OLs), oligodendrocyte precursor cells (OPC), and oligodendrocyte lineage cells are specialized glial cells responsible for the synthesis, wrapping ensheathment, and compacting of myelin in myelinated axons [1–3]. Rudolf Ludwig Virchow (1821–1902) introduced the term myelin and defined it as medullary matter (Markstoff), or myeline, that in extremely large quantity fills up the interval between the axon axis-cylinder and the sheath in primitive nerve-fibers [4].

Michalski and Kothary [1] have set forth a paradigm for development of mature OLs in four distinct phases: (i) the birth, migration and proliferation of OPCs, that occurs in waves; followed by (ii) morphological differentiation with the OL establishing an expansive synthetic network of OL cytoplasmic processes; followed by (iii) axonal contact, which leads to myelin wrapping—ensheathment of targeted neuronal axons with ensuing generation of extremely electron dense and compact myelin with an enduring (iv) long-term trophic and metabolic support system for maintenance and protection of myelinated neurons [1].

As OPCs differentiate into mature OLs they undergo an extensive development of active cytoplasmic reorganization of cytoskeleton proteins and endoplasmic reticulum, which increases their intermediate cytoplasmic electron density and helps to identify them when studying with transmission electron microscopy (TEM) (Figure 1). Identifying characteristics have been presented in Part I Table 1 [5] as follows: Oligodendrocytes are intermediate in size and their thinned cytoplasm also have an intermediate electron density that is helpful when comparing to astrocytes and microglia. They also may occur in groups or nests and are more often found in the white matter regions of the brain. In addition to their small cytoplasmic volume, they have multiple protoplasmic extensions, which allow OLs to concurrently myelinate multiple axons [1–4].

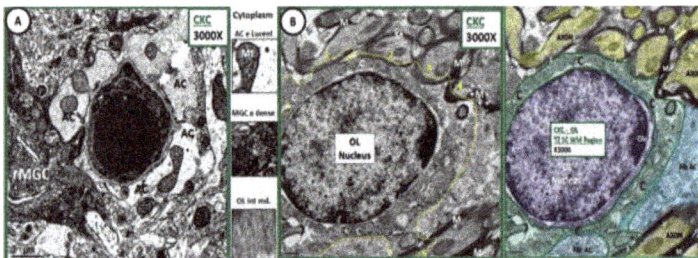

Figure 1. Comparison of astrocyte, ramified microglial cell, and oligodendrocyte to illustrate intermediate electron dense and thin cytoplasm. (**A**) Depicts an astrocyte (AC) with electron lucent cytoplasm and a ramified microglial cell (rMGC) with its electron dense cytoplasm. (**B**) Illustrates a thinned intermediate electron dense cytoplasm of the oligodendrocyte (OL) obtained from the transition zone in subcortical white matter (TZ SCWM) just deep to layer VI as compared to ACs and microglia cells. Note that the OL is in the process of enwrapping at least 5 axons (1–5) with myelin in (**B**) and its pseudo-colored image, far right. Between (**A**,**B**) the cytoplasm has been cut from each cell to further demonstrate the intermediate electron (e) density of the OL cytoplasm. Also note the small amount of cytoplasm as compared to nucleus volume as well as the incorporation of myelin at its outer margins of the cytoplasm plasmalemma. A pseudo-colorized image is inserted far right to aid in identifying OL nucleus (purple); cytoplasm (C green); fibrous astrocyte (fib AC blue); axons (yellow). Magnification ×3000; scale bar = 1 μm in A and 0.5 μm in (**B**). C: cytoplasm; MGC: microglial cell; M: myelin; CKC: age-matched non-diabetic wild type control C57BL/KsJ.

The small cytoplasmic volume of oligodendrocyte may be related to its function of constantly supplying its plasma membrane (up to three-times its volume of plasma membranes) in order to create the multiple myelin lamellar sheaths. These myelin lamella that enwrap multiple unmyelinated axons increase the speed of neuronal transmission of their action potentials via membrane depolarization by high-density voltage-gated sodium channels that creates the saltatory (jumping) conduction of their action potentials and signaling at the nodes of Ranvier (Figure 1B). Importantly, this saltatory conduction allows electrical nerve signals to be propagated long distances at high rates without any degradation of the action potential signaling [1–4].

Myelin also serves as a protective sheath of myelinated neurons in order to provide for long-term axonal integrity and maintenance survival. Myelinated axons are present in the cortical grey matter; however, they are the most abundant within the white matter and give rise to the white matter tracts. The bulk of myelinated axons localizes within the white matter, which are important for carrying large amounts of information from one region of the brain to distant regions and must rapidly transmit this information. This rapid transmission is primarily due to its compacted electron dense myelin sheaths. Therefore, if myelin undergoes any significant abnormal remodeling change there may be a delay in the in the arrival of information to the more distant regional neurons with subsequent cognitive impairment [6,7].

2. Materials and Methods

2.1. Animal Models

As previously presented in Part I [5]: All animal studies were approved by the Institutional Animal Care and Use Committees at the Harry S Truman Memorial Veterans' Hospital and University of Missouri, Columbia, MO, USA (No. 190), and conformed to the Guide for the Care and Use of Laboratory Animals published by the National Institutes of Health (NIH). Eight-week-old female db/db [BKS.Cg-$Dock7^m$ +/+ $Lepr^{db}$/J] (DBC) and wild-type control C57BLKS/J (CKC) mice were purchased from the Jackson Laboratory (Ann Harbor, MI, USA) and were housed under standard laboratory conditions where room temperature was 21–22 °C, and light and dark cycles were 12 h each. Two cohorts of mice were used: lean non-diabetic controls (CKC, $n = 3$), and obese, insulin-resistant, diabetic db/db (DBC, $n = 3$), which were sacrificed for study at 20 weeks of age.

2.2. Tissue Collection and Preparation

Have been previously presented in Part I [5].

3. Results

3.1. Dysmyelination in the Cortical Grey Matter Primarily Layer III

Splitting and separation of myelin lamellar sheaths (dysmyelination) in the cortical grey matter layer III was readily observed in the female diabetic db/db [BKS.Cg$Dock7^m$ +/+ $Lepr^{db}$/J] (DBC) as compared to the nondiabetic age-matched non-diabetic wild type control C57BL/KsJ (CKC) models. Additionally, axonal remodeling was noted, which consisted of aberrant mitochondria and increased axonal cytoplasm electron density as compared to the nondiabetic CKC model (Figures 2 and 3).

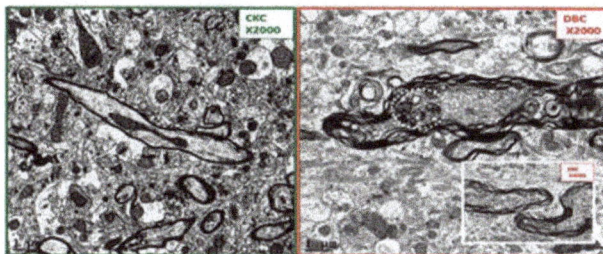

Figure 2. Comparison of control CKC and diabetic diabetic db/db [BKS.Cg$Dock7^m$ +/+ $Lepr^{db}$/J] (DBC) myelination in layer III cortical grey matter. These panels depict the marked difference between the myelination of axons in the cortical grey matter of Layer III. Note in the diabetic DBC panel (to the right) the marked splitting and separation of myelin (dysmyelination) and the grouping of suspected aberrant mitochondria (encircled white dashed line). The insert in the DBC panel is from another model in cortical layer III with dysmyelination. Also note the increased thickness of myelin which measures approximately 0.5 µm in the DBC as compared to the 0.1 µm thickness of the myelin in the CKC model. Also note the elongated axonal mitochondria in the CKC model in contrast to the smaller rounded mitochondria in the DBC. Importantly, note the increase in electron density of the axoplasm of the neuron in the DBC as compared to the CKC. Magnification ×2000; bar = 1 µm. Magnification of insert ×4000 and scale bar = 0.5 µm.

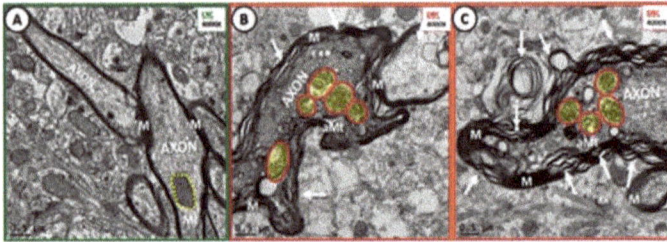

Figure 3. Dysmyelination and aberrant mitochondria in cortical grey matter layer III of diabetic DBC models. (**A**) Depicts the normal compact myelin (M) ensheathing the axons of the nondiabetic control CKC models and note the normal electron dense mitochondria (Mt) (encircled by yellow dashed line). Panels (**B,C**) depict the marked splitting and separation of myelin ensheathment in DBC models (arrows). Also note the aberrant Mt (aMt)—(pseudo-colored yellow with red lines) and increased electron dense cytoplasm in the DBC. Magnification ×4000; bar = 0.5 μm.

Also, ballooning of myelinated axons was detected, but not with the frequency of myelin splitting and separation (Figure 4).

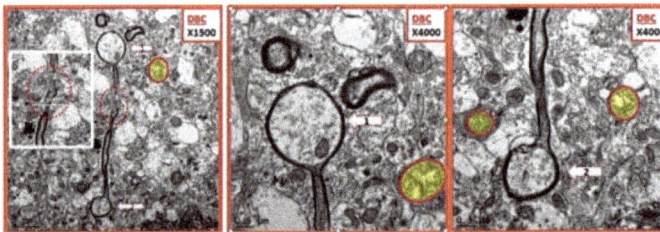

Figure 4. Examples of ballooning in myelinated axons of diabetic DBC models in cortical grey matter. This three-panel image depicts ballooning of myelinated axons that were only observed in the diabetic DBC and did not occur in nondiabetic control CKC. The left-hand panel depicts a myelinated axon with ballooning superiorly (open arrow 1) and a ballooning inferiorly (open arrow 2) and note the interruption of the myelin sheath in mid axon (red dashed oval) and the cropped image insert from this region exploded in Microsoft paint with intact scale bar of 2 μm. Mid panel has open arrow pointing to balloon 1 and right-hand panel has open arrow pointing to balloon 2. Note the aberrant mitochondria pseudo-colored yellow with red outline. Magnification ×1500; scale bar = 2 μm far left, Magnification ×4000; scale bar = 0.5 μm in mid and far right-hand panels.

An unexpected finding within the cortical grey matter consisted of fragmented microtubules—neurofilaments and electron dense proteinaceous aggregations in three different unmyelinated axons at higher magnifications (Figure 5).

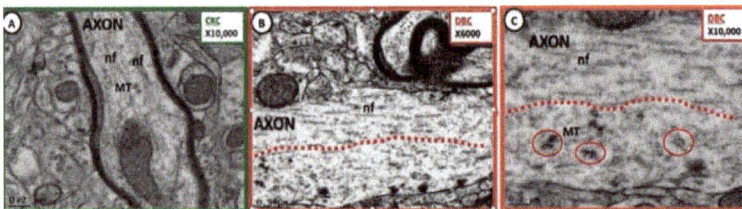

Figure 5. Larger axons, loss of microtubule neurofilament linearity, fragmentation and proteinaceous

aggregation and deposition within axoplasm in some of diabetic DBC models. (**B,C**) Depict a loss of linearity of neurofilaments (nf) with fragmentation and aggregated proteinaceous electron dense deposits (within the lower half, below the red dashed line) axoplasm of diabetic DBC as compared to nondiabetic CKC controls (**A**). Some of the larger electron densities are microtubules (MT), while others could be protein aggregations. (**B,C**) Are from different regions of the same unmyelinated axon. Note that the axon width of the DBC is ~1.5 μm as compared to 0.5 μm in CKC. Magnifications ×10,000 (**A,C**); scale bar = 0.2 μm. (**B**) Magnifications ×6000; scale bar = 0.5 μm.

3.2. Dysmyelination in the Transitional Zone between Cortical Layer VI and White Matter

Due to the observations of splitting and separation of myelin lamellar units in the cortical grey matter, we decided to make deeper cuts to see if the transitional zone (TZ) between cortical layer and subcortical white matter also demonstrated abnormalities in myelinated axons since we were unable to examine any specific white matter tracts. One of the first things we noted was a decrease in neurovascular units in these regions as compared to cortical grey matter. These findings were anticipated, since it is known that the white matter has decreased capillary density as compared to cortical grey matter regions [8].

We noted a marked difference in myelinated axons in the TZ in the DBC models. These regions were observed to have a marked disarray of myelin with splitting—separation and collapse of axons from the myelin lamellar sheaths (Figure 6).

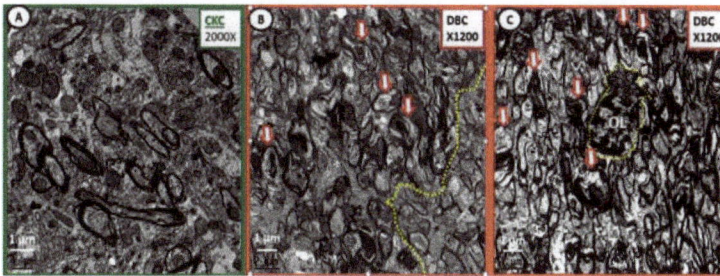

Figure 6. Extensive myelin remodeling disarray in diabetic DBC at deeper transition regions of the subcortical white matter regions. (**A**) Illustrates the normal appearance of the transitional subcortical white matter regions just deep to layer VI grey matter. (**B,C**) Depict markedly abnormal myelin remodeling in the diabetic DBC models. (**B**) Even demonstrates a demarcation between more severe remodeling to the left side of the demarcation (yellow dashed line) with more severe myelin splitting and axonal—axoplasm collapse (open red arrows) within the abnormal myelin lamellar sheaths. (**C**) Depicts a centrally located oligodendrocyte (OL outlined by yellow dashed line) that appears to be in the process of wrapping multiple axons with myelin. Importantly, note the very electron dense chromatin clumping—condensation within the nuclei and the very small amount of cytoplasm. (**B,C**) Depict marked disorganization of myelin lamella—dysmyelination with disordered myelin lamella, which is associated with splitting and separation of the myelin sheath lamella. Also, this region demonstrated marked abnormal remodeling changes of myelinated neurons in the diabetic DBC models as compared to control CKC models. Magnification ×2000; scale bar = 1 μm (**A**). Magnification ×1200; scale bar = 1 μm (**B,C**).

Also, there were abnormalities of OLs in the diabetic DBC models in the transitional zone subcortical white matter between layers VI and deeper white matter (Figures 7 and 8).

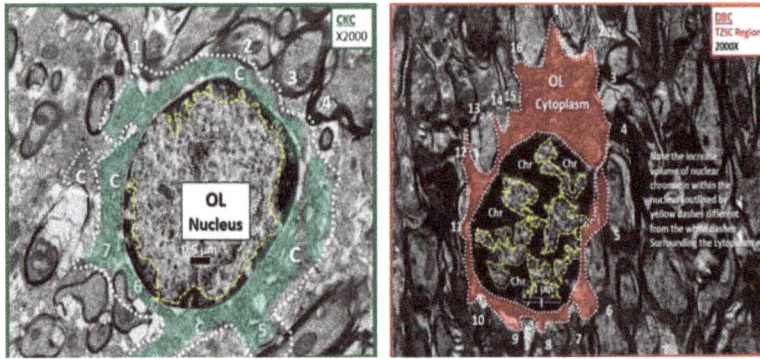

Figure 7. Increased chromatin condensation volume in nuclei of diabetic DBC models in the transitional zone subcortical regions as compared to nondiabetic CKC models. The nondiabetic CKC model to the left (cytoplasm pseudo-colored green and outlined with white dashed line) depicts an OL in the transitional zone subcortical (TZSC) region with surrounding myelinated axons and displays at least 1–7 numbered regions of myelination and maintenance zones. Note that the cytoplasm (C) in control models to the left has approximately seven regions of myelination as compared to diabetic DBC model to the right, which depicts up to 16 regions of myelination and maintenance zones with adjacent numerous electron dense myelinated axons (cytoplasm is pseudo-colored red with white dashed outline). Of great interest in the TZSC regions of the DBC, note that nuclear chromatin (Chr) is markedly increased (outlined by yellow dashed lines) in volume compared to nuclear volume when compared to the CKC nuclear chromatin on the left (outlined by yellow dashed lines). This was a consistent remodeling abnormality in the TZSC regions in the DBC models. Magnification ×2000; bar = 0.5 µm in CKC and 1 µm in DBC.

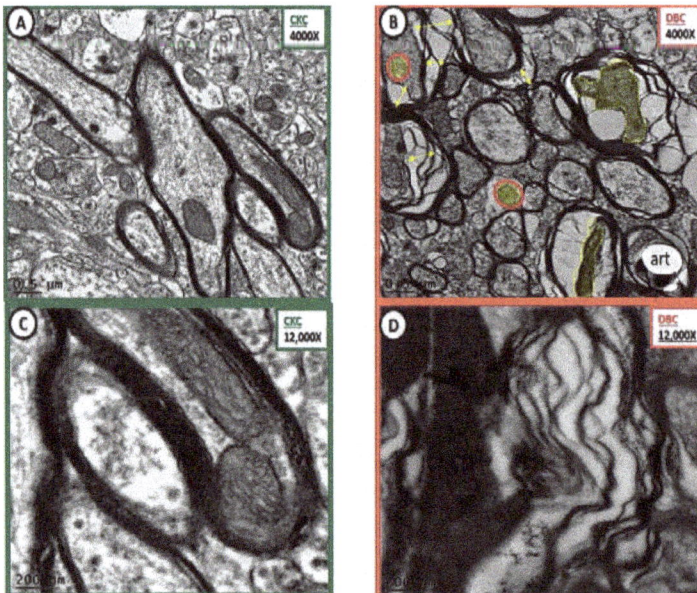

Figure 8. Markedly abnormal subcortical white matter myelin in diabetic DBC models. (**C,D**) Depict marked disorganization—disarrangement of the transitional zone subcortical white matter (SCWM)

myelin and the neuronal axon in the diabetic DBC models. (**B**) Illustrates axon-axoplasm collapse (double arrows) in myelinated neurons. Also note that the neuronal axons become very electron dense once they collapse (pseudo-colored yellow and outlined by yellow dashed lines). Additionally, note the aberrant mitochondria (pseudo-colored yellow and outlined by red lines) as compared to the electron dense Mt with crista in the control CKC models (**A,C**). (**D**) Illustrates the abnormal myelin lamella with marked splitting and separation of myelin lamella. Magnification ×4000; bar = 0.5 µm in (**A,B**). Magnification ×12,000; bar = 200 nm in (**C,D**). art: artifact.

Additionally noted was the collapse of the axons with myelin splitting and separation in the diabetic DBC models (Figures 9 and 10).

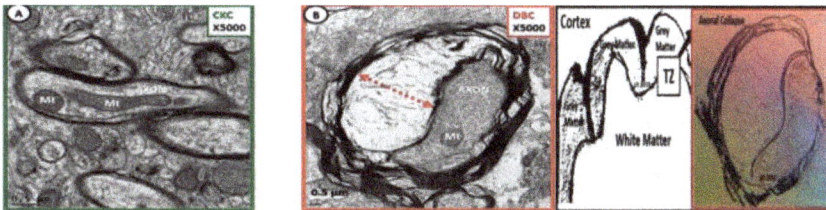

Figure 9. Axonal collapse in dysmyelinated neurons with splitting and separation transitional zones in diabetic DBC. Note in (**B**) that the collapse of the axon within the dysmyelinated neuron with splitting and separation of myelin lamella sheath in the transitional zones (TZ) of the subcortical white matter of the diabetic DBC as compared to the TZ non-collapsed axons in CKC models (**A**). Axonal collapse was markedly increased in the transitional zone regions as compared to the grey matter and not found in any of the CKC models. Note the region of the TZ in artistic rendering to far right of above figure. Magnification ×5000; scale bar = 0.5 µm.

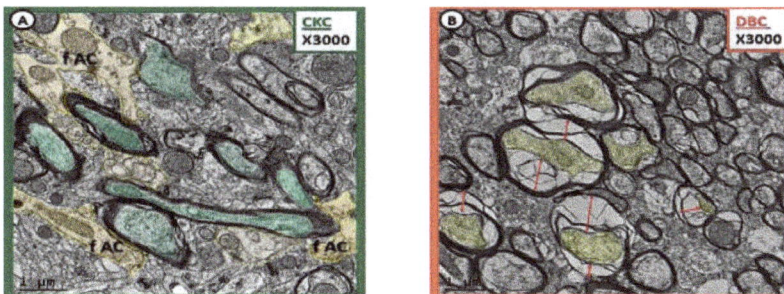

Figure 10. Myelin splitting, separation, and ballooning with axonal collapse in transitional zone in diabetic DBC models. (**A**) Depicts myelinated neurons with pseudo-colored green axons that fully occupy the myelin core. Also note the pseudo-colored yellow fibrous astrocyte (f AC) that are adjacent to the myelinated axons. (**B**) Demonstrates the splitting, separation, and ballooning of the myelin sheath resulting in axonal collapse in the diabetic DBC models in the transitional zone between layers VI and the subcortical white matter. Magnification ×3000; scale bar = 1 µm in (**A,B**).

4. Discussion

White matter is usually thought to be composed primarily by myelinated axons at the gross macroscopic level and is thought to be responsible for imparting a demarcation from the outer grey matter, which contains primarily neuronal cell bodies, glia, synaptic dendrites, and axon terminals of neurons. However, the white matter also contains numerous and varying percentages of unmyelinated axons: for example, the human corpus callosum may have up to 30% unmyelinated axons in contrast to the optic nerve where nearly all axons are myelinated [9].

Myelin wrapping and the final end-product of highly electron dense and compacted myelination of axonal ensheathment is quite complicated and illustrated in a simplified illustration (Figure 11). One can also view a more detailed 3D reconstruction with electron microscopy in the following reference for greater detail [10].

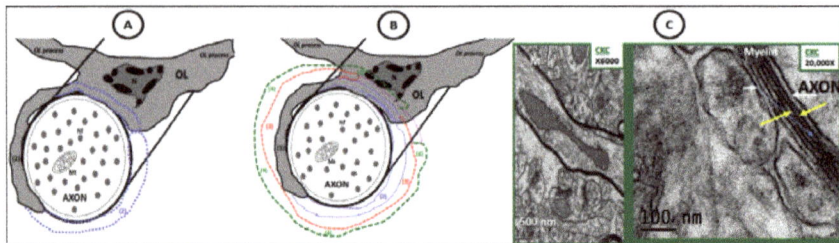

Figure 11. Possible mechanisms for oligodendrocyte myelination. (**A**) Depicts an illustration of the initial engagement of an OL and an unmyelinated axon with a protrusion of an oligodendrocyte cytoplasmic process (grey) beginning to extend and enwrap (blue dashed lines) of an unmyelinated neuron. (**B**) Depicts the possible multi-step process: (1) solid grey oligodendrocyte cytoplasmic process protrusion and engagement of the OL to the unmyelinated axon; (2) extension of the original oligodendrocyte cytoplasmic protrusion—blue dashed line; (3) another wrapping—red dashed line; (4) the most recent extension of wrapping—green dashed line. These previous steps may represent a common OL cellular mechanism of myelination. The multiple wrappings, which result in multilamellar myelin ensheathments are then bound tightly and compacted via the myelin basic protein plus other compacting proteins synthesized and secreted by oligodendrocytes that eventually develop into the highly electron dense tightly wrapped compacted myelinated neurons that we observe in transmission electron microscopic images in control CKC models as depicted in the control CKC model in (**C**). This mechanism does not explain for the lateral extension of the internodal myelin. Note that in (**C**) there is present some separation of myelinated lamella as a result of high magnification ×20,000; scale bar = 100 nm that is not recognized at lower magnification. This higher magnification delineates the electron dense (dense lines—yellow arrows) and the electron lucent (intraperiod lines—white arrows). M: mitochondria; N: nucleus of oligodendrocyte; Nf: neurofilament; OL: oligodendrocyte.

The images in the results section may provide additional concepts and improve our understanding of the oligodendrocyte and myelin formation in both the grey matter and transitional zone between the grey matter and the white matter (Figure 9 far right—artistic rendition) in the DBC models. Indeed, it is obvious that similar to other glial cells, oligodendrocytes respond with cellular and tissue remodeling to the multiple toxicities associated with obesity, insulin resistance, and glucotoxicity when the receptor for leptin is deficient as in the DBC model. Of note, OLs not only effect myelination and their maintenance to individual axons, but also may be important to entire neuronal networks as a result of shape-shifting—remodeling changes of their ultrastructural morphology including myelin splitting, ballooning, and axonal collapse. As a result of leptin receptor deficiency, OLs may remodel their ultrastructure to result in changes of CNS behavioral effects of depression and cognitive impairment. Indeed, OLs are dynamic, adaptive, and plastic and are certainly capable of responding via a response to injury mechanism and even aid in the development of abnormal brain behavior in this diabetic DBC model [11].

The ultrastructural remodeling in the DBC models (Figure 5) could represent an early axoplasm remodeling change of fragmentation of neurofibrillary tangles that are known to be associated with increased possibility of tau pathology in the db/db models of leptin resistance and type 2 diabetes [11].

Additionally, others have shown similar remodeling changes with fragmentation of axonal neurofilaments in both myelinated and unmyelinated axons similar to what we observed (only in unmyelinated neuronal axons) in streptozotocin induced type 1 diabetic rats [12]. However, the unmyelinated axon we demonstrated (Figure 5) may have depicted some proteinaceous aggregation in DBC models in addition to microtubules.

In Figures 2–4 (cortical grey matter) and Figures 6–10 (subcortical white matter transitional zone) we demonstrated splitting, separation, and ballooning of myelinated neurons. These changes have been previously described by others in models of aging [13,14]. Peters et al. state that there are four basic changes in myelin in aged monkey brains, which consist of local splitting, ballooning, redundant myelin, and double myelin sheaths—duplication, which we have depicted in our DBC as compared to the CKC models [13]. These findings seem to also corroborate Parts I and II of this series in that the oligodendrocyte and myelin remodeling changes suggests an accelerated and premature aging process in the diabetic DBC as compared to the control CKC models [14].

In regard to the transitional zone between cortical grey and white matter, the subcortical white matter may represent a region in the brain that is less vascularized [15–17]. Interestingly, our observational findings regarding vascularity in the cortex revealed that there are usually 2–4 neurovascular units (NVU) capillaries per grid examined and in the transitional zone described there was usually only one NVU capillary at the most with a preponderance of no NVU capillaries per grid examined. Additionally, an older paper states the following, "it is possible that the junction between cortex and white matter is relatively avascular, and in this respect this area may be similar to the particular periventricular regions" [18].

Oligodendrocytes and myelination are not static and readily adapt to their environment. The previously described alterations in myelin remodeling in the diabetic DBC models may be detrimental and could impair cognition by the slowing of conduction rates of information—action potential in white matter tracts to distant regions, which could result in a loss of synchronicity not only in individual neurons, but to entire neuronal networks.

4.1. Vascular Stiffness

Vascular stiffness including thoracic aorta or carotid artery not only affects the capillaries of the classical end-organs of diabetes (retinopathy, neuropathy, nephropathy, and cardiomyopathy) due to abnormal pulsatile mechanical forces that are associated with microvascular damage and remodeling but may also affect the brain in diabetic cognopathy. In particular, this same cohort that we studied (db/db—DBC) in these three-part series (Parts I, II, and III) has been previously demonstrated to have aortic vascular stiffening [19]. The capillary neurovascular remodeling changes described in Part I could affect the possible diminished microvessels in the transition zones as well as the ones we demonstrated within the grey matter and could decrease the cerebral blood flow to the transitional zone regions as well as the subcortical white matter [20–22]. These NVU remodeling changes could be an additional risk to the development of dysmyelination as we have observed in both the grey matter and transitional zones as described in this paper. The decreased CBF in the TZ and the subcortical white matter (SCWM) could be even more devastating due the possible decreased capillary density found in these regions in comparison to the grey matter [18] (Figure 12).

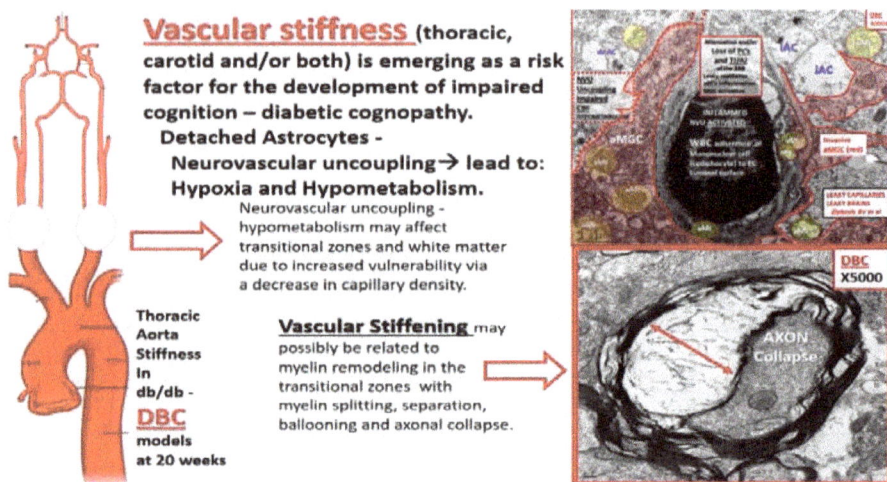

Figure 12. Montage of images demonstrating that vascular stiffness in the thoracic or carotid arteries may result in capillary neurovascular unit remodeling and the possible relationship to the development of dysmyelination in the diabetic DBC models. On the far left are depictions of the thoracic aorta, carotids, and brain circulatory system that are known to experience vascular stiffness in the diabetic DBC model [19]. The open arrow then points to the fact that there may be neurovascular uncoupling, which decreases the cerebral blood flow and could result in hypometabolism not only in the cortical grey matter but also in the vulnerable transitional zone. Cerebral flow pulsatility is augmented in type 2 diabetes mellitus (T2DM) [17] and this has been associated with markers of cerebral damage, such as white matter hyperintensities in T2DM. Thus, thoracic or carotid artery stiffness could result in dysmyelination and in turn the dysmyelination could slow the delivery of information—action potential without proper synchronicity and result in impaired cognition.

Importantly, diabetes is not only a risk factor for stroke, but also a risk factor for the development of white matter lesions [23]. Yotomi Y. et al. have demonstrated that the db/db diabetic model had greater severity of white matter damage that was associated with decreased proliferation and survival of oligodendrocyte progenitor cell [23].

4.2. Axon Initial Segment Shortening in db/db Diabetic DBC Models

Keiichiro Susuki's group has recently demonstrated that diabetic db/db brains (>10 weeks old) are known to abnormally remodel their neuronal axons, which result in axon initial segment (AIS) shortening [24]. While we were unable to demonstrate shortening of the axon initial segment via our ultrastructural observations, we wish to demonstrate the adjacent nanometer proximity of the astrocyte, microglia to the pyramidal neurons. The activation and detachment of the astrocyte and/or activation of microglia provides the potential for cellular crosstalk via ultrastructural astrocyte and microglia, which may be a contributing factor for remodeling change in DBC models (Figure 13). Because of the adjacent nanometer proximity between the glia (astrocytes and microglia) and neurons, we hypothesize that when microglia are activated as in our DBC model their aberrant leaky mitochondria could result in increased oxidative/nitrosative stress such that the AIS could be shortened secondary to excess reactive oxygen/reactive nitrogen species (ROS/RNS) derived from activated microglia, intracellular calcium accumulation, and AIS shortening [24]. Additionally, we observed abnormalities in myelin remodeling—dysmyelination, which could act in synergy with AIS shortening and could contribute to an increased loss of synchronicity of action potential to distant sites and result in dysfunctional signaling to receiving neurons and neuronal networks. These changes could increase the possibility of impaired cognition as noted in the diabetic db/db DBC models [24–27].

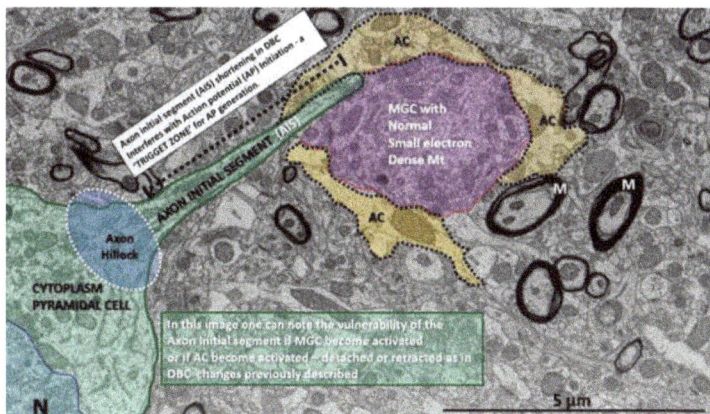

Figure 13. Pyramidal cell demonstrating the normal axon initial segment (AIS) in a control model. Note the cytoplasm of this pyramidal cell has an axon hillock region and also the axon initial segment region as the axon protrudes from the soma of the pyramidal cell. M: myelin; MGC: microglial cell; N: pyramidal nucleus; AP = action potential. Scale bar = 5 µm.

Interestingly, we observed ballooning of some axons with evidence of the neuroprotective astrocyte being detached from the axon and retracted, similar to the neurovascular unit astrocytes in Part I of this series (Figure 14) [5]. Astrocytes are important in protecting the pyramidal neuronal axons in layer III and throughout the cortical grey matter, transitional zones and subcortical white matter [28].

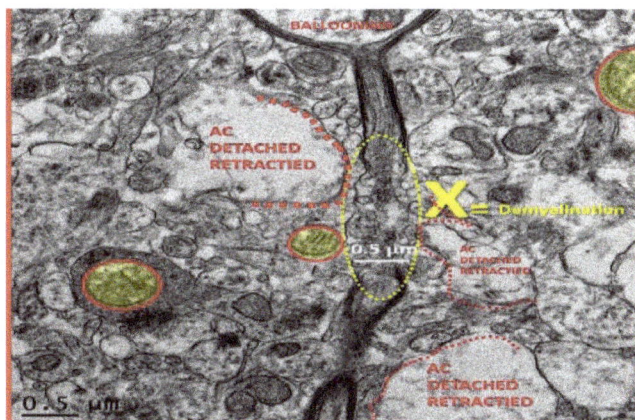

Figure 14. Detached and retracted astrocytes from a ballooning pyramidal neuronal axon in layer III of cortical grey matter. This is a higher magnification of previous image Figure 4 ×1500. In this image one can observe that there is a region marked with the letter X (yellow) where there is an area of myelin loss (demyelination) in a ballooned axon within layer III of the cortical grey matter. Importantly, note the detachment and retraction of astrocytes (AC) from the neuronal axon (defined in red lettering and by dashed lines). Also note the presence of at least three aberrant mitochondria in this region. Magnification ×4000; scale bar = 0.5 µm.

In summary, we have attempted to place this three-part series (Parts I, II, and III) regarding neurovascular unit and glia (astrocyte, microglia, and oligodendrocyte) remodeling changes in perspective to a more clinical setting as they pertain to type 2 diabetes mellitus in humans (Figure 15).

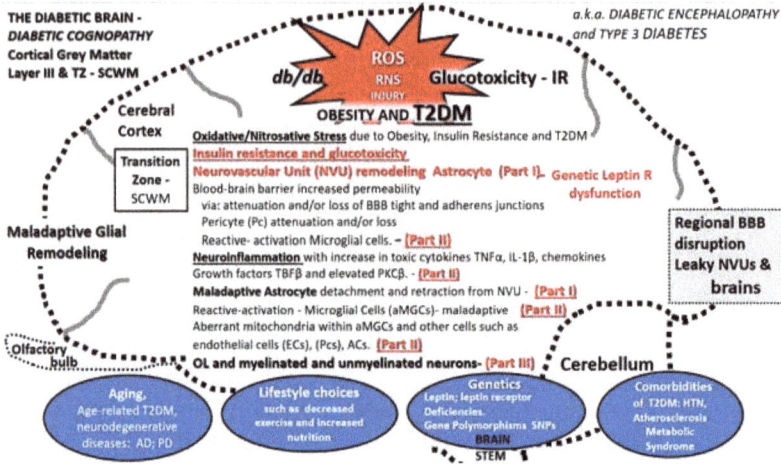

Figure 15. Multiple predisposing risk factors and metabolic and structural defects in DBC models. This figure depicts the multiple predisposing risk factors, metabolic and our ultrastructural remodeling that we have shared regarding the neurovascular unit and glia including the astrocyte (AC), microglia, and oligodendrocyte in this three-part series. The blue ovals at the bottom of the image depict the multiple situations that might give rise to the remodeling changes and how they are related to each of the three-part series as Part I, Part II, and Part III publications as follows: Aging, lifestyle, environment, genetics—particularly the leptin receptor deficiencies in the DBC and also the numerous single nucleotide polymorphisms (SNPs) in humans, and comorbidities associated with obesity (metabolic syndrome and accelerated atherosclerosis). a.k.a: also known as; AD: Alzheimer's disease; aMGC: activated microglia cell; BBB: blood-brain barrier; db/db: DBC; HTN: hypertension; IL-1β: interleukin 1 beta; IR: insulin resistance; NVU: neurovascular unit; OL: oligodendrocyte; PD: Parkinson's disease; PKCβ: protein kinase C beta; R: receptor; ROS/RNS: reactive oxygen/reactive nitrogen species; SCWM: subcortical white matter; T2DM: type 2 diabetes mellitus; TGFβ: transforming growth factor beta; TNFα: tumor necrosis factor alpha; TZ: transition zone.

5. Future Directions

Although we have not yet been able to study oligodendrocyte and myelin extensively with focused ion beam/scanning electron microscopy technology as we have previously done with the microglia in supplement videos in Part II of this series [29], we look forward to this possibility in due time such that we may be able to better understand their 3D stacks to create oligodendrocyte and myelin videos. Additionally, we hope to study oligodendrocytes and myelin remodeling specifically in the corpus callosum and/or optic nerves and how they relate to elongated white matter tracts. Indeed, these are exciting times to study the ultrastructural remodeling changes in the glia.

Author Contributions: M.R.H. and V.G.D. conceptualized the study; M.R.H. performed the image collection and interpretation; D.G.G. prepared the tissue specimens for transmission electron microscopic studies and assisted M.R.H.; M.R.H. prepared the manuscript; A.A. collected tissue specimens; V.G.D., A.A., and D.G.G. assisted in editing.

Funding: This study was supported by an internal grant entitled Excellence in Electron Microscopy grant and issued by the University of Missouri Electron Microscopy Core and Office of Research. No external funding was available.

Acknowledgments: Authors wish to thank Tommi White of the University of Missouri Electron Microscopy Core Facility. Authors also wish to thank our mentor James R. Sowers, who inspired us to interrogate, characterize, and understand the secrets that the tissues behold.

Conflicts of Interest: The authors declare no conflict of interest.

References

1. Michalski, J.P.; Kothary, R. Oligodendrocytes in a nutshell. *Front. Cell. Neurosci.* **2015**, *9*, 340. [CrossRef] [PubMed]
2. Peters, A.; Palay, S.L.; Webster, H. *The Fine Structure of the Nervous System—Neurons and Their Supportive Cells—The Cellular Sheaths of Neurons*, 3rd ed.; Oxford University Press: New York, NY, USA, 1991; pp. 212–261. ISBN 0-19-506571-9.
3. Pukos, N.; Yoseph, R.; McTigue, D.M. To Be or Not to Be: Environmental Factors that Drive Myelin Formation during Development and after CNS Trauma. *Neuroglia* **2018**, *1*, 63–90. [CrossRef]
4. Boullerne, A.I. The history of myelin. *Exp. Neurol.* **2016**, *283*, 431–445. [CrossRef] [PubMed]
5. Hayden, M.R.; Grant, D.; Aroor, A.; Demarco, V.G. Ultrastructural Remodeling of The Neurovascular Unit in The Female Diabetic db/db Model—Part I: Astrocyte. *Neuroglia* **2018**, *1*, 220–244. [CrossRef]
6. Montagne, A.; Nikolakopoulou, A.M.; Zhao, Z.; Sagare, A.P.; Si, G.; Lazic, D.; Barnes, S.R.; Daianu, M.; Ramanathan, A.; Go, A.; et al. Pericyte degeneration causes white matter dysfunction in the mouse central nervous system. *Nat. Med.* **2018**, *24*, 326–337. [CrossRef] [PubMed]
7. Reijmer, Y.D.; Brundel, M.; de Bresser, J.; Kappelle, L.J.; Leemans, A.; Biessels, G.J. Utrecht Vascular Cognitive Impairment Study Group. Microstructural white matter abnormalities and cognitive functioning in type 2 diabetes: A diffusion tensor imaging study. *Diabetes Care* **2013**, *36*, 137–144. [CrossRef] [PubMed]
8. Cavaglia, M.; Dombrowski, S.M.; Drazba, J.; Vasanji, A.; Bokesch, P.M.; Janigro, D. Regional variation in brain capillary density and vascular response to ischemia. *Br. Res.* **2001**, *910*, 81–93. [CrossRef]
9. Walhovd, K.B.; Johansen-Berg, H.; Káradóttir, R.T. Unraveling the secrets of white matter—Bridging the gap between cellular, animal and human imaging studies. *Neuroscience* **2014**, *276*, 2–13. [CrossRef] [PubMed]
10. Snaidero, N.; Möbius, W.; Czopka, T.; Hekking, L.H.; Mathisen, C.; Verkleij, D.; Goebbels, S.; Edgar, J.; Merkler, D.; Lyons, D.A.; et al. Myelin membrane wrapping of CNS axons by PI(3,4,5)P3-dependent polarized growth at the inner tongue. *Cell* **2014**, *156*, 277–290. [CrossRef] [PubMed]
11. Platt, T.L.; Beckett, T.L.; Kohler, K.; Niedowicz, D.M.; Murphy, M.P. Obesity, diabetes, and leptin resistance promote tau pathology in a mouse model of disease. *Neuroscience* **2016**, *315*, 162–174. [CrossRef] [PubMed]
12. Hernández-Fonseca, J.P.; Rincón, J.; Pedreañez, A.; Viera, N.; Arcaya, J.L.; Carrizo, E.; Mosquera, J. Structural and ultrastructural analysis of cerebral cortex, cerebellum, and hypothalamus from diabetic rats. *Exp. Diabetes Res.* **2009**, *2009*, 329632. [CrossRef] [PubMed]
13. Peters, A.; Moss, M.B.; Sethares, C. Effects of aging on myelinated nerve fibers in monkey primary visual cortex. *J. Comp. Neurol.* **2000**, *419*, 364–376. [CrossRef]
14. Wrighten, S.A.; Piroli, G.G.; Grillo, C.A.; Reagan, L.P. A look inside the diabetic brain: Contributors to diabetes-induced brain aging. *Biochim. Biophys. Acta* **2009**, *1792*, 444–453. [CrossRef] [PubMed]
15. Bowley, M.P.; Cabral, H.; Rosene, D.L.; Peters, A. Age changes in myelinated nerve fibers of the cingulate bundle and *corpus callosum* in the rhesus monkey. *J. Comp. Neurol.* **2010**, *518*, 3046–3064. [CrossRef] [PubMed]
16. Sosa, S.M.; Smith, K.J. Understanding a role for hypoxia in lesion formation and location in the deep and periventricular white matter in small vessel disease and multiple sclerosis. *Clin. Sci.* **2017**, *131*, 2503–2524. [CrossRef] [PubMed]
17. Nonaka, H.; Akima, M.; Hatori, T.; Nagayama, T.; Zhang, Z.; Ihara, F. Microvasculature of the human cerebral white matter: Arteries of the deep white matter. *Neuropathology* **2003**, *23*, 111–118. [CrossRef] [PubMed]
18. Brownell, B.; Hughes, J.T. The distribution of plaques in the cerebrum in multiple sclerosis. *J. Neurol. Neurosurg. Psychiatr.* **1962**, *25*, 315–320. [CrossRef]
19. Aroor, A.R.; Das, N.A.; Carpenter, A.J.; Habibi, J.; Jia, G.; Ramirez-Perez, F.I.; Martinez-Lemus, L.; Manrique-Acevedo, C.M.; Hayden, M.R.; Duta, C.; et al. Glycemic control by the SGLT2 inhibitor empagliflozin decreases aortic stiffness, renal resistivity index and kidney injury. *Cardiovasc. Diabet.* **2018**, *17*, 108. [CrossRef] [PubMed]

20. Cooper, L.L.; Mitchell, G.F. Aortic Stiffness, Cerebrovascular Dysfunction, and Memory. *Pulse* **2016**, *4*, 69–77. [CrossRef] [PubMed]
21. Heffernan, K.S. Carotid artery stiffness and cognitive function in adults with and without type 2 diabetes: Extracranial contribution to an intracranial problem? *Atherosclerosis* **2016**, *253*, 268–269. [CrossRef] [PubMed]
22. Lee, K.O.; Lee, K.Y.; Lee, S.Y.; Ahn, C.W.; Park, J.S. Lacunar infarction in type 2 diabetes is associated with an elevated intracranial arterial pulsatility index. *Yonsei Med. J.* **2007**, *48*, 802–806. [CrossRef] [PubMed]
23. Yatomi, Y.; Tanaka, R.; Shimada, Y.; Yamashiro, K.; Liu, M.; Mitome-Mishima, Y.; Miyamoto, N.; Ueno, Y.; Urabe, T.; Hattori, N. Type 2 diabetes reduces the proliferation and survival of oligodendrocyte progenitor cells in ischemia white matter lesions. *Neuroscience* **2015**, *289*, 214–223. [CrossRef] [PubMed]
24. Yermakov, L.M.; Drouet, D.E.; Griggs, R.B.; Khalid, M.; Elased, K.M.; Susuki, K. Type 2 Diabetes Leads to Axon Initial Segment Shortening in db/db Mice. *Front. Cell. Neurosci.* **2018**, *12*, 146. [CrossRef] [PubMed]
25. Benusa, S.D.; George, N.M.; Sword, B.A.; DeVries, G.H.; Dupree, J.L. Acute neuroinflammation induces AIS structural plasticity in a *NOX2*-dependent manner. *J. Neuroinflamm.* **2017**, *14*, 116. [CrossRef] [PubMed]
26. Rasband, M.N. The axon initial segment and the maintenance of neuronal polarity. *Nat. Rev. Neurosci.* **2010**, *11*, 552–562. [CrossRef] [PubMed]
27. Bender, K.J.; Trussell, L.O. The physiology of the axon initial segment. *Annu. Rev. Neurosci.* **2012**, *35*, 249–265. [CrossRef] [PubMed]
28. Bélanger, M.; Magistretti, P.J. The role of astroglia in neuroprotection. *Dialog. Clin. Neurosci.* **2009**, *11*, 281–295.
29. Hayden, M.R.; Grant, D.; Aroor, A.; Demarco, V.G. Ultrastructural Remodeling of The Neurovascular Unit in The Female Diabetic db/db Model—Part II: Microglia and Mitochondria. *Neuroglia* **2018**, *1*, 311–326. [CrossRef]

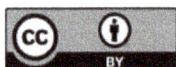

![neuroglia logo] *neuroglia*

MDPI

Article

Putative Receptors Underpinning L-Lactate Signalling in Locus Coeruleus

Valentina Mosienko [1,2], Seyed Rasooli-Nejad [1,3], Kasumi Kishi [1,4], Matt De Both [5], David Jane [1], Matt J. Huentelman [5], Sergey Kasparov [1] and Anja G. Teschemacher [1,*]

[1] Pharmacology and Neuroscience, School of Physiology, University of Bristol, Bristol BS8 1TD, UK; v.mosienko@exeter.ac.uk (V.M.); seyed.rasooli-nejad@charite.de (S.R.-N.); kasumikishi@gmail.com (K.K.); david.jane@bristol.ac.uk (D.J.); Sergey.Kasparov@bristol.ac.uk (S.K.)
[2] Institute of Biomedical and Clinical Sciences, University of Exeter Medical School, Exeter EX4 4PS, UK
[3] Neuroscience Research Centre, Medical University Berlin—Charité, D-10115 Berlin, Germany
[4] Institute of Science and Technology IST Austria, 3400 Klosterneuburg, Austria
[5] Center for Rare Childhood Disorders, Translational Genomics Research Institute, Phoenix, AZ 85004, USA; mdeboth@tgen.org (M.D.B.); mhuentelman@tgen.org (M.J.H.)
[*] Correspondence: Anja.Teschemacher@bristol.ac.uk

Received: 14 October 2018; Accepted: 7 November 2018; Published: 16 November 2018

Abstract: The importance of astrocytic L-lactate (LL) for normal functioning of neural circuits such as those regulating learning/memory, sleep/wake state, autonomic homeostasis, or emotional behaviour is being increasingly recognised. L-Lactate can act on neurones as a metabolic or redox substrate, but transmembrane receptor targets are also emerging. A comparative review of the hydroxy-carboxylic acid receptor (HCA1, formerly known as GPR81), Olfactory Receptor Family 51 Subfamily E Member 2 (OR51E2), and orphan receptor GPR4 highlights differences in their LL sensitivity, pharmacology, intracellular coupling, and localisation in the brain. In addition, a putative Gs-coupled receptor on noradrenergic neurones, LLRx, which we previously postulated, remains to be identified. Next-generation sequencing revealed several orphan receptors expressed in locus coeruleus neurones. Screening of a selection of these suggests additional LL-sensitive receptors: GPR180 which inhibits and GPR137 which activates intracellular cyclic AMP signalling in response to LL in a heterologous expression system. To further characterise binding of LL at LLRx, we carried out a structure–activity relationship study which demonstrates that carboxyl and 2-hydroxyl moieties of LL are essential for triggering D-lactate-sensitive noradrenaline release in locus coeruleus, and that the size of the LL binding pocket is limited towards the methyl group position. The evidence accumulating to date suggests that LL acts via multiple receptor targets to modulate distinct brain functions.

Keywords: L-lactate; hydroxy-carboxylic acid receptor; OR51E2; GPR4; GPR137; cAMP; locus coeruleus; noradrenaline; next generation sequencing; structure–activity relationship

1. Introduction

Astrocytes, the electrically nonexcitable "cousins" of neurones, are strategically placed at the interface between the periphery and neuronal networks of the central nervous system. Among other functions, they handle the import and distribution of glucose, the main energy substrate used by the brain, as well as its storage in the form of glycogen [1]. Glycolytic breakdown of glucose to pyruvate, and its subsequent conversion to L-lactate (LL), yields two units of ATP for intracellular energy transfer or, alternatively, for use as a transmitter. If glycolysis is followed by oxidative phosphorylation, nearly 20 times as much ATP can be produced. This, however, does not mean that almost all ATP in the cell is delivered by mitochondria. In fact, since glycolysis is very fast compared to the mitochondrial oxidation of pyruvate, the contribution of glycolysis to the pool of ATP may be comparable to that originating from oxidative phosphorylation [2], especially during peaks of high metabolic demand. In spite of the obvious discrepancy in energy efficiency, the brain produces large amounts of LL, much of which, surprisingly, is drained into the peripheral circulation [3]. The energetic or functional advantages of this metabolic imbalance are still controversial.

Average physiological extracellular levels of LL reported for the brain are in the sub- to low mM range, but they respond dynamically to plasma LL concentrations, central availability of oxygen, neuronal network activity, or metabolic triggers and can approach ~10 mM under extreme conditions such as seizure or hypoxia [4,5]. In principle, the ability to glycolytically process glucose to LL is shared by astrocytes and neurones, but astrocytes are held to be the main source of LL in the brain, at least under physiological resting conditions where there is a steeper intra-to-extracellular LL gradient in astrocytes as compared to neurones [6]. Astrocytes are known to tolerate hypoxic conditions better than neurones and may more easily upregulate glycolytic activity to bridge periods of oxygen demand exceeding supply [7]. Indeed, they have been shown to switch to aerobic glycolysis while sparing the limited oxygen for neuronal oxidative phosphorylation [8]. According to the astrocyte-to-neuron-lactate-shuttle (ANLS) hypothesis, the astrocyte-derived LL may benefit neurones as an additional energy substrate to sustain periods of elevated activity [6,9,10].

Whether as a valuable energy substrate or a glycolytic waste product, LL has been reported to modulate brain activity and behaviour in various functional contexts [5]. LL was shown to be essential in certain learning and memory paradigms ([11,12]; reviewed in [13]). It is also important for regulating sleep/wake states at the level of the lateral hypothalamic area, as well as negatively correlating with sleep-associated slow wave activity in the cortex [14–16]. Moreover, recent evidence suggests that it acts as an antidepressant in an animal model of depression [17]. Since central cyclic AMP (cAMP) signalling was found to be reduced in depressed patients, this could potentially be explained by the ability of LL to increase cAMP responses in astrocytes and some neuronal phenotypes [18–20].

We have previously reported a mechanism that is consistent with, and may contribute to, LL's overall role as a central activator and regulator of brain state. We found that optogenetically induced release of LL from astrocytes into the extracellular space triggers noradrenaline (NA) release from adjacent noradrenergic neurones [20]. When microinjected into the locus coeruleus (LC) area, LL desynchronised the electroencephalogram activity in the cerebral cortex, indicating that the noradrenergic network was excited [20].

It is becoming increasingly clear that LL utilises a wide variety of signaling mechanisms to influence physiological outputs. These include not only multiple intracellular targets but also effects on putative receptors located on the plasma membrane of the cells.

1.1. Targets and Mechanisms of L-Lactate Signalling in the Brain

Upon import into neurones, LL can be reduced to pyruvate, raising the NADH/NAD+ ratio and switching on NMDA receptor-dependent immediate early gene expression ([21]; Figure 1). This pathway has been suggested to underlie some of the effects of ANLS, for example, memory formation [13]. A distinct pathway that may allow LL to exert long-term effects is via binding to and stabilizing the protein NDRG3 which, in turn, activates kinase activity in favour of Raf-Extracellular signal-regulated kinase signalling to support the tissue response to prolonged hypoxia [22].

In terms of reversible short-term metabolic signalling by LL, ATP-sensitive potassium channels have been suggested as an intracellular target. Analogous to the scenario in pancreatic beta cells, inhibition of these channels by LL-derived ATP increased excitation of orexin neurones in the hypothalamus during arousal [14,23].

In some instances, however, the effects of LL are not consistent with an intracellular action but can only be explained by activation of membrane-associated receptors from the extracellular side. The first specific LL receptor to be characterised was the G-protein coupled receptor (GPR) GPR81, currently known as hydroxy-carboxylic acid receptor 1 (HCA1). Over recent years, further LL membrane receptor candidates have been identified, and the list is likely to lengthen (Figure 1).

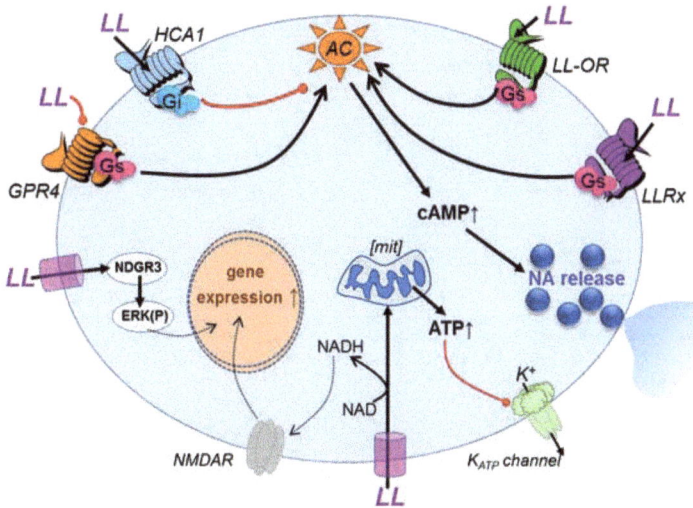

Figure 1. Summary of potential L-lactate (LL)-mediated signalling actions in neurones. L-lactate which is transported into the cell can be metabolised and/or influence gene expression, e.g., via NMDA receptor modulation or ERK pathway activation. Increased ATP production can inhibit K_{ATP} channel activity and increase cell excitability. LL may also act via a range of surface G-protein coupled receptors to stimulate or inhibit cAMP-dependent signalling, such as NA release in noradrenergic neurones. Black arrows indicate stimulatory action, red lines illustrate inhibitory effect. AC—adenylate cyclase; ERK(P)—phosphorylation of extracellular signal–regulated kinases; GPR4—orphan G-protein-coupled receptor 4; HCA1—hydroxy-carboxylic acid receptor; LL-OR—LL-activated olfactory receptor; LLRx—LL receptor on noradrenergic neurones; [mit]—mitochondria; NA—noradrenaline; NMDAR—NMDA receptor.

1.2. Hydroxy-carboxylic acid receptor (HCA1)

HCA1 was the first G-protein-coupled receptor (GPCR) to be described that is activated selectively by LL and a few related monocarboxylates (Table 1). In adipocytes where HCA1 was discovered, this leads to inhibition of lipolysis under conditions of glucose abundance in the fed state [24,25]. It has been reported that HCA1 is also expressed at low levels in the brain, predominantly in neurones, in cerebellum, hippocampus, and neocortex [26]. We carried out RNA sequencing on samples of neurones dissociated from the LC of rats and were unable to confirm its expression in these cells (Table 2). HCA1 is a G_i-protein-coupled receptor and its activation inhibits cAMP production (IC_{50} in vitro according to various sources is between 5–30 mM; [25–27]. The stereoisomer of LL, D-lactate (DL), also a weak agonist at HCA1 (Table 1; [25]).

In spite of its low potency, site-directed mutagenesis and molecular modelling predicts that LL binds specifically as a typical GPCR ligand rather than an allosteric modulator [25]. Being a G_i-coupled receptor, HCA1 should evoke inhibitory effects (hyperpolarisation of the membrane and inhibition of transmitter release), which is opposite to what we found in noradrenergic neurones ([20]; Figure 1). In cultured embryonic cortical neurones, LL inhibited Ca^{2+} signalling in a pertussin toxin-sensitive manner with a half-maximal inhibitory concentration (IC_{50}) of ~5 mM [28]. Since this effect was mimicked by the HCA1 agonist 3,5-dihydroxybenzoic acid (3,5-DHBA), it was indeed consistent with signalling via HCA1.

Table 1. Characteristics of the known L-lactate receptors.

Receptor	LL Potency (Range)	Intracellular Signalling	Other Agonists	Antagonists	References
HCA1	5–30 mM	Gi, cAMP↓	3,5-DHBA; α-HBA; glycolate; γ-HBA	nd	[25,26]
OR51E2	~4 mM	Gs, cAMP↑	Acetate; propionate	nd	[29]
GPR4	1–10 mM	allosteric modulation?	H+	NE 52-QQ57	[30]
LLRx	0.5 mM	Gs, cAMP↑	MPA; aHIBA; HMBA; 2HPA; KA (see Figure 2)	D-lactate	[20]

3,5-DHBA (3,5-dihydroxybenzoic acid), α-HBA (α-hydroxybutyrate), γ-HBA (γ-hydroxybutyrate); aHIBA (α-hydroxyisobutyric acid), HMBA (2-hydroxy-3-methyl-butyric acid), 2HPA ((S)-2-hydroxypentanoic acid, MPA ((S)-(−)-2-methoxy-propionic acid), nd—not determined, LL—L-lactate. LLRx—putative LL receptor on noradrenergic neurones, GPR4—orphan G-protein-coupled receptor 4; OR51E2—LL-sensitive olfactory receptor; HCA1—Hydroxy-carboxylic acid receptor; Gi—Gᵢ-protein activation; Gs—Gₛ-protein activation; KA—kynurenic acid.

Table 2. Expression of known L-lactate receptors in locus coeruleus neurones and astrocytes as determined by RNA sequencing.

Gene Product of Interest	LC (p29)	LC (p7)	LC Neurones	Astrocytes
DbH	43.3	527.7	3556.2	2.5
α₂A-AR	116.8	307.0	268.4	115.9
HCA1	0.0	0.0	0.0	0.0
OR51E2	7.6	21.3	0.0	0.0
GPR4	70.5	26.0	34.6	24.5

Dopamine-β-hydroxylase (DbH), shown for reference as a marker of noradrenergic neurones, is highly expressed in locus coeruleus (LC) tissue from 29- and 7-day-old rats, and in dissociated noradrenergic neurones (area A6) from organotypic brain cultures. Values for a canonical GPCR, α2A-adrenoceptor (α2A-AR), provide a reference for the expression levels of this class of proteins. In comparison, known L-lactate receptors are found at low to negligible levels and not specifically on LC neurones. Numbers represent average FKPM (fragments per kilobase of exon per million fragments mapped) from duplicates. GPR4—orphan G-protein-coupled receptor 4; OR51E2—LL-sensitive olfactory receptor; HCA1—Hydroxy-carboxylic acid receptor.

1.3. Olfactory L-Lactate Receptors

More recently, *OR51E2*, a further LL-activated GPCR, has been reported in the mouse. *OR51E2* belongs to the family of olfactory receptors which invariably couple to a specific subset of G_s-proteins, thereby increasing cAMP levels (Figure 1). The EC_{50} for cAMP elevation in vitro by LL was determined as 4 mM (Table 1; [29]). As expected, the *OR51E2* receptor is found in the rodent olfactory bulb but it is also ectopically expressed in brain and periphery, for example, in glomus cells in the carotid body where its role in activation of carotid sinus nerve activity by LL is currently debated [29,31,32]. Olfactory receptors that are LL-sensitive may be involved in the maladaptive increase in sympathetic drive associated with the progression of chronic heart failure, in a vicious circle that leads to further deterioration of ischemic conditions and lactate acidosis [33,34].

Ectopic localisation of this olfactory receptor also extends to autonomic ganglia and to the brain, predominantly brainstem areas [35,36]. Since we previously showed that G_s-coupling was involved in LL-mediated stimulation of noradrenergic transmission [20], we checked our transcriptomic data and found *OR51E2* expression in LC tissue, but were unable to confirm its expression in isolated LC neurones (Table 2). We suggest that, since expression levels are low and the receptor appears to be not specifically localised to noradrenergic neurones, it is unlikely to account for the central effects of LL we had described earlier.

Nevertheless, in a study to follow up olfactory perception of LL, we discovered that not only mice but also humans can detect the odour of LL. However, *OR51E2* knockout mice were still able to smell it [37]. This points to the existence of one or more additional LL-sensitive olfactory receptors which, if also expressed in the brain, would be expected to contribute to cAMP-mediated LL signalling. At the same time, olfactory receptors are notorious for their broad spectrum of activating ligands and are expected to act cooperatively to identify specific odorants.

1.4. Orphan G-protein-coupled receptor 4 (GPR4)

Since LL is one of the main extracellular organic acids, we investigated whether a proton-sensitive G_s-protein-coupled receptor, GPR4, may mediate or be modulated by LL ([38]; Figure 1, Table 1). Our evidence suggested that GPR4 contributes to the compensatory ventilatory response to increased CO_2 levels in hypercapnic conditions. However, we found that, under physiological blood and brain LL concentrations, GPR4 is partially inhibited by LL and its sensitivity to protons is reduced [30].

GPR4 is prominently expressed in the endothelium of blood vessels, in periphery as well as brain [30]. Localisation in certain neuronal phenotypes such as in retrotrapezoid and raphe nuclei, rostral ventrolateral medulla, septum, and LC in the mature rodent brain has also been demonstrated [30,39]. We detected a low level of expression in the LC (Table 2). However, since LL appears as a negative, presumably allosteric, modulator of GPR4-mediated cAMP production, it cannot be responsible for the effects of LL we observed on noradrenergic neurones [20]. Considering the comparatively minor impact of GPR4 on cardiorespiratory regulation and its wide distribution in the brain, including the raphe nuclei and related areas, it may be modulating processes mediated by these areas, an issue which remains to be investigated [30]. In setting the cAMP tone and levels of neuronal excitability it might, for instance, be involved in regulation of anxiety and depression.

1.5. The L-Lactate Receptor Responsible for Central noradrenaline Release

The receptor that mediates the effect of LL-induced NA release (LLRx) in the brain has not been identified to date. Our previous findings defined several properties for LLRx-mediated NA release ([20]; Figure 1): LL activates LLRx from the extracellular side and does not require entry into the cell. LL has a higher potency, by ~10-fold or more, at LLRx as compared to other so far identified LL receptors and is activated around the physiologically relevant LL concentrations in the healthy brain (0.2–0.5 mM). This makes it suitable for picking up physiologically relevant dynamic changes. The activation of LLRx by LL is inhibited in the extracellular presence of its stereoisomer DL. LLRx is most likely a G_s-coupled receptor as the effect of its activation depended on adenylate cyclase [20].

Since none of the receptors discussed above fits these requirements, our hypothesis is that LL activates one of the orphan G-protein-coupled receptors present in the brain and expressed by noradrenergic neurones. In the current study, we tested an array of LL derivatives for their ability to mimic the LL effect on NA release in order to further characterise the structural requirements for agonists of LLRx. In addition to the primary aim of these experiments, i.e., to establish a structure–activity relationship (SAR) between the LL molecule and LLRx to aid molecular modelling, a second objective was to lay the basis for antagonist and superagonist development. In addition, we carried out next-generation sequencing of neurones in the LC and identified orphan GPCRs which are expressed. We tested a selection of these in heterologous expression systems for their ability to activate G_s-proteins in response to LL stimulation.

2. Materials and Methods

2.1. Chemicals

Analogues of LL in which carboxyl-, hydroxyl-, or methyl groups were modified were obtained from commercial sources: 2-hydroxy-2-propan-sulfonic acid from Alfa Aesar (Heysham, UK); (±)-3-hydroxy-2-methylbutyric acid, 1-hydroxycyclo-propane-carboxylic acid, and (S)-tetrahydro-furoic acid from Acros Organics (Thermo Fisher Scientific, Waltham, MA, USA); and kynurenic acid from Abcam (Cambridge, UK). All other analogues and reagents were obtained from Sigma-Aldrich (Merck, Darmstadt, Germany), unless stated otherwise. L-Lactate and analogues, acetate, and pyruvate were diluted in ddH$_2$O, adjusted to pH 7.4, and used at a final concentration of 2 mM unless otherwise specified. To evaluate blocking by DL, DL was co-applied with LL or LL analogues at a final concentration of 200 µM.

2.2. Organotypic Brain Slice Preparation

All animal procedures were performed in accordance with the UK Animals (Scientific Procedures) Act, 1986, and covered by, PPL 30/3121.

Brainstem slice cultures were prepared as described previously [20]. In brief, 6–7-day-old Wistar rat pups were terminally anaesthetised and decapitated, and the brainstem was immediately removed. Slices of 200 µm thickness were cut at the level of the LC in ice-cold sterile dissection medium (in mM: kynurenic acid 1; Hepes 1; glucose 20; MgCl$_2$ 10) using a vibrating microtome (7000 smz, Campden Instruments, Loughborough, UK). Slices were plated onto cell culture inserts (Millicell PICMORG50, Millipore, Watford, UK) and supplied with 1 mL per well feeding medium (Opti-MEM; 51985-026, Thermo Fisher Scientific, Loughborough, UK) supplemented with 25% fetal bovine serum, 25 mM glucose, and 1% penicillin (10,000 units)/streptavidin (10 mL/L)). To visualise noradrenergic neurones in the LC, we added ~10^9 TU/mL of the adenoviral vector (AVV) AVV-PRSx8-EGFP, which results in green fluorescent protein (EGFP) expression under PRSx8 promoter control [40]. To enable visualisation of astrocytes, an AVV with transcriptionally enhanced glial fibrillary acidic protein (GFAP) promoter was used to express EGFP (AVV-sGFAP-EGFP; [41]). Slices were kept at 37 °C and in 5% CO$_2$ for 7–12 days prior to experiments to allow for AVV-mediated protein expression.

2.3. Fluorescence-Activated Cell Sorting and RNA Sequencing of Locus Coeruleus Neurones and Astrocytes

Organotypic brain slices including LC were transduced with AVV-PRSx8-EGFP or AVV-sGFAP-EGFP. The LC area was dissected, and cells were dissociated as described previously [42], with modifications. The tissue was first digested at 37 °C for 10 min in 5 ml of Hank's Balanced Salt solution (HBS) in mM: 136 NaCl, 5.3 KCl, 4.1 NaHCO$_3$, 1.6 CaCl$_2$, 0.8 MgSO$_4$, 0.44 KH$_2$PO$_4$, 0.13 Na$_2$HPO$_4$, 10 HEPES, 5.5 D-glucose) containing 30 U of papain (Sigma-Aldrich / Merck, Darmstadt, Germany) under orbital shaking, before washing off the papain and triturating with a fire-polished Pasteur pipette. Cells were gently pelleted (3 min, 900 rpm), resuspended in HBS, and filtered through a 50 µm mesh. EGFP-positive cells were sorted using 488 nm laser excitation and 510–550 nm emission in a Becton Dickinson InFlux cell sorter (BD Biosciences, Franklin Lakes, NJ, USA) running BD Software version 1.2. Viable cells were identified based on light scatter and the exclusion of propidium iodide. In addition, single-cell gating was used to exclude doublets and aggregated cells. Following fluorescence-activated cell sorting (FACS), more than 100 cells were collected into 100 µL of 2% Triton in phosphate-buffered saline containing 1 µL RNAseOUT (Invitrogen, Thermo Fisher Scientific, Loughborough, UK), and stored at −80 °C until processed further.

Sequencing libraries for next-generation sequencing (NGS) were prepared with 250 ng of total RNA using Illumina's Truseq RNA Sample Preparation Kit v2 (Illumina, Inc., San Diego, CA, USA) following the manufacturer's protocol. Final PCR-enriched fragments were validated on a 2200 TapeStation (Agilent Technologies, Santa Clara, CA, USA) and quantitated via qPCR using Kapa's Library Quantification Kit (Kapa Biosystems, Wilmington, MA, USA) on the QuantStudio 6 Flex Instrument (Thermo Fisher, Waltham, MA, USA). The final library was sequenced by 50 bp paired-end sequencing on a HiSeq 2500 (Illumina). Illumina BCL files were converted and demultiplexed (bcl2fastq 2.17). FASTQ files were trimmed of adapter sequences (CutAdapt 1.8.3) and aligned to rn5 (STAR 2.5). Aligned reads were summarised as gene-level counts (featureCounts 1.4.4) and as transcripts per million (Kallisto 0.43.0). Sequencing and quality control reports were generated (FastQC 0.11.4 and

Qualimap 2.1.3). Pairwise differential expression analysis was conducted with the R package DESeq2 (1.10.1)

2.4. Measurement of Noradrenaline Release

In our earlier study, we used fast scan cyclic voltammetry to detect NA release in organotypic slices of the LC in response to LL stimulation. Here, in order to expand selection of LL analogues tested and to increase throughput, we implemented an approach based on cell-based neurotransmitter fluorescent engineered reporter cells (CNiFERs; Supplementary Materials Figure S1) [43]. CNiFERs are derived from a HEK293 cell line that stably expresses the Ca^{2+} indicator TN-XXL and a human $\alpha 1$ adrenoreceptor. Binding of NA to the adrenoceptor activates G_q-protein signalling, leading to an increase in cytosolic Ca^{2+} through the phospholipase C-inositol triphosphate pathway which is imaged through the FRET ratio of TN-XXL (Supplementary Materials Figure S1A,B). CNiFERs showed nanomolar sensitivity to NA (EC_{50} = 31 $\pm$ 1.75 nM).

To monitor NA release from organotypic brain slices, 4×10^5 CNiFERs were plated 24 h prior to experiments on a cell culture insert (Supplementary Materials Figure S1C). Imaging experiments were performed at 34 °C under continuous perfusion (150 mL/h) with HEPES-buffered solution (HBS, pH 7.4; in mM: NaCl 138; KCl 5.5; Na_2HPO_4 0.25; KH_2PO_4 0.5; $CaCl_2$ 1.67; $MgSO_4$ 0.8; $NaHCO_3$ 4.25; HEPES 10; Glucose 5.5) in a tissue chamber mounted on a Leica SP5 confocal microscope. Images were collected in a time-lapse mode (0.25 Hz) with excitation at 458 nm and dual emission set to 462–501 nm (Citrine) and 519–595 nm (ECFP). Fluorescence intensities of Citrine and ECFP channels were exported and analysed offline in Excel (Microsoft, Redmond, WA, USA). The FRET ratio (ECFP/Citrine) was calculated, plotted against time, and the area under the curve (AUC) following LL/analogue stimulation was determined as FRET ratio x s. CNiFER responses were calibrated against 100 nM NA to allow evaluation of total NA release in nM x s.

2.5. Patch Clamp of Noradrenergic Neurones

Cultured slices containing the LC and transduced with an AVV-PRSx8-eGFP were transferred to a recording chamber mounted on an upright SP-2 confocal microscope (Leica, Wetzlar, Germany) and continuously superfused with HEPES-buffered solution (in mM: NaCl 137, KCl 5.4, Na_2HPO_4 0.25, KH_2PO_4 0.44, $CaCl_2$ 1.3, $MgSO_4$ 1.0, $NaHCO_3$ 4.2, HEPES 10, Glucose 5.5; pH 7.4) at 34 $\pm$ 1 °C. Current-clamp whole-cell recordings were sampled at 10 kHz using an AxoClamp 2B amplifier (Molecular Devices, San Jose, CA, USA) and a 1401 interface with Spike 2 software (CED, Cambridge, UK). Recording pipettes were pulled with a vertical puller (Narishige PC-10) to 3–5 MΩ resistance and filled with pipette solution (in mM: potassium gluconate 130, HEPES 10, EGTA 5.5, NaCl 4, $MgCl_2$ 2, $CaCl_2$ 1, ATP 2, GTP 1, and glucose 5). After recording 5–10 min of stable baseline in current clamp, LL or its analogues were superfused with the chamber solution for 5–10 min.

2.6. GloSensor Assay of Intracellular cAMP Accumulation

Clones of a selection of human orphan GPCR open reading frames were commercially obtained: GPR61 and GPR176 from cDNA Resource Center (www.cdna.org); GPR81, GPR137, GPR137B, GPR158, GPR180 from SourceBioScience (www.sourcebioscience.com); GPR155 from Origene (www.origene.com); rodent GPR162 was synthesised by Eurofins Scientific (www.eurofins.co.uk). The open reading frames of the receptors were cloned into the expression plasmid pEGFP-N1 under control of the human cytomegalovirus promoter, upstream of a human internal ribosomal entry site, followed by the enhanced green fluorescent protein sequence.

The GloSensor assay was used for cAMP measurements as previously described, with modifications [42]. HEK293 cells were plated in 96-well white polystyrene plates (Greiner Bio-One, Kremsmünster, Austria) in DMEM media (Gibco, Thermo Fisher Scientific, Loughborough, UK) supplemented with 10% fetal bovine serum and 1% penicillin (10,000 units)/streptavidin (10 mL/L)), at a density of 4×10^5 cells/mL to achieve ~70% confluence for transfection. After 20 h, cells were transiently co-transfected with the GloSensor cAMP plasmid GLO22F and a plasmid encoding the GPCR of interest using Trans-IT 293 (Mirus) according to the manufacturer's protocol. Transfection efficiency was confirmed by fluorescent visualisation of EGFP. Twenty-six hours after the transfection, cells were incubated with 850 µM beetle luciferin potassium salt (Promega, Southampton, UK) at pH 7.4 for 2 h in the dark. Prior to adding drugs, media was changed to HBS (Gibco) buffered with 20 mM HEPES and titrated to the desired pH. Cells were incubated with LL for 20 min in a final well volume of 100 µL. Luminescence measurements of cAMP accumulation were obtained using an Infinite M200 PRO microplate reader (Tecan, Männedorf, Switzerland).

2.7. Statistical Analysis

Data are expressed as mean ± standard error of the mean (SEM). Groups were compared using Student's *t*-test or one-way ANOVA as indicated. GraphPad Prism (version 7; La Jolla, CA, USA) was used for data processing and to calculate EC_{50}.

3. Results

3.1. L-*Lactate Releases Noradrenaline from Locus Coeruleus Neurones*

To detect LL-induced release of NA we used a cell-based reporter system developed in D. Kleinfeld's laboratory [43]. These "α1 CNiFER" cells respond with a robust Ca^{2+} increase to NA which is registered through a ratiometric Ca^{2+} indicator which they express. Consistent with our previous observations using fast-scan cyclic voltammetry, a transient change in α1 CNiFER cell signals confirmed that LL (2 mM) evokes NA release from LC neurones in organotypic slices. As we previously reported, this effect was blocked by DL (200 µM) and was independent of the caloric value of LL since neither pyruvate nor acetate (2 mM) triggered NA release [20] (Supplementary Materials Figure S1D).

3.2. Structural Requirements for the Agonistic Action of L-Lactate on Noradrenaline Release

In order to characterise the structural features required for LL binding to LLRx, we chose commercially available LL analogues in which the carboxyl, hydroxyl, or methyl groups were modified (Figure 2A–D). In addition, the effect of chain extension by increasing the distance between the OH and the carboxylate group of LL (e.g., **4**, Figure 2C) or replacing the methyl group of LL with longer alkyl (**9**, **10**) or aralkyl chains (**13–15**, Figure 2D) was studied. Conformational restriction by carbocyclic (**5**) or heterocyclic ring (**7**, **11**) formation was also investigated (Figure 2C,D). Each analogue was tested at 2 mM for its ability to evoke NA release, and the response was normalised to the effect of equimolar LL tested in the same slice (Figure 2E).

L-lactate analogues with modified carboxyl (**1**), hydroxyl (**3**), and methyl groups (**8–10** and **15**) and the heterocyclic analogues (**7** and **11**) stimulated NA release; however, none of these were significantly more efficacious than LL (Figure 2E). All other test compounds (**2**, **4–6**, **12–14**) evoked significantly smaller responses, leading to less than 50% of the NA release triggered by LL application (Figure 2E). We then further focused on the 8 active LL analogues to test for antagonistic properties of DL, and found that analogues (*S*)-(−)-2-methoxypropionic acid (**3**, MPA; Figure 2C), α-hydroxyisobutyric acid (**8**, aHIBA; Figure 2D), 2-hydroxy-3-methylbutyric acid (**9**, HMBA; Figure 2D), (*S*)-2-hydroxyl-pentanoic acid (**10**, 2HPA; Figure 2D), and kynurenic acid (**11**, KA; Figure 2D) fulfilled the criteria for mimicking the effect of LL on NA release (Figure 2F; [20]).

We have previously shown that the effect of LL on NA release was paralleled by depolarisation of noradrenergic neurones, increasing their excitability [20]. In the current set of experiments, we extended this dataset and compared resting membrane depolarisation caused by LL with the effect of LL analogues (Table 3; Supplementary Materials Figure S2). L-lactate, aHIBA (**8**, Figure 2D), and HMBA (**9**, Figure 2D) caused depolarisation in a significant proportion of neurones. However, MPA (**3**, Figure 2C), 2HPA (**10**, Figure 2C), and KA (**11**, Figure 2C), also powerful NA-releasing LL mimetics, evoked no depolarisation (Tables 1 and 3), suggesting that in noradrenergic neurones, depolarisation and cAMP-dependent transmitter release evoked by LL are not coupled in an obligatory way.

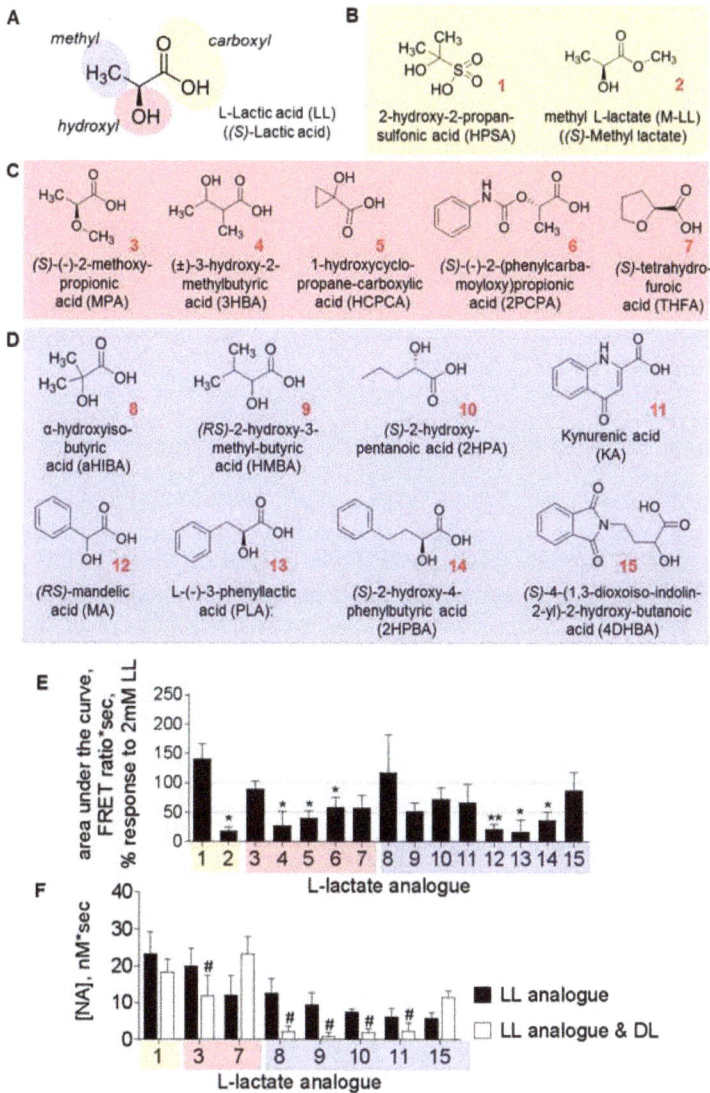

Figure 2. The structure–activity relationship (SAR) between L-lactate analogues and noradrenaline release in locus coeruleus characterises L-lactate binding properties at LLRx. (**A**) Moieties of the L-lactic (LL) acid molecule. The selection of tested LL analogues had alterations in the carboxyl group (**B**) (yellow highlight), in the hydroxyl group (**C**) (red highlight); and in the methyl group (**D**) (blue highlight). (**E**) LL analogues **1**, **3**, **7**, **8–11**, and **15** (2 mM) triggered more than 50% response in noradrenaline-sensitive α1 CNiFER cells as compared to 2 mM LL (100%). The rest of the tested analogues evoked significantly smaller responses compared to LL (** $p < 0.01$, * $p < 0.05$ vs 2 mM LL application for each analogue, paired *t*-test). (**F**) The effect of analogues **3** and **8–11** was blocked by pre-incubation with 200 µM D-lactate (DL; # $p < 0.05$ vs the same analogue without DL, paired *t*-test; E/F—data represented as mean ± SEM).

Table 3. Depolarisation of locus coeruleus neurones evoked by L-lactate and its analogues that cause D-lactate-sensitive noradrenaline release.

LL Analogue (Figure 2)	Cells Analysed (number)	Cells Depolarised (%)	Vm (mV)
LL	94	34	7.3 ± 1.1
3	8	0	
8	28	43	6.2 ± 1.3
9	9	67	5.3 ± 1.0
10	8	25	
11	7	14	

L-lactate (LL) analogue numbers as displayed in Figure 2. Resting membrane potential data (Vm) are displayed as mean ± SEM in cells that showed a response.

3.3. Orphan GPCRs as Putative Targets of L-Lactate

We used the DiscoveRx panel of orphan GPCRs (orphanMAX, LeadHunter; Fremont, CA, USA) to screen for the activity of LL (2–8 mM) and filtered the results for those orphans that were expressed in the LC, based on our NGS data (Table 4).

Only one of the orphan receptors on the panel, GPR162, satisfied the DiscoveRx criteria of >30% for significant activation by LL (at 8 mM). The response of several other receptors, however, exceeded 3 times the standard deviation of the baseline. Note that HCA1 (GPR81) did not respond to the maximum concentration of 8 mM LL as employed in our DiscoveRx screen, indicating that this assay might not be suitable for detection of signalling through these low-affinity receptors.

We considered those orphan GPCRs with likely G_s-protein or unknown coupling that were expressed in noradrenergic neurones of the LC, but not in astrocytes, for further testing (Table 4). Receptors were transiently expressed in HEK293 cells and subjected to the GloSensor cAMP assay to test for the response to LL (Table 4; Figure 3). As expected, HEK293 cells transiently transfected with GPR81 showed a concentration-dependent reduction in cAMP accumulation when stimulated with LL (Figure 3A). Another orphan receptor, GPR180, responded with decrease in cAMP to both 1 mM and 10 mM LL (Figure 3B). The only orphan receptor to significantly increase cAMP production with LL in the range of 1–5 mM was GPR137 (Figure 4A,C). In contrast, its paralogue, GPR137B, which is also highly expressed in noradrenergic cells of the LC, did not respond to 2 mM LL (Figure 4B).

The enantiomer of LL, DL (0.4 mM), did not activate GPR137 to increase cAMP production (Figure 4C). Co-application of 0.4 mM DL with 2 mM LL, which in our previous study blocked LL-evoked effects on NA release, did not significantly affect cAMP accumulation in comparison to 2 mM LL application alone (Figure 4C).

Table 4. Screening of heterologously expressed orphan GPCRs for activation by L-lactate.

GPCR	Coupling?	DiscoveRx Activation (%) by LL (mM)			Expression in LC (NGS)				cAMP Assay: Activation by LL (0.5–10 mM)
		2	4	8	p29	p7	Neuron	Astrocyte	
GPR61	Gs	−2%	16%	19%	97	183	163	0	No response
GPR81	Gi	1%	3%	3%	0	0	0	0	Decrease
GPR137	Gs?	6%	4%	3%	959	628	196	577	Increase
GPR137B	?	nd	nd	nd	226	83	140	125	No response
GPR146	?	−3%	10%	20%	129	49	6	312	nd
GPR155	RGS?	nd	nd	nd	842	412	140	36	No response
GPR158	RGS7	nd	nd	nd	1692	433	613	1	No response
GPR162	?	−9%	15%	30%	1293	1012	282	64	No response
GPR176	Gz	−8%	−2%	9%	193	196	190	9	No response
GPR180	Gi?	nd	nd	nd	768	542	520	83	Decrease

The combination of DiscoveRx panel readout and GloSensor assay for cAMP production suggests further L-lactate (LL)–sensing GPCR candidates. Apart from GPR81, this selection of receptors is expressed in locus coeruleus (LC) neurones at medium to high levels. Coupling information obtained from www.genecards.org. NGS–RNA-Seq by next-generation sequencing; nd—not determined.

A

B

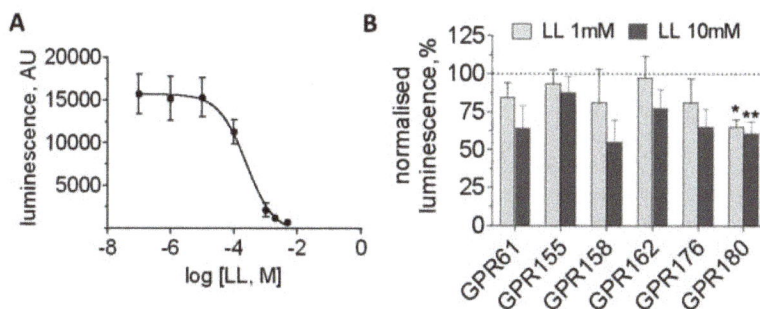

Figure 3. L-lactate activates GPR81- and GPR180-dependent G_i-protein signalling in HEK293 cells. (**A**) L-lactate (LL) concentration-dependently decreases cAMP accumulation in HEK293 cells transiently transfected with GPR81 (0.1 µg/µL; GloSensor assay; EC_{50} 243 µM). In order to create an elevated cAMP baseline level, cells were pretreated with 20 µM NHK 477, a soluble forskolin analogue. (**B**) Selected orphan GPCRs present in locus coeruleus neurones were transiently expressed in HEK293 cells (transfection with 0.1 µg/µL GPCR expression plasmid). Application of LL led to a significant decrease in cAMP only in GPR180-expressing cells. GloSensor assay: luminescence normalised to baseline in absence of LL; data represented as mean ± SEM; ** $p < 0.01$, * $p < 0.05$ vs no LL stimulation; $n = 3$; one-way ANOVA with Dunnett's as post-hoc test.

4. Discussion

This study aimed to further characterise LLRx, the LL receptor which mediates the communication between activated astrocytes and noradrenergic neurones [20]. Our previous evidence had suggested that LL acts at an extracellular site and was not consistent with the modulation of K_{ATP} channels. Based on the sensitivity of the effect to inhibition of adenylate cyclase or protein kinase A, we hypothesised that LLRx is most likely a GPCR that activates G_s-protein signalling, suggestive of an orphan GPCR or one of the olfactory receptors.

The potency of LL via its action on LLRx (EC_{50} ~0.5 mM) should be low compared to that of other endogenous GPCR ligands. For example, NA acting at β-adrenoceptors is around three orders of magnitude more potent (see Supplement in [44]). It is, however, fully consistent with a specific response based on low-affinity binding, given the high physiological extracellular LL concentration in the brain. Indeed, in comparison to the other LL receptors reported to date, HCA1 and OR51E2, the EC_{50} of LL at LLRx is around 10-fold lower and appears well correlated with the operational range of brain LL concentrations. It is, therefore, most suitable for mediating a dynamic physiological response to LL.

The experimental disadvantage of a low-affinity ligand–receptor interaction is that it rules out specific pull-down approaches to concentrate and biochemically analyse the receptor. Hence, we adopted an alternative approach to evaluate the properties of the LL–LLRx interaction and to determine an agonist profile for the LLRx-mediated stimulation of NA release.

The carboxyl group seems to be essential for LL's agonist activity as it was intact in all NA-releasing analogues, and methylation of the carboxyl group to form the ester analogue M-LL abolished the effect (**2**, Figure 2B,E,F). Replacement of the carboxyl group by a more acidic sulfonate group in HPSA (**1**, Figure 2B) did result in triggering NA release, but eliminated the antagonist effect of DL. This suggests that HPSA acts via a different mechanism than by activation of LLRx. Indeed, it may be that HPSA is decomposing into acetone and sulphuric acid, leading to a false positive result.

The 2-hydroxyl group was intact in most of the active LL analogues, indicating its importance for NA release. Most analogues with 2-OH deletion or modifications, particularly addition of large groups, were inactive, apart from MPA, THFA, and KA (**3, 7** Figure 2C, **11**, Figure 2D, respectively). The DL-sensitive effect of MPA indicates that the hydroxyl group may act as a hydrogen bond acceptor, but hydrogen bond donation is not necessary to trigger NA release. THFA (**7**, Figure 2C) can be thought of as a conformationally restricted analogue of LL and MPA (**3**, Figure 2C), while HCPCA

(**5**, Figure 2C) is a conformationally restricted analogue of LL and aHIBA (**8**, Figure 2D). THFA and HCPCA were less active than the parent molecules MPA and aHIBA, respectively, suggesting that the conformations of THFA and HCPCA are not optimal for interaction with LLRx. Kynurenic acid (KA, **11**, Figure 2D) can be thought of as a conformationally restricted analogue of LL in which the NH group acts as a mimic of the OH group of LL and the methyl group of LL is incorporated into the ring structure. The 4-oxo group of KA, which is a hydrogen bond acceptor, may also play a role in interacting with LLRx. Future SAR studies are needed to explore this possibility.

Addition of a second methyl group in the α-position, as in aHIBA (**8**, Figure 2D), or extension of the carbon chain from the methyl group as in HMBA and 2HPA (**9**, **10**, Figure 2D), supports activation of LLRx. However, large lipophilic residues replacing or added as substituents to the methyl group prevent DL-sensitive NA release (**12–15**, Figure 2D), indicating a limitation of size in the binding pocket.

The comparison of the analogues that cause NA release and those that evoke membrane depolarisation shows that, in noradrenergic neurones, NA release can be evoked without necessarily increasing the cells' electrical excitability. This is unsurprising, given previous evidence for cAMP-mediated increase in exocytosis [45]. In fact, extensive evidence indicates that depolarisation should not be the primary mechanism regulating NA release, because noradrenergic neurones are characteristically depolarised at rest. Membrane potentials of LC neurones, in vitro as well as in vivo, are typically near -50 mV (Supplementary Materials Figure S2; [20,46–48]. Moreover, LC neurones in vivo and in slices tend to generate a constant low-frequency stream of action potentials while their excitation by a sensory stimulus triggers only a very short (~20 ms) barrage of 3–5 additional action potentials which is followed by a long period of quiescence lasting hundreds of milliseconds [49,50]. Therefore, the conventional logic of neuronal networks where high-frequency action potential activity triggers release of a neurotransmitter, such as glutamate, does not apply to noradrenergic neurones. A mechanism which sensitises the NA release machinery and potentiates NA release to the steady-state level of intracellular Ca^{2+} (with or without additional depolarisation) should be a much more effective way to control NA release.

It is also important to note that the chemicals tested here can affect multiple targets. Kynurenic acid, for example, while effectively triggering DL-sensitive NA release, is also a well-known glutamate receptor antagonist [51]. Blocking of glutamate receptors theoretically should lead to a decrease rather than an increase in neuronal excitability, but KA nevertheless triggered release of NA.

Whilst beyond the scope of the current study, analogues that failed to produce a positive response in the NA release assay may have antagonist or weak partial agonist properties. If such compounds are identified and optimised, they may be expected to facilitate future studies to characterise the physiological and pathophysiological roles of this astrocytic signalling pathway.

The DiscoveRx panel screening is based on β-arrestin-induced internalisation and should be independent of the type of G-protein the receptor couples with. The approach is not very sensitive and, in the case of low-potency agonists such as LL, relatively high concentrations of agonist need to be employed, potentially leading to nonspecific effects. Only few concentration-dependent responses to LL (2–8 mM) were detected. When following up on the effect of LL on GPR162, we were unable to confirm a LL-induced change in cAMP production in transiently transfected HEK293 cells. This suggests that GPR162 does not signal via G_s-proteins and is therefore not consistent with LLRx function.

We acknowledge that we selected orphan candidates with medium to high expression levels in LC and with either unknown or proposed G_s-coupling in order to determine their cAMP response to LL (Table 4). Of these, only GPR137 produced a concentration-dependent but DL-insensitive increase in cAMP, making it an interesting candidate for further study. GPR137 has two paralogues, GPR137B and GPR137C, which are located on different chromosomes. Unusually for GPCRs, all three paralogues contain introns, raising the possibility of multiple variants through alternative splicing. GPR137 has been suggested to play a role in the proliferation of malignant tumours, but its functional significance for the brain has not yet been explored [52,53]. Neither ligands nor physiological actions of

GPR137B and GPR137C are currently established. However, as the cAMP response was not inhibited by co-application of DL, GPR137 does not fulfil all properties proposed for "LLRx" (Figure 4C).

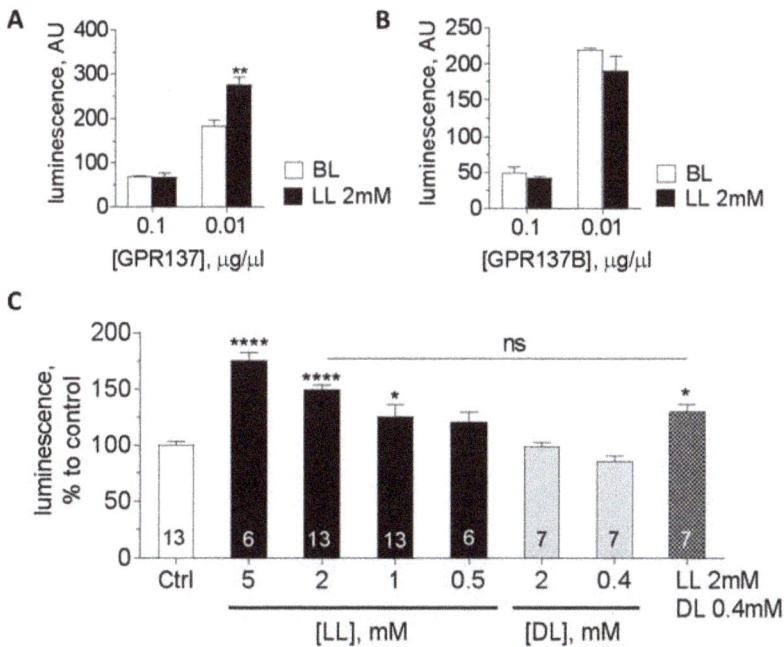

Figure 4. L-lactate stimulates GPR137-dependent cAMP accumulation in HEK293 cells. (**A**) HEK293 cells transiently transfected with GPR137 (0.01 µg/µL) respond to 2 mM L-lactate (LL) with cAMP accumulation (GloSensor assay, $n = 3$, ** $p < 0.01$ vs baseline (BL), one-way ANOVA with Tukey's post-hoc test). (**B**) HEK293 cells expressing GPR137B do not respond to 2 mM LL. (**C**) Concentration range of LL and DL effects on cAMP in HEK293 cells transiently transfected with GPR137 (0.01 µg/µL). LL significantly increases cAMP at concentrations ≥ 1 mM. D-lactate (DL) elicits no response and does not significantly inhibit the effect of 2 mM LL (data are shown as mean ± SEM; n values for each dataset are represented in the respective columns; **** $p < 0.0001$, * $p < 0.05$ vs control, one-way ANOVA with Tukey's post-hoc test).

Looking into the future, the list of potential LL receptor candidates is by no means complete if we include orphan GPCRs with low to medium expression levels such as GPR146 and others (not shown) to explore further as targets for LL-mediated signalling. Since LL-mediated release of NA is implicated in regulation of sleep/wake and attention states, learning and memory, and cardiorespiratory control, a better understanding of—and pharmacological tools to control—this signalling axis may have significant health implications.

Supplementary Materials: The following are available online at http://www.mdpi.com/2571-6980/1/2/25/s1, Figure S1. L-lactate evokes noradrenaline release from organotypic brain slices cultures as confirmed by using α1 CNiFER cells. Figure S2. L-lactate and analogues excite noradrenergic LC neurones.

Author Contributions: Conceptualisation: S.K., A.G.T.; data acquisition and analysis: V.M., S.R.-N., K.K., M.D.B.; advice on LL analogue chemistry: D.J.; NGS—M.D.B., M.J.H.; manuscript writing and editing: A.G.T., V.M., S.K.

Funding: This work was supported by grants from BBSRC BB/L019396/1, and MRC MR/L020661/1.

Acknowledgments: David Kleinfeld for his gift of CNiFER cells, Lesley Arberry for expert technical support, Andrew Herman for support with FACS sorting.

Conflicts of Interest: The authors declare no conflict of interest.

References

1. Oe, Y.; Baba, O.; Ashida, H.; Nakamura, K.C.; Hirase, H. Glycogen distribution in the microwave-fixed mouse brain reveals heterogeneous astrocytic patterns. *GLIA* **2016**, *64*, 1532–1545. [CrossRef] [PubMed]

2. Locasale, J.W.; Cantley, L.C. Metabolic flux and the regulation of mammalian cell growth. *Cell. Metab.* **2011**, *14*, 443–451. [CrossRef] [PubMed]

3. Dienel, G.A. Lack of appropriate stoichiometry: Strong evidence against an energetically important astrocyte-neuron lactate shuttle in brain. *J. Neurosci. Res.* **2017**, *95*, 2103–2125. [CrossRef] [PubMed]

4. Abi-Saab, W.M.; Maggs, D.G.; Jones, T.; Jacob, R.; Srihari, V.; Thompson, J.; Kerr, D.; Leone, P.; Krystal, J.H.; Spencer, D.D.; et al. Striking differences in glucose and lactate levels between brain extracellular fluid and plasma in conscious human subjects: Effects of hyperglycemia and hypoglycemia. *J. Cereb. Blood Flow Metab.* **2002**, *22*, 271–279. [CrossRef] [PubMed]

5. Mosienko, V.; Teschemacher, A.G.; Kasparov, S. Is L-lactate a novel signaling molecule in the brain? *J. Cereb. Blood Flow Metab.* **2015**, *35*, 1069–1075. [CrossRef] [PubMed]

6. Machler, P.; Wyss, M.T.; Elsayed, M.; Stobart, J.; Gutierrez, R.; von Faber-Castell, A.; Kaelin, V.; Zuend, M.; San Martin, A.; Romero-Gomez, I.; et al. In Vivo Evidence for a Lactate Gradient from Astrocytes to Neurons. *Cell Metab.* **2016**, *23*, 94–102. [CrossRef] [PubMed]

7. Supplie, L.M.; Duking, T.; Campbell, G.; Diaz, F.; Moraes, C.T.; Gotz, M.; Hamprecht, B.; Boretius, S.; Mahad, D.; Nave, K.A. Respiration-Deficient Astrocytes Survive as Glycolytic Cells In Vivo. *J. Neurosci.* **2017**, *37*, 4231–4242. [CrossRef] [PubMed]

8. Fernandez-Moncada, I.; Ruminot, I.; Robles-Maldonado, D.; Alegria, K.; Deitmer, J.W.; Barros, L.F. Neuronal control of astrocytic respiration through a variant of the Crabtree effect. *Proc. Natl. Acad. Sci. USA* **2018**, *115*, 1623–1628. [CrossRef] [PubMed]

9. Pellerin, L.; Magistretti, P.J. Sweet sixteen for ANLS. *J. Cereb. Blood Flow Metab.* **2011**, *32*, 1152–1166. [CrossRef] [PubMed]

10. Weber, B.; Barros, L.F. The Astrocyte: Powerhouse and Recycling Center. *Cold Spring Harb. Perspect. Biol.* **2015**, *7*, a020396. [CrossRef] [PubMed]

11. Suzuki, A.; Stern, S.A.; Bozdagi, O.; Huntley, G.W.; Walker, R.H.; Magistretti, P.J.; Alberini, C.M. Astrocyte-neuron lactate transport is required for long-term memory formation. *Cell* **2011**, *144*, 810–823. [CrossRef] [PubMed]

12. Newman, L.A.; Korol, D.L.; Gold, P.E. Lactate produced by glycogenolysis in astrocytes regulates memory processing. *PLoS ONE* **2011**, *6*, e28427. [CrossRef] [PubMed]

13. Alberini, C.M.; Cruz, E.; Descalzi, G.; Bessieres, B.; Gao, V. Astrocyte glycogen and lactate: New insights into learning and memory mechanisms. *GLIA* **2017**, *66*, 1244–1262. [CrossRef] [PubMed]

14. Clasadonte, J.; Scemes, E.; Wang, Z.; Boison, D.; Haydon, P.G. Connexin 43-Mediated Astroglial Metabolic Networks Contribute to the Regulation of the Sleep-Wake Cycle. *Neuron* **2017**, *95*, 1365–1380. [CrossRef] [PubMed]

15. Naylor, E.; Aillon, D.V.; Barrett, B.S.; Wilson, G.S.; Johnson, D.A.; Johnson, D.A.; Harmon, H.P.; Gabbert, S.; Petillo, P.A. Lactate as a biomarker for sleep. *Sleep* **2012**, *35*, 1209–1222. [CrossRef] [PubMed]

16. Rempe, M.J.; Wisor, J.P. Cerebral lactate dynamics across sleep/wake cycles. *Front Comput. Neurosci.* **2014**, *8*, 174. [CrossRef] [PubMed]

17. Carrard, A.; Elsayed, M.; Margineanu, M.; Boury-Jamot, B.; Fragniere, L.; Meylan, E.M.; Petit, J.M.; Fiumelli, H.; Magistretti, P.J.; Martin, J.L. Peripheral administration of lactate produces antidepressant-like effects. *Mol. Psychiatry* **2018**, *23*, 392–399. [CrossRef] [PubMed]

18. Reiach, J.S.; Li, P.P.; Warsh, J.J.; Kish, S.J.; Young, L.T. Reduced adenylyl cyclase immunolabeling and activity in postmortem temporal cortex of depressed suicide victims. *J. Affect Disord.* **1999**, *56*, 141–151. [CrossRef]

19. Vardjan, N.; Chowdhury, H.H.; Horvat, A.; Velebit, J.; Malnar, M.; Muhic, M.; Kreft, M.; Krivec, S.G.; Bobnar, S.T.; Mis, K.; et al. Enhancement of Astroglial Aerobic Glycolysis by Extracellular Lactate-Mediated Increase in cAMP. *Front Mol. Neurosci.* **2018**, *11*, 148. [CrossRef] [PubMed]

20. Tang, F.; Lane, S.; Korsak, A.; Paton, J.F.; Gourine, A.V.; Kasparov, S.; Teschemacher, A.G. Lactate-mediated glia-neuronal signaling in the mammalian brain. *Nat. Commun.* **2014**, *5*, 3284. [CrossRef] [PubMed]

21. Yang, J.; Ruchti, E.; Petit, J.M.; Jourdain, P.; Grenningloh, G.; Allaman, I.; Magistretti, P.J. Lactate promotes plasticity gene expression by potentiating NMDA signaling in neurons. *Proc. Natl. Acad. Sci. USA* **2014**, *111*, 12228–12233. [CrossRef] [PubMed]
22. Lee, D.C.; Sohn, H.A.; Park, Z.Y.; Oh, S.; Kang, Y.K.; Lee, K.M.; Kang, M.; Jang, Y.J.; Yang, S.J.; Hong, Y.K.; et al. A lactate-induced response to hypoxia. *Cell* **2015**, *161*, 595–609. [CrossRef] [PubMed]
23. Parsons, M.P.; Hirasawa, M. ATP-sensitive potassium channel-mediated lactate effect on orexin neurons: Implications for brain energetics during arousal. *J. Neurosci.* **2010**, *30*, 8061–8070. [CrossRef] [PubMed]
24. Cai, T.Q.; Ren, N.; Jin, L.; Cheng, K.; Kash, S.; Chen, R.; Wright, S.D.; Taggart, A.K.; Waters, M.G. Role of GPR81 in lactate-mediated reduction of adipose lipolysis. *Biochem. Biophys. Res. Commun.* **2008**, *377*, 987–991. [CrossRef] [PubMed]
25. Liu, C.; Wu, J.; Zhu, J.; Kuei, C.; Yu, J.; Shelton, J.; Sutton, S.W.; Li, X.; Yun, S.J.; Mirzadegan, T.; et al. Lactate inhibits lipolysis in fat cells through activation of an orphan G-protein-coupled receptor, GPR81. *J. Biol. Chem.* **2009**, *284*, 2811–2822. [CrossRef] [PubMed]
26. Lauritzen, K.H.; Morland, C.; Puchades, M.; Holm-Hansen, S.; Hagelin, E.M.; Lauritzen, F.; Attramadal, H.; Storm-Mathisen, J.; Gjedde, A.; Bergersen, L.H. Lactate receptor sites link neurotransmission, neurovascular coupling, and brain energy metabolism. *Cereb. Cortex* **2014**, *24*, 2784–2795. [CrossRef] [PubMed]
27. Morland, C.; Lauritzen, K.H.; Puchades, M.; Holm-Hansen, S.; Andersson, K.; Gjedde, A.; Attramadal, H.; Storm-Mathisen, J.; Bergersen, L.H. The lactate receptor, G-protein-coupled receptor 81/hydroxycarboxylic acid receptor 1, Expression and action in brain. *J. Neurosci. Res.* **2015**, *93*, 1045–1055. [CrossRef] [PubMed]
28. Bozzo, L.; Puyal, J.; Chatton, J.Y. Lactate modulates the activity of primary cortical neurons through a receptor-mediated pathway. *PLoS ONE* **2013**, *8*, e71721. [CrossRef] [PubMed]
29. Chang, A.J.; Ortega, F.E.; Riegler, J.; Madison, D.V.; Krasnow, M.A. Oxygen regulation of breathing through an olfactory receptor activated by lactate. *Nature* **2015**, *527*, 240–244. [CrossRef] [PubMed]
30. Hosford, P.S.; Mosienko, V.; Kishi, K.; Jurisic, G.; Seuwen, K.; Kinzel, B.; Ludwig, M.G.; Wells, J.A.; Christie, I.N.; Koolen, L.; et al. CNS distribution, signalling properties and central effects of G-protein coupled receptor 4. *Neuropharmacology* **2018**, *138*, 381–392. [CrossRef] [PubMed]
31. Conzelmann, S.; Levai, O.; Bode, B.; Eisel, U.; Raming, K.; Breer, H.; Strotmann, J. A novel brain receptor is expressed in a distinct population of olfactory sensory neurons. *Eur. J. Neurosci.* **2000**, *12*, 3926–3934. [CrossRef] [PubMed]
32. Torres-Torrelo, H.; Ortega-Saenz, P.; Macias, D.; Omura, M.; Zhou, T.; Matsunami, H.; Johnson, R.S.; Mombaerts, P.; Lopez-Barneo, J. The role of Olfr78 in the breathing circuit of mice. *Nature* **2018**, *561*, E33–E40. [CrossRef] [PubMed]
33. McBryde, F.D.; Abdala, A.P.; Hendy, E.B.; Pijacka, W.; Marvar, P.; Moraes, D.J.; Sobotka, P.A.; Paton, J.F. The carotid body as a putative therapeutic target for the treatment of neurogenic hypertension. *Nat. Commun.* **2013**, *4*, 2395. [CrossRef] [PubMed]
34. Marina, N.; Tang, F.; Figueiredo, M.; Mastitskaya, S.; Kasimov, V.; Mohamed-Ali, V.; Roloff, E.; Teschemacher, A.G.; Gourine, A.V.; Kasparov, S. Purinergic signalling in the rostral ventro-lateral medulla controls sympathetic drive and contributes to the progression of heart failure following myocardial infarction in rats. *Basic Res. Cardiol.* **2013**, *108*, 317. [CrossRef] [PubMed]
35. Yuan, T.T.; Toy, P.; McClary, J.A.; Lin, R.J.; Miyamoto, N.G.; Kretschmer, P.J. Cloning and genetic characterization of an evolutionarily conserved human olfactory receptor that is differentially expressed across species. *Gene* **2001**, *278*, 41–51. [CrossRef]
36. Weber, M.; Pehl, U.; Breer, H.; Strotmann, J. Olfactory receptor expressed in ganglia of the autonomic nervous system. *J. Neurosci. Res.* **2002**, *68*, 176–184. [CrossRef] [PubMed]
37. Mosienko, V.; Chang, A.J.; Alenina, N.; Teschemacher, A.G.; Kasparov, S. Rodents and humans are able to detect the odour of L-Lactate. *PLoS ONE* **2017**, *12*, e0178478. [CrossRef] [PubMed]
38. Ludwig, M.G.; Vanek, M.; Guerini, D.; Gasser, J.A.; Jones, C.E.; Junker, U.; Hofstetter, H.; Wolf, R.M.; Seuwen, K. Proton-sensing G-protein-coupled receptors. *Nature* **2013**, *425*, 93–98. [CrossRef] [PubMed]
39. Kumar, N.N.; Velic, A.; Soliz, J.; Shi, Y.; Li, K.; Wang, S.; Weaver, J.L.; Sen, J.; Abbott, S.B.; Lazarenko, R.M.; et al. PHYSIOLOGY. Regulation of breathing by CO_2 requires the proton-activated receptor GPR4 in retrotrapezoid nucleus neurons. *Science* **2015**, *348*, 1255–1260. [CrossRef] [PubMed]

40. Teschemacher, A.G.; Wang, S.; Lonergan, T.; Duale, H.; Waki, H.; Paton, J.F.; Kasparov, S. Targeting specific neuronal populations in the rat brainstem using adeno- and lentiviral vectors: Applications for imaging and studies of cell function. *Exp. Physiol.* **2005**, *90*, 61–69. [CrossRef] [PubMed]

41. Figueiredo, M.; Lane, S.; Stout, R.F., Jr.; Liu, B.; Parpura, V.; Teschemacher, A.G.; Kasparov, S. Comparative analysis of optogenetic actuators in cultured astrocytes. *Cell Calcium* **2014**, *56*, 208–214. [CrossRef] [PubMed]

42. Lobo, M.K.; Karsten, S.L.; Gray, M.; Geschwind, D.H.; Yang, X.W. FACS-array profiling of striatal projection neuron subtypes in juvenile and adult mouse brains. *Nat. Neurosci.* **2006**, *9*, 443–452. [CrossRef] [PubMed]

43. Muller, A.; Joseph, V.; Slesinger, P.A.; Kleinfeld, D. Cell-based reporters reveal in vivo dynamics of dopamine and norepinephrine release in murine cortex. *Nat. Methods* **2014**, *11*, 1245–1252. [CrossRef] [PubMed]

44. Liu, B.; Mosienko, V.; Vaccari, C.B.; Prokudina, D.; Huentelman, M.; Teschemacher, A.G.; Kasparov, S. Glio- and neuro-protection by prosaposin is mediated by orphan G-protein coupled receptors GPR37L1 and GPR37. *GLIA* **2018**. [CrossRef] [PubMed]

45. Chavez-Noriega, L.E.; Stevens, C.F. Increased transmitter release at excitatory synapses produced by direct activation of adenylate cyclase in rat hippocampal slices. *J. Neurosci.* **1994**, *14*, 310–317. [CrossRef] [PubMed]

46. Williams, J.T.; Bobker, D.H.; Harris, G.C. Synaptic potentials in locus coeruleus neurons in brain slices. *Prog. Brain Res.* **1991**, *88*, 167–172. [PubMed]

47. Pepper, C.M.; Henderson, G. Opiates and opioid peptides hyperpolarize locus coeruleus neurons in vitro. *Science* **1980**, *209*, 394–395. [CrossRef] [PubMed]

48. Aghajanian, G.K.; Vandermaelen, C.P. α 2-adrenoceptor-mediated hyperpolarization of locus coeruleus neurons: Intracellular studies in vivo. *Science* **1982**, *215*, 1394–1396. [CrossRef] [PubMed]

49. Cedarbaum, J.M.; Aghajanian, G.K. Activation of locus coeruleus neurons by peripheral stimuli: Modulation by a collateral inhibitory mechanism. *Life Sci.* **1978**, *23*, 1383–1392. [CrossRef]

50. Foote, S.L.; Aston-Jones, G.; Bloom, F.E. Impulse activity of locus coeruleus neurons in awake rats and monkeys is a function of sensory stimulation and arousal. *Proc. Natl. Acad. Sci. USA* **1980**, *77*, 3033–3037. [CrossRef] [PubMed]

51. Alt, A.; Weiss, B.; Ogden, A.M.; Knauss, J.L.; Oler, J.; Ho, K.; Large, T.H.; Bleakman, D. Pharmacological characterization of glutamatergic agonists and antagonists at recombinant human homomeric and heteromeric kainate receptors in vitro. *Neuropharmacology* **2004**, *46*, 793–806. [CrossRef] [PubMed]

52. Zong, G.; Wang, H.; Li, J.; Xie, Y.; Bian, E.; Zhao, B. Inhibition of GPR137 expression reduces the proliferation and colony formation of malignant glioma cells. *Neurol. Sci.* **2014**, *35*, 1707–1714. [CrossRef] [PubMed]

53. Mager, L.F.; Koelzer, V.H.; Stuber, R.; Thoo, L.; Keller, I.; Koeck, I.; Langenegger, M.; Simillion, C.; Pfister, S.P.; Faderl, M.; et al. The ESRP1-GPR137 axis contributes to intestinal pathogenesis. *Elife* **2017**, *6*, e28366. [CrossRef] [PubMed]

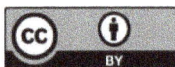

![neuroglia logo] *neuroglia*

MDPI

Article

Role for Astroglia-Derived BDNF and MSK1 in Homeostatic Synaptic Plasticity

Ulyana Lalo [1], Alexander Bogdanov [2], Guy W. J. Moss [3], Bruno G. Frenguelli [1] and
Yuriy Pankratov [1,*]

[1]   School of Life Sciences, University of Warwick, Gibbet Hill Campus, Coventry CV4 7AL, UK;
      laloulya@yahoo.com (U.L.); b.g.frenguelli@warwick.ac.uk (B.G.F.)
[2]   Institute for Chemistry and Biology, Immanuel Kant Baltic Federal University 2 Universitetskaya str.,
      Kaliningrad 236040, Russia; axebogdanov@gmail.com
[3]   Department of Neuroscience, Physiology and Pharmacology, University College London,
      London WC1E 6BT, UK; g.moss@ucl.ac.uk
*   Correspondence: y.pankratov@warwick.ac.uk

Received: 5 November 2018; Accepted: 12 November 2018; Published: 22 November 2018

Abstract: Homeostatic scaling of synaptic strength in response to environmental stimuli may underlie the beneficial effects of an active lifestyle on brain function. Our previous results highlighted a key role for brain-derived neurotrophic factor (BDNF) and mitogen- and stress-activated protein kinase 1 (MSK1) in experience-related homeostatic synaptic plasticity. Astroglia have recently been shown to serve as an important source of BDNF. To elucidate a role for astroglia-derived BDNF, we explored homeostatic synaptic plasticity in transgenic mice with an impairment in the BDNF/MSK1 pathway (MSK1 kinase dead knock-in (KD) mice) and impairment of glial exocytosis (dnSNARE mice). We observed that prolonged tonic activation of astrocytes caused BDNF-dependent upregulation of excitatory synaptic currents accompanied by enlargement of synaptic boutons. We found that exposure to environmental enrichment (EE) and caloric restriction (CR) strongly upregulated excitatory but downregulated inhibitory synaptic currents in old wild-type mice, thus counterbalancing the impact of ageing on synaptic transmission. In parallel, EE and CR enhanced astrocytic Ca^{2+}-signalling. Importantly, we observed a significant deficit in the effects of EE and CR on synaptic transmission in the MSK1 KD and dnSNARE mice. Combined, our results strongly support the importance of astrocytic exocytosis of BDNF for the beneficial effects of EE and CR on synaptic transmission and plasticity in the ageing brain.

Keywords: aging; dendritic spines; synaptic strength; glia–neuron interactions; ion conductance microscopy; synaptic scaling; diet; enriched environment; GABA receptors; AMPA receptors; TrkB receptors; Arc/Arg3.1; calcium signalling

1. Introduction

The ability of neurons to autonomously scale their synaptic strength in response to hyper- or hypoexcitability of their neighbours is instrumental for brain adaptation to environmental challenges during development, adulthood, and ageing [1–3]. Such forms of adaptive changes in synaptic strength are generally termed homeostatic synaptic plasticity [2]. The responsiveness of synapses and neuronal networks to environmental stimuli has been linked to the potential beneficial effects of an active lifestyle on the ageing brain [4–8].

Brain-derived neurotrophic factor (BDNF) has emerged as an important mediator of synaptic adaptation to both activity deprivation and environmental enrichment [1,9,10]. Increased production of BDNF has been observed in rodents in response to environmental enrichment [1,3], which, via the

BDNF tropomyosin receptor kinase B (TrkB receptor), promotes dendritic growth, and increased spine density [11].

The role of BDNF in synaptic adaptation relies on a number of proteins, including the cytoskeletal-associated protein Arc/Arg3.1 and mitogen- and stress-activated protein kinase 1 (MSK1). In particular, our previous data have shown a quintessential role for MSK1 in BDNF-mediated homeostatic synaptic scaling in vitro, and the effects of environmental enrichment (EE) on synaptic transmission in hippocampus in vivo [9]. Since the release of BDNF can be increased by various environmental stimuli, such as physical activity or a change in diet [9,12,13], the BDNF/MSK1 pathway might play an important role in the beneficial effects of both physical activity and caloric restriction (CR) on synaptic function, in particular in the ageing brain.

Recent data has highlighted an important role for astroglia as a source of BDNF [14,15]. It has been recently demonstrated that astrocytes can release BDNF via Ca^{2+}-dependent exocytosis [14]. In addition, astrocytes, which mediate neurovascular coupling and orchestrate metabolic support of neurons [16–18], are strategically positioned to mediate the effects of enhanced physical activity and CR. Our recent results show that EE and CR can both enhance astroglial Ca^{2+}-signalling [19]. Thus, we hypothesise that astroglia-derived BDNF could be instrumental for homeostatic synaptic scaling and experience-dependent synaptic plasticity.

To verify this hypothesis, we explored the effects of tonic activation of astrocytes in situ and in vivo (via environmental stimuli) on synaptic scaling in transgenic mice with an impairment of BDNF/MSK1 signalling (MSK1 kinase dead knock-in mice) and an impairment of glial exocytosis (dnSNARE mice).

2. Materials and Methods

All animal work was carried out in accordance with UK legislation and "3R" strategy; research did not involve non-human primates. This project was approved by the University of Warwick Animal Welfare and Ethical Review Body (AWERB), approval number G13-19, and regulated under the auspices of the UK Home Office Animals (Scientific Procedures) Act licenses P1D8E11D6 and I3EBF4DB9. Experiments were performed in astrocytes and neurons of the hippocampus and somatosensory cortex of dn-SNARE transgenic mice [19–22], their wild-type littermates (WT), and transgenic mice with MSK1 kinase dead knock-in (MSK1 KD mice) [9]; the MSK1 KD mice had the same genetic background as dnSNARE mice (C57/Bl6). We used mice of two age groups, 6–12 (average 7.8) weeks and 9–15 (average 12.7) months. We compared animals kept under standard housing conditions (SH) vs. animals exposed to the EE from birth [9], including ad libitum access to the running wheel, or kept on mild CR diet (food intake individually regulated to maintain the body weight loss of 10–15%) for 4 to 6 weeks.

2.1. Slice and Cell Preparation

Mice were anaesthetized by halothane and then decapitated, in accordance with UK legislation. Brains were removed rapidly after decapitation and placed into ice-cold physiological saline containing (mM): NaCl 130, KCl 3, $CaCl_2$ 0.5, $MgCl_2$ 2.5, NaH_2PO_4 1, $NaHCO_3$ 25, glucose 15, pH of 7.4 gassed with 95% O_2–5% CO_2. Transverse slices (260 μm) were cut at 4 °C and then placed in physiological saline containing (mM): NaCl 130, KCl 3, $CaCl_2$ 2.5, $MgCl_2$ 1, NaH_2PO_4 1, $NaHCO_3$ 22, glucose 15, pH of 7.4 gassed with 95% O_2–5% CO_2 and kept for 1.5 to 5 h prior to cell isolation and recording.

Astrocytes were identified by their morphology under differential contrast observation, green fluorescent protein (GFP) fluorescence (astrocytes from dn-SNARE mice) or staining with sulforhodamine 101 (astrocytes from WT and MSK1 KD mice). After recording, the identification of astrocytes was confirmed via their functional properties (high potassium conductance, low input resistance, and strong activity of glutamate transporters) as described previously [20–23]. To facilitate high-quality whole-cell recordings in the brain tissue slices of old mice, tissue slices were treated with a vibrating glass ball to remove the upper layer of dead cells and expose healthy neurons [24].

Hippocampal cultures were prepared from WT and MKS1 KD mice as described previously [9]. Briefly, hippocampi were dissected, recovered by enzymatic digestion with trypsin and dissociated through a Gilson pipette. For immunocytochemistry and for miniature excitatory postsynaptic currents (mEPSC) recordings, cells were plated at a density of approximately 100,000 per dish onto 22-mm glass coverslips coated with poly-L-lysine. Cultures were maintained at 37 °C in neurobasal medium (Gibco, Themo Fisher Scientific, UK) containing 1% L-glutamine (Gibco), 1% penicillin–streptomycin (Gibco) and 2% B27 supplement (Gibco) in a 95% O_2/5% CO_2-humidified incubator. Neurons were used between 12 to 16 days in vitro.

2.2. Electrophysiological Recordings

Whole-cell voltage-clamp recordings from cortical neurones and astrocytes were made with patch pipettes (4–5 MΩ) filled with intracellular solution (in mM): 110 CsCl, 10 NaCl, 10 HEPES, 5 MgATP, 1 D-Serine, 0.1 EGTA, pH 7.35. Currents were monitored using an MultiClamp 700B patch-clamp amplifier (Axon Instruments, Union City, CA, USA) filtered at 2 kHz and digitized at 4 kHz. Experiments were controlled by a Digidata1440A data acquisition board (Axon Instruments) and WinWCP software (Strathclyde University, Edinburgh, UK); data were analysed by custom lab software. Liquid junction potentials were compensated with the patch-clamp amplifier. The series and input resistances were 5–7 MΩ and 700–1200 MΩ, respectively; both series and input resistance varied by less than 20% in the cells accepted for analysis.

2.3. High-Resolution Scanning of Synaptic Boutons

Synaptic morphology was imaged in the neuronal cultures using the super-resolution hopping probe ion conductance microscopy, an advanced version of scanning ion conductance microscopy (SICM) [25]. The identification of synaptic boutons and SICM 3D topographical imaging were carried out using a custom-modified SICM scanner ICNano (Ionoscope, London, UK), as described previously [25]. Briefly, the sample was positioned in the X-Y directions with a nanopositioning stage (Physik Instrumente, Karlsruhe, Germany) and the scanning pipette was positioned in Z-direction with a piezoelectric actuator (PI). The fine-tipped scanning nanopipettes were pulled from borosilicate glass (outer/internal diameter 1/0.5 mm) with a horizontal laser puller P-2000 (Sutter Instruments, Novato, CA); pipette resistance was in the range of 80 to 100 MΩ corresponding to the estimated tip diameter of 90–120 nm. Nanopipettes were held in voltage-clamp mode with an Axopatch 200B patch-clamp amplifier (Axon Instruments); the amplifier head-stage was mounted on the z-scanning head. The amplifier output signal was monitored by the SICM electronics, which simultaneously controlled sample and pipette positioning.

The scan system was mounted onto an inverted microscope Nikon TE2000-U (Nikon Instruments, Kingston, UK) equipped with epifluorescence illumination. The sample was preloaded with the fluorescent synaptic marker FM1-43 (3 µM, 15 min loading followed by 15 min washout). FM1-43 fluorescence was imaged 100X 1.3 numerical aperture (NA) oil immersion objective and an EM-CCD camera (Andor iXon3, Andor Technology, Belfast, UK). Synaptic boutons were identified by matching the tentative boutons in topography and FM1-43 fluorescence [25]. The raw SICM data were processed using Gwyddion 5.0 microscopy analysis software (Czech Metrology Institute, Brno, Czech Republic) [26]. After constructing a 3D topographical image of identified synaptic varicosities, their maximal span in X-Y-Z dimensions (Δx, Δy and Δz) was determined and the effective size was calculated as the square root of ($\Delta x^2 + \Delta y^2 + \Delta z^2$) quotient. The synaptic varicosity volume was estimated as the volume of an ellipsoid of Δx, Δy and Δz dimensions.

2.4. Multiphoton Fluorescent Ca^{2+}-Imaging in Astrocytes

To monitor the cytoplasmic free Ca^{2+} concentraton ($[Ca^{2+}]_i$) in situ, astrocytes of neocortical slices were loaded via 30 min incubation with 1 µM of Rhod-2AM (dnSNARE mice) or Oregon Green Bapta-2AM and sulphorhodamine 101 (wild-type and MSK1 KD mice) at 33 °C. Two-photon images of neurons and astrocytes were acquired at 5 Hz frame rate using a Zeiss LSM-7MP multiphoton microscope (Carl Zeiss, Jena, Germany) coupled to a MaiTai (SpectraPhysics, Santa Clara CA, USA) pulsing laser; experiments were controlled by ZEN LSM software (Carl Zeiss). Images were further analysed offline using ZEN LSM (Carl Zeiss) and ImageJ 1.52 (NIH) software [27]. The $[Ca^{2+}]_i$ levels were expressed as $\Delta F/F$ ratio averaged over a region of interest (ROI). For analysis of spontaneous Ca^{2+}-transients in astrocytes, three ROIs located over dendrites and one ROI located over the soma were chosen. Overall Ca^{2+}-response to receptors agonists or synaptic stimulation was quantified using an ROI covering the whole cell image.

2.5. Data Analysis

All data are presented as mean $\pm$ standard deviation (SD) and the statistical significance of differences between data groups was tested by two-tailed unpaired *t*-test, unless indicated otherwise. For all cases of statistical significance reported, the statistical power of the test was between 0.8 and 0.9.

The spontaneous transmembrane currents recorded in neurons were analysed offline using methods described previously [20,21]. The amplitude distributions of spontaneous and evoked currents were analysed with the aid of probability density functions and likelihood maximization techniques; all histograms shown were calculated as probability density functions. The amplitude distributions were fitted with either multiquantal binomial model or bimodal function consisting of two Gaussians with variable peak location, width and amplitude. Parameters of models were fit using likelihood maximization routine.

3. Results

3.1. Astroglia-Induced Homeostatic Synaptic Scaling in Cultured Neurons

A conventional approach to test molecular mechanisms of homeostatic synaptic plasticity is exposure of primary neuronal cultures to conditions of chronic inhibition or enhancement of neuronal firing, e.g., 24 h-long incubation with tetrodotoxin or picrotoxin [9,10]. To probe the specific role of astrocytes, we modified this approach and selectively enhanced astroglial Ca^{2+}-signalling with TFLLR, an agonist of PAR-1 receptors [20]. The efficiency and specificity of PAR-1 receptor-mediated activation of astrocytes and lack of such action in neurons have been verified previously [20].

The 24 h-long incubation with TFLLR (3 μM) caused a considerable increase in the amplitude of mEPSCs in wild-type hippocampal pyramidal neurons (Figure 1A) suggesting that enhancement of astrocytic signalling can induce synaptic scaling. The average mEPSC amplitude increased from 14.01 ± 2.77 pA ($n = 11$) to 26.7 ± 6.55 pA ($n = 9$, $p < 0.01$).

To confirm that the observed synaptic scaling was BDNF-dependent, we incubated wild-type cultured neurones in TFLLR with Cyclotraxin-B (CTX-B, 10 nM), a selective and potent TrkB receptor inhibitor which has been shown to block the actions of BDNF [28]. Addition of the TrkB receptor inhibitor blocked the TFFLR-induced enhancement of mEPSCs (Figure 1A). Furthermore, the glia-induced synaptic scaling was impaired in cell cultures derived from MSK1 KD mice (Figure 1B,C) indicating the crucial role for BDNF-MSK1 pathway in this phenomenon.

Analysis of amplitude distributions of mEPSCs (Figure 1B) showed that the increase in the average amplitude occurred due to an increase in the unitary quantal size of synaptic response (manifested as the main peak of the amplitude distribution). The incubation with TFLLR alone caused a robust increase in the quantal size of mEPSCs recorded in wild type neurons, whereas there was no significant change in mEPSC frequency (Figure 1B,C). These results imply that glia-induced BDNF-dependent homeostatic synaptic scaling occurs mainly via postsynaptic mechanisms, similar to previous reports on various forms of homeostatic synaptic plasticity.

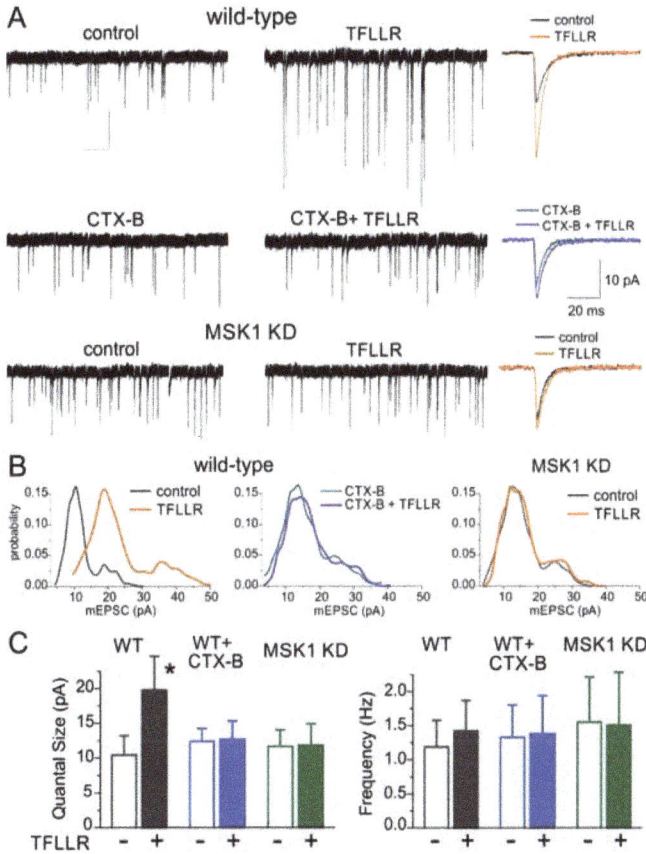

Figure 1. Mitogen- and stress-activated protein kinase 1 and brain-derived neurotrophic factor mediate astroglia-induced synaptic scaling in hippocampal neurons. (**A**) Synaptic scaling was induced in cultured hippocampal pyramidal neurons via incubation with the selective astroglia activator TFLLR (PAR-1 receptor agonist). Upper and middle panels show representative mEPSCs from wild-type neurons in control media (upper left) and after 24 h incubation with either 3 µM TFLLR alone (upper right) or the TrkB inhibitor Cyclotraxin B (CTX B) alone (middle left) or TFLLR and Cyclotraxin B together (middle right). Bottom panels show mEPSCs recorded in neurons of MSK1 KD mice. The insets on the right show corresponding average mEPSC waveforms. Note that incubation with TFLLR upregulated only mEPSCs recorded in the wild-type mice under control conditions. Synaptic currents were recorded at a membrane potential of −80 mV in the presence of picrotoxin (100 µM), TTX (1 µM), and PPADS (10 µM). (**B**) Corresponding amplitude distributions recorded in the same neurons as in (**A**). Note that the unitary quantal size, indicated by the position of the main peak in the amplitude distribution, undergoes a considerable increase, suggesting a postsynaptic effect of exposure to TFLLR in the wild-type, but not MSK1 KD neurons or in the WT neurons in the presence of BDNF TrkB receptor blocker. (**C**) Bar graphs show the quantal size and average frequency of mEPSCs recorded as described above. Data show mean ± SD for 9–12 neurons from three to four primary neuronal cultures. Note the significant increase ($p < 0.005$, unpaired t-test) in the quantal mEPSC amplitude in wild-type neurones after incubation with TFLLR. The lack of significant changes in the mEPSC frequency supports the postsynaptic origin of the effect. In contrast, activation of astrocytes with TFLLR did not cause significant alterations in mEPSCs in MSK KD1 neurons or WT neurons in the presence of BDNF TrkB receptor blocker. * $p < 0.005$.

3.2. Astroglia-Induced Homeostatic Changes in Synaptic Morphology

An enhancement of strength of excitatory synapses at postsynaptic locus can occur via two principle pathways: an increase in efficacy of neurotransmitter receptors (i.e., permeability and open time of glutamate receptor-associated ion channels) or an increase in their surface expression. These functional alterations are often accompanied by changes in synaptic morphology, in particular an increase in the size of dendritic spines. Brain-derived neurotrophic factor has been previously implicated in the regulation of synaptic morphology via induction of *Arc/Arg3.1* gene [9,29,30].

To elucidate whether this cascade is involved in the TFFLR-induced synaptic scaling, we assessed the alterations in the size and shape of postsynaptic sites using SICM. This technique is based on decrease in the ionic current passing through a glass microelectrode in close proximity of cells (or any other obstacles). The SICM method enables the imaging of live cells at nanoscale resolution and adequately maps the shape and size of small subcellular structures, such as dendrites, axons and synaptic boutons [25]. This technique has been successfully used before in the structure–function studies of synaptic networks of cultured hippocampal neurons and mechano-sensory stereocilia of cochlear hair cells [25,31].

To test for the effects of astroglia-derived BDNF on synaptic morphology, we examined live neurons from wild-type mice hippocampal cultures incubated with TFLLR alone, TFLLR with the inhibitor of TrkB receptors, or BDNF (Figure 2A). To identify functional synapses, neurons were labelled with FM1-43, an activity-dependent marker of synaptic vesicles, prior to SICM imaging (Figure 2A). Whenever a FM1-43 signal was observed, varicosities could be mapped at the SICM images; with the size and shape of varicosities consistent with the geometry expected of synaptic boutons. We targeted fluorescently-labelled varicosities located on distal dendrites to increase the probability of encountering excitatory synapses. Upon 3D-mapping of identified synaptic boutons (Figure 2B), their volume and effective size were evaluated as described in Methods (Figure 2C).

Consistent with our observations of astroglia-induced increase in synaptic strength, 24 h-incubation with TFLLR caused significant, up to 60%, increase in the average size of synapses (from 0.798 ± 0.223 μm to 1.248 ± 0.345 μm, $p < 0.01$). Correspondingly, the average volume of synaptic boutons showed >2.5-fold increase, from 0.218 ± 0.208 μm^3 to 0.569 ± 0.489 μm^3 ($n = 31$, $p < 0.01$).

The effect of TFLLR was effectively antagonized by Cyclotraxin-B (average size increased by just 10%) and reproduced by incubation with BDNF (Figure 3C).

Combined with data on the changes in mEPSC amplitude (Figure 1), these results demonstrate that activation of astrocytes can engage the BDNF-dependent molecular cascade, which is instrumental for homeostatic regulation of synaptic strength.

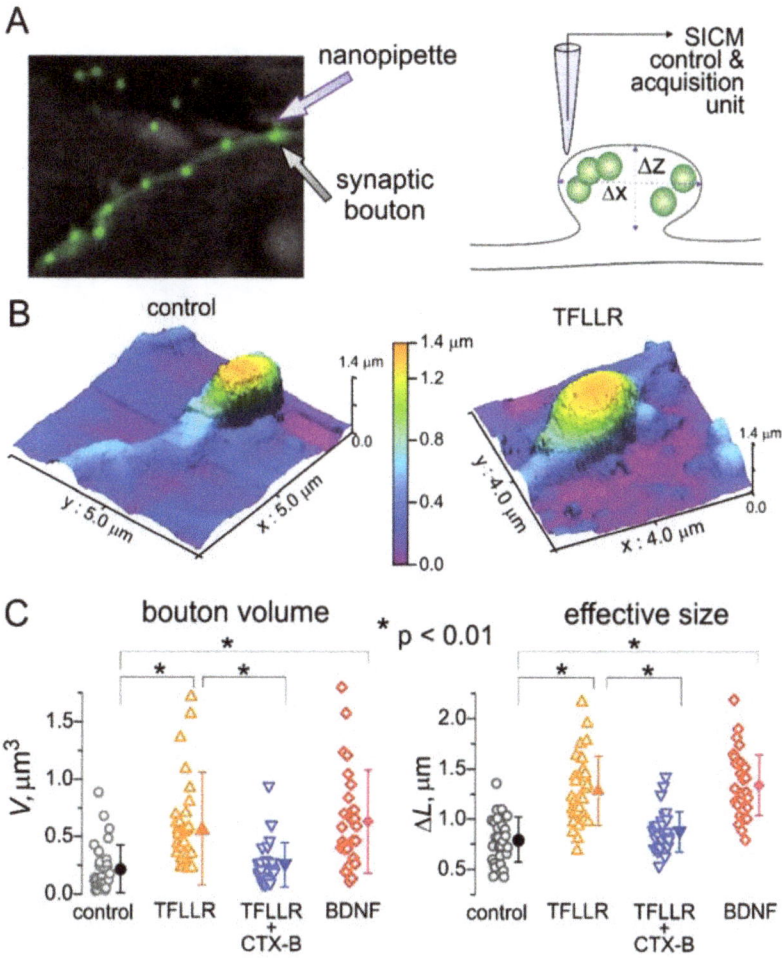

Figure 2. Astroglia and brain-derived neurotrophic factor (BDNF) regulate synaptic size. (**A**) The principle of tomographic imaging of synaptic boutons using high-resolution hopping probe scanning ion conductance microscopy (SICM). Synapses of live hippocampal neurons were prestained with synaptic vesicle marker FM1-43. (**B**) High-resolution SICM 3D images of hippocampal synapses of wild-type neurons in control and after 24 h incubation with 3 μM TFLLR. The X- and Y-scales are indicated on the images, the Z-scale is indicated as pseudo-colour (same scale for both graphs). (**C**) The pooled data on the volume (V; μm^3) and size (ΔL, μm) of synaptic boutons of wild-type neurons in control and after 24 h-incubation with the PAR1 agonist TFLLR alone, TFLLR and the TrkB antagonist Cyclotraxin B (CTX B), and BDNF. Open symbols indicate individual boutons, the closed symbols show mean ± standard deviation for the whole group (n = 30–35 boutons for three preparations). Note the significant increase in the size and volume of synapses after incubation with either TFLLR or BDNF.

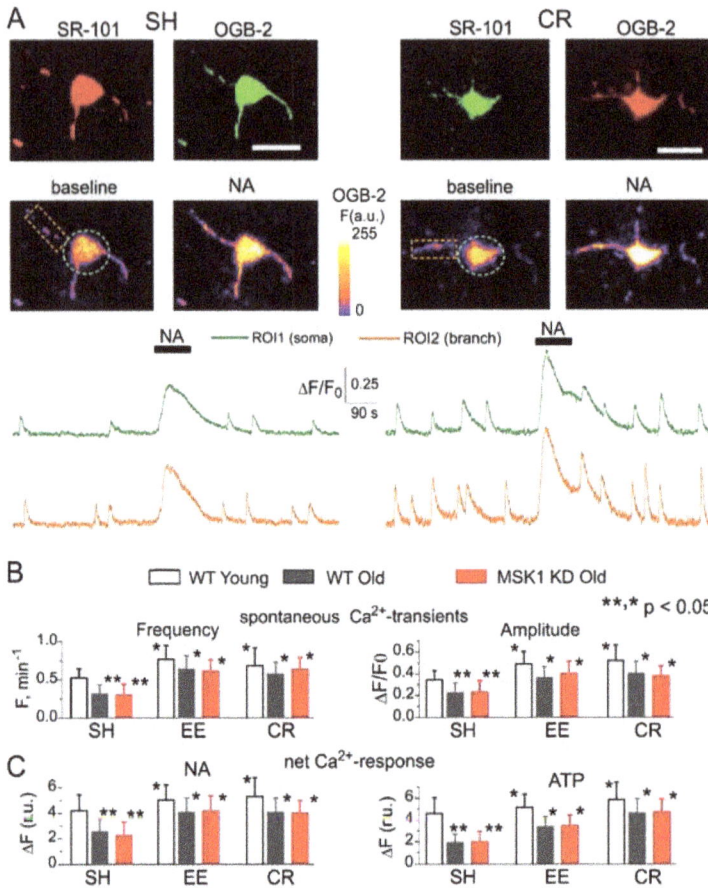

Figure 3. Age- and experience-dependent changes in astrocytic Ca^{2+} signalling. Astroglial Ca^{2+}-signalling was evaluated in the neocortex of 6–12 week-old (young) and 9–15 month-old mice (old) as described previously [26–28]. The MSK1 KD and their wild-type littermates were kept either in standard housing (SH) or exposed to environmental enrichment (EE) or caloric restriction (CR) as described in the Methods. (**A**) Representative multiphoton images of astrocytes of old MSK1 KD mouse preloaded with Oregon Green BAPTA-2 AM (OGB-2) and stained with fluorescent astroglial marker SR101 and pseudo-colour images of OGB-2 fluorescence recorded before and after application of noradrenaline (NA, 1 μM). Graphs below show the time course of OGB-2 fluorescence averaged over regions indicated in the fluorescent images. Note the increase in the amplitude and frequency of spontaneous Ca^{2+}-elevations and in response to NA. (**B**) The pooled data on peak amplitude and frequency of the baseline spontaneous Ca^{2+}-transients recorded in astrocytes of WT, MSK1, and dn-SNARE mice of different ages and treatments. Number and size of spontaneous events were pooled for the whole cell image. (**C**) The pooled data on the net responses to application of 1 μM noradrenaline and 10 μM ATP. Net response was evaluated as an integral Ca^{2+}-signal measured within 3 min after stimulation, averaged over the whole cell image and normalized to the baseline integral Ca^{2+} signal. Data in the panels (B, C) are shown as mean ± SD for the 6 to 12 astrocytes from 3 to 4 animals. Asterisks (*, **) correspondingly indicate statistical significance ($p < 0.05$) of the effect of EE or CR treatment (as compared to SH) and difference between the old and young mice of the same treatment group and genotype. Note the significant increase in spontaneous and evoked Ca^{2+}-signalling in astrocytes of mice exposed to EE and CR, and the lack of difference in Ca^{2+}-signalling in the WT, MSK1 KD, and dnSNARE mice.

3.3. Astrocytes Participate in Homeostatic Plasticity In Vivo

BDNF-mediated homeostatic synaptic scaling has been implicated in the positive effects of environmental enrichment on synaptic transmission [9]. There is also evidence that an increase in BDNF can underlie the beneficial effects of a low-calorie diet on brain function [12,32]. Previously, we demonstrated that environmental enrichment and caloric restriction can enhance Ca^{2+}-signalling in neocortical astrocytes [19]. Hence, one might predict that an increase in astroglial Ca^{2+}-dependent BDNF release plays a key role in the beneficial effects of EE and CR on synaptic transmission in the aging brain. To explore the role of this signalling mechanism in a behavioural model of experience-dependent synaptic plasticity, we examined the effect of environmental enrichment and caloric restriction on excitatory and inhibitory synaptic transmission in the neocortex.

First, we verified that EE and CR can enhance Ca^{2+}-signalling in neocortical astrocytes of MSK1 KD mice. Astroglial Ca^{2+}-signalling was monitored using multiphoton fluorescence microscopy as described previously [20,22,23]. We measured spontaneous cytosolic Ca^{2+} transients in the branches and soma of neocortical astrocytes of 6–12 week-old (young adults) and 9–15 months old (old) mice (Figure 3). There was no significant difference in Ca^{2+}-signalling between neocortical astrocytes of old wild-type and MSK1 KD mice (Figure 3). Similar to our previous reports, the amplitude and frequency of spontaneous astrocytic Ca^{2+}-transients in old WT and MSK1 KD mice raised in standard housing (SH) were significantly lower than those measured in the young SH WT mice. Most importantly, EE and CR significantly increased spontaneous astroglial Ca^{2+}-signalling in the old WT and MSK1 KD mice to a similar extent (Figure 3A,B).

We also assessed the responses of astrocytes to exogenous activation of NA and ATP receptors since these neurotransmitters are released during enhanced neuronal and physical activity [21,33,34] and potentially can mediate a link between environmental enrichment and the function of astrocytes. There is also growing evidence of the importance of α1AR and P2Y receptors for astrocytic Ca^{2+}-signalling and glia–neuron interactions [21,22,33,34]. EE and CR had a moderate effect on the amplitudes of astrocytic responses to NA (3 μM) and ATP (30 μM) in the young mice, but caused a significant enhancement of astroglial responses at the older age, both in the WT and MSK1 KD mice (Figure 3C).

These results have verified that Ca^{2+}-signalling in astrocytes, and especially the effects of EE and CR, are not affected by MSK1 KD knock-in. We have previously demonstrated that astroglial Ca^{2+}-signalling is not altered in the dnSNARE mice either [19,20,23]. Hence, if any difference in the impact of EE and CR on synaptic transmission in the dnSNARE and MSK1 KD mice were observed, they should be attributed not to the deficit in astroglial Ca^{2+}-elevation, but rather to the impairment of downstream signalling cascades, namely astroglial exocytosis and BDNF-mediated regulation of neuronal synaptic strength.

To test this, we recorded AMPA receptor-mediated mEPSCs in neocortical pyramidal neurons in the presence of the GABA$_A$ receptor antagonist picrotoxin (100 μM), and the P2 Receptor antagonist PPADS (10 μM). Exposure of wild-type mice to EE from birth to 6–12 weeks increased the average amplitude of mEPSCs to 18.6 $\pm$ 6.04 pA (n = 12), as compared to 21.3 $\pm$ 5.97 (n = 13) in the SH mice. The difference between the EE and SH mice was even larger for the older mice (Figure 4A,B), which might be related to the age-related decline in the amplitude of excitatory synaptic currents. In the older mice, the mEPSC amplitude increased from 10.86 $\pm$ 3.55 pA (SH, n = 10) to 14.34 $\pm$ 3.47 pA (EE, n = 8).

Exposure to CR had similar positive effect on mEPSCs (Figure 4B). The observed effects of both EE and CR were, most likely, of postsynaptic origin since they were accompanied by a significant increase in quantal size, whereas the frequency of mEPSCs did not undergo considerable changes (Figure 4C).

In stark contrast to the WT mice, mEPSCs recorded from MSK1 KD mice undergo the same age-related decline, but did not exhibit the EE- or CR-induced increase in amplitude (Figure 4A,B). In line with data obtained in the MSK1 KD mice, the dnSNARE mice showed only modest EE- and CR-induced increase in the average mEPSCs amplitude. The difference in the quantal size of mEPSCs in the WT and dnSNARE mice was statistically significant only for the EE in the younger age ($p < 0.05$). The incomplete inhibition of EE-induced plasticity in the young dnSNARE mice could be attributed to the mosaic (50–60% of cells) expression of dnSNARE and therefore incomplete loss of glial exocytosis. In addition, neuronal release of BDNF cannot be excluded.

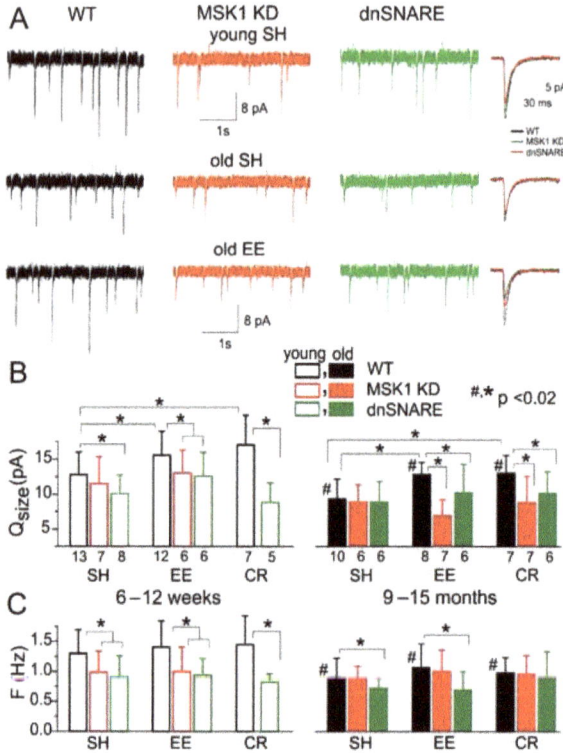

Figure 4. Experience-dependent alterations in excitatory synaptic transmission. AMPA receptor-mediated spontaneous miniature excitatory postsynaptic currents (mEPSCs) were recorded in neocortical layer 2/3 pyramidal neurons at −80 mV in the presence of 100 μM picrotoxin, 1 μM TTX and 10 μM PPADS. (**A**) Representative whole-cell currents recorded in young (top row) and old SH (middle row) and EE (bottom row) WT, MSK1 KD and dnSNARE mice (left, middle, and right columns, respectively). The inserts on the right shows average mEPSC waveforms. Note the significant decrease in mEPSC amplitude in the old WT mice of standard housing, and upregulation of mEPSCs in the EE mice of the same age. The effect of EE is impaired in the MSK1 KD and dnSNARE mice. (**B, C**) Pooled data on the quantal size (B) and frequency (C) of mEPSCs in mice of different age and experience groups. Data are shown as mean ± SD for the number of neurons indicated in (B). The statistical significance (2-population unpaired *t*-test) for the difference between young and old mice of same genotype and experience is indicated by (#) symbols; asterisks (*) indicate statistical significance of the difference between different genotype and experience groups as indicated.

The dependence of EE- and CR-induced upscaling of excitatory synaptic currents on the MSK1 signalling pathway and astrocytic exocytosis closely agrees with our results obtained in cell cultures (Figures 1 and 2). Combined together, our in vitro and ex vivo data strongly support the crucial importance of astroglial release of BDNF for homeostatic plasticity of excitatory synaptic transmission.

Finally, we explored the experience-dependent plasticity of inhibitory synaptic signalling. We recorded GABA receptor-mediated miniature inhibitory synaptic currents (mIPSCs) at a membrane potential of −80 mV in the presence of glutamate and P2X receptor antagonists (DNQX and PPADS, respectively). The pattern of age- and environment-related alterations in the GABAergic synaptic currents was different to the changes exhibited by mEPSCs. Firstly, both the quantal size and frequency of mIPSCs undergo dramatic increase in older WT and the MSK1 KD mice (Figure 5). In addition, GABAergic currents were upregulated in the dnSNARE mice of both age groups as compared to their WT-littermates (Figure 5A,B); this result is in line with our previous observations [19]. Secondly, exposure of the wild-type mice to EE and CR efficiently downregulated inhibitory synaptic signalling, especially in the neurons of older mice (Figure 5A,B). In contrast to mEPSCs, the EE- and CR-induced downscaling of mIPSCs was absent in the dnSNARE but not in the MSK1 KD mice. This might be explained by participation of other gliotransmitters, in particular ATP [19], in astroglial-driven modulation of GABA receptors.

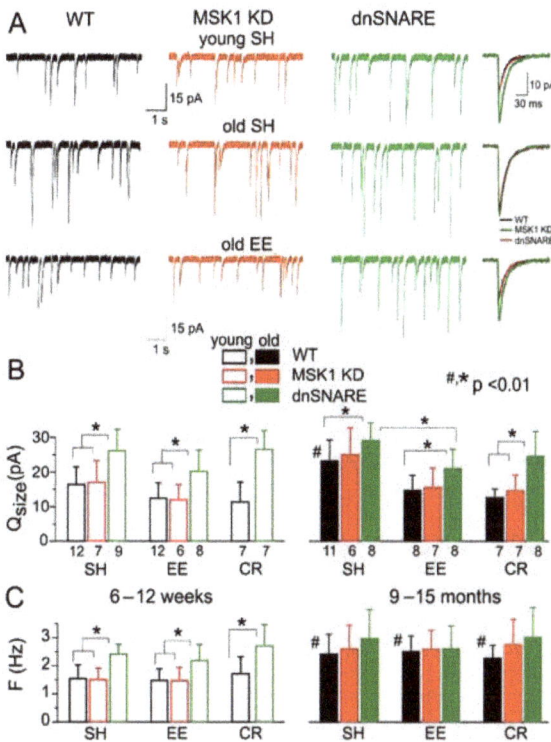

Figure 5. Experience-dependent alterations in inhibitory synaptic transmission. GABA$_A$ receptor-mediated miniature inhibitory postsynaptic currents (mIPSCs) were recorded in neocortical layer 2/3 pyramidal neurons at −80 mV in the presence of 30 µM DNQX, 1 µM TTX, and 10 µM PPADS. (**A**) Representative whole-cell currents recorded in young (top row) and old SH (middle row) and EE (bottom row) WT, MSK1 KD, and dnSNARE mice (left, middle, and right columns, respectively). The inserts on the right shows average mIPSCs waveforms. (**B**, **C**) Pooled data on the quantal size (B) and frequency (C) of mIPSCs in mice of different age and experience groups. Data are shown as mean ± SD for the number of neurons indicated in (B). The statistical significance (2-population unpaired *t*-test) for the difference between young and old mice of same genotype and experience is indicated by (#) symbols; asterisks (*) indicate statistically significance of the difference between different genotype and experience groups as indicated. Note the significant increase in mIPSC amplitude in the old standard housed WT mice and down-regulation of mIPSCs in the EE mice of the same age. The effect of EE is impaired in the MSK1 KD and dnSNARE mice.

Combined, our data strongly support the importance of astrocytic exocytosis and BDNF/MSK1-mediated signalling for the beneficial effects of EE and CR on synaptic transmission in the ageing brain.

4. Discussion

Our experiments in cultured neurons demonstrated that long-term enhancement of astrocytic Ca^{2+}-signalling can lead to neuronal synaptic scaling that engages the same BDNF/MSK1 cascade that has been shown to underlie homeostatic synaptic plasticity induced by alterations in neuronal firing [9,10]. The astrocyte-induced alterations in synaptic strength (Figure 1) and morphology (Figure 2) depend on the activity of BDNF TrkB receptors and MSK1. Combined with recently reported data unequivocally showing the ability of astrocytes to release BDNF via exocytosis [14], our results strongly suggest that astrocyte-derived BDNF can modulate homeostatic synaptic scaling.

Our ex vivo data also highlighted the importance of astroglial-derived BDNF and the BDNF/MSK1 pathway for experience-dependent homeostatic synaptic plasticity. Firstly, we observed that exposure of mice to EE and CR can induce an increase in glutamatergic (Figure 4), and a decrease in GABAergic synaptic transmission (Figure 5). The impact of EE and CR was significantly reduced in dnSNARE mice, indicating the critical importance of astrocytic exocytosis, which is very likely the main pathway of BDNF release [14]. Secondly, the effects of EE and CR on synaptic transmission and plasticity differed significantly in the wild-type and MSK1 KD mice (Figures 4 and 5), where one of the main pathways of BDNF-mediated homeostatic plasticity was impaired [9]. Finally, the exposure to EE and CR led to significant upregulation of Ca^{2+}-signalling in astrocytes, which did not differ in the WT and transgenic mice. The most likely explanation for all our observations of changes in glutamatergic mEPSCs would be the enhancement of Ca^{2+}-dependent release of BDNF from astrocytes which, in turn, upregulates the strength of excitatory synapses via MSK1-dependent cascade.

As for the homeostatic plasticity of GABAergic transmission, it was only weakly affected by the impairment of the BDNF/MSK1 pathway, but was critically dependent on astroglial exocytosis. These results highlight an important difference in astroglial-driven homeostatic regulation of excitatory and inhibitory synaptic transmission: the former is modulated mainly via the BDNF/MSK1 pathway whereas the latter is modulated, most likely, by other gliotransmitters. As our previous results suggest, the vesicular release of ATP can play an important role in astroglial-driven modulation of GABA receptors [20].

Our data highlighted interesting trends in age-related alterations in synaptic transmission: a decrease in the efficacy of excitatory synapses, and an increase in the efficacy of inhibitory synapses, but neither were accompanied by marked change in the frequency of synaptic events. These observations suggest that, at least at early stages of ageing, neurons retain a significant number of functional synapses, and cognitive decline can be associated with dysregulation, rather than complete loss of synapses. Furthermore, our present (Figure 3) and previous data [19,35,36] on age-related decline in astroglial Ca^{2+}-signalling and the release of gliotransmitters suggest a very plausible reason of such dysregulation—impairment of glia-driven modulation of synaptic activity. This hypothesis is strongly supported by observation that manipulations which facilitate astroglial signalling, e.g., EE, CR, reversed the changes in excitatory and inhibitory synaptic signalling back to a "younger" state (Figures 4 and 5). Also, the notion of impairment of glial regulation of balance between the excitatory and inhibitory signals onto principal neurons as a putative cause of age-related cognitive decline agrees with our previous observation that enhancement of astrocytic Ca^{2+}-signalling, including EE- and CR-induced, can rescue long-term synaptic plasticity in old mice [19,35,36]. Nonetheless, this model of age-related alterations of synaptic function needs to be explored further, in particular in relation to neurodegenerative disorders.

To conclude, our results strongly support the physiological importance of astroglial exocytosis, in particular the release of BDNF, for communication between astrocytes and neurons and experience-related synaptic plasticity across a lifetime.

Author Contributions: Conceptualization, B.G.F. and Y.P.; Data Curation, U.L., G.W.J.M., and Y.P.; Formal Analysis, U.L., A.B., and Y.P.; Investigation, U.L. and A.B.; Methodology, G.W.J.M., B.G.F., and Y.P.; Resources, G.W.J.M. and B.G.F.; Supervision, Y.P.; Writing—original draft, U.L. and Y.P.

Funding: This work was supported by the BBSRC UK grants number BB/K009192/1 to Y.P. and BB/F021445/1 to B.G.F. and Y.P. and BB/D01817X/1 to G.W.J.M.

Acknowledgments: The authors thank Professor J. Simon Arthur (University of Dundee) for developing and providing MSK1 KD mice.

Conflicts of Interest: Authors declare no conflicts of interests

References

1. Baroncelli, L.; Braschi, C.; Spolidoro, M.; Begenisic, T.; Sale, A.; Maffei, L. Nurturing brain plasticity: Impact of environmental enrichment. *Cell Death Differ.* **2010**, *17*, 1092–1103. [CrossRef] [PubMed]
2. Nelson, S.B.; Turrigiano, G.G. Strength through diversity. *Neuron* **2008**, *60*, 477–482. [CrossRef] [PubMed]
3. Nithianantharajah, J.; Hannan, A.J. Enriched environments, experience-dependent plasticity and disorders of the nervous system. *Nat. Rev. Neurosci.* **2006**, *7*, 697–709. [CrossRef] [PubMed]
4. Hillman, C.H.; Erickson, K.I.; Kramer, A.F. Be smart, exercise your heart: Exercise effects on brain and cognition. *Nat. Rev. Neurosci.* **2008**, *9*, 58–65. [CrossRef] [PubMed]
5. Mercken, E.M.; Carboneau, B.A.; Krzysik-Walker, S.M.; de Cabo, R. Of mice and men: The benefits of caloric restriction, exercise, and mimetics. *Ageing Res. Rev.* **2012**, *11*, 390–398. [CrossRef] [PubMed]
6. Merzenich, M.M.; Van Vleet, T.M.; Nahum, M. Brain plasticity-based therapeutics. *Front. Hum. Neurosci.* **2014**, *8*, 385. [CrossRef] [PubMed]
7. Nithianantharajah, J.; Hannan, A.J. The neurobiology of brain and cognitive reserve: Mental and physical activity as modulators of brain disorders. *Prog. Neurobiol.* **2009**, *89*, 369–382. [CrossRef] [PubMed]
8. Van Praag, H. Exercise and the brain: Something to chew on. *Trends Neurosci.* **2009**, *32*, 283–290. [CrossRef] [PubMed]
9. Correa, S.A.; Hunter, C.J.; Palygin, O.; Wauters, S.C.; Martin, K.J.; McKenzie, C.; McKelvey, K.; Morris, R.G.; Pankratov, Y.; Arthur, J.S.; et al. MSK1 regulates homeostatic and experience-dependent synaptic plasticity. *J. Neurosci.* **2012**, *32*, 13039–13051. [CrossRef] [PubMed]
10. Turrigiano, G.G.; Leslie, K.R.; Desai, N.S.; Rutherford, L.C.; Nelson, S.B. Activity-dependent scaling of quantal amplitude in neocortical neurons. *Nature* **1998**, *391*, 892–896. [CrossRef] [PubMed]
11. Cowansage, K.K.; LeDoux, J.E.; Monfils, M.H. Brain-derived neurotrophic factor: A dynamic gatekeeper of neural plasticity. *Curr. Mol. Pharmacol.* **2010**, *3*, 12–29. [CrossRef] [PubMed]
12. Rothman, S.M.; Griffioen, K.J.; Wan, R.; Mattson, M.P. Brain-derived neurotrophic factor as a regulator of systemic and brain energy metabolism and cardiovascular health. *Ann. N. Y. Acad. Sci.* **2012**, *1264*, 49–63. [CrossRef] [PubMed]
13. Song, J.H.; Yu, J.T.; Tan, L. Brain-Derived Neurotrophic Factor in Alzheimer's Disease: Risk, Mechanisms, and Therapy. *Mol. Neurobiol.* **2015**, *52*, 1477–1493. [CrossRef] [PubMed]
14. Stenovec, M.; Lasic, E.; Bozic, M.; Bobnar, S.T.; Stout, R.F., Jr.; Grubisic, V.; Parpura, V.; Zorec, R. Ketamine Inhibits ATP-Evoked Exocytotic Release of Brain-Derived Neurotrophic Factor from Vesicles in Cultured Rat Astrocytes. *Mol. Neurobiol.* **2016**, *53*, 6882–6896. [CrossRef] [PubMed]
15. Vignoli, B.; Battistini, G.; Melani, R.; Blum, R.; Santi, S.; Berardi, N.; Canossa, M. Peri-Synaptic Glia Recycles Brain-Derived Neurotrophic Factor for LTP Stabilization and Memory Retention. *Neuron* **2016**, *92*, 873–887. [CrossRef] [PubMed]
16. Rodriguez-Arellano, J.J.; Parpura, V.; Zorec, R.; Verkhratsky, A. Astrocytes in physiological aging and Alzheimer's disease. *Neuroscience* **2015**. [CrossRef] [PubMed]
17. Verkhratsky, A.; Nedergaard, M. Astroglial cradle in the life of the synapse. *Philos. Trans. R. Soc. Lond. B Biol. Sci.* **2014**, *369*. [CrossRef] [PubMed]
18. Rodriguez, J.J.; Terzieva, S.; Olabarria, M.; Lanza, R.G.; Verkhratsky, A. Enriched environment and physical activity reverse astrogliodegeneration in the hippocampus of AD transgenic mice. *Cell Death Dis.* **2013**, *4*, e678. [CrossRef]
19. Lalo, U.; Bogdanov, A.; Pankratov, Y. Diversity of Astroglial Effects on Aging- and Experience-Related Cortical Metaplasticity. *Front. Mol. Neurosci.* **2018**, *11*, 239. [CrossRef] [PubMed]

20. Lalo, U.; Palygin, O.; Rasooli-Nejad, S.; Andrew, J.; Haydon, P.G.; Pankratov, Y. Exocytosis of ATP from astrocytes modulates phasic and tonic inhibition in the neocortex. *PLoS Biol.* **2014**, *12*, e1001747. [CrossRef] [PubMed]

21. Lalo, U.; Palygin, O.; Verkhratsky, A.; Grant, S.G.; Pankratov, Y. ATP from synaptic terminals and astrocytes regulates NMDA receptors and synaptic plasticity through PSD-95 multi-protein complex. *Sci. Rep.* **2016**, *6*, 33609. [CrossRef] [PubMed]

22. Pankratov, Y.; Lalo, U. Role for astroglial alpha1-adrenoreceptors in gliotransmission and control of synaptic plasticity in the neocortex. *Front. Cell. Neurosci.* **2015**, *9*, 230. [CrossRef] [PubMed]

23. Rasooli-Nejad, S.; Palygin, O.; Lalo, U.; Pankratov, Y. Cannabinoid receptors contribute to astroglial Ca^{2+}-signalling and control of synaptic plasticity in the neocortex. *Philos. Trans. R. Soc. Lond. B Biol. Sci.* **2014**, *369*, 20140077. [CrossRef] [PubMed]

24. Lalo, U.; Pankratov, Y. Exploring the Ca2+-dependent synaptic dynamics in vibro-dissociated cells. *Cell Calcium* **2017**, *64*, 91–101. [CrossRef] [PubMed]

25. Novak, P.; Li, C.; Shevchuk, A.I.; Stepanyan, R.; Caldwell, M.; Hughes, S.; Smart, T.G.; Gorelik, J.; Ostanin, V.P.; Lab, M.J.; et al. Nanoscale live-cell imaging using hopping probe ion conductance microscopy. *Nat. Methods* **2009**, *6*, 279–281. [CrossRef] [PubMed]

26. Sikora, A.; Rodak, A.; Unold, O.; Klapetek, P. The development of the spatially correlated adjustment wavelet filter for atomic force microscopy data. *Ultramicroscopy* **2016**, *171*, 146–152. [CrossRef] [PubMed]

27. Schneider, C.A.; Rasband, W.S.; Eliceiri, K.W. NIH Image to ImageJ: 25 years of image analysis. *Nat. Methods* **2012**, *9*, 671–675. [CrossRef] [PubMed]

28. Zhong, P.; Liu, Y.; Hu, Y.; Wang, T.; Zhao, Y.P.; Liu, Q.S. BDNF interacts with endocannabinoids to regulate cocaine-induced synaptic plasticity in mouse midbrain dopamine neurons. *J. Neurosci.* **2015**, *35*, 4469–4481. [CrossRef] [PubMed]

29. Messaoudi, E.; Kanhema, T.; Soule, J.; Tiron, A.; Dagyte, G.; da Silva, B.; Bramham, C.R. Sustained Arc/Arg3.1 synthesis controls long-term potentiation consolidation through regulation of local actin polymerization in the dentate gyrus in vivo. *J. Neurosci.* **2007**, *27*, 10445–10455. [CrossRef] [PubMed]

30. Waung, M.W.; Pfeiffer, B.E.; Nosyreva, E.D.; Ronesi, J.A.; Huber, K.M. Rapid translation of Arc/Arg3.1 selectively mediates mGluR-dependent LTD through persistent increases in AMPAR endocytosis rate. *Neuron* **2008**, *59*, 84–97. [CrossRef] [PubMed]

31. Korchev, Y.E.; Negulyaev, Y.A.; Edwards, C.R.; Vodyanoy, I.; Lab, M.J. Functional localization of single active ion channels on the surface of a living cell. *Nat. Cell Biol.* **2000**, *2*, 616–619. [CrossRef] [PubMed]

32. Lopez-Otin, C.; Galluzzi, L.; Freije, J.M.; Madeo, F.; Kroemer, G. Metabolic Control of Longevity. *Cell* **2016**, *166*, 802–821. [CrossRef] [PubMed]

33. Paukert, M.; Agarwal, A.; Cha, J.; Doze, V.A.; Kang, J.U.; Bergles, D.E. Norepinephrine controls astroglial responsiveness to local circuit activity. *Neuron* **2014**, *82*, 1263–1270. [CrossRef] [PubMed]

34. Rudolph, R.; Jahn, H.M.; Courjaret, R.; Messemer, N.; Kirchhoff, F.; Deitmer, J.W. The inhibitory input to mouse cerebellar Purkinje cells is reciprocally modulated by Bergmann glial P2Y1 and AMPA receptor signaling. *Glia* **2016**, *64*, 1265–1280. [CrossRef] [PubMed]

35. Lalo, U.; Palygin, O.; North, R.A.; Verkhratsky, A.; Pankratov, Y. Age-dependent remodelling of ionotropic signalling in cortical astroglia. *Aging Cell* **2011**, *10*, 392–402. [CrossRef] [PubMed]

36. Lalo, U.; Rasooli-Nejad, S.; Pankratov, Y. Exocytosis of gliotransmitters from cortical astrocytes: Implications for synaptic plasticity and aging. *Biochem. Soc. Trans.* **2014**, *42*, 1275–1281. [CrossRef] [PubMed]

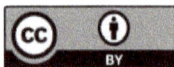

MDPI

St. Alban-Anlage 66

4052 Basel

Switzerland

Tel. +41 61 683 77 34

Fax +41 61 302 89 18

www.mdpi.com

Books Editorial Office

E-mail: books@mdpi.com

www.mdpi.com/journal/books

www.ingramcontent.com/pod-product-compliance
Lightning Source LLC
Chambersburg PA
CBHW051705210326
41597CB00032B/5382